Infosys Science Foundation Series

Infosys Science Foundation Series in Mathematical Sciences

The *Infosys Science Foundation Series in Mathematical Sciences,* a Scopus-indexed book series, is a sub-series of the *Infosys Science Foundation Series.* This sub-series focuses on high-quality content in the domain of mathematical sciences and various disciplines of mathematics, statistics, bio-mathematics, financial mathematics, applied mathematics, operations research, applied statistics and computer science. With this series, Springer and the Infosys Science Foundation hope to provide readers with monographs, handbooks, professional books and textbooks of the highest academic quality on current topics in relevant disciplines. Literature in this sub-series will appeal to a wide audience of researchers, students, educators, and professionals across mathematics, applied mathematics, statistics and computer science disciplines.

More information about this subseries at http://www.springer.com/series/13817

Praveen Agarwal · Juan J. Nieto ·
Michael Ruzhansky · Delfim F. M. Torres
Editors

Analysis of Infectious Disease Problems (Covid-19) and Their Global Impact

Springer

Editors
Praveen Agarwal
Anand International College of Engineering
Jaipur, Rajasthan, India

Michael Ruzhansky
Department of Mathematics: Analysis, Logic and Discrete Mathematics
Ghent University
Ghent, Belgium

Mathematical Sciences
Queen Mary University of London
London, UK

Juan J. Nieto
Institute of Mathematics
University of Santiago de Compostela
Santiago, Spain

Delfim F. M. Torres
Department of Mathematics
University of Aveiro
Aveiro, Portugal

ISSN 2363-6149 ISSN 2363-6157 (electronic)
Infosys Science Foundation Series
ISSN 2364-4036 ISSN 2364-4044 (electronic)
Infosys Science Foundation Series in Mathematical Sciences
ISBN 978-981-16-2449-0 ISBN 978-981-16-2450-6 (eBook)
https://doi.org/10.1007/978-981-16-2450-6

Mathematics Subject Classification (2010): 26A33, 42A38, 42B10, 46F12, 65R10, 65F35, 65J05, 26A18

This Springer imprint is published by the registered company Springer Nature Singapore Pte Ltd.
The registered company address is: 152 Beach Road, #21-01/04 Gateway East, Singapore 189721, Singapore

Preface

Any condition which interferes with the normal functioning of the body and which causes discomfort or disability or impairment of the health of a living organism is called a *disease*. The *disease agent* is a factor (substance or force) which causes a disease by its excess or deficiency or absence. The impact of severe diseases on people is a real concern in terms of suffering as well as social and economic implications. In recent era, there are several communicable diseases, namely Covid-19, malaria, dengue fever, HIV/AIDS, tuberculosis, cholera, Zika virus, chickenpox, influenza, pneumonia, and so on, which impair the health of the human population around the globe. Some of these communicable diseases carry from person to person by viral diseases and their pathogens, which impact the human body through sexual intercourse.

In recent years, the control of these acute diseases has been a great concern for bio-mathematicians and medical experts. It has been approved that these infectious diseases are fatal to billions of people and also cause the loss of their worth. Mathematical modeling plays a crucial role in the study of these adverse types of diseases. The basic ambition to evaluate and eradicate these diseases through mathematical models is to minimize their effects by understanding their mechanism and the agents that cause the spread of these diseases, so that it gives a better chance to predict these diseases and their impacts and also give a way to control them. Mathematical models allow us to extrapolate from current information about the state and progress of an outbreak to predict the future and, most importantly, to quantify the uncertainty in these predictions. Most of these mathematical models contain ordinary or partial differential equations. In some cases, instead of integer order, fractional order can be used to analyze the real phenomena behind the problems. In one way or another, researchers encounter different kinds of nonlinear ordinary or partial differential equations.

The aim of this edited volume is to collect original research articles that focus on recent results, which can be obtained from the novel methods constructed by many researchers, for all types of infection diseases, as well as developments in recent methods with new operators or new approximations. It is also involving the review articles discussing the current state of the art.

In this book, we are happy to have 30 chapters in two parts. Part I is based on "general analysis," and Part II contains papers on "country-specific analysis on Covid-19." All chapters are contributed from eminent researchers around the globe who are internationally known experts in their fields. Throughout this book, the analysis of infectious disease problems (Covid-19) and their global impact have been explained very carefully in the simplest possible terms and illustrated by a number of complete workout examples. This book contains some useful theorems and their proofs.

The book is organized as follows.

In Part I, chapter "Continued and Serious Lockdown Could Have Minimized Many Newly Transmitted Cases of Covid-19 in the U.S.: Wavelets, Deterministic Models, and Data" discusses model-based estimates of Covid-19 in the USA during April–June 2020. Model-based predictions of Covid-19 for the low and high range of transmission rates and with varying degrees of preventive measures including the lockdowns have been provided. It is shown how 10 cases that do not adhere to proper care and do not comply with the lockdown on April 30, 2020, result, at the end of May and at the end of June, in 50,000 and 55,000 new cases, respectively. These values for the months of May and June would be 251,000 and 511,000, respectively, in the case of a worse adherence rate of 50 infected (but unidentified) individuals. Continued and serious lockdown measures bring the average daily rate of new cases to lower figures, with a range of 4,300 per day to 8,000 per day in May.

In chapter "Dynamical Analysis of a Caputo Fractional Order SIR Epidemic Model with a General Treatment Function," a fractional-order SIR epidemic model is proposed. We first prove the existence, uniqueness, non-negativity, and boundedness of solutions to the considered model. We also study the existence of equilibrium points. Some sufficient conditions are derived to ensure, in terms of the basic reproduction number, the global asymptotic stability of the disease-free equilibrium point and endemic equilibrium point. Finally, numerical simulations are illustrated to verify the validity of our theoretical results.

In chapter "Protective Face Shield Effectiveness: Mathematical Modelling," a 3D mathematical model of the airflow distribution near the cylindrical surface of a face shield was explored. The model is based on a numerical solution of the Navier–Stokes gas dynamics equations. The simulation results are compared with full-scale experiments. A probability model is also considered. Quantitative conclusions are made about the effectiveness of the protective face shields.

Chapter "On the Evolution Equation for Modelling the Covid-19 Pandemic" introduces and discusses the evolution equation and, based exclusively on this equation, considers random walk models for the time series available on the daily confirmed Covid-19 cases for different countries. It is shown that a conventional random walk model is not consistent with the current global pandemic time series data, which exhibits non-ergodic properties. We therefore consider a self-affine random walk field model which provides the non-ergodic fields that are evident in the available data. This is based on using a spectral scaling relationship of the type $1/\omega^{\alpha}$, where ω is the angular frequency and $\alpha \in (0, 1)$ conforms to a zero-mean Gaussian distribution. It is then shown that α is a primary parameter for evaluating the global status of the pandemic in the sense that the pandemic will become extinguished as $\alpha \to 0$ for all countries. For this reason, and, based on the data currently available, a study is made of the variations for 100 randomly selected countries. Finally, in the context of the bio-dynamic hypothesis, a parametric model is considered for simulating the three-dimensional structure of a spike protein which may be of value in the development of a vaccine.

Chapter "Modelling the Dynamics of Fake News Spreading Transmission During Covid-19 Through Social Media" discusses the transmission of fake news to understand the rate of spreading. Therefore, the objective of this paper is to propose a mathematical model that can describe the dynamics of the spread of fake news through social media along the period of MCO through different social media platforms. This study also suggests some measures that can be taken by different parties, such as individuals, society, and government to solve the issue of fake news transmission.

In chapter "Generalized Logistic Equations in Covid-Related Epidemic Models," we discuss how to develop a simple computable model for infection propagation, based on vicinity and interaction time conditions, between healthy and infectious persons. This simple and robust model can be adapted for realistic simulations. The three use cases studied in detail are as follows:

(1) An elderly care home, where contamination at joint meals is considered,
(2) A household in lockdown, stay at home, with contamination at joint meals considered, and
(3) A large venue event with lots of interaction between participants and crowd effects.

Each use case is presented in its phenomenology, with some illustrative references, facts, and data, of interest for practical simulation and model adaptation, scenarios, and corresponding interpretations. Then, the agent-based model conditional to vicinity and interaction time between healthy and infected persons within this use case is established, with its hypotheses. An active stochastic contagion propagation model is developed, deriving the probability of infection from the presence of infectious persons in the vicinity of a healthy person, during an interaction time. Numerical examples are discussed. Bounds and limits are established in some specific cases of interest.

Chapter "A Transition of Shared Mobility in Metro Cities—A Challenge Post-Lockdown Covid-19" brings a contribution to the foundational basic research on the logistic equation and its generalizations which hopefully have repercussions for epidemiologic applications.

In chapter "Analysis of Covid-19 Virus Spreading Statistics by the Use of a New Modified Weibull Distribution," we use a Bureau of Public Road (BPR) model to combat this issue endangering the environment and public health. We exploit the BPR function to relate average travel time to the estimated number of commuters traveling by car. We collect mode share data from the NITI Aayog, state resource centres, which give unique figures of the impact of shared mobility in India and how, in its absence, various sectors will be affected. Using the given data and the BPR, we evaluate increased vehicle volumes on the road if different portions of transit and carpool users switch to single-occupancy vehicles and its effect on multiple other factors. Based on this study, we predict that cities with significant transit ridership are at risk for extreme traffic and pollution unless transit systems can resume safe with effective protocols.

In chapter "Lifting Lockdown Control Measure Assessment: From Finite- to Infinite-Dimensional Epidemic Models for Covid-19," in anticipation of substantial fatal effects on the health of people following this human-to-human spread, we aim to propose a new six-parameter modified Weibull distribution to analyze the spread of Covid-19. We apply this model to study the cumulative cases infected in some countries, we give a global analysis of the statistical data of the pandemic, and we prove that our new distribution efficiently generalizes some existing models and fits correctly some data registered from February to June 2020. We use these results to assess the potential for human-to-human spread to occur around the globe.

The main focus of chapter "Introduction to the Grey Systems Theory and Its Application in Mathematical Modeling and Pandemic Prediction of Covid-19" is on public health control strategies, which are currently the main way to mitigate the Covid-19 pandemic. We introduce and compare compartmental models of increasing complexity for Covid-19 transmission to describe the dynamics of the disease spread. We begin by considering an SEAIR model including basic characteristics related to Covid-19. Next, we shall pay attention to age structure modeling to emphasize the role of age-group individuals on the disease spread. A model with constant delay is also formulated to show the impact of the latency period on the severity of Covid-19. Since there is evidence that for Covid-19 disease, important relationships exist between what is happening in the host and what is occurring at the population level, we shall link the basic model to in-host dynamics through the so-called threshold-type delay models. Finally, we will include demographic effects to the most complex models and we will conduct rigorous bifurcation analysis to quantify possible factors responsible for disease progression.

Chapter "Mathematical Analysis of Diagnosis Rate Effects in Covid-19 Transmission Dynamics with Optimal Control" is devoted to present the scientific background for the appearance of gray systems in the 1980s. Then, the history of astonishing development, along with the main components and fundamental principles of the gray systems, is also introduced. Currently, a gray system is an emerging research area with strong possibilities to transect across and apply to a wide range of scientific areas, including industry, agriculture, geology, ecology, medicine, education, etc. However, most applications of the systems are from Chinese-speaking researchers, while the theory itself is still uncommon in uncertainty mathematics. Finally, the representative models with high accuracy are put into practice by predicting and handling the outbreak of the Covid-19 pandemic. Not only can the systems predict the total number of positive cases, but they can also be applied in various other medical practices, including telecare and data management. Their performances are also compared with other uncertainty models, including machine learning, which has proven that gray system models have the ability to perform equally well, or even better, especially in the context of limited data.

Many countries around the world are trying to fight Covid-19, and their main methods are lockdown, quarantine, isolation, and awareness programs to encourage people to adopt social distancing and maintain personal hygiene. The lockdown is aimed to restrict the movement of humans from or to certain places. Quarantine is aimed toward separating the susceptible humans from infected or exposed humans as much as possible, whereas isolation is aimed toward keeping the confirmed cases of infected humans away from the rest of the population. The confirmed cases are mainly identified through the diagnosis of individuals who showed symptoms of Covid-19 and sometimes through random checking of individuals hoping to identify either asymptomatic or pre-symptomatic cases, which is generally an expensive method. In this chapter, we develop a mathematical model to investigate the role of diagnosis rate in the transmission dynamics of Covid-19 together with the combined effects of quarantine and isolation.

Chapter "Development of Epidemiological Modeling RD-Covid-19 of Coronavirus Infectious Disease and Its Numerical Simulation" discusses a model which is fully analyzed both qualitatively and quantitatively in order to gain insight about the role of different model parameters in the disease transmission dynamics, especially those related to diagnosis and quarantine. The analysis will include the estimation of both the basic and the control reproduction numbers and sensitivity analysis of the reproduction numbers to the corresponding model parameters. The optimal control theory will be also applied to the model to examine the role of some other optimal control strategies and to study the effect of diagnosis and quarantine rates in the effectiveness of these controls.

In chapter "Mediterranean Diet—A Healthy Dietary Pattern and Lifestyle for Strong Immunity," we have developed a new epidemiological dynamical model named RD-Covid-19 (version 1.0) model. The traditional epidemiological model of an infectious disease known as susceptible–exposed–infected–recovered–dead (SEIRD) is modified to develop this new model. RD-Covid-19 is a networked epidemiological model in which a data-driven logistic model and traditional models such as susceptible, infected, and recovered (SIR), SEIR, and SEIQRDP are interlinked. The completer model forecasts the spread of the Covid-19. For the model, the parameters are estimated by fitting the model with real data.[1] The Levenberg–Marquardt nonlinear least-squares optimization technique is applied for the estimation of the parameters and for the fitting of the model. Numerical simulation of the model carried out with the estimated values of the parameters and outcome of the model generates the temporal profile of infected, recovered, and death cases. The severity of the model is measured by computing the basic reproduction number ($R0$). Data (real-time data) used in the model RD-Covid-19 related to the public are categorized as confirmed, recovered, and death cases. The model is executed to explore the corona outbreak in China, India, Brazil, and Russia. The estimated value of the basic reproduction number, $R0$, is well in agreement with that obtained from the outcome of traditional models SIR and SEIR. Implementation of lockdown impacts the model and its innovation, showing the advantage to make decisions on risk management

[1] Source: John Hopkins University and WHO dashboard.

by the competent authority. The verification and validation (V&V) process of our model is carried out by comparing its results with an analogical logistic model.

Chapter "Rate-Induced Tipping Phenomena in Compartment Models of Epidemics" is based on a Mediterranean diet. The health and the overall well-being are greatly affected by an individual diet, lifestyle, age, and genetics, as well as the individual's response to stress, pathogens, and environmental pollution, which is mainly dictated by the immune system. A healthy gut microbiota plays a crucial role in the development and maintaining of a healthy immune system. Numerous studies have shown that nutrients including vitamins, such as A, B6, B12, C, D, E, and folate; trace elements, such as zinc, iron, selenium, magnesium, and copper; and omega-3 fatty acids are complementary in maintaining a strong immune system. Besides nutrition, a healthy lifestyle including successful management of stress and anxiety, adequate sleep and rest, and physical activity is also crucial for boosting the immune system. A strong immune system would effectively respond to the attacks of pathogens (viruses and bacteria), such as the current coronavirus. The Mediterranean way of living seems an optimal dietary pattern and a lifestyle that could help in maintaining a healthy and diverse gut microbiota and, thus, strong immunity. Mediterranean diet is mainly plant-based dietary pattern, which emphasizes consumption of fruits, vegetables, whole grains, nuts, legumes, and seeds followed by moderate consumption of fish, poultry, fermented dairy products, and extra virgin olive oil as a main source of healthy fats, while the use of processed red meat products and refined sugars is low. Plenty of water, fruit juices, and herb teas are also consumed with frequent, but moderate consumption of red wine usually with the meals. Taking rests, daily physical exercises, leisure activities, and being a part of the community are also common features of the Mediterranean lifestyle. Therefore, the Mediterranean diet rich in valuable phytonutrients, such as vitamins, minerals, dietary fibers, and antioxidant polyphenols, could help in building a healthy gut and a strong immune system to effectively respond to the Covid-19 pandemic.

Chapter "Analysis of Impact of Covid-19 Pandemic on Financial Markets" aims to explore non-autonomous compartment models of epidemics, like SIR models with time-dependent transmission and recovery rates as parameters, and particularly the occurrence of rate-induced tipping phenomena. Specifically, we are interested in the question, whether there can exist parameter paths that do not cross any bifurcation points, but yet give rise to tipping when the parameters vary over time. From the literature, it is known that such rate-induced tipping occurs, for example, in two-dimensional models of ecosystems or predator–prey systems. We show in this chapter that rate-induced tipping can also occur in compartment models of epidemics. Thus, regarding the Covid-19 crisis, not only the measures established in a lockdown and the moment of the lockdown, but also the rate by which lockdown measures are implemented may have a drastic influence on the number of infectious.

Chapter " Symptom-Based Testing in a Compartmental Model of Covid-19" discusses the impact of the Covid-19 pandemic on the North American financial markets and proposes a framework for stress testing and financial scenario generation of market indicators. This framework includes the following main components:

- Epidemiological dynamic model describing the evolution of the number of susceptible, infected, recovered, and death cases with social distancing,
- Dynamical model describing dependence between financial indicators and growth of the pandemic in different geographical areas, and
- Conditional stress scenario generation and financial portfolio analysis.

In chapter "Challenges in Modeling of an Outbreak's Prediction, Forecasting and Decision Making for Policy Makers," testing and isolation of cases is discussed which is an important component of our strategies to fight SARS-CoV-2. In this chapter, we consider a compartmental model for Covid-19 including a nonlinear term representing symptom-based testing. We analyze how the considered clinical spectrum of symptoms and the testing rate affect the outcome and the severity of the outbreak.

In chapter "Dynamics of Inter-community Spread of Covid-19," an attempt has been made to review the current state of the art in epidemiological modeling, assessment of predictive models as well as forecasting of a new pathogen. The primary concern is the containment of the outbreak from the widespread of the disease among the whole population. This article also focuses on the development of management tools and techniques in decision making for policy makers that are based on scientific evidence. Moreover, the identification, detection, and reporting for the outbreak of an infectious disease particularly a new pathogen in a timely manner are quite challenging and tedious. Apparently understanding and reporting of such events commonly rely on statistical and mathematical tools, and both these approaches commonly depend upon a priory estimate as well as some reliable data. For example, statistical models require a sizable number of events to develop predictive models, which is impossible at the outset of an outbreak of the disease to collate enough number of samples, whereas the mathematical models are reliable as well as have better predictive behavior, but they also require better initial guess apart from some rigid constraints to fully satisfy the model's assumptions. Apart from these issues, the other important features to study in the epidemiology of the disease is how fast and quickly the scientific community promptly can pinpoint and able to address any causal factor which may sucre to account for the magnitude and severity of the epidemics of new pathogen that may have been taken place to any geographic locations. Hence in this chapter, first of all the SIR model (susceptible: S, infected: I, and recovered: R) will be outlined, as it is the most commonly used model in the epidemiology of infectious diseases. Moreover, the applicability and utilization of $R0$ in the public health domain especially adaptive policy with management tools will be developed for the healthcare workers as well as the higher management of the healthcare facility.

In chapter "Similarity Measure of q-Rung Orthopair Fuzzy Soft Sets and Its Application in Covid-19 Problem," we have developed a model for the spread of Covid-19 within a community, and we pay attention to the sensitivity of the derived basic reproduction number to each model parameter. This model was extended to investigate the impact of migration between two communities on the spread of the disease. Three special cases, unidirectional migration, unrestricted bidirectional migration, and partial bidirectional migration, were considered. Covid-19 data for two Nigerians states, namely Lagos (high-burden community) and Ogun (low-burden community), were obtained from the Web site of the Nigeria Centre for Disease Control for parameter estimation and simulation. Our results show that the basic reproduction number of the original model is most sensitive to the recovery rate of symptomatic infectious individuals. From the inter-community spread model, we find that the rate of coupling plays a vital role in the control of the pandemic. Our results project the different possible scenarios based on different lockdown and infection rates in two different communities.

In chapter "Local Fractional Calculus to Design the Growth System of Covid-19 Using Measure of Non-compactness," we introduce q-rung orthopair fuzzy soft sets (q-ROFSSs) and some basic properties. Also, we define a similarity measure of q-ROFSSs, and their properties are studied. Finally, we provide an application of q-ROFSSs in Covid-19.

In chapter "Social Opinion Influence on Epidemic Scenarios," we use the concept of local fractional calculus and measure of non-compactness to design the growth system of Covid-19. To achieve this, we establish a fixed-point and coupled fixed-point theorems for a new μ-set contraction condition in partially ordered Banach spaces, whose positive cone K is normal. We provide adequate examples to validate the epidemic dynamics with graphical presentations. We also use presently available data to validate it.

In chapter "Modelling the Significant Effect of Public Health Interventions on Covid-19 Transmission," we have considered different scenarios describing the eagerness of the population to accept the confinement policies and propose a way to directly include this information into an epidemic model.

In chapter "Optimal Control of Vaccination and Plasma Transfusion with Potential Usefulness for Covid-19," we use susceptible–exposed–infected–recovered (SEIR) model to predict the outbreak of the disease. SEIR model was chosen because exposed individuals who are asymptomatic or having mild symptoms contribute to the increase of a number of infections. We also work on modeling the transmission dynamics of Covid-19 in the presence of three intervention measures. The proposed model describes the evolution of the disease in the population when preventive measures, active case-finding, and hospitalization interventions are implemented as strategies to control and eradicate the disease. Variation in the effectiveness of combined interventions for infectious individuals is observed and analyzed by simulating the Covid-19 model with interventions. Our simulation results show that more rigorous and stringent public health interventions would reduce the risk of Covid-19 spreading. It is of great importance and practical significance to ensure early prevention, early detection, and early treatment to combat Covid-19.

In Part II, in chapter "Optimal Control of Vaccination and Plasma Transfusion with Potential Usefulness for Covid-19," we introduce two control functions in the compartmental SEIR model representing vaccination and plasma transfusion. Optimal control problems are proposed to study the effects of these two control measures on the reduction of infected individuals and increase of recovered individuals with minimal costs. Up to our knowledge, the plasma transfusion treatment has never been considered as a control strategy for epidemics mitigation. The proposed vaccination and treatment strategies may have a real application in the challenging and hard problem of controlling the Covid-19 pandemic.

In chapter "Fractional Diffusion Equation as a Mathematical Model of the Incidence of Coronavirus Disease Covid-19," we provide the statistical analysis of the numerical indicators of the incidence in the Russian Federation in 2020 of Covid-19. These were constructed corresponding histograms and theoretical distribution densities and found estimates of the distribution parameters by the maximum likelihood method. Based on the statistical analysis of the data, we verified the parameters of the differential equation containing fractional differentiation operator in Caputo sense. In connection with the spread of coronavirus infection (Covid-19), it seems helpful to build a mathematical model of the number of infected persons to predict the spread of infection.

In chapter "An SEIR Epidemic Model of Fractional Order to Analyze the Evolution of the Covid-19 Epidemic in Argentina," we present a case study by using a susceptible–exposed–infected–recovered (SEIR) diffusion model of fractional order in time to analyze the evolution of the epidemic in Buenos Aires and neighboring areas (Región Metropolitana de Buenos Aires, (RMBA)) comprising about 15 million inhabitants. In the SEIR model, individuals are divided into four classes, namely susceptible (S), exposed (E), infected (I), and recovered (R). The SEIR model of fractional order allows for the incorporation of memory, with hereditary properties of the system, being a generalization of the classic SEIR first-order system, where such effects are ignored. Furthermore, the fractional model provides one additional parameter to obtain a better fit of the data. The parameters of the model are calibrated by using as data the number of casualties officially reported. Since infinite solutions honor the data, we show a set of cases with different values of the lockdown parameters, fatality rate, and incubation and infectious periods. The different reproduction ratios $R0$ and infection fatality rates (IFRs) so obtained indicate the results may differ from recently reported values, constituting possible alternative solutions. A comparison with results obtained with the classic SEIR model is also included. The analysis allows us to study how isolation and social distancing measures affect the time evolution of the epidemic.

Chapter "Modeling Effectiveness of Partial Lockdown in Breaking Covid-19 Transmission Chain in Malaysia" focuses on the Covid-19 which was first reported in Wuhan, China, in early December 2019. On March 11, 2020, the World Health Organization declared Covid-19 a worldwide pandemic. Within six months, this highly infectious disease has rapidly spread over 200 countries in six continents, infecting more than 12 million and killing more than 560,000. Malaysia recorded, as of July 12, a total of 8,718 persons tested positive for Covid-19, with 122 deaths, and 8,519 fully recovered, out of a population of 32.4 million. Unprecedented public health and socioeconomic policy have been formulated by the Malaysian government to control the catastrophic pandemic spread and to resolve deep socioeconomic disruptions and uncertainties. For Malaysia, a major pandemic control policy measure is the Movement Control Order (MCO) over a period of 24 weeks from March 18 to August 31, 2020. This MCO decision is facilitated by the use of epidemiology models such as the susceptible–infected–recovered (SIR) model. This MCO has resulted in major socioeconomic disruptions and uncertainty. To overcome these immense economic disruptions and uncertainty, several major economic stimulation packages amounting to RM 250 billion, equivalent to 17% of Malaysia 2019 GDP, are formulated to revitalize Malaysia's economy. Epidemiology models are widely used worldwide to formulate socially acceptable policy measures for breaking the infection transmission chain and for enhancing economic resilience. Since the start of Covid-19 outbreak in Malaysia, we use and continuously calibrate the existing SIR-based in-house FluSiM@USM model to examine the effectiveness of various intervention and mitigation measures in reducing the pandemic burden, the result of which is presented in this chapter. Our epidemic model analysis suggests that MCO has managed to effectively control the spread of Covid-19 by significantly reducing the effective reproduction number *Rt*, from 3.5 to 0.2 over a period of 12 weeks. The constantly evolving knowledge of Covid-19 transmission dynamics requires regular data updates and model enhancements. Collaboration and communication between modelers and public health authorities are essential to formulating and supporting complex public health policy decision. This chapter highlights the effectiveness of MCO in controlling Covid-19 spread. It discusses major socioeconomic disruptions and uncertainties caused by Covid-19 and MCO to the Malaysian and world economy. Guided by the Sendai Framework for Disaster Risk Reduction developed by the United Nations, this chapter will focus the deliberation on the trade-offs between saving life and saving the economy.

In chapter "An Extensive Time Series Analysis of Covid-19 Data Sets on the Indian States," transmission dynamics of the disease is analyzed mathematically with the help of the epidemic compartmental model. The dimensionless number—basic reproduction number, *R*0—is computed by using the next-generation matrix method. Moreover, the local and global stability of the equilibrium points of the model is discussed. The occurrence of bifurcation in the model is investigated. Simulations are made to observe the mathematical results graphically.

Chapter "Modeling the Spread of Covid-19 Pandemic in Morocco" proposes a delayed mathematical model to predict the epidemiological trend of Covid-19 in Morocco. Parameter estimation and sensitivity analysis of the proposed model are rigorously studied. Moreover, numerical simulations are presented in order to test the effectiveness of the preventive measures and strategies were imposed by the Moroccan authorities and also help policy makers and public health administration to develop these strategies.

In chapter "Study of Transmission Dynamics of Covid-19 Virus Using Fractional Model: Case of Morocco," a generalized fractional-order SEIR model is proposed, denoted by SEIRP, in order to study the dynamic behavior of Covid-19 and the effect of lockdown of susceptible population. Some conditions are established to ensure the local asymptotic stability of disease-free and endemic equilibrium points. We apply our results to the case of Morocco country. The theoretical results are validated by some numerical simulations.

Jaipur, India Praveen Agarwal
Santiago, Spain Juan J. Nieto
London, Belgium Michael Ruzhansky
Aveiro, Portugal Delfim F. M. Torres

Acknowledgements

It is our pleasure to express our thanks to all the contributors of chapters in this book who participated in this collective effort. The editors would like to thank the anonymous referees for their valuable comments and suggestions.

We would like to acknowledge the superb assistance that the staff of Springer has provided for the publication of this work. Here, we specially thank Mr. Shamim Ahmad (**Senior Editor**, Mathematical Sciences, Springer) for his valuable support from the beginning to end of this project.

Praveen Agarwal was very thankful to the SERB (project TAR/2018/000001), DST (project DST/INT/DAAD/P- 21/2019 and INT/RUS/RFBR/308), and NBHM (DAE)(project 02011/12/2020 NBHM(R.P)/R&D II/7867) and Nonlinear Dynamics Research Center (NDRC), Ajman University, Ajman, UAE, for their necessary support. Delfim F. M. Torres is grateful to the support of FCT through project UIDB/04106/2020 (CIDMA).

India & UAE	Praveen Agarwal
Santiago, Spain	Juan J. Nieto
London, Belgium	Michael Ruzhansky
Aveiro, Portugal	Delfim F. M. Torres

Contents

Country Specific Analysis

About the Editors

Praveen Agarwal is Associate Professor at the Department of Mathematics, Anand International College of Engineering, Jaipur, India. He completed his Ph.D. in Mathematics from the Malviya National Institute of Technology, Jaipur, India. His areas of research include special functions, fractional calculus, numerical analysis, differential and difference equations, inequalities, and fixed point theorems. He has authored 7 research monographs and edited volumes and over 150 research articles with approximately 100 mathematicians from around the world in prestigious national and international journals. He has delivered invited talks in universities and institutions around the world as well as guided various research students over the years. He is the recipient of the Most Outstanding Researcher (2018) award for his outstanding contribution to mathematics by the then Union Minister of Human Resource Development of India, Prakash Javadekar.

Juan J. Nieto is Professor of Mathematical Analysis at the University of Santiago de Compostela, Spain, since 1991 and a fellow of the Royal Galician Academy of Sciences. He received his Ph.D. in Mathematics from the University of Santiago de Compostela, Spain, in 1983. His most influential contributions to date are in the area of differential equations, and his research interests are in fractional calculus, fuzzy equations and epidemiological models. He is one of the most cited mathematicians in the world according to the Web of Knowledge and appears in the Thompson Reuters Highly Cited Researchers list. His works have been published in various journals and conference proceedings of repute.

Michael Ruzhansky is Senior Full Professor at the Department of Mathematics, Ghent University, Belgium, and Professor at the School of Mathematical Sciences, Queen Mary University of London, UK. He received his Ph.D. in Mathematics from Utrecht University, The Netherlands, in 1998, with the thesis titled "Singular Fibrations with Affine Fibers, with Applications to the Regularity Properties of Fourier

Integral Operators." He completed his M.Sc. in Mathematics and Education at St. Petersburg State University, Russia, in 1995, with the thesis titled "Linear Optimal Filtering Theory with the Generalized Quadratic Quality Functional." He is a recipient of several awards, including Ferran Sunyer I Balaguer Prize (2018), Odysseus I Project (2018), Ferran Sunyer I Balaguer Prize (2014) and Daiwa Adrian Prize (2010).

Delfim F. M. Torres is Full Professor of Mathematics at the Department of Mathematics, the University of Aveiro (UA), Portugal. He received his Ph.D. in mathematics from the University of Aveiro, in 2002. He is also the Director of the FCT Doctoral Programme Consortium in Mathematics and Applications (MAP-PDMA) of the Universities of Minho, Aveiro and Porto, Portugal. His main research areas are calculus of variations and optimal control, optimization with emphasis on the regularity of solutions and necessary optimality conditions, fractional derivatives and integrals, dynamic equations on time scales or measure chains, and mathematical biology. He has published over 400 scientific and pedagogical publications, including research papers in reputed international journals, refereed conference proceedings, chapters in books, and books (as an author and editor). Having guided 21 Ph.D. Torres has a strong experience in graduate and postgraduate student supervision and teaching mathematics, both in Portugal and abroad. Moreover, he has led teams and has been a member of several national and international R&D projects, including EU projects and networks. He was a key scientist of the European Marie Curie Project SADCO (Sensitivity Analysis for Deterministic Controller Design), Network for Initial Training, under the 7th Framework Programme FP7-PEOPLE-2010-ITN.

General Analysis

Continued and Serious Lockdown Could Have Minimized Many Newly Transmitted Cases of Covid-19 in the U.S.: Wavelets, Deterministic Models, and Data

Arni S. R. Srinivasa Rao and Steven G. Krantz

Abstract We have provided model-based estimates of Covid-19 in the U.S. during April–June 2020. The newly reported Covid-19 cases of April in the U.S. have not acquired the virus in the same month. We estimate that there was an average of 29,000/day Covid-19 cases in the U.S. transmitted from infected to susceptible during April 1–24, 2020, after adjusting for under-reported and under-diagnosed. We have provided model-based predictions of Covid-19 for the low and high range of transmission rates and with varying degrees of preventive measures including the lockdowns. We predict that even if 10% of the susceptible and 20% of the infected who were not identified as of April 30, 2020 do not adhere to proper care or do not obey lockdown, then by the end of May and by end of June 50,000 and 55,000 new cases, respectively, will emerge. These values for the months of May and June with worse adherence rates of 50% by susceptible and infected (but not identified) will be 251,000 and 511,000, respectively. Continued and serious lockdown measures could bring this average daily rate of new cases to a further low with a range of 4,300/day to 8,000/day in May.

Keywords Covid-19 · Modeling · Wavelets

Both the authors contributed in writing. ASRS Rao designed the study, developed the methods, models, collected data, performed analysis, computing, creating Figures and Tables, wrote the first draft. SG Krantz participated in the design, interpretation of results, and contributed in editing the draft, approving the methods. Both the authors approved the final manuscript.

A. S. R. S. Rao (✉)
Laboratory for Theory and Mathematical Modeling, Department of Medicine-Division of Infectious Diseases, Medical College of Georgia, Augusta, GA 30912, USA
e-mail: arrao@augusta.edu

Department of Mathematics, Augusta University, Augusta, GA 30912, USA

S. G. Krantz
Department of Mathematics, Washington University in St. Louis, One Brookings Drive, Campus Box 1146, St. Louis, MO 63130, USA

P. Agarwal et al. (eds.), *Analysis of Infectious Disease Problems (Covid-19) and Their Global Impact*, Infosys Science Foundation Series,
https://doi.org/10.1007/978-981-16-2450-6_1

1 Introduction

The current growth rate of Covid-19 in the world and in the U.S. as of August 10, 2020, is still alarming. We have provided here retrospective model-based estimates for the period April–June 2020 in the US, i.e. for the period just after the lifting of serious lockdown. The cumulative number of novel coronavirus cases in the U.S. is still very high at more than 1,062,466 as of April 30, 2020, and more than 876,000 of these cases were reported during April 1–30, 2020 [1]. We have asked a couple of questions: namely, did the lockdown implemented by various states in the U.S. by the end of March 2020 had any impact so far, especially in preventing the new Covid-19 cases in the recent weeks in the U.S.? Was there any degree of damage in further controlling the spread of Covid-19 in the U.S. by relaxing the lockdown measures to keep-up the economy? We found that relaxing ongoing efforts on controlling the pandemic in the U.S. could have striking impact on the number of new cases for the months of May and June 2020. A 50% relaxed approach in the lockdown or poor preventive measures in the U.S. could had led to additional new Covid cases up to 200,000 to 370,000. We provide several other scenarios too which are in Tables 1–6.

It is not always easy to conduct experiments to get the parameters of transmissions during the lockdowns [2]. One can indirectly obtain the number of people who were infected in a geographical area within a specified time and obtain population-level incidence rates based on the newly reported cases. But we know that often not all cases are reported or diagnosed or both [3]. That means a true incidence rate in the population is not easy to obtain unless we adjust the reported cases with the number not reported and retrospectively adjust the past reported data [3].

Table 1 Predicted Covid-19 cases in the U.S. under the varying degrees of adhering to lockdown and other preventive measures from May 1 to June 30, 2020 (Medium range)

End of the month in 2020	Predicted new Covid-19 cases by age groups (medium range) (with percentage of people among infected but not yet detected who are not adhering lockdown and other preventive measures is = 20)				Percentage of susceptible people not adhering to lockdown and other preventive precautions
	<18	**18–64**	**65+**	**Total**	
May	259	37,876	12,275	50,410	10
June	312	41,275	13,701	55,288	
May	326	42,123	14,054	56,503	20
June	455	50,215	17,407	68,077	
May	402	46,929	16,048	63,379	30
June	605	61,294	21,971	83,870	
May	489	52,340	18,285	71,114	40
June	860	75,018	27,600	103,478	
May	588	58,432	20,796	79,816	50
June	1,142	92,011	34,542	127,695	
May	700	65,289	23,614	89,603	60
June	1,493	113,043	43,111	157,647	
May	827	73,007	26,778	100,612	70
June	1931	139,067	53,690	194,688	

Table 2 Predicted Covid-19 cases in the U.S. under the varying degrees of adhering to lockdown and other preventive measures from May 1 to June 30, 2020 (high range)

End of the month in 2020	Predicted new Covid-19 cases by age groups (high range) (with percentage of people among infected but not yet detected who are not adhering lockdown and other preventive measures is = 20)				Percentage of susceptible people not adhering to lockdown and other preventive precautions
	<18	**18–64**	**65+**	**Total**	
May June	315 430	38,012 41,961	13,918 16,923	52,245 59,314	10
May June	460 775	42,991 53,741	17,684 25,234	61,135 79,750	20
May June	642 1,277	49,186 70,781	22,104 36,482	71,932 108,540	30
May June	866 1,992	56,818 95,007	27,315 51,854	84,999 148,853	40
May June	1,140 3,002	66,151 129,108	33,484 72,982	100,775 205,092	50
May June	1,475 4,418	77,507 176,827	40,807 102,126	119,789 283,371	60
May June	1,882 6,396	91,270 243,366	49,521 142,408	142,673 392,170	70

Table 3 Predicted Covid-19 cases in the U.S. under the varying degrees of adhering to lockdown and other preventive measures from May 1 to June 30, 2020 (Low range)

End of the month in 2020	Predicted new Covid-19 cases by age groups (low range) (with percentage of people among infected but not yet detected who are not adhering lockdown and other preventive measures is = 50)				Percentage of susceptible people not adhering to lockdown and other preventive precautions
	<18	**18–64**	**65+**	**Total**	
May June	647 781	94,637 103,182	30,687 34,248	125,971 138,211	10
May June	815 1,138	105,303 125,521	35,131 43,506	141,249 170,165	20
May June	1,006 1,587	117,315 153,203	40,115 54,908	158,436 209,698	30
May June	1,223 2,150	130,840 187,486	45,705 68,962	177,768 258,598	40
May June	1,470 2,854	146,065 229,525	51,979 86,295	199,514 318,674	50
May June	1,750 3,732	163,201 282,440	59,020 107,679	223,971 393,851	60
May June	2,067 4,824	182,486 347,401	66,925 134,072	251,478 486,297	70

Table 4 Predicted Covid-19 cases in the U.S. under the varying degrees of adhering to lockdown and other preventive measures from May 1 to June 30, 2020 (high range)

End of the month in 2020	Predicted new Covid-19 Cases by age groups (high range) (with percentage of people among infected but not yet detected who are not adhering lockdown and other preventive measures is = 50)				Percentage of susceptible people not adhering to lockdown and other preventive precautions
	<18	**18–64**	**65+**	**Total**	
May June	787 1,075	95,029 104,893	34,791 42,290	130,607 148,258	10
May June	1,150 1,937	107,472 134,318	44,199 63,033	152,821 199,288	20
May June	1,604 3,189	122,953 176,861	55,238 91,092	179,795 271,142	30
May June	2,164 4,975	142,020 237,308	68,253 129,403	212,437 371,686	40
May June	2,850 7,493	165,336 322,333	83,657 182,010	251,843 511,836	50
May June	3,683 11,020	193,699 441,204	101,938 254,480	299,320 706,704	60
May June	4,702 159,40	228,070 606,754	123,685 354,478	356,457 961,232	70

Table 5 Predicted Covid-19 cases in the U.S. under the varying degrees of adhering to lockdown and other preventive measures from May 1 to June 30, 2020 (medium range)

End of the month in 2020	Predicted new Covid-19 cases by age groups (medium range)				Percentage of susceptible people not adhering to lockdown and other preventive precautions
	<18	**18–64**	**65+**	**Total**	
May June	1293 1562	189,270 206,345	61,370 68,482	251,933 276,389	10
May June	1629 2274	210,594 250,987	70,254 86,976	282,477 340,237	20
May June	2012 3172	234,608 306,295	80,215 109,746	316,835 419,213	30
May June	2447 4297	261,664 374,772	91,388 137,801	355,499 516,870	40
May June	2940 5703	292,078 459,510	103,924 172,386	398,942 637,599	50
May June	3500 7455	326,328 564,324	117,993 215,034	447,821 786,813	60
May June	4133 9636	364,869 693,920	133,786 267,638	502,788 971,194	70

Table 6 Predicted Covid-19 cases in the U.S. under the varying degrees of adhering to lockdown and other preventive measures from May 1 to June 30, 2020 (high range)

End of the month in 2020	Predicted new Covid-19 cases by age groups (high range)				Percentage of susceptible people not adhering to lockdown and other preventive precautions
	<18	**18–64**	**65+**	**Total**	
May	1,573	190,051	69,566	261,190	10
June	2,148	209,755	84,521	296,424	
May	2,300	214,924	88,360	305,584	20
June	3,870	268,519	125,895	398,284	
May	3,206	245,862	110,407	359,475	30
June	6,370	353,414	181,803	541,587	
May	4,325	283,959	136,393	424,677	40
June	9,929	473,922	258,039	741,890	
May	5,696	330,535	167,137	503,368	50
June	14,942	643,223	362,546	1,020,711	
May	7,366	387,176	203,612	598,154	60
June	21,954	879,549	506,202	1,407,715	
May	9,393	455,793	246,982	712,168	70
June	31,716	1,208,000	703,876	1,943,592	

2 Methods, Models and Data

We want to understand through simple transmission dynamic principles what fraction of these cases were possibly acquired during April. We want to understand these numbers by adjusting for under-reporting including the under-diagnosis during the period. Further, we develop age-structured population models of Covid-19 spread, and combining the outcomes with wavelet analysis, we have determined the impact of not adhering to lockdown and other preventive measures combined in the U.S. for the period May–June, 2020. Our methods, models and the data are described in the next paragraphs (Fig. 1).

Let f_n be the cumulative number of Covid-19 cases reported at the end of the nth day and $f_0 = 0$ be the number of Covid-19 cases at the beginning. Let f_1 be the number of cases at the end of 1st day. Let $I_i = f_{i+1} - f_i$ for $i = 0, 1, 2, ..., n-1$ be the new cases on the each day. Let $c_i \in (0, 1)$ be the fraction of I_i of those infected on the ith day such that

$$c_i I_i d = 1, \tag{1}$$

where d is the average incubation period. That is,

$$c_i I_i + c_i I_i + \ldots c_i I_i (d \text{ times}) = I_i, \tag{2}$$

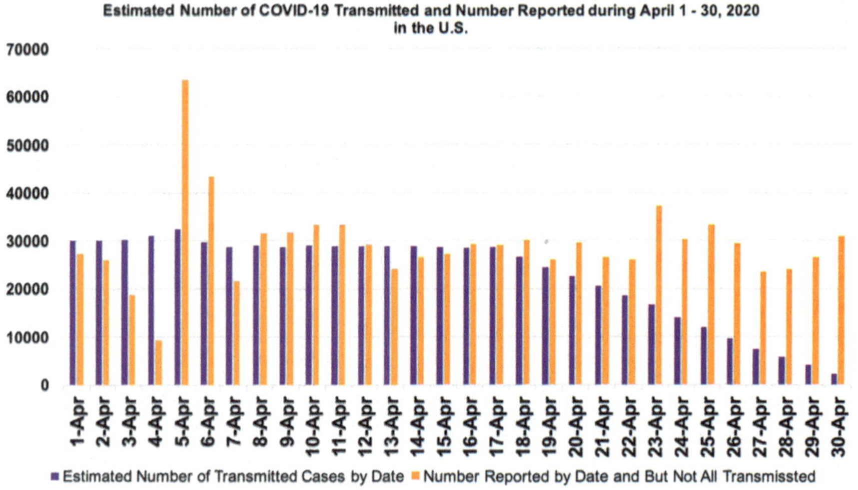

Fig. 1 Estimated transmissions occurred during each day and the number of reported per day during April 1–23, 2020. The estimated cases are skewed because some of the transmission occurred before April 19 might be reported at a later date

is satisfied. Through Eq. (1), we have distributed newly reported cases on the ith day into ith day cases and cases from $d-1$ number of days prior to ith day. We assumed that c_i is constant in (1), so that, I_i is uniformly distributed during [ith day, d days prior]. Instead of uniform distribution of I_i as considered in (1), one can consider a skewed or nonuniform or some random distribution if there is strong evidence of the same. Under such nonuniform situations as well we will have $\sum_{i=1}^{d} c_i I_i = I_i$ and $\sum_{i=1}^{d} c_i = 1$. Once each I_i value is partitioned into $d-1$ days prior to the ith day, then the number of transmuted cases in each day is computed using the below set of equations:

$$\begin{aligned} c_1 I_1 + c_1 I_2 + \ldots + c_1 I_d &= A(I_1) \\ c_2 I_2 + c_2 I_3 + \ldots + c_2 I_{d+1} &= A(I_2) \\ &\vdots \\ c_d I_d + c_d I_{d+1} + \ldots + c_d I_{2d-1} &= A(I_d) \end{aligned} \tag{3}$$

$$\begin{aligned} c_{d+1} I_{d+1} + c_{d+1} I_{d+2} + \ldots + c_{d+1} I_{2d} &= A(I_{d+1}) \\ c_{d+2} I_{d+2} + c_{d+2} I_{d+3} + \ldots + c_{d+2} I_{2d+1} &= A(I_{d+2}) \\ &\vdots \\ c_{2d} I_{2d} + c_{2d} I_{2d+1} + \ldots + c_{2d} I_{3d-1} &= A(I_{2d}) \end{aligned} \tag{4}$$

These continue until the last reported cases are available for a given population. For the computations in this article, we considered uniform c_i values over d days by assuming $c_i = c$ within the period of study. Then, we assumed that the daily new cases April 1–13 were uniformly distributed into 1/14th, 2/14th, 3/14th and so on until 13/14th fractions of the reported, and we assumed all the cases from April 14 were the result of those transmitted during the month of April. A similar backward adjustment of reported cases was theoretically demonstrated in our earlier article with advanced network structures [5].

Let Y be the total number of newly infected cases which were not traced into the system. Let $Y = Y_1 + Y_2 + Y_3$, where Y_k is the number of infected in the age group k for k = 0–17, 18–64, 65 +, respectively. Let X be the total number of susceptible individuals and $X = \sum_{k=1}^{3} X_k$, where X_k is the size of susceptible in the age group k. Let $L(X_k) = \varnothing_k X_k$ be the fraction $\varnothing_k$ of susceptible X_k who do not practice lockdown or other preventive measures in the age group k, such that

$$L(X) = L(X_1 + X_2 + X_3) = \phi_1 X_1 + \phi_2 X_2 + \phi_3 X_3, \tag{5}$$

where $\varnothing = \sum_{k=1}^{3} \varnothing_k$ is the total fraction of susceptibles in the population who do not adhere to any preventive measures including the lockdown. Similarly, we will assume that

$$L(Y) = L(Y_1 + Y_2 + Y_3) = \psi_1 Y_1 + \psi_2 Y_2 + \psi_3 Y_3, \tag{6}$$

where $\psi = \sum_{k=1}^{3} \psi_k$ is the total fraction of infected (who are not traced) in the population who do not adhere to any preventive measures including the lockdown. The differential equations describing the transmission dynamics from infected to susceptible are given below:

$$\frac{dL(X_1)}{dt} = -\left[L(X_1) \sum_{k=1}^{3} \beta_{k1} L(Y_k)\right]$$

$$\frac{dL(X_2)}{dt} = -\left[L(X_2) \sum_{k=1}^{3} \beta_{k2} L(Y_k)\right]$$

$$\frac{dL(X_3)}{dt} = -\left[L(X_3) \sum_{k=1}^{3} \beta_{k3} L(Y_k)\right]$$

$$\frac{dL(Y_1)}{dt} = \left[L(X_1) \sum_{k=1}^{3} \beta_{k1} L(Y_k)\right] - \gamma_1 L(Y_1)$$

$$\frac{dL(Y_2)}{dt} = \left[L(X_2) \sum_{k=1}^{3} \beta_{k2} L(Y_k)\right] - \gamma_2 L(Y_2)$$

$$\frac{dL(Y_3)}{dt} = [L(X_3)\sum_{k=1}^{3}\beta_{k3}L(Y_k)] - \gamma_3 L(Y_3) \tag{7}$$

Here, β_{kl} is the average transmission rate from an infected in the age group k to a susceptible in the age group l and γ_k is the recovery rate for the age group k. Similar age structure population models for the Covid-19 were developed by us in predicting the U.S. population aged 65 + with underlying medical conditions [7]. Once we obtain predicted values of new Covid-19 cases, we will use Meyer's wavelets to demonstrate the difference of magnitudes between observed and predicted cases and wavelets for the difference among various degrees of not adhering to lockdown or other preventive measures. Meyer's wavelets are a natural improvement over the Fourier series and transforms. A Fourier series $f(x)$ is written in terms of coefficients a_0, a_n and b_n for $n \in \mathrm{N}$, the set of natural numbers and with trigonometric functions as below

$$f(x) = \frac{a_0}{2} + \sum_{n=1}^{\infty}(a_n \cos nx + b_n \sin nx), \tag{8}$$

where $\cos nx + i \sin nx = e^{inx}$. Further, if $f(x)$ is Lebesgue integrable on an interval $[0, a]$ with a period a, then we write

$$f(x) = \frac{a_0}{2} + \sum_{n=1}^{\infty}\left(a_n \cos\frac{2\pi nx}{a} + b_n \sin\frac{2\pi nx}{a}\right),$$

where

$$a_n = \frac{2}{a}\int_0^a f(s)\cos\frac{2\pi ns}{a}\, ds,$$

$$b_n = \frac{2}{a}\int_0^a f(s)\sin\frac{2\pi ns}{a}\, ds.$$

Once we have Fourier series, one can obtain Fourier transformations, f_T, through (9), written as

$$f_T(z) = \int_{-\infty}^{\infty} e^{-izs} f(s)\, ds, \tag{9}$$

where z is a complex numbers and $f(s)$ is a Fourier series function (8).

The Meyer wavelets $\psi(\omega)$ also use trigonometric functions which are infinitely differentiable on a certain domain. Several useful resources on wavelets are available in [8–14]. We have used such wavelets in Covid-19 modeling [3, 5, 7, 15]. These wavelets when plotted helps us to distinguish the degree of difference in the magnitude between various levels of relaxation of lockdown and other preventive measures during Covid-19 lockdowns. The Meyer wavelets $U(\omega)$ together with accompanying function v are given below.

What is interesting about this new wavelet technique is the following. The traditional trigonometric functions sine and cosine do not localize well. Once we know a trigonometric function on a small interval, then it is uniquely determined on the entire real line. But wavelets localize nicely in both the space and the phase variables. This makes them particularly useful for image compression, signal processing and data analysis. Wavelets are the key to our new approach to understanding the corona pandemic. Let

$$U(\omega) = \begin{cases} \frac{1}{\sqrt{2\pi}} \sin\left(\frac{\pi}{2} v\left(\frac{3|\omega|}{2\pi} - 1\right)\right) e^{\frac{i\omega}{2}} & \text{if } 2\pi/3 < |\omega| < 4\pi/3 \\ \frac{1}{\sqrt{2\pi}} \cos\left(\frac{\pi}{2} v\left(\frac{3|\omega|}{2\pi} - 1\right)\right) e^{\frac{i\omega}{2}} & \text{if } 4\pi/3 < |\omega| < 8\pi/3 \cdot \\ 0 & \text{otherwise} . \end{cases} \tag{10}$$

Here $v(x) = 0$ For $x < 0$ and

$$v(x) = \begin{cases} x & \text{for } x \in (0, 1) \\ 1 & \text{for } x > 1 \end{cases} \tag{11}$$

General population age structure models are well-known in epidemiology, population biology, ecology, see for example [16–25]. However, the novelty of our work lies in linking the wavelets in conceptualizing the differences between the magnitudes of $L(Y_1)$, $\left[L(Y_2), L(Y_3)\right.$ with varying $\varnothing$ and ψ values. Such exposure of Meyer's wavelets or other wavelets were done earlier. For a more general application potential and beauty of applicability of wavelets, one can refer to [31].

3 Data

For the modeling purpose, we have used the reported data that was available as of April 23, 2020, the date we have designed the study, developed models and have started calibrating to predict until June 30, 2020. As of April 23, 2020, the age distribution of the Covid-19 cases in the U.S. among those whose age can be ascertained are as follows: 2,791 (aged < 18), 475,659 (aged 18–64), 149,243 (aged 65 +). The number of infected during April 1–22, 2020, who were not reported are estimated at 224,785 by our previous calculation of under-reporting in the U.S. [6]. These new cases of April, we have divided into the age groups as per the CDC data above. This would provide us with $Y_1 = 999$, $Y_2 = 170,339$, and $Y_3 = 53,446$. Demographic data from census.gov [26] with adjustment for annual growth that was observed over the past decadal growth gives us susceptible populations X_1,X_2,X_3. We considered the lack of adherence from 10 to 70% for both susceptible and infected. We could provide combinations of these and provide more predictions, but we prepared for these finite number of combinations. One can try all other permutations and combinations. Distributing $\varnothing$ and ψ within each age groups, we have considered the following ratio [10% : 60% : 30%]. The β values for low range of predictions considered are

$$\beta\,(\text{low}) = \begin{Bmatrix} 2.0833 \times 10^{-10} & 1.84615 \times 10^{-10} & 2.0833 \times 10^{-10} \\ 2.0833 \times 10^{-10} & 1.84615 \times 10^{-10} & 2.0833 \times 10^{-10} \\ 2.0833 \times 10^{-10} & 2.0833 \times 10^{-10} & 2.0833 \times 10^{-10} \end{Bmatrix}$$

These low range of predictions are calibrated just as in our previous medium range of values in the study [7]. Originally, these transmission rates were calibrated earlier for the U.S. data on reported Covid-19 cases during March 1–14 and March 15–April 6, 2020, which were calibrated from our paper [3]. The high-range transmission parameters considered are

$$\beta\,(\text{high}) = \begin{Bmatrix} 4.1667 \times 10^{-10} & 2.3077 \times 10^{-11} & 4.1667 \times 10^{-10} \\ 2.3077 \times 10^{-11} & 2.3077 \times 10^{-11} & 4.1667 \times 10^{-10} \\ 4.1667 \times 10^{-10} & 4.1667 \times 10^{-10} & 4.1667 \times 10^{-10} \end{Bmatrix}$$

4 Results

Out of the 876,000 Covid-19 cases newly reported during April 1–30, 2020, we have estimated that 684,027 cases were the result of transmissions within this period. To do this, we have assumed a few things, the first being the average incubation period as per CDC as 2–14 days [4]. Adjusting the reported cases with the not reported cases computed as of April 6, 2020, in the ratio of 1:1.5 as noted in [6], the true acquired estimated number during April 1–30 stands at 684,027. According to the CDC data released on April 30, 23% of the cases are in the age group 65 + [1]. This implies that 23% of 684,027, that is, 235,989 number of new cases who are aged 65 + occurred during the period. This number is consistent with another modeling study on 65+ [7] which predicts the number of new cases during April–June 2020 (Fig. 2).

In addition to backward computation of newly transmitted cases in the month of April 2020 explained above and also in the Appendix, we have also developed dynamics models to understand the spread of Covid-19 for the immediate months in the U.S. We further used wavelets to demonstrate the difference in the spread that could occur due to varying degrees of seriousness of the lockdown implementation by susceptible and infected (who are not aware of their status). We assumed all the detected cases are been either self-quarantined or adhering to the preventive measures.

Serious preventive measures and continued lockdown could bring down the new cases in May in addition to the main results of our study mentioned in the introduction. We also note that a relaxed approach toward lockdown and other preventive measures might be a burden on the hospital system (Fig. 3).

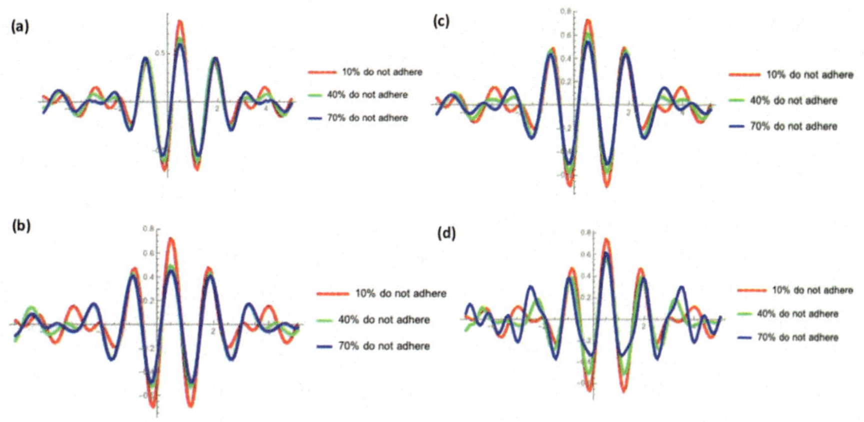

Fig. 2 Meyer wavelets for the difference between magnitudes of predicted new Covid-19 cases in the U.S. for the months of May and June, 2020. All four sets are drawn based on ψ=20% with $\phi = 10\%, 40\%, 70\%$. We have provided details of terminology and methods adopted in the Appendix and actual predicted values are in Tables 1 through Table 6. **a** Difference of magnitude in the month of May for low-range predictions, **b** difference of magnitude in the month of June for low-range predictions, **c** difference of magnitude in the month of May for high-range predictions, **d** difference of magnitude in the month of June for high-range predictions.

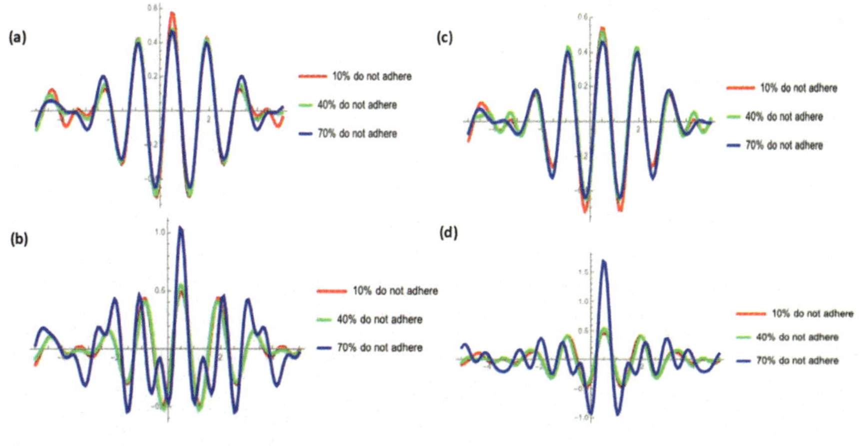

Fig. 3 Meyer wavelets for the difference between magnitudes of predicted new Covid-19 cases in the U.S. for the months of May and June, 2020. All the four sets are drawn based on $\psi = 50\%$ with $\phi = 10\%,\ 40\%\ ,70\%$. **a** Difference of magnitude in the month of May for low-range predictions, **b** difference of magnitude in the month of June for low-range predictions, **c** difference of magnitude in the month of May for high-range predictions, **d** difference of magnitude in the month of June for high-range predictions

5 Concluding Remarks

In summary, we see that on average about 34,000/day new cases occurred that were transmitted during April 1–30, 2020. This is very high. This possibly indicates that the lockdowns and prevention measures have not been adhered to at the fullest. A complete lockdown could bring new infections to a much lower level in the next few weeks. Average daily cases with strict measures can be brought down to a range of 4,300/day to 8,000/day in May. There is reason to believe that under-reporting is skewing our understanding of coronavirus infection and spread. It can be shown that lockdown measures are among the most effective for controlling virus development and spread. Premature lifting of the lockdown could lead to disaster.

As an ending remark, we want to emphasize that one could build more complex models for the transmission dynamics of Covid-19 in the U.S. or for any population if there is strong evidence of transmission-level parameters at the sub-population level. Making models more complex unnecessarily without any supportive evidence would not yield any better results and sometimes such exercises could bring misleading results [33]. There are two levels of complexities one can introduce, one at the level of the parameters and another at the sub-population selection level but that needs very careful assessment of the situation, and modeling should not stand as a mere mathematical exercise.

Funding None to report to this study.

Conflicts None.

References

1. CDC.: https://www.cdc.gov/coronavirus/2019-ncov/cases-updates/cases-in-us.html. Assessed 20 April 2020
2. Boccia, S., Ricciardi, W., Ioannidis, J.P.A.: What other countries can learn from Italy during the COVID-19 pandemic. JAMA Intern. Med. (2020). https://doi.org/10.1001/jamainternmed.2020.1447
3. Krantz, S.G, Rao, A.S.R.S.: Level of under-reporting including under-diagnosis before the first peak of COVID-19 in various countries: preliminary retrospective results based on wavelets and deterministic modeling. Infect. Control Hosp. Epidemiol. 1–8 (2020). https://doi.org/10.1017/ice.2020.116
4. CDC Clinical Questions about COVID-19: Questions and Answers. https://www.cdc.gov/coronavirus/2019-ncov/hcp/faq.html
5. Krantz, S.G., Polyakov, P.G., Rao, A.S.R.S.: True epidemic growth construction through harmonic analysis. J. Theor. Biol. (Elsevier) **494**, 110243 (2020)
6. Mathematical modeling draws more accurate picture of coronavirus cases by Toni Baker. https://www.eurekalert.org/pub_releases/2020-04/mcog-mmd041020.php. Accessed 20 April 2020
7. Rao, A.S.R.S., Miller, D.D., Berman, A.E., Hess, D., Krantz, S.G.: Immediate and near future prediction of COVID-19 patients in the U.S. Population Aged 65+ with the prior medical

conditions of hypertension, cardiovascular and lung diseases: methods, models and acute care estimates. medRxiv (2020). https://doi.org/10.1101/2020.04.12.20062166
8. Meyer, Y., Ryan, R.D.: Wavelets: Algorithms and Applications. Society for Industrial and Applied Mathematics, Philadelphia (1993)
9. Krantz, S.G.: A Panorama of Harmonic Analysis, Carus Mathematical Monographs, 27. Mathematical Association of America, Washington (1999)
10. Hernández, E., Weiss, G.: A First Course on Wavelets. CRC Press, LLC, Boca Raton (1996)
11. Labate, D., Weiss, G., Wilson, E.: Wavelets. Not. Am. Math. Soc. **60**, 66–76 (2013)
12. Meyer, Y.: Wavelets, Vibrations and Scalings. With a preface in French by the author. CRM Monograph Series, 9. American Mathematical Society, Providence, RI (1998)
13. Kaiser, G.: A Friendly Guide to Wavelets, pp. xviii + 300. Birkh¨auser, Basel and Boston, MA (1994). ISBN 0-8176-3711-7
14. Krantz, S.G.: Differential Equations A Modern Approach with Wavelets. CRC Press, Boca Raton (2020)
15. Rao, A.S.R.S., Krantz, S.G., Kurien, T., Bhat, R., Sudhakar, K.: Model-based retrospective estimates for COVID-19 or coronavirus in India: continued efforts required to contain the virus spread. Curr. Sci. **118**(7), 1023–1025 (2020)
16. Shukla, J., Dubey, B.: Modelling the depletion and conservation of forestry resources: effects of population and pollution. J. Math. Biol. **36**, 71–94 (1997). https://doi.org/10.1007/s00285 0050091
17. Anderson, R., May, R.: Population biology of infectious diseases: part I. Nature **280**, 361–367 (1979). https://doi.org/10.1038/280361a0
18. Kakehashi, M.: A mathematical analysis of the spread of HIV/AIDS in Japan. Math. Med. Biol.: A J. IMA **15**(4), 299–311 (1998). https://doi.org/10.1093/imammb/15.4.299
19. Rao, A.S.R.S., Anderson, R.M.: Helminth dynamics: mean number of worms, reproductive rates. Handb. Statist. **36**, 397–404 (2017)
20. Bauch, C.T., Rao, A.S.R.S, Pham, B.Z., Krahn, M., Gilca, V., Duval, B., Chen, M.H., Tricco, A.C.: A dynamic model for assessing universal Hepatitis A vaccination in Canada. Vaccine **25**(10), 1719–1726 (2007)
21. Rao, A.S.R.S.: Population stability and momentum. Not. Am. Math. Soc. **9**, 1062–1065 (2014)
22. Rao, A.S.R.S., Carey, J.R.: On the three properties of stationary populations and knotting with non-stationary populations. Bull. Math. Biol. (Springer) **81**(10), 4233–4250 (2019)
23. Srinivasu, P.D.N., Prasad, B.S.R.V., Venkatesulu, M.: Biological control through provision of additional food to predators: a theoretical study. Theor. Popul. Biol. **72**(1), 111–120 (2007)
24. Castillo-Chavez, C., Hethcote, H.W., Andreasen, V., Levin, S.A., Liu, W.: Cross-immunity in the dynamics of homogeneous and heterogeneous populations. In: Gross, L., Hallam, T.G., Levin, S.A. (eds.) Mathematical ecology. Proceedings, Autumn Course Research Seminars, Trieste 1986, pp. 303–316. World Scientific Publ. Co., Singapore (1988)
25. Dey, S., Joshi, A.: Two decades of drosophila population dynamics: modeling, experiments, and implications. Handb. Stat. **39**, 275–312 (2017)
26. Levin, S.A.: Ecology in theory and application. In: Levin S.A., Hallam T.G., Gross L.J. (eds.) Applied Mathematical Ecology. Biomathematics, vol 18. Springer, Berlin, Heidelberg (1989)
27. Rao, A.S.R.S., Thomas, K., Kurapati, S., Bhat, R.: Improvement in survival of people living with HIV/AIDS and requirement for 1st-and 2nd-line art in India: a mathematical model. Not. Am. Math. Soc. **59**(4), 560–562 (2012)
28. Mandal, S., Bhatnagar, T., Arinaminpathy, N., et al.: Prudent public health intervention strategies to control the coronavirus disease 2019 transmission in India: a mathematical model-based approach. Indian J. Med. Res. **151** (2020). https://doi.org/10.4103/ijmr.IJMR_504_20
29. Rao, A.S.R.S., Thomas, K., Sudhakar, K., Maini, P.K.: HIV/AIDS epidemic in India and predicting the impact of the national response: mathematical modeling and analysis. Math. Biosci. Eng. **4**, 779–813 (2009)
30. www.census.gov
31. Hubbard, B.B.: The World According to Wavelets: The Story of a Mathematical Technique in the Making, 2nd edn (2010)

32. Walker, J.S.: A Primer on Wavelets and Their Scientific Applications (Studies in Advanced Mathematics), 2nd edn, Kindle Edition (2008)
33. Jewell, N.P., Lewnard, J.A., Jewell, B.L.: Predictive mathematical models of the COVID-19 pandemic: underlying principles and value of projections. JAMA. Published online April 16 (2020). https://doi.org/10.1001/jama.2020.6585

Dynamical Analysis of a Caputo Fractional Order SIR Epidemic Model with a General Treatment Function

A. Lamrani Alaoui, M. Tilioua, M. R. Sidi Ammi, and P. Agarwal

Abstract In this work, a fractional order SIR epidemic model is proposed. We first prove the existence, uniqueness, non-negativity and boundedness of solutions to the considered model. We also study the existence of equilibrium points. Some sufficient conditions are derived to ensure, in terms of the basic reproduction number, the global asymptotic stability of the disease free equilibrium point and endemic equilibrium point. Finally, numerical simulations are illustrated to verify the validity of our theoretical results.

Keywords Fractional derivative · Global stability · Nonlinear incidence function · Lyapunov functionals

1 Introduction

Recently, fractional derivatives have attracted a great attention and has known a big development [4, 5, 20, 31, 44]. Therefore, it is well known that fractional differential

A. L. Alaoui · M. Tilioua
Moulay Ismail University of Meknes, FST Errachidia, MAIS Laboratory, MAMCS Group, Meknes, Morocco
e-mail: abdesslemalaoui@gmail.com

M. Tilioua
e-mail: m.tilioua@umi.ac.ma

M. R. Sidi Ammi (✉)
Moulay Ismail University of Meknes, FST Errachidia MAIS Laboratory, AMNEA Group, Meknes, Morocco
e-mail: m.sidiammi@umi.ac.ma

P. Agarwal
Department of Mathematics, Anand International College of Engineering, Jaipur 303012, Rajasthan, India
e-mail: goyal.praveen2011@gmail.com

Nonlinear Dynamics Research Center (NDRC), Ajman University, Ajman, UAE

P. Agarwal et al. (eds.), *Analysis of Infectious Disease Problems (Covid-19) and Their Global Impact*, Infosys Science Foundation Series,
https://doi.org/10.1007/978-981-16-2450-6_2

equations are suitable tools and more effective and valuable in many fields of science and engineering as economics, biology, physics due to its naturally relation to system with memory which is a common feature of many phenomena. For more details see [27, 33, 38]. Fractional derivatives generalize to a certain extent ordinary derivatives. Thus, there is no field left untouched by this new derivatives.

In many works [1, 17, 23, 26, 41–43], the transmission of the infection in the population is modelled by an incidence function taking many forms in the literature. Most of epidemiological models focus on incidence function without delay assuming that infection could occur instantaneously once there is a contact between an infectious individual and a susceptible individuals.

In general, it is often to use Lyapunov's second method also called direct method of Lyapunov to analyze the local or global asymptotic stability properties. It is a robust tool that allows to determine the stability of a system without explicitly integrating the differential equation. For further details see [6, 16, 21, 22, 25, 40, 47]. The stability study of differential equations is still one of the most important problems. This problem has changed significantly over the years. Nowdays, many authors have more interest in the stability analysis of fractional differential systems. The first study trials of this kind of problems dates back many years ago. Afterwards, many researchers devoted enough time to the stability analysis and related questions. For nonlinear fractional differential systems, stability analysis presents much more difficult comparing with integer differential models [2, 3, 11, 30, 32]. Caputo's fractional derivative is considered among well known different definitions of fractional derivatives that have been used more than others. It has the advantage that it conserves the fact that Caputo derivative of a constant is equal to zero, which is not the case for others derivatives.

We are convinced that the treatment policy is a powerful tool and plays a crucial role in controlling or decreasing the spread of infectious diseases as measles, tuberculosis, Covid-19, etc. We can see, for instance, [8, 12, 13, 24, 29, 34].

We provide a brief review of some previous works that have studied a dynamical processes with fractional derivatives. In [10], a fractional-order of HIV infection of CD4 + T-cells has introduced. It is shown that the model possesses non-negative solutions and that the equilibrium points are locally asymptotically stable. The authors have discussed in [14] the stability of equilibrium points of a fractional-order SIR and SIRS epidemic models with variable population size. In [18], a fractional SIR model has been analyzed using the modified Riemann Liouville derivative. The unique global positive solution for the fractional SIR model has been obtained and the asymptotic stability of the positive solution is analyzed. In [39], the stability analysis of a fractional-order epidemics model with multiple equilibriums was studied. By applying fractional calculus, it was given a detailed analysis of the equilibrium points of the model. In [28], a fractional order predator-prey model incorporating a prey refuge was proposed. Some sufficient conditions were derived to ensure the global asymptotic stability of the predator-extinction equilibrium point and coexistence equilibrium point.

The paper is organized as follows. The mathematical model is formulated in Sect. 2. In Sect. 3, preliminaries on the Caputo fractional calculus are presented. In

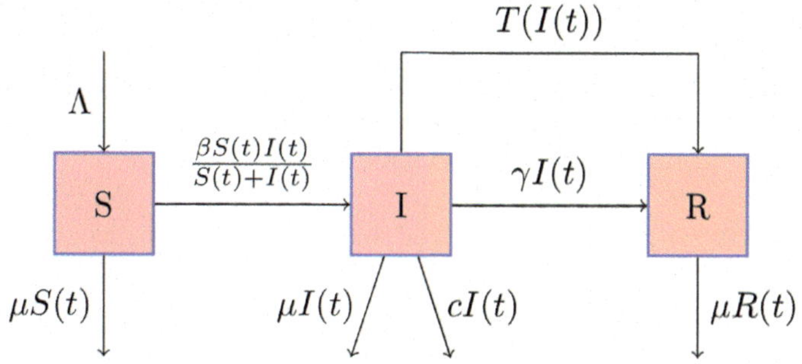

Fig. 1 Flow diagram of the disease transmission

Sect. 4, we shall study the well-posedness of the considered model. More precisely, the positivity and boundedness of the solution are established and the basic reproduction number and equilibria are determined. In Sects. 5 and 6, a local and global analysis of the considered model is investigated, respectively. The usefulness of our model is then illustrated by a numerical example in Sect. 7. We finish the paper by providing some concluding remarks and a perspective for future contributions.

2 Mathematical Model and Preliminaries

We are interested in a general SIR epidemic model with general treatment function. The dynamics of the Caputo fractional-order system is presented by the following flowchart (Fig. 1).

From the diagram, we have the following fractional-order SIR model

$$\begin{cases} {}_{t_0}^{C}D_t^{\alpha} S(t) = \Lambda - \mu S(t) - \beta \dfrac{S(t)I(t)}{S(t)+I(t)}, \\ {}_{t_0}^{C}D_t^{\alpha} I(t) = \beta \dfrac{S(t)I(t)}{S(t)+I(t)} - (\mu + c + \gamma)I(t) - T(I), \\ {}_{t_0}^{C}D_t^{\alpha} R(t) = T(I) + \gamma I(t) - \mu R(t), \end{cases} \tag{1}$$

where $S(t)$, $I(t)$ and $R(t)$ denote the numbers of susceptible, infected and recovered individuals at time t respectively. ${}_{t_0}^{C}D_t^{\alpha}$ stands for the Caputo fractional derivative described below. Here, Λ is the recruitment rate of the population. μ is the natural death. Moreover, individuals leave the susceptible compartment at a rate $\beta \frac{S(t)I(t)}{S(t)+I(t)}$. The transmission of infectious individuals to the recovered compartment is governed by γ, while c represents the disease-related death rate.

In what follows, let $T : \mathbb{R}_+ \to \mathbb{R}_+$ be a continuously differentiable function satisfying the following hypotheses:

($\mathbf{T}_1$) $T(0) = 0$.

($\mathbf{T}_2$) The treatment rate $\dfrac{T(I)}{I}$ is monotone increasing.

The hypothesis ($\mathbf{T}_1$) is natural: no treatment if there is no infected individuals while the hypothesis ($\mathbf{T}_2$) reflects the increasing effort needed from the public health authorities to provide treatment during the time of the infection.

Since the two first equations of system (1) are uncoupled to the third remaining equation, system (1) can be easily reduced to the following equivalent system:

$$\begin{cases} {}_{t_0}^{C}D_t^{\alpha} S(t) = \Lambda - \mu S(t) - \beta \dfrac{S(t)I(t)}{S(t)+I(t)}, \\ {}_{t_0}^{C}D_t^{\alpha} I(t) = \beta \dfrac{S(t)I(t)}{S(t)+I(t)} - (\mu + c + \gamma)I(t) - T(I), \end{cases} \quad (2)$$

3 Preliminaries

In this section, we introduce notations, definitions, and preliminary facts needed in the remaining of this paper.

Definition 3.1 Let $a > 0, t > a, \alpha, t \in \mathbb{R}$. The Caputo fractional derivative of order α of function $f \in \mathbb{C}^n$ is given by

$${}_{a}^{C}D_t^{\alpha} f(t) = \frac{1}{\Gamma(n-\alpha)} \int_a^t \frac{f^{(n)}(\xi)}{(t-\xi)\alpha + 1 - n} d\xi, n-1 < \alpha < n \in \mathbb{N}.$$

Proposition 3.1 *[9] Let $f(t),\ g(t) : [a,b] \longrightarrow \mathbb{R}$ be such that ${}_{a}^{C}D_t^{\alpha} f(t)$ and ${}_{a}^{C}D_t^{\alpha} g(t)$ exist almost everywhere and let $c_1, c_2 \in \mathbb{R}$. Then, ${}_{a}^{C}D_t^{\alpha}(c_1 f(t) + c_2 g(t))$ exists almost everywhere, and*

$${}_{a}^{C}D_t^{\alpha}(c_1 f(t) + c_2 g(t)) = c_1\, {}_{a}^{C}D_t^{\alpha} f(t) + c_2\, {}_{a}^{C}D_t^{\alpha} g(t)$$

Proposition 3.2 *The Caputo fractional derivative of a constant function is zero.*

Definition 3.2 [37] The Mittag-Leffler function in two parameters is defined as $E_{\alpha,\beta}(z) = \sum_{i=0}^{\infty} \dfrac{z^i}{\Gamma(i\alpha+\beta)}$, $z \in \mathbb{C}$, where $\alpha > 0, \beta > 0$, $\mathbb{C}$ denotes the complex plane.

Lemma 3.1 (Generalized Mean Value Theorem) *[36] Suppose that $w(t) \in C[a,b]$ and ${}_{t_0}^{C}D_t^{\alpha} w(t) \in C[a,b]$ for $0 < \alpha \leq 1$, then we have*

$$w(t) = w(a) + \frac{1}{\Gamma(1+\alpha)}\, {}_{t_0}^{C}D_\xi^{\alpha} w(\xi) \Delta (t-a)^{\alpha},$$

with $a \leq \xi \leq t$, $\forall t \in (a,b]$.

Remark 3.1 Let $0 < \alpha \leq 1$. Suppose that $w(t) \in C[a,b]$ and ${}_{t_0}^{C}D_t^{\alpha} w(t) \in C[a,b]$. It follows from Lemma 3.1 that if ${}_{t_0}^{C}D_t^{\alpha} f(t) > 0$ for all $t_0 \in [a,b]$, then there is a neighborhood N of t_0 such that $w(t) > w(a)$, and if ${}_{t_0}^{C}D_t^{\alpha} w(t) < 0$ for all $t_0 \in (a, b)$, then there is a neighborhood N of t_0 such that $w(t) < w(a), \forall t \in N$.

Let us consider the following general fractional differential equation in the Caputo sense

$$\begin{cases} {}_{a}^{C}D_t^{\alpha} x(t) = f(t, x(t)), \quad \alpha \in (0, 1), \\ x_0 = x(t_0). \end{cases} \tag{3}$$

Definition 3.3 The constant x^* is an equilibrium point of the Caputo fractional dynamic system (3) if and only if $f(t, x^*) = 0$.

Lemma 3.2 *[28] Let $u(t)$ be a continuous function on $[t_0, +\infty)$and satisfying*

$$\begin{cases} {}_{t_0}^{C}D_t^{\alpha} u(t) \leq \Lambda - \mu u(t), \quad \alpha \in (0, 1), \\ u(t_0) = u_0. \end{cases}$$

where $0 < \alpha \leq 1$, $(\Lambda, \mu) \in \mathbb{R}^2$ and $\mu \neq 0$, and $t_0 \geq 0$ is the initial time. Then

$$u(t) \leq (u_{t_0} - \frac{\Lambda}{\mu})E_{\alpha}(-\mu(t - t_0)^{\alpha}) + \frac{\Lambda}{\mu}.$$

We now introduce the fractional LaSalle's invariance principle.

Lemma 3.3 *[19] Suppose D is a bounded closed set. Every solution of ${}_{t_0}^{C}D_t^{\alpha} x(t) = f(x)$ starts from a point in D and remains in D for all time. If $\exists V(x) : D \to \mathbb{R}$ with continuous first partial derivatives satisfies the following condition:*

$${}_{t_0}^{C}D_t^{\alpha} V|_{{}_{t_0}^{C}D_t^{\alpha} x(t) = f(x)} \leq 0$$

If $E = \{x, \ {}_{t_0}^{C}D_t^{\alpha} V|_{{}_{t_0}^{C}D_t^{\alpha} x(t) = f(x)} = 0\}$ and M be the largest invariant set of E. Then every solution $x(t)$ originating in D tends to M as $t \to \infty$. Particularly, when $M = 0$, then $x \to 0$ as $t \to \infty$.

4 The Well-Posedness of the Model and Equilibria

In this section, we will discuss existence, uniqueness, boundedness and non-negativity of the solution of system (2). To this end, we need the following results.

Theorem 4.1 *For any given nonnegative initial conditions, there exists a unique solution of system (2) defined on $[0, +\infty)$, and this solution remains non-negative and bounded for all $t \geq 0$.*

Proof It is not hard to see that the right side of system (2) satisfies the first condition of Lemma 4 in [7]. Denote $X(t) = (S(t), I(t))^T$, then system (2) can be reformulated as follows:

$$ {}_{t_0}^{C}D_t^{\alpha} X(t) = \xi + A_1 X(t) + \frac{S(t)}{S(t)+I(t)} A_2 X(t) + F(X(t)), $$

where

$$ A_1 = \begin{pmatrix} -\mu & 0 \\ 0 & -(\mu + c + \gamma) \end{pmatrix}, \quad A_2 = \begin{pmatrix} 0 & -\beta \\ 0 & \beta \end{pmatrix}, $$

and

$$ \xi = \begin{pmatrix} \Lambda \\ 0 \end{pmatrix}, \quad F(X(t)) = \begin{pmatrix} 0 \\ -T(I) \end{pmatrix}. $$

Since T is a continuously differentiable function in the interior of $\mathbb{R}_+$, it follows that there exists $L > 0$ such that

$$ \|F(X(t))\| \leq L\|X(t)\|. $$

Then

$$ \|{}_{t_0}^{C}D_t^{\alpha} X(t)\| \leq \|\xi\| + (\|A_1\| + \|A_2\| + L)\|X(t)\|. $$

By virtue of Lemma 4 in [7], there exists a unique solution $X(t)$ of system (2) with initial condition $X(t_0)$. Now, we will prove that the solution $(S(t), I(t))$ of (2) belongs to $\mathbb{R}_+^2$, for all $t \geq 0$. Let us assume, by absurd, that there exists an instant time where the condition fails. Let

$$ t_1 := \inf\{t > 0, (S(t), I(t)) \notin \mathbb{R}_+^2\}. $$

Thus, $(S(t_1), I(t_1)) \in \mathbb{R}_+^2$ and one of the quantities $S(t_1)$ or $I(t_1)$ is zero. Suppose that $S(t_1) = 0$. Since

$$ {}_{t_0}^{C}D_t^{\alpha} S(t_1) = \Lambda > 0, $$

by continuity of ${}_{t_0}^{C}D_t^{\alpha}$, we conclude that ${}_{t_0}^{C}D_t^{\alpha}([t_1, t_1 + \xi[) \subseteq \mathbb{R}_+$, for some $\xi > 0$. It follows from Lemma 3.1 that $S([t_1, t_1 + \xi[) \subseteq \mathbb{R}_+$ which is a contradiction. Then, $S(t)$ is nonnegative. In an analogous way we can prove that $I(t)$ is nonnegative. Finally, it remains to establish the boundedness of the solution. By summing all the equations of system (2), we obtain

$$ {}_{t_0}^{C}D_t^{\alpha} N(t) = \Lambda - \mu S(t) - (\mu + c)I(t) \leq \Lambda - \mu N(t). $$

It follows from Lemma 3.2 that

$$N(t) \leq (N(0) - \frac{\Lambda}{\mu})E_\alpha(-\mu t^\alpha) + \frac{\Lambda}{\mu}.$$

Since $0 \leq E_\alpha(-\mu t^\alpha) \leq 1$, we have

$$N(t) \leq N(0) + \frac{\Lambda}{\mu}.$$

This implies that the solution is bounded. The proof of Theorem is now complete.

The feasible region of system (1) is given by

$$\Gamma = \left\{(S, I, R) \in \mathbb{R}^3_+, S(t) + I(t) + R(t) \leq \frac{\Lambda}{\mu}\right\}.$$

Let $\mathring{\Gamma}$ be the interior of Γ. In this stage, we use the next generation method [45] to give the basic reproduction number for our model which is considered among the most significant thresholds when studying the asymptotically stability of infectious disease models.

Lemma 4.1 *The basic reproduction number for the model (2) is given by*

$$R_0 = \frac{\beta}{(\mu + c + \gamma) + T'(0)},$$

4.1 Existence of Endemic Equilibrium

System (2) always has a disease-free equilibrium $E_0 = (S_0, 0)$ where $S_0 = \dfrac{\Lambda}{\mu}$. We have the following result.

Lemma 4.2 *If $R_0 > 1$, the system (2) admits a unique endemic equilibrium $E^* = (S^*, I^*)$.*

To prove the unique endemic equilibrium $E^* = (S^*, I^*)$ we introduce the following auxiliary lemma.

Lemma 4.3 *[15] The equation*

$$b - au(t) - T(u(t)) = 0,$$

where $a > 0$ and $b > 0$ has a unique positive solution.

Proof We look for solutions (S^*, I^*) of the equations ${}^C_{t_0}D^\alpha_t S(t) = 0$ and ${}^C_{t_0}D^\alpha_t I(t) = 0$. First note that ${}^C_{t_0}D^\alpha_t S(t) + {}^C_{t_0}D^\alpha_t I(t) = 0$ implies

$$\Lambda - \mu S^* - (\mu + c + \gamma)I^* - T(I^*) = 0,$$

and so

$$S^* = \frac{\Lambda - (\mu + c + \gamma)I^* - T(I^*)}{\mu}.$$

Let H be a function defined from $\mathbb{R}^+$ to $\mathbb{R}$ by

$$H(I) = \frac{\beta(\Lambda - (\mu + c + \gamma)I(t) - T(I(t)))}{\Lambda - (\mu + c + \gamma)I(t) - T(I(t)) + \mu I(t)} - (\mu + c + \gamma) - \frac{T(I(t))}{I(t)}.$$

We have

$$\lim_{I \to 0^+} H(I) = \beta - (\mu + c + \gamma) - T^{'}(0) = \Big((\mu + c + \gamma) + T^{'}(0)\Big)(R_0 - 1) > 0,$$

and

$$H\big(I_0\big) = -\Big((\mu + c + \gamma) + \frac{T(I_0)}{I_0}\Big) < 0,$$

where I_0 is the unique solution of equation $\Lambda - (\mu + c + \gamma)I(t) - T(I(t)) = 0$. Then there exists a unique positive solution $I = I^*$. Now, we proceed to the analysis of the local properties of the model (2).

5 Local Stability Analysis

In this section, we show the local asymptotic stability of both the disease-free equilibrium E_0 and the endemic E^* of system (2).

Theorem 5.1 *If $R_0 < 1$, then the disease-free equilibrium E_0 of the system (2) is locally asymptotically stable. If $R_0 > 1$, the disease-free equilibrium E_0 is unstable.*

Proof The Jacobian matrix of system (2) is given by

$$J = \begin{pmatrix} -\Big(\mu + \dfrac{\beta I^2}{(S+I)^2}\Big) & -\dfrac{\beta S^2}{(S+I)^2} \\ \dfrac{\beta I^2}{(S+I)^2} & \dfrac{\beta S^2}{(S+I)^2} - \Big((\mu + c + \gamma) + T'(I)\Big) \end{pmatrix}.$$

Then the Jacobian matrix of system (2) at E_0 is

$$J(E_0) = \begin{pmatrix} -\mu & -\beta \\ 0 & \beta - \Big((\mu + c + \gamma) + T'(0)\Big) \end{pmatrix}.$$

with the eigenvalues $\lambda_1 = -\mu$ and $\lambda_2 = \beta - \Big((\mu + c + \gamma) + T'(0)\Big) = \Big((\mu + c + \gamma) + T'(0)\Big)(R_0 - 1)$.

If $R_0 < 1$, all eigenvalues are negative. Namely, $|\arg(\lambda_i)| = \pi, i = 1, 2$. Since all eigenvalues $\lambda_i, i = 1, 2$ of Jacobian matrix $J(E_0)$ satisfy $|\arg(\lambda_i)| > \frac{\alpha\pi}{2}$, then E_0 is locally asymptotically stable. If $R_0 > 1$, then $\lambda_2 > 0$ and $|arg(\lambda_2)| = 0 < \frac{\alpha\pi}{2}$. Therefore, E_0 is unstable.

Now, we explore the stability of the endemic equilibrium E^*. The Jacobian matrix of system (2) at the endemic equilibruim E^* is

$$J = \begin{pmatrix} -\left(\mu + \frac{\beta(I^*)^2}{(S^*+I^*)^2}\right) & -\frac{\beta(S^*)^2}{(S^*+I^*)^2} \\ \frac{\beta(I^*)^2}{(S^*+I^*)^2} & \frac{\beta(S^*)^2}{(S^*+I^*)^2} - \left((\mu+c+\gamma) + T'(I^*)\right) \end{pmatrix}.$$

It yields that the characteristic equation of $J(E^*)$ is

$$P(\lambda) = \lambda^2 + a_1\lambda + a_2 = 0, \tag{4}$$

where

$$a_1 = \left(\mu + \frac{\beta(I^*)^2}{(S^*+I^*)^2}\right) - \frac{\beta(S^*)^2}{(S^*+I^*)^2} + (\mu+c+\gamma) + T'(I^*),$$

and

$$a_2 = \left(\mu + \frac{\beta(I^*)^2}{(S^*+I^*)^2}\right)\left(-\frac{\beta(S^*)^2}{(S^*+I^*)^2} + (\mu+c+\gamma) + T'(I^*)\right) + \frac{\beta^2(S^*)^2(I^*)^2}{(S^*+I^*)^4}.$$

We have

$$(\mu+c+\gamma) = \beta\frac{S^*}{S^*+I^*} - \frac{T(I^*)}{I^*}.$$

It follows that

$$a_1 = \left(\mu + \frac{\beta(I^*)^2}{(S^*+I^*)^2}\right) + \frac{\beta S^* I^*}{(S^*+I^*)^2} - \left(\frac{T(I^*)}{I^*} - T'(I^*)\right),$$

$$a_2 = \left(\mu + \frac{\beta(I^*)^2}{(S^*+I^*)^2}\right)\left(\frac{\beta S^* I^*}{(S^*+I^*)^2} - \left(\frac{T(I^*)}{I^*} - T'(I^*)\right)\right) + \frac{\beta^2(S^*)^2(I^*)^2}{(S^*+I^*)^4}.$$

From hypothesis **(T2)** we have

$$T'(I^*) \geq \frac{T(I^*)}{I^*}.$$

$a_1 > 0$ and $a_2 > 0$. Hence, we obtain the following theorem.

Theorem 5.2 *If $R_0 > 1$, then the endemic equilibrium E^* is locally asymptotically stable.*

6 Global Stability Analysis

6.1 Infection-Free Equilibrium

Theorem 6.1 *Assume that the hypotheses* ($\mathbf{T}_1$) *and* ($\mathbf{T}_2$) *hold. Then the disease free equilibrium E_0 of the system (2) is globally asymptotically stable, if and only if $R_0 \leq 1$.*

To prove this theorem we need the following lemma which can be found in [2].

Lemma 6.1 *Let $x(t) \in \mathbb{R}$ be a continuous and derivable function. Then, for any time instant $t \geq t_0$*

$$\frac{1}{2}{}^{C}_{t_0}D^{\alpha}_{t}x^2(t) \leq x(t){}^{C}_{t_0}D^{\alpha}_{t}x^2(t), \forall\alpha \in (0, 1)$$

Proof Let

$$V(S, I) = \frac{1}{2}I^2(t). \tag{5}$$

We have

$$\begin{aligned}
{}^{C}_{t_0}D^{\alpha}_{t}V(S, I) &\leq I(t)\Big(\beta\frac{S(t)I(t)}{S(t)+I(t)} - (\mu + c + \gamma)I(t) - T(I)\Big)\\
&\leq I^2(t)\frac{S(t)I(t)}{S(t)+I(t)}\Big(\beta S(t) - (\mu + c + \gamma)I(t)\\
&- (\mu + c + \gamma)S(t) - \frac{T(I(t))}{I(t)}(S(t) + I(t))\Big)\\
&\leq I^2(t)\frac{S(t)I(t)}{S(t)+I(t)}\Big((\beta - (\mu + c + \gamma) - T^{'}(0))S(t)\\
&- (\mu + c + \gamma)I(t) - T(I(t))\Big)\\
&\leq I^2(t)\frac{S(t)I(t)}{S(t)+I(t)}\Big((\beta - (\mu + c + \gamma) - T^{'}(0))S(t)\\
&- (\mu + c + \gamma)I(t) - T(I(t))\Big)\\
&\leq -I^2(t)\frac{S(t)I(t)}{S(t)+I(t)}((\mu + c + \gamma) + T^{'}(0))\Big((1 - R_0)S(t)\\
&+ (\mu + c + \gamma)I(t) + T(I(t))\Big).
\end{aligned}$$

We conclude that ${}^{C}_{t_0}D^{\alpha}_{t}V(S, I) \leq 0$. Hence, V is a Lyapunov function for system (2). Namely, ${}^{C}_{t_0}D^{\alpha}_{t}V(S, I) \leq 0$ for all $(S, I) \in \mathring{\Gamma}$. Therefore, ${}^{C}_{t_0}D^{\alpha}_{t}V(S, I) = 0$ if and only if $(S, I) = (S_0, 0)$. One can show that the largest invariant subset where ${}^{C}_{t_0}D^{\alpha}_{t}V(S, I) = 0$ is the singleton $\{E_0\}$. Due to LaSalle's Invariance Principle, E_0 is globally asymptotically stable. This completes the proof.

6.2 Endemic Equilibrium

Theorem 6.2 *Assume that the hypotheses* ($\mathbf{T}_1$) *and* ($\mathbf{T}_2$) *hold. If* $R_0 > 1$, *then* E^* *is the only endemic equilibrium and is globally asymptotically stable.*

The next lemma plays an important role in the proof of the above theorem.

Lemma 6.2 *[46] Let* $y(.)$ *be a continuous and differentiable function with* $y(t) \in \mathbb{R}_+$. *Then, for any time instant* $t \geq t_0$, *one has*

$$ {}_{t_0}^{C}D_t^{\alpha}(y(t) - y^* - y^* \ln(\frac{y(t)}{y^*})) \leq (1 - \frac{y(t)}{y^*}) {}_{t_0}^{C}D_t^{\alpha} y(t),\ y^* \in \mathbb{R}^+, \forall \alpha \in (0, 1) \quad (6)$$

Proof Introducing the following Lyapunov functional

$$V(S, I) = I^*\Big(S(t) - S^* - S^* \ln\Big(\frac{S(t)}{S^*}\Big)\Big) + S^*\Big(I(t) - I^* - I^* ln\Big(\frac{I(t)}{I^*}\Big)\Big).$$

Then

$$\begin{aligned} {}_{t_0}^{C}D_t^{\alpha} V(S, I) \leq\ & I^*\Big(1 - \frac{S^*}{S(t)}\Big)\Big(\Lambda - \mu S(t) - \beta \frac{S(t)I(t)}{S(t) + I(t)}\Big) \\ & + S^*\Big(\frac{I(t) - I^*}{I(t)}\Big)\Big(\beta \frac{S(t)I(t)}{S(t) + I(t)} - (\mu + c + \gamma)I(t) - T(I(t)\Big). \end{aligned}$$

We have

$$\begin{cases} \Lambda = \mu S^* + \beta \dfrac{S^* I^*}{S^* + I^*}, \\ (\mu + c + \gamma) = \beta \dfrac{S^*}{S^* + I^*} - \dfrac{T(I^*)}{I^*}. \end{cases}$$

Then we get

$$\begin{aligned} {}_{t_0}^{C}D_t^{\alpha} V(S, I) \leq\ & I^*\Big(1 - \frac{S^*}{S(t)}\Big)\Big(\mu S^* + \beta \frac{S^* I^*}{S^* + I^*} - \mu S(t) - \beta \frac{S(t)I(t)}{S(t) + I(t)}\Big) \\ & + S^*\Big(I(t) - I^*\Big)\Big(\beta \frac{S(t)}{S(t) + I(t)} - (\mu + c + \gamma) - \frac{T(I(t))}{I(t)}\Big) \\ \leq\ & -\mu I^* \frac{(S(t) - S^*)^2}{S(t)} - \beta I^* \frac{(S(t) - S^*)}{S(t)}\Big(\frac{S(t)I(t)}{S(t) + I(t)} - \frac{S^* I^*}{S^* + I^*}\Big) \\ & + \beta S^*\Big(I(t) - I^*\Big)\Big(\frac{S(t)}{S(t) + I(t)} - \frac{S^*}{S^* + I^*}\Big) \\ & - \beta S^*\Big(I(t) - I^*\Big)\Big(\frac{T(I(t))}{I(t)} - \frac{T(I^*)}{I^*}\Big). \end{aligned}$$

Using the two inequalities

$$\begin{cases} \dfrac{S^*I^*}{S^*+I^*} - \dfrac{S(t)I(t)}{S(t)+I(t)} = \dfrac{-S(t)S^*(I(t)-I^*) - I(t)I^*(S(t)-S^*)}{(S^*+I^*)(S(t)+I(t))}, \\ \dfrac{S(t)}{S(t)+I(t)} - \dfrac{S^*}{S^*+I^*} = \dfrac{I^*(S(t)-S^*) - S^*(I(t)-I^*)}{(S^*+I^*)(S(t)+I(t))}, \end{cases}$$

imply

$$\begin{aligned} {}_{t_0}^{C}D_t^{\alpha} V(S,I) \leq & -\Big(\frac{\beta I(t)(I^*)^2}{(S^*+I^*)(S(t)+I(t))} + \mu I^*\Big)\frac{(S(t)-S^*)^2}{S(t)} \\ & - \beta (S^*)^2 \frac{(I(t)-I^*)^2}{(S^*+I^*)(S(t)+I(t))} \\ & - S^*\Big(I(t)-I^*\Big)\Big(\frac{T(I(t))}{I(t)} - \frac{T(I^*)}{I^*}\Big). \end{aligned}$$

The hypothesis **(T1)** ensures that

$$S^*\Big(I(t)-I^*\Big)\Big(\frac{T(I(t))}{I(t)} - \frac{T(I^*)}{I^*}\Big) \geq 0.$$

Hence, ${}_{t_0}^{C}D_t^{\alpha} V(S,I) \leq 0$. We conclude that the endemic equilibrium of system (2) is globally asymptotically stable provided that $R_0 > 1$.

7 Numerical Simulations

In this section, we carry out numerical simulations to support the theoretical analysis. We solve the initial value fractional order problem (7) using an algorithm proposed in [35] and based on the modified trapezoidal rule and fractional Euler's method. We have chosen this algorithm because it is used in a direct way without using linearization, perturbation or restrictive assumptions. It is a powerful method employed by several authors to compute numerical solutions of their mathematical models. We consider, without loss of generality, different values of fractional order derivatives $\alpha = 0.82, 0.85, 0.9$ and 1.0. The simulation results confirm, numerically, the stability result of Theorems 6.1 and 6.2.

Consider the following fractional SIR epidemic model with treatment:

$$\begin{cases} {}_{t_0}^{C}D_t^{\alpha} S(t) = \Lambda - \mu S(t) - \beta \dfrac{S(t)I(t)}{S(t)+I(t)}, \\ {}_{t_0}^{C}D_t^{\alpha} I(t) = \beta \dfrac{S(t)I(t)}{S(t)+I(t)} - (\mu + c + \gamma)I(t) - \dfrac{rI^2(t)}{a+I(t)}, \\ {}_{t_0}^{C}D_t^{\alpha} R(t) = \gamma I(t) + \dfrac{rI^2(t)}{a+I(t)} - \mu R(t). \end{cases} \tag{7}$$

with the initial conditions

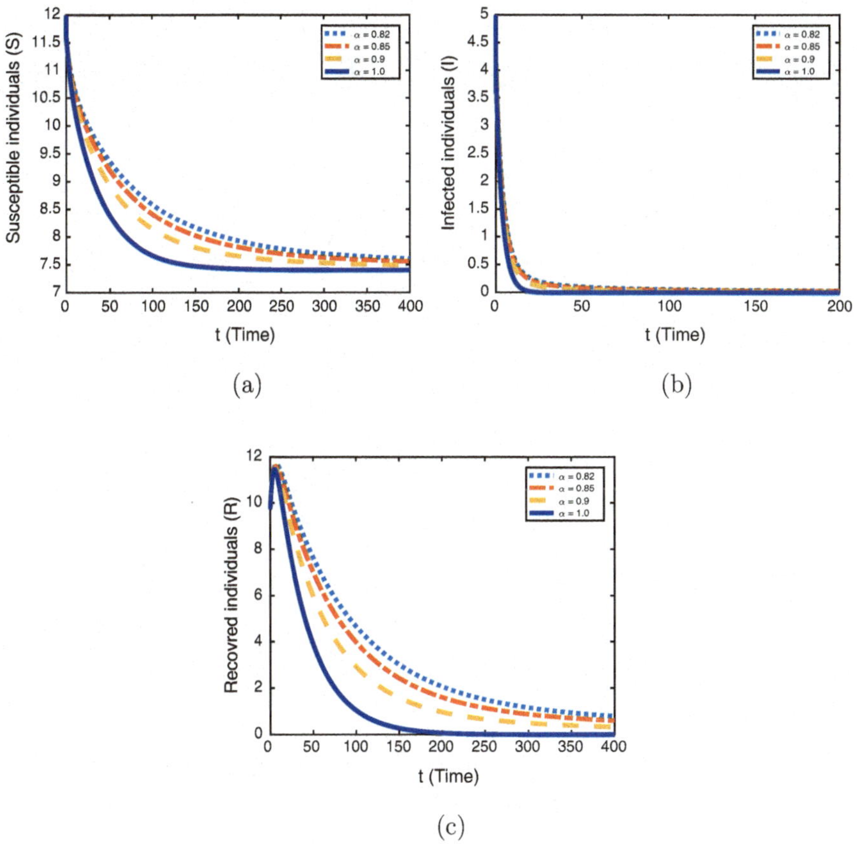

Fig. 2 The time series of the model (7), with Figures **a**, **b** and **c** represent (respectively) S(t), I(t) and R(t), with the above parameters

$$S(0) = 12.0, \quad I(0) = 5.0, \quad R(0) = 9.0.$$

The parameters are chosen as $\Lambda = 0.2$, $r = 0$, $a = 0.4$, $\mu = 0.027$, $\beta = 0.048$, $c = 0.062$ and $\gamma = 0.3$. It is easy to check that $R_0 = 0.9140 < 1$ and $E_0 = (7.4074, 0, 0)$. The treatment term takes the following form

$$T(I) = \frac{rI^2(t)}{a + I(t)}$$

Let us make some comments on the obtained results. It is obvious from Fig. 2 and 3 that the solution for a large t converges to the disease free equilibrium E_0 and to the endemic equilibrium E^*, respectively. However, we find that the treatment decreases the number of infectious individuals (see Fig. 4).

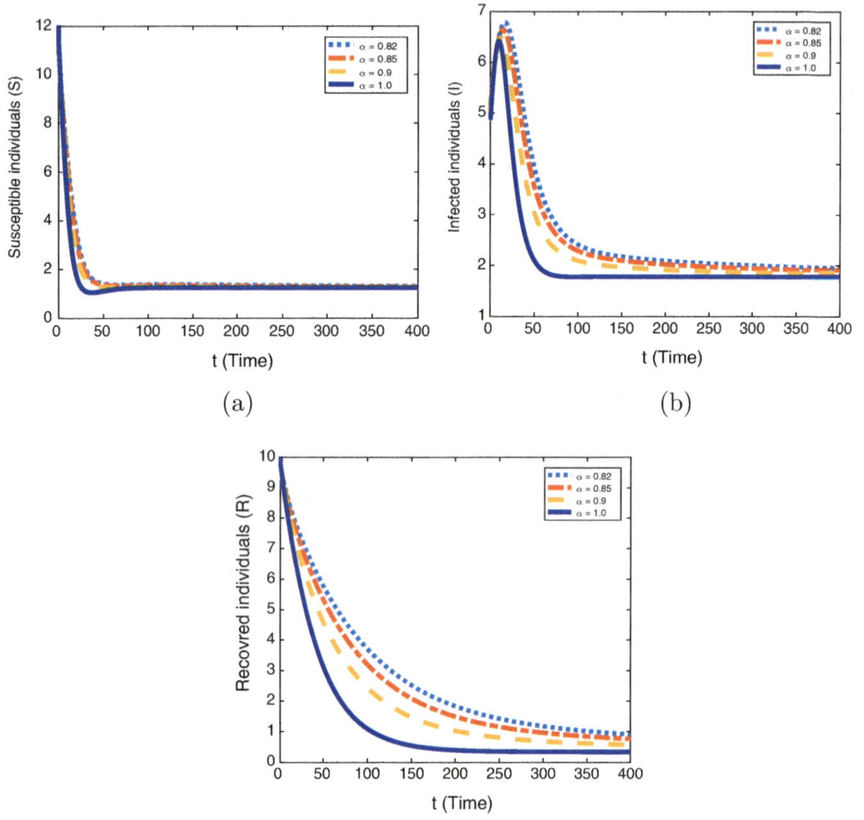

(c)

Fig. 3 The time series of the model (7), with Figures **d**, **e** and **f** represent (respectively) S(t), I(t) and R(t). With the same parameters as in Fig. 2 except $\beta = 0.23$, $\gamma = 0.005$, $a = 0.092$. In this case, $R_0 = 18.1245 > 1$

8 Concluding Remarks

In summary, the basic reproduction number R_0 determines the existence of the equilibrium for the model (2). When $R_0 \leq 1$, model (2) has one unique disease-free equilibrium E_0. While for $R_0 > 1$, model (2) has a disease free equilibrium E_0 and one unique endemic equilibrium E^*. We proved by means of Lyapunov method that all steady state of the model (2) are globally asymptotically stable. We showed that the disease free equilibrium state is globally asymptotically stable for $R_0 \leq 1$. When $R_0 > 1$, we have shown that the existence of a unique endemic equilibrium, which is globally asymptotically stable. As future work we can study the purposed model with general incidence rate and delay, and this is currently a work in progress.

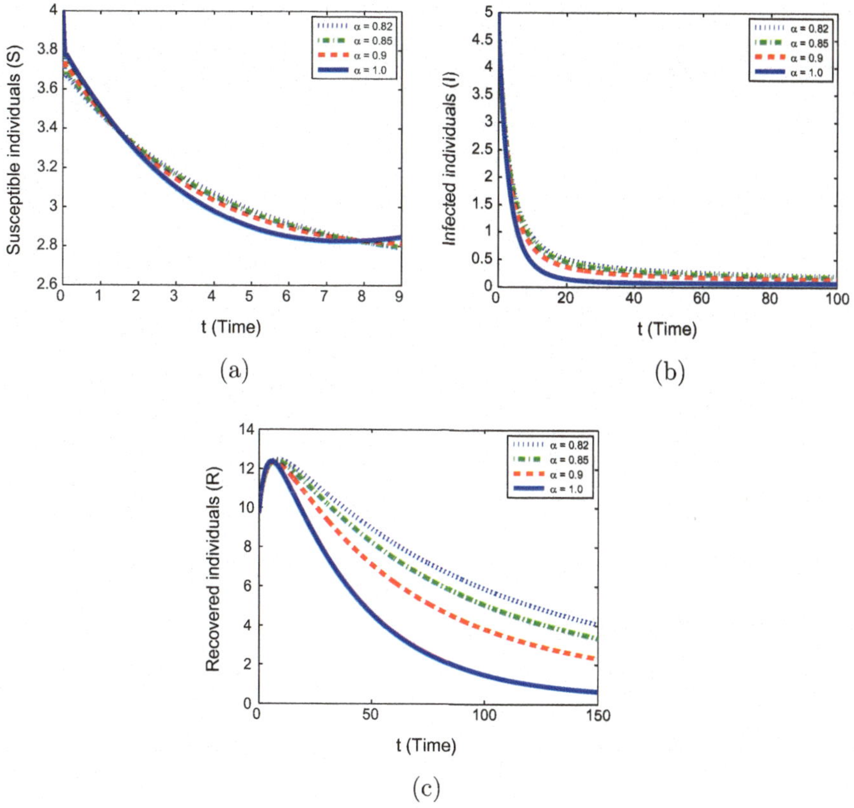

Fig. 4 The time series of the model (7), with Figures **g**, **h** and **i** represent (respectively) S(t), I(t) and R(t). With the same parameters as in Fig. 3 except $r = 0.15$. In this case, $R_0 = 0.4370 < 1$

Acknowledgements The authors wish to thank the reviewers for careful reading and valuable suggestions to improve the quality of the paper.The support from Moulay Ismail University of Meknes (project UMI 2018) and Covid-19 project (Analyse épidémique du Covid-19 au Maroc par modélisation dynamique et intelligence artificielle) jointly funded by CNRST and the Moroccan Ministry of Higher Education and Scientific Research, is acknowledged. P. Agarwal was very thankful to the SERB (project TAR/2018/000001), DST (project DST/INT/DAAD/P-21/2019, INT/RUS/RFBR/308) and NBHM (project 02011/12/ 2020NBHM(R.P)/R& D II/7867) for their necessary support for providing the necessary facility.

References

1. Abdo, M.S., Shah, K., Wahash, H.A., Panchal, S.K.: On a comprehensive model of the novel coronavirus (covid-19) under mittag-leffler derivative. Chaos, Solid. & Fractals **135** (2020)
2. Aguila-Camacho, N., Duarte-Mermoud, M.A., Gallegos, J.A.: Lyapunov functions for fractional order systems. Commun. Nonlinear Sci. Numer. Simul. **19**(9), 2951–2957 (2014)

3. Ahmed, E., El-Sayed, A., El-Saka, H.A.: On some Routh-Hurwitz conditions for fractional order differential equations and their applications in Lorenz, Rössler, Chua and Chen systems. Phys. Lett. A **358**(1), 1–4 (2006)
4. Ahmed, I., Baba, I.A., Yusuf, A., Poom, K., Wiyada, K.: Analysis of caputo fractional-order model for covid-19 with lockdown. Adv. Differ. Equ. **394** (2020)
5. Almeida, R., Cruz, A.M.C.B., Martins, N., Monteiro, M.T.T.: An epidemiological MSEIR model described by the Caputo fractional derivative. Int. J. Dyn. Control **7**, 776–784 (2019)
6. Beretta, E., Hara, T., Ma, W., Takeuchi, Y.: Global asymptotic stability of an SIR epidemic model with distributed time delay. Nonlinear Anal.: Theory, Methods Appl. **47**(6), 4107–4115 (2001)
7. Boukhouima, A., Hattaf, K., Yousfi, N.: Dynamics of a fractional order HIV infection model with specific functional response and cure rate. Int. J. Differ. Equ. **332** (2017)
8. Chauhan, S., Bhatia, S.K., Gupta, S.: Effect of pollution on dynamics of SIR model with treatment. Int. J. Biomath. **08**(06), 1550083 (2015)
9. Diethelm, K.: The analysis of fractional differential equations an application-oriented exposition using differential operators of Caputo type. Springer, Berlin Heidelberg (2010)
10. Ding, Y., Ye, H.: A fractional-order differential equation model of HIV infection of CD4+ T-cells. Math. Comput. Model. **50**(3–4), 386–392 (2009)
11. Duarte-Mermoud, M.A., Aguila-Camacho, N., Gallegos, J.A., Castro-Linares, R.: Using general quadratic lyapunov functions to prove Lyapunov uniform stability for fractional order systems. Commun. Nonlinear Sci. Numer. Simul. **22**(1), 650–659 (2015)
12. Dubey, B., Dubey, P., Dubey, B.: Dynamics of an SIR model with nonlinear incidence and treatment rate. 10:718–737 (2016)
13. Eckalbar, J.C., Eckalbar, W.L.: Dynamics of an epidemic model with quadratic treatment. Nonlinear Anal.: Real World Appl. **12**(1), 320–332 (2011)
14. El-Saka, H.: The fractional-order SIR and SIRS epidemic models with variable population size. Math. Sci. Lett. **2**, 195–200 (2013)
15. Elazzouzi, A., Lamrani Alaoui, A., Tilioua, M., Tridane, A.: Global stability analysis for a generalised delayed sir model with vaccination and treatment. Adv. Differ. Equ. 532 (2019)
16. Enatsu, Y., Messina, E., Nakata, Y., Muroya, Y., Russo, E., Vecchio, A.: Global dynamics of a delayed SIRS epidemic model with a wide class of nonlinear incidence rates. J. Appl. Math. Comput. **39**(1), 15–34 (2012)
17. Enatsu, Y., Nakata, Y., Muroya, Y.: Global stability of SIRS epidemic models with a class of nonlinear incidence rates and distributed delays. Acta Math. Sci. Ser. B Engl. Ed. **32**(3), 851–865 (2012)
18. Guo, Y.: The stability of the positive solution for a fractional SIR model. Int. J. Biomath. **10**, 06 (2016)
19. Huo, J., Zhao, H., Zhu, L.: The effect of vaccines on backward bifurcation in a fractional order HIV model. Nonlinear Anal.: Real World Appl. **26**, 289–305 (2015)
20. Karaji, P., Nyamoradi, N.: Analysis of a fractional SIR model with general incidence function. Appl. Math. Lett. (2020)
21. Korobeinikov, A.: Lyapunov functions and global stability for SIR and SIRS epidemiological models with non-linear transmission. Bull.Math. Biol. **68**(3), 615 (2006)
22. Korobeinikov, A., Maini, P.K.: A lyapunov function and global properties for SIR and SEIR epidemiological models with nonlinear incidence. Math. Biosci. Eng. **1**(1), 57–60 (2004)
23. Kuang, Y.: Delay differential equations with applications in population dynamics. Mathematics in Science and Engineering, vol. 191. Academic Press Inc, Boston, MA (1993)
24. Kumar, A., Nilam: Stability of a time delayed SIR epidemic model along with nonlinear incidence rate and Holling type-ii treatment rate. Int. J. Comput. Methods **15**(06), 1850055 (2018)
25. LaSalle, J., Artstein, Z.: The Stability of Dynamical Systems. CBMS-NSF Regional Conference Series in Applied Mathematics. Society for Industrial and Applied Mathematics (1976)
26. Li, C.-H., Tsai, C.-C., Yang, S.-Y.: Analysis of the permanence of an SIR epidemic model with logistic process and distributed time delay. Commun. Nonlinear Sci. Numer. Simul. **17**(9), 3696–3707 (2012)

27. Li, H.-L., Zhang, L., Hu, C., Jiang, Y.-L., Teng, Z.: Dynamic analysis of a fractional-order single-species model with diffusion. Nonlinear Anal.: Modell. Control **22**, 303–316, 05 (2017)
28. Li, H.-L., Zhang, L., Hu, C., Jiang, Y.-L., Teng, Z.: Dynamical analysis of a fractional-order predator-prey model incorporating a prey refuge. J. Appl. Math. Comput. **54**(1-2), 435–449, 5 (2017)
29. Li, J., Teng, Z., Wang, G., Zhang, L., Hu, C.: Stability and bifurcation analysis of an SIR epidemic model with logistic growth and saturated treatment. Chaos, Solit. Fractals **99**, 63–71 (2017)
30. Li, Y., Chen, Y., Podlubny, I.: Mittag-Leffler stability of fractional order nonlinear dynamic systems. Automatica **45**(8), 1965–1969 (2009)
31. Lin, W.: Global existence theory and chaos control of fractional differential equations. J. Math. Anal. Appl. **332**(1), 709–726 (2007)
32. Liu, K., Jiang, W.: Stability of nonlinear Caputo fractional differential equations. Appl. Math. Model. **40**(5), 3919–3924 (2016)
33. Mainardi, F.: Fractional relaxation-oscillation and fractional diffusion-wave phenomena. Chaos, Solit. Fractals **7**(9), 1461–1477 (1996)
34. Majeed, S.N.: Dynamical study of an SIR epidemic model with nonlinear incidence rate and regress of treatment. Ibn AL- Haitham J. Pure Appl. Sci., 384–396 (2018)
35. Odibat, Z., Momani, S.: An algorithm for the numerical solution of differential equations of fractional order. J. Appl. Math. Inf. **26**, 01 (2008)
36. Z. Odibat and N. Shawagfeh. Generalized Taylor's formula. *Applied Mathematics and Computation*, 186:286–293, 03 2007
37. Podlubny , I., Thimann, K.V.: Fractional differential equations: an introduction to fractional derivatives, fractional differential equations, to methods of their solution and some of their applications (1998)
38. Rossikhin, Y., Shitikova, M.: Applications of fractional calculus to dynamic problems of linear and nonlinear hereditary mechanics of solids. Appl. Mech. Rev. **50**, 01 (1997)
39. Rostamy, D., Mottaghi, E.: Stability analysis of a fractional-order epidemics model with multiple equilibriums. Adv. Differ. Equ. **2016**(1), 170 (Jun 2016)
40. Salle , J.L., Lefschetz, S.: Stability by Liapunov's Direct Method with Applications, vol. 4 of Mathematics in Science and Engineering. Elsevier (1961)
41. Sarbaz, H.K., Muhammad, S., Mehboob, A., Faisal, S.: A quantitative and qualitative analysis of the covid-19 pandemic model. Chaos, Solit. Fractals **138**, 109932 (2020)
42. Shaikh, A.S., Shaikh, I.N., Nisar, K.S.: A mathematical model of covid-19 using fractional derivative: outbreak in india with dynamics of transmission and control. Adv. Differ. Equ. **373** (2020)
43. Soniya, L., Gunjan, S., Bhawna, M., Rajesh, K.: Predicting optimal lockdown period with parametric approach using three-phase maturation SIRD model for covid-19 pandemic. Chaos, Solit. Fractals **138**, 109939 (2020)
44. Tuan, N.H., Mohammadi, H., Rezapour, S.: A mathematical model for covid-19 transmission by using the caputo fractional derivative. Chaos, Solit. Fractals **140**, 110107 (2020)
45. Van den Driessche, P., Watmough, J.: Reproduction numbers and sub-threshold endemic equilibria for compartmental models of disease transmission. Math. Biosci. **180**, 29–48 (2002)
46. Vargas-De-León, C.: Volterra-type Lyapunov functions for fractional-order epidemic systems. Commun. Nonlinear Sci. Numer. Simul. **24**, 75–85 (July 2015)
47. Yasuhiro, T., Wanbiao, M., Edoardo, B.: Global asymptotic properties of a delay SIR epidemic model with finite incubation times. Nonlinear Anal. **42**(6), 931–947 (2000)

Protective Face Shield Effectiveness: Mathematical Modelling

Zalimkhan Nagoev, Viktor Narozhnov, Arsen Pskhu, and Sergo Rekhviashvili

Abstract A face shield is a type of the personal protective equipment that is used to protect a person's face from various external hazardous influences—splashes, drops and aerosols, thermal and optical radiation. It is believed that face shields effectively prevent contamination of the mucous membranes of the human body. According to the World Health Organization (WHO) recommendations, social and medical personnel in contact with Covid-19 patients should use similar protective equipment, including protective face shields. In the present work, a 3D mathematical model of the airflow distribution near the cylindrical surface of a face shield was explored. The model is based on a numerical solution of the Navier–Stokes gas dynamics equations. The simulation results are compared with full-scale experiments. A probability model is also considered. Quantitative conclusions are made about the effectiveness of the protective face shields.

Keywords Face shield · Mathematical modelling · Navier–Stokes equations · Numerical solution · Probability model

Z. Nagoev · V. Narozhnov · A. Pskhu (✉) · S. Rekhviashvili
Kabardino-Balkarian Scientific Center of the Russian Academy of Sciences, Nalchik, Russia
e-mail: pskhu@list.ru

Z. Nagoev
e-mail: zaliman@mail.ru

S. Rekhviashvili
e-mail: rsergo@mail.ru

P. Agarwal et al. (eds.), *Analysis of Infectious Disease Problems (Covid-19) and Their Global Impact*, Infosys Science Foundation Series,
https://doi.org/10.1007/978-981-16-2450-6_3

1 Introduction

A newly emerged and rapidly spread infectious disease Covid-19 made experts in diverse fields of medicine, biology, chemistry, sociology, physics and even mathematics unite to combat it. It is only through the joint efforts of all specialists and a comprehensive approach that this problem can be effectively tackled.

The development, testing and deployment of personal protective equipment for facial and respiratory protection are crucial elements of the anti-pandemic measures. We believe that mathematical modelling can play a rather constructive role in this. It is well known that mathematical methods have long been widely used in biology and medicine [1]. Among them are probability theory, statistics, combinatorics, ordinary and partial differential equations, control theory and linear programming. Nowadays, for instance, it is impossible to imagine the genetic science without modern mathematical and computer science methods.

Mathematical modelling is an effective tool for studying qualitative properties of various phenomena or processes. The modelling process consists of the following steps: a mathematical model construction, software implementation, numerical experiment and verification. A mathematical model is based on an analysis of a phenomenon and experimental results. The analysis allows us to determine the main characteristics and parameters, obtain theoretical and empirical formulas, as well as derive relevant differential, integral or integro-differential equations (or systems of equations). Next, a software implementation of the constructed model is carried out. For this, as a rule, various high-level programming languages or suitable computing environments (computer mathematics systems), as well as a problem-oriented software (which is designed to solve a problem in a specific area) are used. Then numerical calculation is carried out to identify some unknown parameters that give an idea of certain properties of the objects that are modelled. Finally, verification is performed. For this, qualitative or quantitative results of modelling are compared with experimental or observation data.

The aim of this work is to evaluate the effectiveness of protective face shields in preventing the transmission of airborne infections. In particular, we construct a mathematical model of an airflow around the surface of a protective face shield. The model is based on the stationary Navier–Stokes equation. Moreover, we describe and analyse the results of full-scale experiments conducted with a protective face shield, including visualization of airflow at various angles of attack. We also consider a probability model of the process under study.

The theoretical and experimental results of this work allow us to draw encouraging conclusions regarding the protective properties of the face shield equipment under discussion.

2 Practical Application of Face Shields

Covid-19 is primarily transmitted between people through respiratory droplets [2–6]. Apparently, a contact transmission is also possible [7, 8], for example, through household items. It is also known that viruses can enter a human body through the eyes [9–11]. This danger cannot be excluded in the case of Covid-19 [3].

An adult human has about 15,000 L of ambient air passing through the respiratory system per day. The bacterial and viral content of the air is filtered and settles on the surface of epithelial cells. Particles of moisture, saliva, mucus, sputum with pathogenic microflora, including Covid-19, are ejected from the nasopharynx of a patient, or a virus carrier. For a short period of time, an infected area is generated around the patient with a maximum concentration of aerosol particles. Particles larger than 100 microns (large droplet phase) settle rapidly. The dispersion range usually does not exceed 2–3 m. The degree of the virus concentration and the duration of its suspension in the air depends on the size of the airborne particles generated by people's breathing, talking, sneezing and coughing.

It has been established that the Covid-19 is sufficiently stable in the environment [12, 13]. So, the virus can remain viable in the air for several hours to several days. Therefore, an infection can occur through household items, dishes and door handles of public institutions long after they have been touched by an ill person. There is another factor that influences the occurrence of the coronavirus infection—the number of viral particles that enter the body. The smaller is the number of them, the less likely the body's protective barriers will be overcome, and a disease will occur. The enclosed spaces, especially with a large gathering of people such as offices, schools, kindergartens, public transport, shops suggest high viruses concentration. For protection against viruses and bacteria, it is effective to use medical or respirator masks in combination with a protective face shield [14] (Fig. 1).

According to the World Health Organization's guidance [15], during the outbreak of Covid-19, it is very important to use appropriate personal protective equipment, including a medical mask and eye or face protection (face shield). In addition to standard precautions, wearing a medical mask and a face shield would avoid infection through contamination of mucous membranes.

An effective face shield must cover the sides of the face and go below the chin. A protective face shield with good safety properties should provide good visibility. This is achieved by proper operation, which includes: orderly cleaning of the rim and the shield surface with soap/detergent and water, and disinfection with 70% alcohol or 0.1% sodium hypochlorite [15], followed by a thorough washing with clean water; avoidance of mechanical damage; proper storage. Hand hygiene is also important before putting on and after removing a protective face shield. A protective face shield prevents a direct airflow, splash of chemicals, infectious substances or body fluids from getting on a person's face. In addition, the use of a face shield helps to avoid random face-and-mask touching by reflex.

In [16], one can find a systematic review and a meta-analysis of how physical distancing, face masks and eye protection prevent transmission of SARS-CoV-2

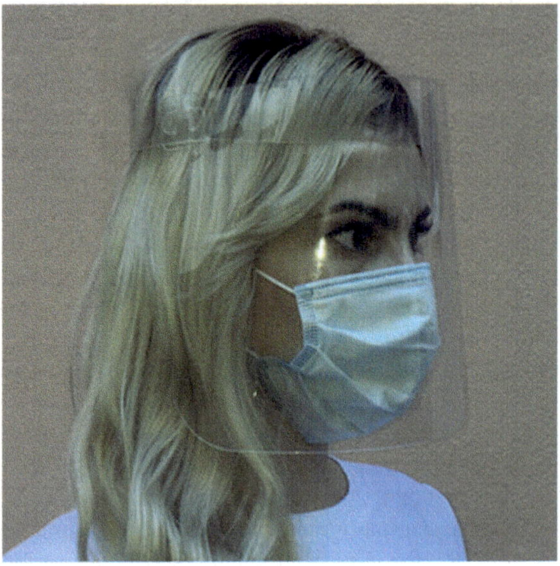

Fig. 1 A medical mask and a protective face shield combination

and Covid-19. In particular, it was shown that transmission of viruses is lower with physical distancing of 1 m or more. Moreover, wearing of a face mask could result in a large reduction in risk of infection. Eye protection also was associated with less infection. Therefore, the problem of evaluating the effectiveness of a face shield is relevant.

3 Mathematical Modelling

We use the theory of viscous gas flow [17]. The basic principle of macroscopic gas dynamics is that a medium consisting of a large number of individual particles is regarded as a continuous medium that provides a framework for equations of motion. In general, the medium may be viscous, compressible and thermally conductive. In our case, this approach means that aerosol particles generate a rarefied gas, which is considered as a continuous medium due to its small-sized particles.

The system of equations consists of equations for a gas flow density, velocity and energy. In addition, we employ an equation of state describing the thermodynamic properties of a medium. The gas dynamics equations can be written in two different forms: with respect to the Euler coordinates, i.e. fixed in space, and with respect to the Lagrangian coordinates associated with the motion of a continuous medium. Below we give a derivation of these equations.

3.1 Euler Form of Equations

The continuity equation. Consider a cavity of volume V into which a gas flow enters through surface S. The mass of the incoming substance through the surface S per unit time is

$$\int_S \mathbf{j}\, d\mathbf{S},$$

$$d\mathbf{S} = \mathbf{n}\, dS,$$

where $\mathbf{j}$ is the flux density, $\mathbf{n}$ is the unit normal vector and dS is the square element. The flow entering the cavity reduces the amount of gas. The moving gas in terms of units of mass per unit time is

$$-\frac{\partial}{\partial t}\int_V \rho\, dV,$$

where ρ is the bulk density of the gas. Equating these expressions, we get

$$\int_S \mathbf{j}\, d\mathbf{S} = -\frac{\partial}{\partial t}\int_V \rho\, dV. \tag{1}$$

On the other hand, the Ostrogradsky–Gauss theorem gives

$$\int_S \mathbf{j}\, d\mathbf{S} = \int_V (\nabla,\, \mathbf{j})\, dV, \tag{2}$$

where $(\cdot,\, \cdot)$ stands for a dot product. Comparing (1) and (2), we obtain the continuity equation:

$$\frac{\partial \rho}{\partial t} + (\nabla,\ \mathbf{j}) = 0. \tag{3}$$

By definition, the flux density is

$$\mathbf{j} = \rho\, \mathbf{v}, \tag{4}$$

where $\mathbf{v}$ is the vector of velocity. Once having substituted (4) into (3), we get

$$\frac{\partial \rho}{\partial t} + \rho\, (\nabla,\ \mathbf{v}) + (\mathbf{v},\ \nabla\rho) = 0. \tag{5}$$

The equation of motion. Applying Newton's equations of motion to the gas, we can derive the equation of motion:

$$\rho \frac{d\mathbf{v}}{dt} = -\nabla\, p, \tag{6}$$

where p is the pressure. Despite possible local or non-local compression, the total mass of the gas conserved. Therefore, the density in (6) is not under the sign of differentiation. For the differential of velocity, we can write

$$d\mathbf{v} = \frac{\partial \mathbf{v}}{\partial t} dt + \frac{\partial \mathbf{v}}{\partial \mathbf{r}} d\mathbf{r}.$$

Now we introduce the material derivative

$$\frac{d\mathbf{v}}{dt} = \frac{\partial \mathbf{v}}{\partial t} + (\mathbf{v},\, \nabla)\, \mathbf{v}, \tag{7}$$

where

$$(\mathbf{v},\, \nabla) = v_x \frac{\partial}{\partial x} + v_y \frac{\partial}{\partial y} + v_z \frac{\partial}{\partial z}.$$

By (6) and (7), we get

$$\frac{\partial \mathbf{v}}{\partial t} + (\mathbf{v},\, \nabla)\, \mathbf{v} = -\frac{1}{\rho} \nabla p. \tag{8}$$

The equation of energy balance. Kinetic energy E per unit volume of gas is defined by

$$E = \frac{\rho \mathbf{v}^2}{2} + \rho u,$$

where u is the internal energy per unit mass. Taking into account the equations of continuity and motion, and differentiating with respect to time, we obtain the energy balance equation

$$\frac{\partial E}{\partial t} = -(\nabla,\, \mathbf{Q}), \tag{9}$$

$$\mathbf{Q} = \rho \mathbf{v} \left(\frac{\mathbf{v}^2}{2} + u + \frac{p}{\rho} \right),$$

where $\mathbf{Q}$ is the energy flux density.

3.2 *Lagrangian Form of Equations*

In terms of the material derivative

$$\frac{d}{dt} = \frac{\partial}{\partial t} + (\mathbf{v},\, \nabla),$$

the equations of hydrodynamics can be written in the Lagrangian form. In this case, the equations take a simple form:

the equation of continuity

$$\frac{d\rho}{dt} = -\rho\,(\nabla,\ \mathbf{v}), \tag{10}$$

the equation of motion

$$\rho\frac{d\mathbf{v}}{dt} = -\nabla\, p, \tag{11}$$

and the equation of energy balance

$$\frac{dE}{dt} = (\nabla,\ \mathbf{v}\,E - \mathbf{Q}) = -(\nabla,\ \mathbf{v}\,p) = -p(\nabla,\ \mathbf{v}) - (\mathbf{v},\ \nabla p). \tag{12}$$

For the system of equations to be closed, it should be supplemented by the gas equation of state:

$$E = E(p,\ \rho). \tag{13}$$

There are many equations that can be applied to a wide range of temperatures and pressures [18]. The choice of the equation of state depends on the specific physical problem for which a mathematical model is being developed. The simplest model is the ideal gas model with

$$E = \frac{p}{\rho\,(\gamma - 1)}, \tag{14}$$

where γ is the heat capacity ratio.

3.3 Model Description

The inclusion of gas viscosity in the equation of motion leads to the Navier–Stokes equation:

$$\rho\left[\frac{\partial\,\mathbf{v}}{\partial\,t} + (\mathbf{v},\ \nabla)\,\mathbf{v}\right] = -\nabla\, p + \eta\,\nabla^2\mathbf{v} + \left(\xi + \frac{\eta}{3}\right)\,\nabla(\nabla,\ \mathbf{v}), \tag{15}$$

where ξ and η are the viscosity coefficients.

Let the gas flow have low flow velocities and be incompressible, i.e.

$$(\nabla,\ \mathbf{v}) = 0. \tag{16}$$

This allows us to simplify the Eq. (15); we can write

$$\frac{\partial\,\mathbf{v}}{\partial\,t} + (\mathbf{v},\ \nabla)\,\mathbf{v} = -\frac{1}{\rho}\nabla\, p + \frac{\eta}{\rho}\,\nabla^2\mathbf{v}. \tag{17}$$

It should be noted that in this case we may not take into account Eqs. (9) and (12). Because all four unknown functions (three velocity components and pressure) can be found from the three equations of motion corresponding to the three velocity components and the solenoidality condition.

In case of steady-state flow, by (17) we can finally obtain

$$(\mathbf{v},\ \nabla)\mathbf{v} = -\frac{1}{\rho}\nabla p + \frac{\eta}{\rho}\nabla^2\mathbf{v}. \tag{18}$$

The boundary condition on the surface Ω has the form

$$\mathbf{v}|_\Omega = 0. \tag{19}$$

Aerodynamic equations can be reduced to a dimensionless form by introducing some specific numbers. The Reynolds, Prandtl, Euler and Mach numbers are principle and are defined as:

$$\mathrm{Re} = \frac{v_0 l_0}{\nu},\quad \mathrm{Pr} = \frac{\nu}{a},\quad \mathrm{Eu} = \frac{p}{\rho\, v_0^2},\quad \mathrm{M} = \frac{v_0}{v_s},$$

where v_0 and l_0 are the characteristic flow velocity and geometric size, a is the thermal diffusivity, ν is the kinematic viscosity, p is the pressure, and v_s is the speed of sound in the environment. In the dimensionless form, the equations are universal, since they can describe the nature of infinite number of different flows with the same numbers. For example, if two stationary gas flows have different velocities and different kinematic viscosities, but their Reynolds numbers are the same, then the motion of these flows can be described by the same dimensionless equation. This constitutes the essence of the law of similarity for aerodynamics and hydrodynamics.

The law of similarity in aerodynamics is of extreme practical importance, since it allows us to simulate various phenomena. Thus, in our problem of incompressible flow around the face shield, all the values to be determined depends only on the angle of attack α and the Reynolds number Re. Consequently, the conditions for physical similarity are $\alpha = const$ and $\mathrm{Re} = const$. When simulating this phenomenon, the experimental results can be used only for the similar values of α and Re.

Depending on the Reynolds number, a flow can be either laminar or turbulent. For small Reynolds numbers, the flow is laminar. In this case, the fluid layers do not mix. Turbulence arises spontaneously when Reynolds number exceeds the critical value. Local pressure gradients, conservative forces and flows around the shield surface can cause neighbouring layers to move randomly and mix up. As a consequence, in a turbulent flow, one can observe nonlinear waves with a geometric structure of self-similarity (fractals) at different spatial scales. These waves occupy a finite volume, and therefore some part of the flow is always laminar. In the mathematical sense, turbulence means the appearance of strange attractors in the phase space of the system of aerodynamic equations. The description of turbulence is closely related to the existence and smoothness of solutions to the Navier–Stokes equation.

Developed turbulence occurs if the Reynolds numbers are large and chaotic velocity pulsations happen. Important information about the local structure of developed turbulence can be obtained using the concepts of similarity and dimension. As the Reynolds number increases, turbulences of smaller scales arise and redistribute energy between all scales. In this case, as a rule, when pulsation is of smaller scales, energy dissipation occurs due to viscous forces. Let v_0 and l_0 be speed and size of a turbulent vortex, and ε be the energy dissipated per unit mass per unit time (dimension is $[\varepsilon] = \mathrm{L}^2\mathrm{T}^{-3}$). If a small scale is selected, the velocity should depend only on ε and l_0. This gives the only relationship between the size and velocity:

$$v_0 = C\,(\varepsilon\, l_0)^{1/3},$$

where C is an unknown constant. This formula is known as the Kolmogorov–Obukhov law. This law is reliably confirmed experimentally by measurements of developed turbulence spectra. As was repeatedly obtained from experiments, C is 1.44±0.6.

3.4 Numerical Methods

The system of equations (16), (18) together with the boundary condition (19) (the Dirichlet problem) is used for simulating stationary air flows at the surface of a protective face shield. The gas flow problem has been solved numerically using the finite element method and the Newton–Raphson algorithm [19]. The method has a quadratic convergence.

The essence of the finite element method is as follows. First, we subdivide the considered domain into small simple parts, i.e. into finite elements. For each of these elements, we consider an approximating function, which, as a rule, is a polynomial and is zero outside the element [20, p.21]. Assuming that approximating functions are equal at the points of the boundary of neighbour elements, we obtain a system for finding unknown coefficients.

Let

$$\min_{\mathbf{v}} \left\{ \Phi(\mathbf{v}) = \int_V \varphi\left(\mathbf{r},\ \mathbf{v}(\mathbf{r}),\ \frac{d\mathbf{v}(\mathbf{r})}{d\mathbf{r}}\right) d^3\mathbf{r} \right\}$$

be the variational form of the problem (18) and (19). Here $\mathbf{v}(\mathbf{r})$ is an unknown flow velocity. The functional $\Phi(\mathbf{v})$ contains information about the external source functions and boundary values. The integral over V can be rewritten as a sum for each element

$$\Phi(\mathbf{v}) = \sum_{k=1}^{N} \Phi_k(\mathbf{v}),$$

where N is a number of subdivision elements. Now, for each element, we replace the function $\mathbf{v}(\mathbf{r})$ by its approximation

$$\mathbf{v}(\mathbf{r}) = P(\mathbf{v}_k, \mathbf{r})$$

with unknown coefficients $\mathbf{v}_1, ..., \mathbf{v}_M$ to be determined. Thus, we obtain $\Phi(\mathbf{v})$ as a function of parameters $\mathbf{v}_1, ..., \mathbf{v}_M$.

Next, the problem of finding an optimum of $\Phi(\mathbf{v})$ leads to the system of equations

$$\frac{\partial \Phi}{\partial \mathbf{v}_1} = 0, \ldots, \frac{\partial \Phi}{\partial \mathbf{v}_M} = 0 \tag{20}$$

that consists of M equations with M unknowns $\mathbf{v}_1, ..., \mathbf{v}_M$.

To solve the obtained system, the Newton–Raphson method can be used. This method, as a rule, provides fast convergence. Let us rewrite the system (20) as

$$\begin{cases} f_1(\mathbf{v}_1, ..., \mathbf{v}_M) = 0, \\ \vdots \\ f_M(\mathbf{v}_1, ..., \mathbf{v}_M) = 0, \end{cases}$$

where $f_i(\mathbf{v}_1, ..., \mathbf{v}_M)$: $V \to \mathbb{R}$ are given continuously differential functions ($i = \overline{1, M}$, $V \subset \mathbb{R}^M$).

Let $\mathbf{v}_1^*, ..., \mathbf{v}_M^*$ be a desired solution. Expanding f_i as the Taylor series about the points $\mathbf{v}_1^*, ..., \mathbf{v}_M^*$ gives

$$\begin{cases} f_1(\mathbf{v}_1, ..., \mathbf{v}_M) = f_1(\mathbf{v}_1^*, ..., \mathbf{v}_M^*) + \frac{\partial f_1}{\partial \mathbf{v}_1}(\mathbf{v}_1^* - \mathbf{v}_1) + \frac{\partial f_1}{\partial \mathbf{v}_1}(\mathbf{v}_1^* - \mathbf{v}_1) + \ldots, \\ \vdots \\ f_M(\mathbf{v}_1, ..., \mathbf{v}_M) = f_M(\mathbf{v}_1^*, ..., \mathbf{v}_M^*) + \frac{\partial f_M}{\partial \mathbf{v}_M}(\mathbf{v}_M^* - \mathbf{v}_M) + \frac{\partial f_M}{\partial \mathbf{v}_M}(\mathbf{v}_M^* - \mathbf{v}_M) + \ldots. \end{cases}$$

Assuming that $\mathbf{v}_1, ..., \mathbf{v}_M$ are close enough to $\mathbf{v}_1^*, ..., \mathbf{v}_M^*$, we get a linearized system (written in matrix form)

$$F(\overline{\mathbf{v}}) \approx F(\overline{\mathbf{v}}^*) + J(\overline{\mathbf{v}} - \overline{\mathbf{v}}^*),$$

$$\overline{\mathbf{v}} = (\mathbf{v}_1, ..., \mathbf{v}_M)^T, \overline{\mathbf{v}}^* = (\mathbf{v}_1^*, ..., \mathbf{v}_M^*)^T,$$

$$F(\overline{\mathbf{v}}) = (f_1(\overline{\mathbf{v}}), \ldots, f_M(\overline{\mathbf{v}}))^T,$$

$$F(\overline{\mathbf{v}}^*) = (f_1(\overline{\mathbf{v}}^*), \ldots, f_M(\overline{\mathbf{v}}^*))^T,$$

where

$$J = \begin{pmatrix} \frac{\partial f_1}{\partial \mathbf{v}_1} & \cdots & \frac{\partial f_1}{\partial \mathbf{v}_M} \\ \vdots & \ddots & \vdots \\ \frac{\partial f_M}{\partial \mathbf{v}_1} & \cdots & \frac{\partial f_M}{\partial \mathbf{v}_M} \end{pmatrix},$$

is the Jacobian matrix.

Solution of the linearized system can be obtained by iterations

$$\overline{\mathbf{v}}^{j+1} = \overline{\mathbf{v}}^{j} - J^{-1} F(\overline{\mathbf{v}}^{j}).$$

The iterative process continues until the condition

$$\left\| \overline{\mathbf{v}}^{j+1} - \overline{\mathbf{v}}^{j} \right\| \leq \varepsilon$$

is satisfied. Here, ε is a required accuracy of the solution. It should be noted that the main difficulty in applying this method is to find the inverse Jacobian matrix. To solve this problem, the Gauss–Jordan method [21] can be used.

3.5 Computer Simulation

Now we present the results of computer simulation. The object of modelling is a face shield designed in the form of a thin semi-cylindrical shell. The shield has a thickness of 1 mm, an outer radius of 9 cm and a height of 21 cm. Modelling was carried out for the following air parameters: temperature 293.15 K, density 1.204 kg/m^3, bulk viscosity $1.088 \cdot 10^{-5}$ Pa · s. The initial flow velocity is 2 m/s that corresponds to the average normal human breathing [22]. In Fig. 2, there are simulation results of a flow around the face shield at different angles of attack α.

The airflow around the face shield deforms creating an area with variable velocities and pressure. The flow parallel to the vertical plane of symmetry is symmetric. For shields that are nearly flat, the flow direction changes very sharply. Therefore, the flows slow down in front of the shield surface, contract at the edges and form rarefaction regions beyond the edges. There is a jet wake flow behind the shield. In front of the shield, the pressure is higher than in an undisturbed flow. Behind the shield, due to rarefaction, the pressure decreases. The rounded shield makes the flow around the front and rear parts smoother.

A non-zero angle of attack results in an asymmetric flow. In this case, the greater deformation of the flow is observed in a spot of greater curvature of the body surface. In this area, the flow is compressed, and due the condition (16), then it spreads out in a thin current layer. A less curved surface has little effect on the flow pattern. At the place of the greater contraction, the flow velocity increases locally while the pressure decreases. Behind the shield, the flow deforms less and, therefore, the flow velocity and pressure also change less. In general, the flow deformation substantially depends on the shield configuration and its position against the flow.

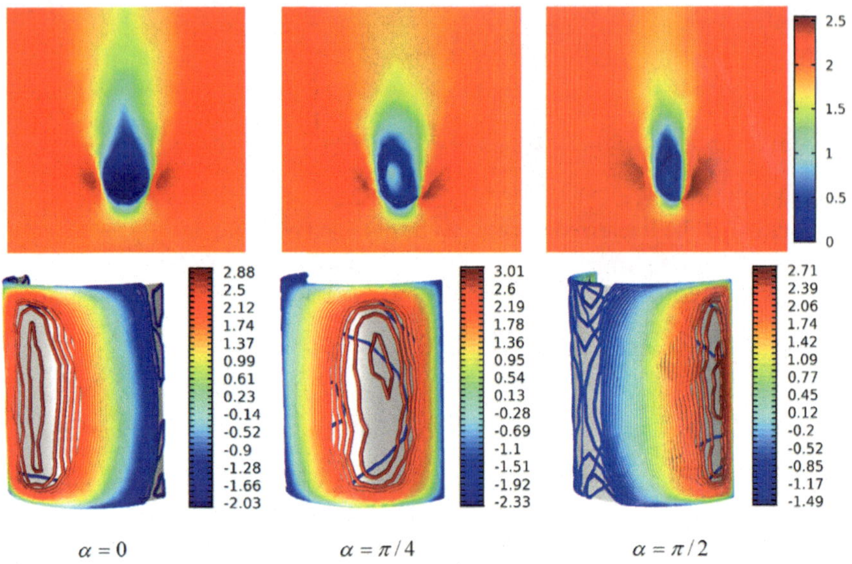

Fig. 2 Simulation results of the flow around a semi-cylindrical face shield. The top images are velocity fields (m/s). The lower images are pressure distributions (Pa)

4 Full-Scale Experiment

Here, we present the results of an experiment with aerosol flows around a face shield. In the experiment, an ultrasonic humidifier and CPU fan were used. With the help of the humidifier, water vapour was produced with particles less than 5 microns in size, and the fan was used for directing the vapour flow. The fan speed—and therefore the flow velocity—was controlled by the power supply. The testing results at various angles of attack around a face shield are presented in Fig. 3.

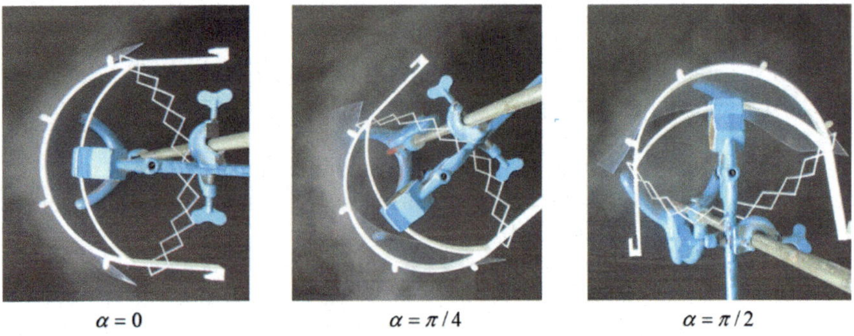

Fig. 3 Flows near the protective face shield functional surface

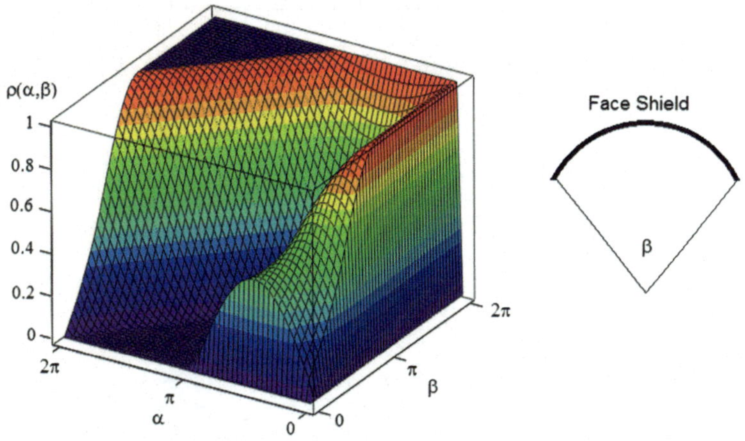

Fig. 4 Protective face shield effectiveness function

At $\alpha = 0$, the vapour flow directed towards the shield is almost entirely dissipated. In this case, the face shield provides maximum protection. When the angle of attack is not zero, some of the flow can penetrate into the zone behind the shield reducing the protection effectiveness. Depending on the flow velocity, turbulent swirling flow may occur at the leading edge of the shield, what contributes to the additional flow infiltration into the geometric shadow region. Frontal flow ($\alpha = \pi/2$) is divided into two approximately equal parts. One part of the flow gets reflected back into the external space, and the other part, with a lower velocity, enters the zone behind the shield. Such flow distribution seems most undesirable.

In reality, the airflows are of a random nature; therefore, for assessing the possibility of air flows entering the protected zone, it is appropriate to use the probabilistic approach. The results of modelling and experimental studies show that if the flows have low velocities and there is no turbulence, then the effectiveness of a face shield can be determined by the area of its projection (shadow) on the plane perpendicular to the direction of flow.

As above, we assume that the protective face shield is a cylindrical surface, the base of which is a circular arc with an angle of β, where $\beta \in [0, 2\pi]$ (see Fig. 4). Consider

$$\rho(\alpha, \beta) = \frac{1}{S_0} S(\alpha, \beta),$$

where $S(\alpha, \beta)$ is the 'shadow' area protected from the flow, S_0 is the maximum projected area of the shield and α is the angle of attack. Hence,

$$\rho(\alpha, \beta) = \frac{1}{2 \sin\left(\min\{\frac{\pi}{2}, \beta\}\right)} \times$$

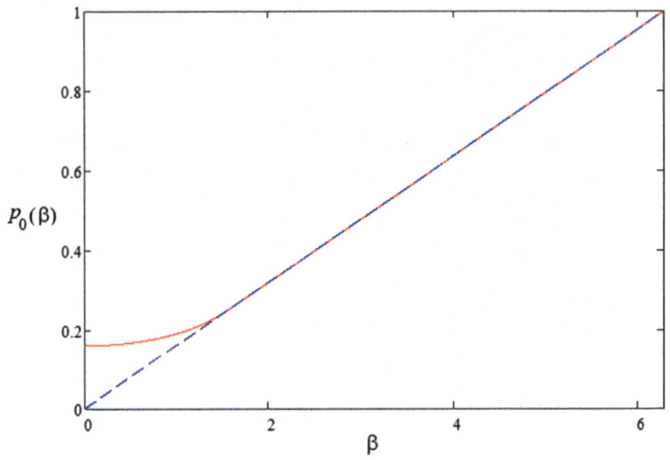

Fig. 5 Face shield effectiveness depending on the angle β. The dashed line corresponds to the function $y(x) = x/(2\pi)$

$$\times \begin{cases} \cos(\min\{\pi, \alpha\}) - \cos(\min\{\pi, \beta + \alpha\}), \alpha \in [0, 2\pi - \beta], \\ 2 + \cos(\min\{\pi, \alpha\}) - \cos(\min\{\pi, \beta + \alpha - 2\pi\}), \alpha \in [2\pi - \beta, 2\pi], \end{cases} \tag{21}$$

where $\min\{a, b\}$, as usual, denotes the minimum of a and b.

Figure 4 presents a three-dimensional graph of the function $\rho(\alpha, \beta)$ given by (21). Averaging (21) for all angles of attack, we obtain the effectiveness estimation:

$$p_0 = \frac{1}{2\pi} \int_0^{2\pi} \rho(\alpha, \beta) d\alpha = \frac{\beta}{2\pi \sin\left(\min\{\frac{\pi}{2}, \beta\}\right)}, \tag{22}$$

which does not depend on α. The result is predictable: for a given radius, the effectiveness of a protective face shield is proportional to the base arc angle β. For example, if a shield is flat (i.e. $\beta = 0$) then $p_0 = 1/(2\pi) \approx 0.159$. Under the random air flow, such a shield is the least effective compared to others with the same linear sizes and $\beta > 0$. It should be noted that formula (22) is obtained without taking into account the influence exerted by the head of a person equipped with the protective face shield. As a matter of fact, formula (22) gives a lower estimate for the worst case. Indeed, the performances p of the protective face shield should apparently satisfy $p > p_0$. Figure 5 shows a graph of the function $p_0(\beta)$.

5 Conclusion

The paper studies the effectiveness of a protective face shield in prevention the direct contact with the air flows, which may pose a risk of infection. We have considered two mathematical models. The first model is based on the flow problem and the numerical solutions of the Navier–Stokes system of equations. The second model is based on the probabilistic approach, with the air flows randomly directed towards the protective shield. In addition, face shields have been tested using steam flows *in vivo*. The obtained results reveal that effectiveness of a protective face shield increases with increasing bending, i.e. base arc angle (for the same linear sizes).

In should be added that a face shield and a medical or respirator mask complement each other. The simultaneous use of these two protective agents improves the safety properties of each of them. However, the following should be taken into account. A face shield restricts the air penetration into the respiratory system (as can be inferred from the results of Sect. 4), just as well as a medical mask can make respiration difficult [23, 24]. Therefore, in order to avoid undesirable consequences, care must be taken when using these two protective agents together. This is especially relevant for their indoor use and also for the use by people with poor health. It should also be borne in mind that materials in contact with the human skin can cause allergic reactions in sensitive individuals [25].

References

1. Edelstein-Keshet, L.: Mathematical models in biology. SIAM (2005)
2. Borak, J.: Airborne transmission of COVID-19. Occup. Med. (2020). https://doi.org/10.1093/occmed/kqaa080
3. Han, Q., Lin, Q., Ni, Z., You, L.: Uncertainties about the transmission routes of 2019 novel coronavirus. Influenza Other Respir. Viruses. (2020). https://doi.org/10.1111/irv.12735
4. Bonato, G., Dioscoridi, L., Mutignani, M.: Faecal-oral transmission of SARS-COV-2: practical implications. Gastroenterology (2020). https://doi.org/10.1053/j.gastro.2020.03.066
5. Qu, G., Li, X., Hu, L., Jiang, G.: An imperative need for research on the role of environmental factors in transmission of novel coronavirus (COVID-19). Environ. Sci. Technol. (2020). https://doi.org/10.1021/acs.est.0c01102
6. Ren, Y., Li, L., Jia, Y.-M.: New method to reduce COVID-19 transmission - the need for medical air disinfection is now. J. Med. Syst. (2020) https://doi.org/10.1007/s10916-020-01585-8
7. Household transmission investigation protocol for 2019-novel coronavirus (COVID-19) infection. Geneva: World Health Organization, (2020)
8. Wei, L., Bo, Z., Jianhua, L., Shihua, L., Zhiqiang, C., et al.: Characteristics of Household Transmission of COVID-19. Clin. Infect. Dis. (2020). https://doi.org/10.1093/cid/ciaa450
9. Kenneth, F.M.: The transmission of infection through the eye. JAMA (1919). https://doi.org/10.1001/jama.1919.02610090020005
10. Belser, J.A., Gustin, K.M., Maines, T.R., Pantin-Jackwood, M.J., Katz, J.M., Tumpey, T.M.: Influenza virus respiratory infection and transmission following ocular in oculation in ferrets. PLoS Pathog. (2012). https://doi.org/10.1371/journal.ppat.1002569
11. Belser, J.A., Lash, R.R., Garg, Sh., Tumpey, T.M., Maines, T.R.: The eyes have it: influenza virus infection beyond the respiratory tract. Lancet Infect. Dis. (2018). https://doi.org/10.1016/S1473-3099(18)30102-6

12. Morawska, L., Cao, J.: Airborne transmission of SARS-CoV-2: The world should face the reality. Environ Int. (2020). https://doi.org/10.1016/j.envint.2020.105730
13. Van Doremalen, N., Bushmaker, T., Morris, D., Holbrook, M.: Aerosol and surface stability of HCoV-19 (SARS-CoV-2) compared to SARS-CoV-1. N. Engl. J. Med. (2020). https://doi.org/10.1101/2020.03.09.20033217
14. Roberge, R.J.: Face shields for infection control. A review. J. Occup. Environ Hyg. (2016). https://doi.org/10.1080/15459624.2015.1095302
15. Infection prevention and control during health care when coronavirus disease (COVID-19) is suspected or confirmed. Geneva: World Health Organization, (2020)
16. Chu, D.K., Akl, E.A., Duda, S., Solo, K., Yaacoub, S., Schüemann, H. J. et al.: Physical distancing, face masks, and eye protection to prevent person-to-person transmission of SARS-CoV-2 and COVID-19: a systematic review and meta-analysis. Lancet (2020) https://doi.org/10.1016/S0140-6736(20)31142-9
17. Loitsyanskii, L.G.: Mechanics of Liquids and Gases. Pergamon Press (1966)
18. Eliezer, Sh., Ghatak, A., Hora, H.: Fundamentals of Equations of State. World Scientific (2002)
19. Kim, N.-H.: Introduction to Nonlinear Finite Element Analysis. Springer (2015)
20. Sabonnadiere, J.-C., Coulomb, J.-L.: Finite Element Methods in CAD: Electrical and Magnetic Fields. Springer-Verlag (1987)
21. Lipschutz, S., Lipson, M.: Linear Algebra. McGraw-Hill (2009)
22. Lei, Z., Yang, J., Zhuang, Z., Roberge, R.: Simulation and Evaluation of Respirator Faceseal Leaks Using Computational Fluid Dynamics and Infrared Imaging. Ann. Occup. Hyg. (2012). https://doi.org/10.1093/annhyg/mes085
23. Wizner, K., Nasarwanji, M., Fisher, E., Steege, A.L., Boiano, J.M.: Exploring respiratory protection practices for prominent hazards in healthcare settings. J. Occup. Environ Hyg. (2018). https://doi.org/10.1080/15459624.2018.1473581
24. Advice on the use of masks in the context of COVID-19. Geneva: World Health Organization, (2020)
25. Foo, C.C., Goon, A.T., Leow, Y.H., Goh, C.L.: Adverse skin reactions to personal protective equipment against severe acute respiratory syndrome-a descriptive study in Singapore. Contact Derm. (2006). https://doi.org/10.1111/j.1600-0536.2006.00953.x

On the Evolution Equation for Modelling the Covid-19 Pandemic

J. M. Blackledge

Abstract The paper introduces and discusses the evolution equation, and, based exclusively on this equation, considers random walk models for the time series available on the daily confirmed Covid-19 cases for different countries. It is shown that a conventional random walk model is not consistent with the current global pandemic time series data, which exhibits non-ergodic properties. A self-affine random walk field model is investigated, derived from the evolutionary equation for a specified memory function which provides the non-ergodic fields evident in the available Covid-19 data. This is based on using a spectral scaling relationship of the type $1/\omega^\alpha$ where ω is the angular frequency and $\alpha \in (0, 1)$ conforms to the absolute values of a normalised zero mean Gaussian distribution. It is shown that α is a primary parameter for evaluating the global status of the pandemic in the sense that the pandemic will become extinguished as $\alpha \to 0$ for all countries. For this reason, and based on the data currently available, a study is made of the variations in α for 100 randomly selected countries. Finally, in the context of the Bio-dynamic Hypothesis, a parametric model is considered for simulating the three-dimensional structure of a spike protein which may be of value in the development of a vaccine.

Keywords Einstein's Evolution equation · Self-Affine random walk fields · Pandemic time series analysis · Bio-dynamics hypothesis · Fractal geometry of spike proteins.

J. M. Blackledge (✉)
School of Mathematics, Statistics and Computer Science, University of KwaZulu-Natal, KwaZulu-Natal, South Africa
e-mail: jonathan.blackledge@TUDublin.ie

School of Electrical and Electronic Engineering, Technological University Dublin, Dublin, Ireland

Department of Computer Science, University of Western Cape, Western Cape, South Africa

Faculty of Arts, Science and Technology, Wrexham Glyndrw University of Wales, Wales, UK

Centre for Advanced Studies, Warsaw University of Technology, Warsaw, Poland

Science Foundation Ireland, Dublin, Ireland

P. Agarwal et al. (eds.), *Analysis of Infectious Disease Problems (Covid-19) and Their Global Impact*, Infosys Science Foundation Series,
https://doi.org/10.1007/978-981-16-2450-6_4

1 Introduction

Coronaviruses are a family of viruses that can cause illnesses from the common cold to severe acute respiratory syndrome. In late 2019, a new coronavirus was identified as the cause of a disease outbreak that originated in China. The virus is now known as the severe acute respiratory syndrome coronavirus 2 (SARS-CoV-2). The disease it causes is called coronavirus disease 2019 (Covid-19), and, in March 2020, the World Health Organisation declared the Covid-19 outbreak a pandemic [1]. A pandemic is an epidemic of an infectious disease that spreads across large regions such as multiple continents or worldwide, affecting a substantial number of people. They are a natural occurrence of human evolution, made more probable by the increasing size of the human population and its propensity to localisation in urban centres. Past pandemics were caused by diseases such as Small Pox and Tuberculosis. The most fatal pandemic in recorded history was the Black Death (The Plague), which killed an estimated 75–200 million people in the 14th Century. The most notable pandemic of the last century occurred over 100 years ago, namely the influenza pandemic (Spanish flu) which killed an estimated 50–100 million people worldwide.

The 1918 Spanish flu pandemic initiated some of the earliest work on the mathematical modelling of infectious diseases. Since the pioneering work of Kermack and McKendrick in 1926-27 [2], modelling the dynamics of disease transmission has been based on the development of increasingly complex systems of differential equations. A fundamental property of such models is the Basic Reproduction Number which is a threshold value, below which an infectious disease cannot spread in a susceptible population. This number needs to be less than one for an infectious disease to be extinguished.

In the context of any infectious disease, and, an associated vaccination program (if one exists), the concept of herd immunity is fundamental [3]. This is because with herd immunity, it is not necessary to vaccinate an entire population in order to reduce the progress and possibly eliminate an infectious disease, a concept that proved its value during the eradication of Smallpox in the1970 s, for example. Since then, mathematical modelling has become increasingly important for public health policy making. This has included the control of the human immunodeficiency viruses in terms of predicting the further course of the epidemic and trying to identify the most effective prevention strategies. With further infectious disease outbreaks such as the Severe Acute Respiratory Syndrome virus of 2002, Swine Flu in 2009, and, more recently, the outbreak of Covid-19, infectious disease models have become increasingly sophisticated, e.g. [4, 5].

Mathematical models that are based on systems of differential equation are examples of deterministic models where each term in the equation plays a part in modelling a specific component of a dynamical process. Such models depend on multiple parameters (coefficients and initial conditions, for example) that affect the solutions obtained. This is because each term that is included is usually predicated on some coefficient which needs to be known relatively accurately and may vary in time. In the absence of accurate values for these coefficients, some of which may be known unknown's, these models can output error prone results in terms of predicted outcomes as a function of time. In the current Covid-19 pandemic, the sophistication of such models has been extended further to incorporate more and more effects in line with the policies and practices implemented by central government and local health authorities. The sophistication of such models increases further the parameter sets whose values require increasingly accurate estimates. This problem is typical of situations in mathematical modelling where deterministic models become too complex to provide future forecasts that are accurate enough to be of significance [6]. Further, if these models include nonlinear terms, it is likely that the output(s) may be become chaotic. In this case, the determinism of such models becomes an irrelevance and we must turn to the application of stochastic modelling methods which is the subject of this work.

In this paper, an approach is explored whose aim it to model a set of time series (Covid-19 daily cases, for example) but not in terms of predicting a specific outcome for a specific country at a point in time. Instead we focus on modelling the global random walk field for the current Covid-19 pandemic. This is where the assembly of all time series for all countries is treated as a set of random walks to produce a 'random walk field'. The aim is to simulate this field in a way that is representative of the known data and to show that it is analogous to the interaction of a canonical ensemble of particles each undergoing random motion over a period of time. In this context, it is assumed that the pandemic will eventually diffuse throughout the world population and become a steady state effect rather than be fully eradicated, and, that any intervention in this process will only delay the final steady state condition rather than extinguish it.

A random walk model is developed which illustrates that the Covid-19 data fields available (i.e. the set of time series data on daily cases) are not representative of classical diffusion [7] but of fractional diffusion [8]. The development of this model is predicated on an analysis of the evolution equation as are all the results presented in the paper. This allows the models developed to be understood in the context of a fundamental field equation of statistical physics as discussed in the following section. We then use this field equation to develop models for ergodic random and non-ergodic self-affine random walk fields which is the subject of Sect. 3 and Sect. 4, respectively. This is followed by the introduction of a parametric solution for modelling the structural complexity of the viral spike protein which may have ramifications in the development of a vaccine subject to the Bio-dynamics Hypothesis as presented in Sect. 5.

The Bio-dynamics Hypothesis is the result of asking a simple question: why are so many biological entities, irrespective of their physical scale or origin, composed of self-affine structures? In the context of this question, the hypothesis states that: If replication is a self-affine process of time, then the geometrical structure of the result is also self-affine [9]. The hypothesis attempts to relate the dynamical behaviour of replication, mutation and evolutionary biology to the self-affine structure (the fractal structure) of biological entities. In this paper, we present some results from an analysis of Covid-19-based data assuming that the pandemic is a self-organising processes, a result that is derived specifically from the evolution equation. This approach complements the analysis of the pandemic based on self-organising maps, for example [10].

2 The Evolution Equation

Let $p(\mathbf{r})$ denote a Probability Density Function (PDF) where

$$\int_{-\infty}^{\infty} p(\mathbf{r})d^n\mathbf{r} = 1$$

which characterises the position of particles in a n-dimensional space $\mathbf{r} \in \mathbb{R}^n$ ($n = 1, 2, 3$). At any instant in time t, the particles are distributed in space as a result of some 'random walk' process involving elastic interactions or 'elastic scattering' (with other like particles in the same n-dimensional space, when, in all cases, both momentum and energy are conserved). Let $u(\mathbf{r}, t)$ denote the density function (i.e. the number of particles per unit of an n-dimensional space) associated with a canonical assemble of particles all undergoing the same random walk processes.

Consider an initial condition where we have an infinitely small concentration of such particles at a time $t = 0$ located at an origin $\mathbf{r} = \mathbf{0}$. The density function at $t = 0$ is then given by $u(\mathbf{r}, 0) = \delta^n(\mathbf{r})$ where $\delta^n(\mathbf{r})$ is the n-dimensional Dirac delta function. At some short time later $t << 1$, it can be expected that the density function will be determined by the PDF governing the distribution of particles after a (short duration) random walk. Thus we can write

$$u(\mathbf{r}, t) = p(\mathbf{r}) \otimes u(\mathbf{r}, 0) = p(\mathbf{r}) \otimes \delta^n(\mathbf{r}) = p(\mathbf{r})$$

where $\otimes$ denotes the convolution integral over $\mathbf{r}$. The PDF $p(\mathbf{r})$ therefore represents the response (in a statistical sense) to a short time random walk process, and, in this context, can be taken to be is a distributional Impulse Response Function (IRF). Thus, for any time t, the density field at some later time $t + \tau$ will be given by

$$u(\mathbf{r}, t + \tau) = p(\mathbf{r}) \otimes u(\mathbf{r}, t) \tag{1}$$

For any instant in time t, Eq. (1) shows that the spatial behaviour of the density field at some future time τ is given by the convolution of the density of particles at a previous time with the PDF of the system that governs its 'statistical evolution'. In this sense, $p(\mathbf{r})$ is analogous to the IRF of a linear stationary system when, for an initial condition $u_0(\mathbf{r}) \equiv u(\mathbf{r}, t = 0)$, say,

$$u(\mathbf{r}, t) = g(r, t) \otimes u_0(\mathbf{r})$$

where $g(r, t)$ is the characteristic Green's function of the system. However, in this case $u(\mathbf{r}, t)$ denotes a deterministic function associated with the behaviour of a deterministic system, whereas in Eq. (1), $u(\mathbf{r}, t)$ is the density function associated with the evolution of a distribution for a stochastic system. This 'system' is taken to be stationary in a statistical sense because it is assumed that $p(\mathbf{r})$ does not vary in time and the time evolution model given by Eq. (1) is referred to as being 'Ergodic'. Further, we note that if the PDF is symmetric, then $p(\mathbf{r}) \equiv p(r)$ where $r =\mid \mathbf{r} \mid$.

Equation (1) is an evolution equation first derived by Albert Einstein in 1905 [11]. It is the principal field equation for elastic scattering processes in statistical mechanics and is an example of a continuous time random walk model where $p(\mathbf{r})$ is the PDF for the displacement $\mathbf{r}$ of a particles position over time interval τ. For some stochastic source function $s(\mathbf{r}, t)$, the evolution equation is generalised further to the form

$$u(\mathbf{r}, t + \tau) = p(\mathbf{r}) \otimes u(\mathbf{r}, t) + s(\mathbf{r}, t) \tag{2}$$

This equation describes the evolution of the density function $u(\mathbf{r}, t)$ when the initial particle concentration is replenished in space and/or time and can be extended further to include a decay factor over time when it is required to consider an evolution equation of the type (for decay rate factor λ, say)

$$u(\mathbf{r}, t + \tau) = p(\mathbf{r}) \otimes u(\mathbf{r}, t) + s(\mathbf{r}, t) - \lambda u(\mathbf{r}, t)$$

In this paper, we focus exclusively on the application of Eq. (2) for modelling and analysing time series data associated with the Covid-19 pandemic. In this application, the density field u is taken to be the number of infections divided by the number of those at risk to infection.

One of the purposes of this paper is to bring to the attention of the reader the value of using Eq. (2) to develop a unified framework for stochastic modelling in public health medicine. In this context, there are two other equations which, although essentially different ways of writing Eq. (2), are nevertheless informative, especially in regard to understanding some of the consequences of imposing certain condition on Eq. (2) and the interpretation of the results that follow. These equations are discussed in the following sections.

2.1 *The Classical Kolmogorov–Feller Equation*

Consider the following Taylor series for the function $u(\mathbf{r}, t + \tau)$ in Eq. (2):

$$u(\mathbf{r}, t + \tau) = u(\mathbf{r}, t) + \tau \frac{\partial}{\partial t} u(\mathbf{r}, t) + \frac{\tau^2}{2!} \frac{\partial^2}{\partial t^2} u(\mathbf{r}, t) + \ldots$$

For $\tau << 1$

$$u(\mathbf{r}, t+\tau) \simeq u(\mathbf{r}, t) + \tau \frac{\partial}{\partial t} u(\mathbf{r}, t)$$

and from Eq. (2), we obtain the Classical Kolmogorov–Feller Equation (CKFE), [13, 14]

$$\tau \frac{\partial}{\partial t} u(\mathbf{r}, t) = -u(\mathbf{r}, t) + u(\mathbf{r}, t) \otimes p(\mathbf{r}) + s(\mathbf{r}, t) \quad (3)$$

which is a representation of Eq. (2) when $\tau << 1$.

Equation (3) is based on a critical assumption which is that the time evolution of the density field $u(\mathbf{r}, t)$ is influenced only by short term events and that longer term events have no influence on the behaviour of the field at any later time. This is to say that the 'system' described by Eq. (3) has no 'memory'. This statement is the physical basis upon which the condition $\tau << 1$ is imposed, thereby facilitating the Taylor series expansion of the function $u(\mathbf{r}, t+\tau)$ to first order alone. It means that if a time series is taken to be described by $u(t)$ (for some fixed position in space) then the behaviour of this time series at any time t is not influenced by its behaviour at some earlier time less that t. This is the basis for understanding classical diffusion, for example, when Eq. (3) can be used to derive the classical diffusion equation given that $p(\mathbf{r})$ is a Gaussian distribution. For $\mathbf{r} \in \mathbb{R}^n$, this can be shown by approximating the Characteristic Function for a Gaussian distribution (which is itself Gaussian). For example, if we consider the case when the source function is zero and apply the approximation $\exp(- \mid \mathbf{k} \mid^2) \simeq 1 - k^2$, then, in Fourier space, Eq. (3) is given by

$$\tau \frac{\partial}{\partial t} U(\mathbf{k}, t) = -k^2 U(\mathbf{k}, t)$$

which is a Fourier space representation of the classical diffusion equation

$$\frac{\partial}{\partial t} u(\mathbf{r}, t) = D \nabla^2 u(\mathbf{r}, t)$$

where $D = 1/\tau$ is the diffusivity, i.e. a measure of the rate at which particles can spread. The Green's function solution to the diffusion equation is [15]

$$u(\mathbf{r}, t) = g(r, t) \otimes u_0(\mathbf{r})$$

where $g(r, t)$ is the Green's function given by

$$g(r, t) = \left(\frac{1}{4\pi D t} \right)^{\frac{n}{2}} \exp\left(-\frac{r^2}{4Dt} \right), \quad t \geq 0$$

and $u_0(\mathbf{r}) = u(\mathbf{r}, t = 0)$ is the initial condition. On the basis of this solution, we can infer that as τ increases, the speed of diffusion decreases, i.e. the distribution of $u(\mathbf{r}, t)$ in time is slower for larger values of τ. The equivalent solution to Eq. (3) which is inclusive of the source function is

$$u(\mathbf{r},t) = g(r,t) \otimes u_0(\mathbf{r}) + \int_0^t g(\mathbf{r},t-\tau) \otimes s(\mathbf{r},t) d\tau$$

Thus, if we consider an asymptotic solution when $r \to 0$, then for $u_0(\mathbf{r}) = 0$ we obtain

$$u(t) = \left(\frac{1}{4\pi Dt}\right)^{\frac{n}{2}} \otimes s(t), \ \ s(t) \equiv s(0,t)$$

where $\otimes$ denotes the casual convolution integral in time. This result is an example of a continuous time random walk model for a stochastic time source $s(t)$ which, for classical diffusion, is characterised by scaling factor $1/t^{n/2}$.

2.2 *The Generalised Kolmogorov–Feller Equation*

Given that Eq. (3) is memory invariant, the question arises as to how longer temporal influences can be modelled, other than by taking an increasingly larger number of terms in the Taylor expansion of $u(\mathbf{r}, t + \tau)$ which is not analytically consequential, i.e. writing Eq. (2) in the form

$$\tau \frac{\partial}{\partial t} u(\mathbf{r},t) + \frac{\tau^2}{2!} \frac{\partial^2}{\partial t^2} u(\mathbf{r},t) + \ldots = -u(\mathbf{r},t) + u(\mathbf{r},t) \otimes p(r) + s(\mathbf{r},t)$$

The key to solving this problem is to consider the idea of expressing the Taylor series on the left-hand side of the equation above in terms of a 'memory function' $m(t)$ and write

$$\tau m(t) \otimes \frac{\partial}{\partial t} u(\mathbf{r},t) = -u(\mathbf{r},t) + u(\mathbf{r},t) \otimes p(r) + s(\mathbf{r},t) \quad (4)$$

This is the generalised Kolmogorov–Feller equation (GKFE). In addition to specifying the source function and the PDF in order to develop a solution for u, this equation also requires a memory function to be specified. In this case, if a time series is taken to be described by $u(t)$ (for a fixed position in space) then the behaviour at a time t is influenced by the behaviour at some earlier time according to the characteristics of the memory function. This is an example of a stochastic process in which the past influences the future. The time scale over which this effect is possible then depends on the 'width' in time of the memory function where it is noted that the GKFE reduces to the CKFE when $m(t) = \delta(t)$ which is equivalent to imposing the condition $\tau << 1$.

2.3 Orthonormal Memory Functions

For any inverse function or class of inverse functions of the type $n(t)$, say, such that

$$n(t) \otimes m(t) = \delta(t)$$

the GKFE can be written in the form

$$\tau \frac{\partial}{\partial t} u(\mathbf{r}, t) = -n(t) \otimes u(\mathbf{r}, t) + n(t) \otimes u(\mathbf{r}, t) \otimes p(\mathbf{r}) + n(t) \otimes s(\mathbf{r}, t) \quad (5)$$

where the CKFE is again recovered when $n(t) = \delta(t)$ given that $\delta(t) \otimes \delta(t) = \delta(t)$. The function $n(t)$ is a orthonormal function of $m(t)$. Writing the GKFE in this form facilitates the development of solutions for $u(\mathbf{r}, t)$ given that $n(t)$ can be derived from $m(t)$. In principle, this is possible, given that in Fourier space, the orthonormality relationship between $m(t)$ and $n(t)$ is (using the convolution theorem)

$$N(\omega) = \frac{1}{M(\omega)} \quad (6)$$

where $N(\omega)$ and $M(\omega)$ are the Fourier transforms of $n(t)$ and $m(t)$, respectively.

2.4 Time Series Models

Equation (5) is a description for a density field that is dependent on both space and time. Given that we are interested in analysing data that are time series alone, it is necessary to develop a time-only series model. A conditional example of this is to note that when $p(\mathbf{r}) = \delta^n(\mathbf{r})$, we can write Eq. (5) as

$$\tau \frac{d}{dt} u(t) = n(t) \otimes s(t) \quad (7)$$

where

$$u(t) = \int u(\mathbf{r}, t) d^n \mathbf{r} \text{ and } s(t) = \int s(\mathbf{r}, t) d^n \mathbf{r}$$

To generalise this result further, we consider an asymptotic result for the spatial component of Eq. (5). To do this, we note that using a Taylor expansion for the convolution integral over $\mathbf{r}$, we can write

$$u(\mathbf{r}, t) \otimes p(\mathbf{r}) = \int p(\mathbf{r} - \mathbf{s}) u(\mathbf{s}, t) d^n \mathbf{s} = \int [p(\mathbf{r}) - \mathbf{s} \cdot \nabla p(\mathbf{r}) + \ldots] u(\mathbf{s}, t) d^n \mathbf{s}$$

$$= p(\mathbf{r})\int u(\mathbf{s},t)d^n\mathbf{s} + \nabla p(\mathbf{r})\cdot\left[\int \mathbf{s}u(\mathbf{s},t)d^n\mathbf{s}\right] + \ldots \sim p(\mathbf{r})\int u(\mathbf{s},t)d^n\mathbf{s}$$

If the PDF is such that $p(\mathbf{r}) \to 0$ as $r \to \infty$, and, in addition, we can assume that the gradient of $p(\mathbf{r})$ and all higher-order gradients approach zero in the same limit, then, given the above series, we can consider the case where

$$u(\mathbf{r},t) \otimes p(\mathbf{r}) \sim 0, \quad r \to \infty$$

The contribution of the term $n(t) \otimes u(\mathbf{r},t) \otimes p(\mathbf{r})$ in Eq. (5) then becomes insignificant, and we can consider the time-only dependent asymptotic equation

$$\tau\frac{d}{dt}u(t) = -n(t) \otimes u(t) + n(t) \otimes s(t) \tag{8}$$

where $u(t) \equiv u(\mathbf{r},t), \ r \to \infty$ and $s(t) \equiv s(\mathbf{r},t), \ r \to \infty$.

The essential difference between Eqs. (8) and (7) is compounded in the inclusion or otherwise of the term $-n(t) \otimes u(t)$, respectively. In the latter case, i.e. Eq. (8), the spectral response of $u(t)$ to $s(t)$ is determined by the transfer function

$$T(\omega) = \frac{N(\omega)}{N(\omega) + i\omega\tau}$$

In the former case, i.e. Eq. (7), the transfer function is

$$T(\omega) = \frac{N(\omega)}{i\omega\tau}$$

In both cases, the stochastic behaviour of the density field $u(t)$ depends on the source function $s(t)$ and the memory function $m(t)$.

2.5 *Logarithmic Scale Analysis*

If we let $u = \log w$, then Eq. (7) becomes

$$\tau\frac{d}{dt}\log w(t) = n(t) \otimes s(t)$$

By way of an example, consider case when $n(t) = \delta(t)$ and

$$\tau\frac{d}{dt}\log w(t) = s(t)$$

Then, for a constant value of $s(t) = \pm s_0 \forall t$ say, we obtain the standard exponential growth/decay model when, for some initial condition $w_0 = w(t = 0)$,

$$w(t) = w_0 \exp(\pm s_0 t/\tau)$$

Thus, we observe that this most basic of time evolution models (exponential growth/decay) is in fact, just a conditional model of the evolution equation when $p(\mathbf{r}) = \delta^n(\mathbf{r})$ and $n(t) = \delta(t)$ where the density field is taken to be on a logarithmic scale. For a time varying source function, over some interval of time t, the solution is

$$w(t) = \exp\left[\frac{1}{\tau}\int^{t} s(\xi)d\xi\right]$$

3 Random Walk Fields

Consider the example data given in Fig. 1 which shows the daily new confirmed Covid-19 cases (for approximately 200 days) on a linear scale for different countries [16]. The plots provide the rolling 7-day average where the number of confirmed cases is taken to be lower than the number of actual cases due to limited testing. One of the purposes of applying a rolling average is to eliminate the characteristic and

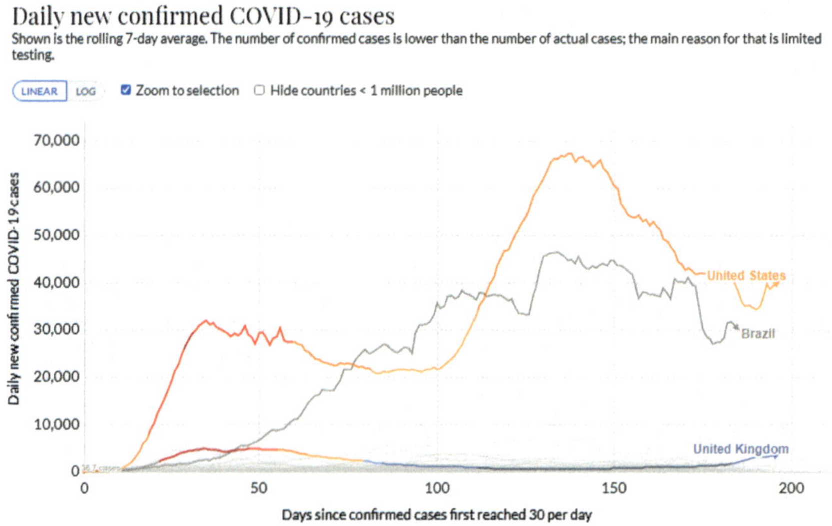

Fig. 1 Daily confirmed Covid-19 cases (for approximately 200 days) on a linear scale for a range of different countries with highlights for the UK, the USA and Brazil [16]

periodic decrease on the daily rates that occurs over the weekends, at least for the majority of countries when a Saturday and a Sunday are non-working days for the majority of the population. The data must be considered to contain a wide range of errors (e.g. false negatives and false positives), and, on a country by country basis, to have substantial differences in accuracy, consistency and relevance. In this context, Fig. 1 highlights three specific times series for cases in the UK, the USA and Brazil to illustrated some extreme example differences in the progression of the disease for three different countries.

The reasons for the differences in the growth (and decay) of the disease on a country-by-country basis are multifaceted. They are due to differences in the health systems of each country, their social-economic characteristics, the genetic dispositions of the population, age range and immunity signatures, etc. as well as the production and management of the data and the different policies adopted by central governments to control the disease. Thus, the data provided in Fig. 1 cannot be assumed to be an fully accurate representation for any case or to have a uniformity in its inaccuracies across the range of countries given. In this regard, the purpose of this section is to show that in a global context, the behaviour of the pandemic from one country to another appears to reflect a random walk process (a stochastic time series). Taking all the times series given in Fig. 1 produces a random walk field. It is this field that is a focus of the mathematical modelling considered in this work.

In terms of Eq. (7), the random walk model that is now considered is predicated on a one-dimensional model when $\tau << 1$, i.e. the system has no memory so that $n(t) = \delta(t)$. It therefore represents a model in which the simulation of the results given in Fig. 1 are based on the assumption that any interventions imposed or otherwise by a central authority are irrelevant and that the evolution of the pandemic is independent of any other factors such a asymmetry, herd immunity and the effects of a vaccination program, for example. In this case, Eq. (7) reduces to the simplest of evolution equations, namely,

$$\tau \frac{d}{dt} u(t) = s(t) \tag{9}$$

Fig. 2 provides an example of a typical set of random walks—a random walk field consisting of 15 trajectories over 200 steps re-scaled to 1. This results are based on using Euler's method and forward differencing the gradient in time for Eq. (9) to produce the difference equation

$$u_{n+1} = u_n + \Delta s_n, \; n = 1, 2, ..., N - 1$$

with $\Delta = 0.001$. Each trajectory follows a different random path from a common initial condition $u_1 = 0$. In this case, s_n is taken to be a Gaussian distributed (discrete) variable with a mean of zero. The random walks therefore have both positive and negative amplitudes.

The random walk field illustrated in Fig. 2 spreads out over time, the difference from one trajectory to the next being due to different initial conditions used to seed the Gaussian random number generator (in this example, the MATLAB function

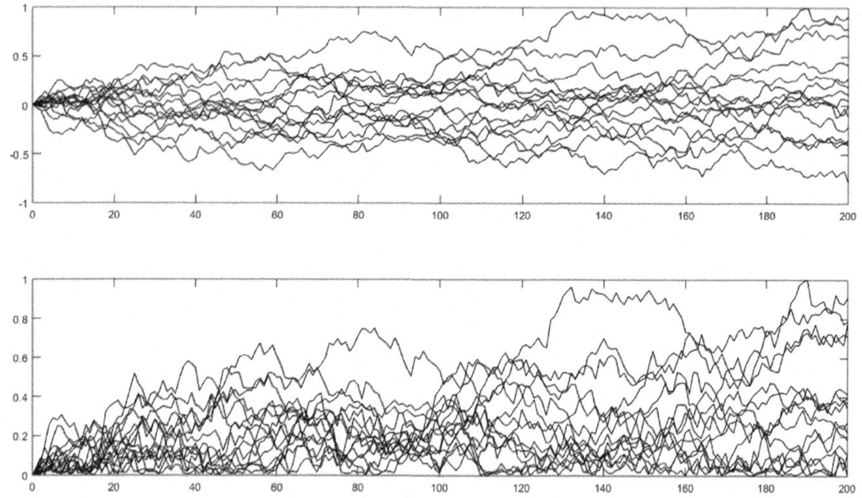

Fig. 2 Simulation of a random walk field illustrating random walks for u_n (above) and $| u_n |$ based on Eq. (9) for a random Gaussian distributed source s_n

randn has been applied). The result is to produce a random walk field whose spatial dissipation is not as diverse as is evident in Fig. 1 (for the time series given by $| u(t) |$). The principal reason for this is that the distribution in amplitudes of the trajectories given in Fig. 2 are within a common range and thus the distribution of gradients for any trajectory is the same, i.e. given Eq. (9), the derivative of $u(t)$ must be zero mean Gaussian distributed if $s(t)$ is so distributed. The principal difference between a random walk field based on Eq. (9) and that given in Fig. 1 is that in the former case, the field is ergodic [17] from one trajectory to the next.

For a system to be ergodic, any collection of random samples from a process must represent the average statistical properties of the entire process. In other words, regardless of what the individual samples are, a broad view of the collection of samples must represent the whole process. In the case of Fig. 1, it is clear that the statistical properties of the time series vary significantly from one country to another, specifically in regard to the standard deviation of the daily case time differences, i.e. the gradients of each time series. In this context, Eq. (9), and, the model it is predicated upon, fails to account for the differences in the infection rates that are observed. The solution to this issue is explored in the section that follows.

4 Self-Affine Random Walk Fields

The solution to Eq. (7) requires the distribution of the source term to be quantified and the memory function to be specified. In the latter case, let the memory function be given by

$$m(t) = \frac{1}{\Gamma(1-\alpha)t^{\alpha}}, \quad \alpha \in (0, 1) \tag{10}$$

where Γ is the Gamma function. The reason for adopting this particular function is that, as shall now be shown, the solution to Eq. (7) can be shown to yield a self-affine time series which is characteristic of many natural random processes including those presented in Fig. 1. In this context, the aim is to both simulate and quantify the data field in Fig. 1, the quantification being compounded in the parameter α. To do this, we note a key result which is that

$$\frac{1}{(i\omega)^{\alpha}} \leftrightarrow \frac{1}{\Gamma(\alpha)t^{1-\alpha}}$$

where $\leftrightarrow$ denotes Fourier transformation. Thus,

$$m(t) \leftrightarrow \frac{1}{(i\omega)^{1-\alpha}} \Rightarrow N(\omega) = (i\omega)^{1-\alpha}$$

given Eq. (6).

4.1 Solution for Eq. (7)

In Fourier space, Eq. (7) is given by (using the Convolution Theorem)

$$i\omega\tau U(\omega) = N(\omega)S(\omega)$$

where $U(\omega)$ and $S(\omega)$ are the Fourier transforms of $u(t)$ and $s(t)$, respectively. Thus, we can write

$$U(\omega) = \frac{1}{i\omega\tau}(i\omega)^{1-\alpha}S(\omega)$$

or, using the convolution theorem again,

$$u(t) = \frac{1}{\tau\Gamma(\alpha)t^{1-\alpha}} \otimes s(t) \tag{11}$$

The solution for $u(t)$ is then expressed in terms of the Riemann–Liouville (fractional) integral which is an icon of the fractional calculus, Liouville having been one of the first to consider the possibility of fractional calculus in 1832. The integral may be considered to be the anti-derivative of a fractional differential and one of its principal properties is its scale invariance, given that for some scale length $\lambda > 0$ (in this case, a scale in time) and using a change of variable, it can be shown that

$$u_\lambda(t) = \frac{1}{\tau\Gamma(\alpha)t^{1-\alpha}} \otimes s(\lambda t) = \frac{u(\lambda t)}{\lambda^\alpha}$$

and we can therefore write

$$u(\lambda t) = \lambda^\alpha u_\lambda(t)$$

For this reason, the function $u(t)$ is a random scaling fractal and has a power spectral density function which scales with frequency as $1/\mid \omega \mid^{2\alpha}$ assuming that the power spectral density function for $s(t)$ is a constant, i.e. $s(t)$ is a 'white noise' source. This scaling law is a principal 'signature' for stochastic time series that exhibit random self-affine properties, the relationship between α and the fractal dimension $D \in (1, 2)$ for such a time series being [18]

$$\alpha = \frac{5}{2} - D$$

4.2 *Solution for Eq. (8)*

Given Eq. (10), and, following the analysis given in Sect. 4.1, Eq. (8) becomes

$$u(t) = -\frac{1}{\tau\Gamma(\alpha)t^{1-\alpha}} \otimes u(t) + \frac{1}{\tau\Gamma(\alpha)t^{1-\alpha}} \otimes s(t) \tag{12}$$

which has the transfer function

$$T(\omega) = \frac{1}{1 + \tau(i\omega)^\alpha} \tag{13}$$

One approach to solving Eq. (12) is to apply iteration when

$$u^{(k+1)}(t) = -\frac{1}{\tau\Gamma(\alpha)t^{1-\alpha}} \otimes u^{(k)}(t) + \frac{1}{\tau\Gamma(\alpha)t^{1-\alpha}} \otimes s(t),\ k = 0, 1, 2, ...$$

where

$$u^{(1)}(t) = \frac{1}{\tau\Gamma(\alpha)t^{1-\alpha}} \otimes s(t)$$

The first iteration is then equivalent to Eq. (11). In this case, a condition for the convergence of the solution must be investigated and obtained. Another approach to the problem is to consider the relationship between Eqs. (11) and (12) in terms of their respective transfer functions. This is the approach that is considered here, as shall now be addressed.

Since the transfer function for Eq. (11) is $1/\tau(i\omega)^\beta,\ \beta \in (0, 1)$, if we can relate α to β, then it becomes possible to compare the solution given by Eq. (11) and the

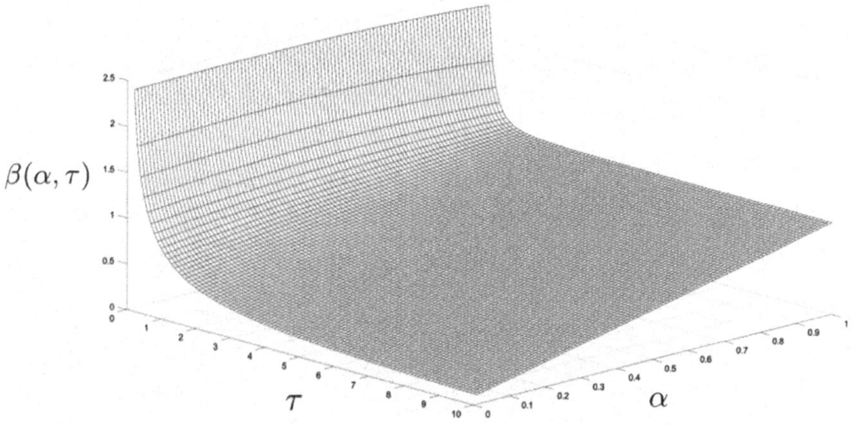

Fig. 3 Surface plot of $\beta(\alpha, \tau)$, $\alpha \in (0, 1)$, $\tau \in (0, 10]$ based on Eq. (14) illustrating that for $\tau >> 1$, there is a linear relationship between α and β.

solution we now require to Eq. (12). To do this, we equate the power spectra of the two transfer functions. This yields a relationship between α and β for τ given by

$$\tau^2 \mid \omega \mid^{2\beta} = 1 + \tau^2 \mid \omega \mid^{2\alpha} + 2\tau \mid \omega \mid^{\alpha} \cos(\alpha\pi/2)$$

so that upon setting $\omega = e$ we can write

$$\beta = \frac{1}{2}\log[1 + \tau^2 \exp(2\alpha) + 2\tau \exp(\alpha)\cos(\alpha\pi/2)] - \log\tau \tag{14}$$

Figure 3 shows a plot of β for $\alpha \in (0, 1)$ and $\tau \in (0, 10]$ based on Eq. (14) and illustrates that as $\tau > 1$ increases, there develops a linear relationship between α and β. In particular, for $\tau = 10$, a linear fit between the two parameters yields $\beta = 0.9016\alpha + 0.09393$. Since Eqs. (11) and (12) are both scaled by $1/\tau$, this result implies that for $\tau >> 1$ the two equations are equivalent. Thus, the solution for $u(t)$ given by Eq. (11) is equivalent to the solution for $u(t)$ given by Eq. (12) with $\alpha \simeq 1.1\beta - 0.1$. Moreover, any estimate for α given $u(t)$ based on Eq. (11) through application of a regression analysis is simply related to an estimate for α, given Eq. (12). For this reason, in the following section, we focus on the time series model compounded in Eq. (11).

4.3 Random Walk Analysis

Equation (11) can be written in the form

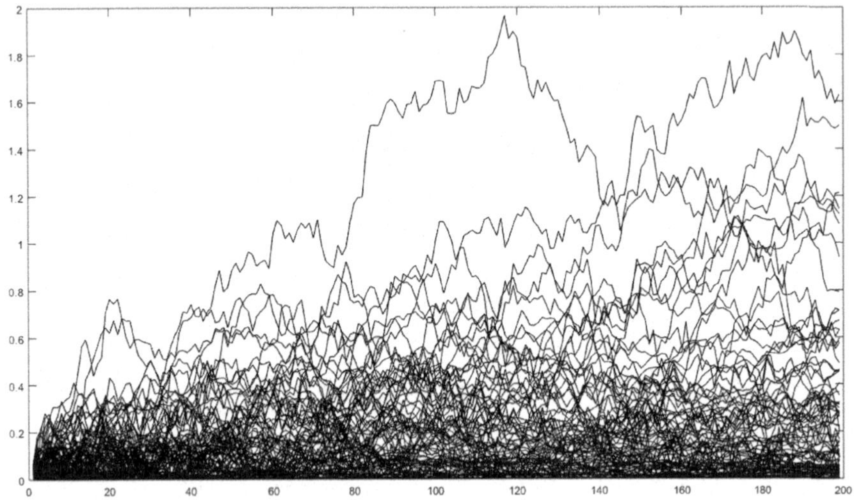

Fig. 4 Example simulation of a self-affine random walk field $| u(t) |$ for $\tau = 10$ using Eq. (15) when $\alpha \in (0, 1)$ is assumed to be a random Gaussian distributed variable

$$\tau \frac{d}{dt} u(t) = \frac{d}{dt} \left(\frac{1}{\Gamma(\alpha) t^{1-\alpha}} \right) \otimes s(t) = \frac{1}{\Gamma(\alpha) t^{1-\alpha}} \otimes \frac{d}{dt} s(t) \qquad (15)$$

This provides an equation that is compatible with Eq. (9) so that, on comparing Eq. (9) with Eq. (15), it is apparent that if α is the same for all random walk trajectories the random walk field will be ergodic. However, if α varies randomly from one country to another, a non-ergodic random walk field will result of the type that is evident in Fig. 1. In this regard, the value of α determines the relative rate of growth of a trajectory and it is clear that as $\alpha \to 0$, any rate of growth becomes increasing suppressed because $\Gamma(\alpha) \to \infty$ as $\alpha \to 0$. This characteristic is reflected in Fig. 4 which shows an example random walk field $| u(t) |$ for $\tau = 10$ based on Eq. (15) where $\alpha \in (0, 1)$ is chosen from a zero mean Gaussian distributed source (by taking the absolute value of the output array and normalising the result) .

An essential difference between this model and that presented in Sect. 3 is that the non-ergodic characteristics of random walk field—specifically, the standard deviation of the gradients of $u(t)$ - are a measure of the random changes in the value of $\alpha \in (0, 1)$ for each country. This is a consequence of the self-affine model developed through the application of the memory function given by Eq. (10).

4.4 Example Results

Based on the model for the memory function given by Eq. (10), α determines the memory of the system. The memory decays faster as $\alpha \to 1$ when one can intuitively expect the random walk field to have greater dispersion. In this sense, α can be interpreted as a measure of 'control' on the rate of infection which in turn, is related to issues such a lock-down and herd immunity. Thus, in the context of the self-affine random walk model being considered, the infection will be suppressed when $\alpha \to 0$ for all countries (assuming travel continues form one country to another). Consequently, the evaluation of α on a country by country basis using available data is informative as given in Fig. 5 for 100 randomly selected countries. The basis for these results is the application of a least squares regression method to compute α given that (for a constant C)

$$\log \mid U(\omega) \mid^2 = C - 2\alpha \log(\omega), \quad \omega > 0$$

where $\mid U(\omega) \mid^2$ is the power spectrum of the data plotted in Fig. 1 for each country.

The results in Fig. 5 illustrate some important features that include the following:

(i) The values of α are not confined to the condition $\alpha \in (0, 1)$;
(ii) there is a significant diversity in the values of α computed;
(iii) the distribution of values for α decays with higher values;
(iv) the mean value of α is 0.5746.

The reasons for point (i) above are that the quantity of data currently available is not significant enough to provide accuracy on the computation of α through the regression method used (i.e. a least squares estimate of α). Another issue is that for some countries, the model for $u(t)$ being considered may not conform to the data. Hence, the results shown in Fig. 5 should not be taken to be statistically significant. It is expected that the significance of such results will improve as further data becomes available. Nevertheless, in regard to point (ii) above, the results illustrate that there is, as would be expected, significant diversity in the random walk fields given in Fig. 1 for the Covid-19 pandemic, irrespective of directives from the World Health Organisation, for example.

By way of some specific examples, compared to Sweden, α is larger for both the USA and the UK, for example, that have introduced lock-down policies [19]. Sweden has endorsed a policy not to lock down the country in response to the global pandemic. Thus, on the basis of Eq. (11), and its interpretation with regard to the pandemic, Sweden is better served by the policies the Health authorities have introduced [20], as predicated on the self-affine random walk approach being considered in this work.

It should be noted that as α approaches 0, the memory function given by Eq. (10) becomes constant in time, i.e. $m(t) \to 1$ as $\alpha \to 0$ when $\Gamma(1-\alpha) = 1$. A memory function that is constant in time implies that the density field u is time invariant. This is because, from Eq. (4),

$$\tau m(t) \otimes \frac{\partial}{\partial t} u(\mathbf{r}, t) = \tau u(\mathbf{r}, t) \otimes \frac{d}{dt} m(t) = 0, \quad \text{if} \quad m(t) = 1 \forall t$$

and we are then left with the time-independent equation

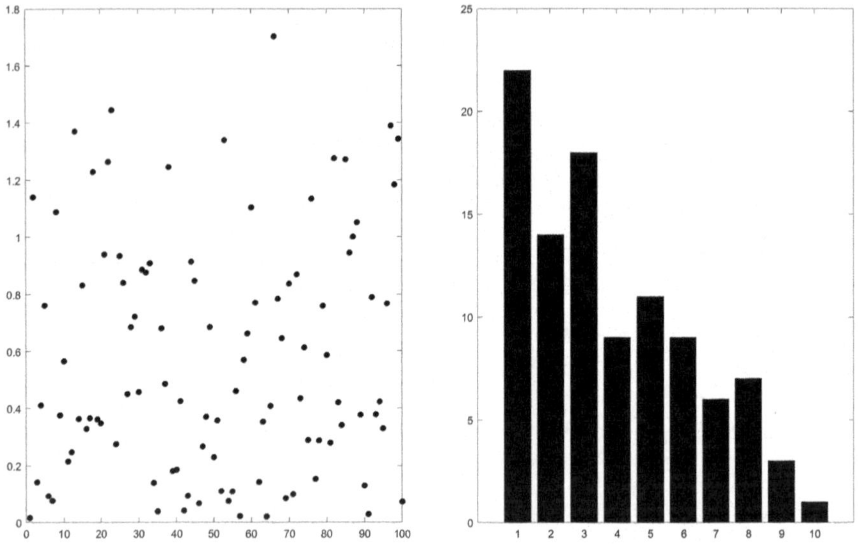

Fig. 5 Values of α for 100 randomly selected countries (left) and the associated 10-bin distribution (right)

$$u(\mathbf{r}) \otimes p(\mathbf{r}) + s(\mathbf{r}) = u(\mathbf{r}) \tag{16}$$

From Eq. (11), it is clear that $u(t) \to 0 \; \forall t$ as $\alpha \to 0$ when the density field ceases to evolve in time, its spatial distribution being determined by the solution to Eq. (16). In this context, if $p(\mathbf{r}) = \delta^n(\mathbf{r})$, then $s(\mathbf{r}) = 0$. On the other hand, for a Lévy distribution with approximated Characteristic Function (for Lévy Index γ)

$$P(\mathbf{k}) = \exp(- \mid k \mid^\gamma) \sim 1 - \mid k \mid^\gamma, \; \gamma \in (0, 2)$$

we can write Eq. (16) in terms of the fractional Poisson equation

$$\nabla^\gamma u(\mathbf{r}) = s(\mathbf{r}) \tag{17}$$

where $\nabla^\gamma u(\mathbf{r}) \leftrightarrow - \mid \mathbf{k} \mid^\gamma U(\mathbf{k})$. The relationship between γ and the fractal dimension is given by [18]

$$\gamma = \frac{3}{2}n + 1 - D, \; \mathbf{r} \in \mathbb{R}^n$$

Thus, for example, when $n = 2$, Eq. (17) is the equation for a Mandelbrot surface [18].

5 The Bio-Dynamics Hypothesis

The Bio-dynamics Hypothesis is concerned with the connectivity between the dynamical behaviour of bio-organisms in regard to their replication and growth and the geometrical structures of the physical forms that result. It states that if the growth of a bio-organism is self-affine, then the geometry of the organism will also be self-affine.

In this section, we consider a similar model to that discussed in Sect. 4 but with a focus on developing a parametric representation whose aim is to reflect the self-affine structures of proteins. The reason for this is that understanding and interpreting the structure (geometric configuration) of the spike protein on a coronavirus is the key to developing a vaccine. This is because it is through the spike protein that the virus attaches, fuses and gains entry to cells. Therefore, analysis of the spike protein 'architecture' coupled with its mechanics is vital in revealing information that can prompt the discovery of countermeasures against the virus.

In this context, the basic principle for developing a vaccine is well known. If a protein can be found that has the same structure as the spike protein and is introduced into the body prior to infection, then anti-bodies will be generated by the body that will destroy the virus by suppressing its ability to replicate through elimination of the spike protein. On this basis, what is required is a search and/or fabrication of proteins whose self-affine structure is the same as the spike protein.

5.1 Self-affine Structures of a Virus

It is well known that there is a correlation between the effect (in particular, its fatalness) of a virus and its fractal geometry. This refers primarily, but not exclusively, to the surface roughness of a virus and its metabolic rate. In turn, the surface roughness is related to the structural complexity of the spike proteins and their density on the surface of the virus. For a single near spherical cell, its metabolic rate, M_R, scales as $M_R \sim r^2$ where r is the radius of the cell but for a virus, its metabolic rate scales as $M_R \sim r^D$ where $D \in (2, 3)$ is the fractal dimension of the surface and r is the characteristics radius of the virus [21].

Figure 6 shows a comparison of the simulated structures for the spike proteins of the Covid-19 virus, the influenza virus and the Human Immunodeficiency Virus (HIV). In each case, the spike protein is not one continuous feature but is composed of specific protein strands which are colour coded. While the Covid-19 spike protein displays structural similarities to the spike proteins of influenza virus and HIV, it is, by comparison, the largest class I fusion protein known to date. Given that Covid-19 is new and there is no general immunity to it, this is why it is so relatively dangerous.

Use of Eq. (17) to model such structures is not relevant. This is due to the following:

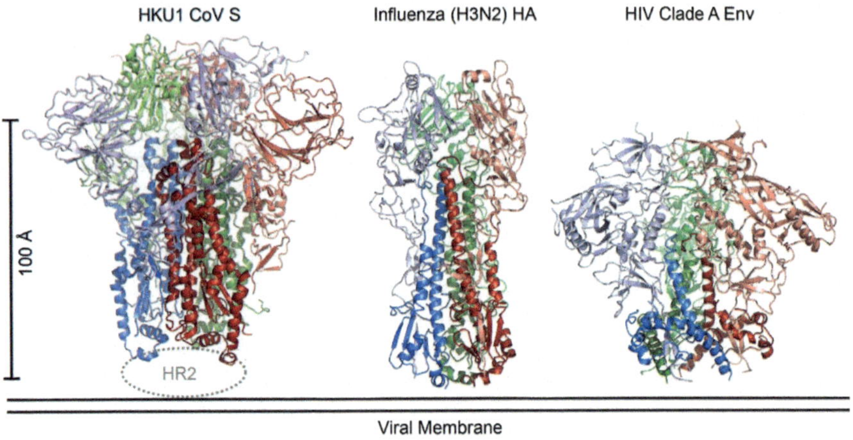

Fig. 6 Comparison of the simulated structural complexity of the spike protein's for coronavirus (CoV S), the influenza virus and HIV [22]

- the equation assumes that the evolution process is time-independent;
- it is not compatible with modelling a self-affine field that is based on long continuous strands of which proteins are an important example.

Instead, we consider a parametric self-affine model which is discussed in the following section.

5.2 A Parametric Self-affine Model

For $p(\mathbf{r}) = \delta^n(\mathbf{r})$, Eq. (5) reduces to

$$\tau \frac{\partial}{\partial t} u(\mathbf{r}, t) = n(t) \otimes s(\mathbf{r}, t)$$

Consider a solution to this equation based on an additive separation of variables when

$$u(\mathbf{r}, t) = u_x(t) + u_y(t) + u_z(t) \text{ and } s(\mathbf{r}, t) = s_x(t) + s_y(t) + s_z(t).$$

The source function is taken to model a system characterised by a set of additive spatial sources which may have independent stochastic properties. We are then interested in the evolution of a density field in a three-dimensional space that is taken to be described by the parametric curve $[u_x(t), u_y(t), u_z(t)]$.

Following the solution method discussed in Sect. 4 for the memory function given by Eq. (10), we can write the solution for each component of the parametric curve as

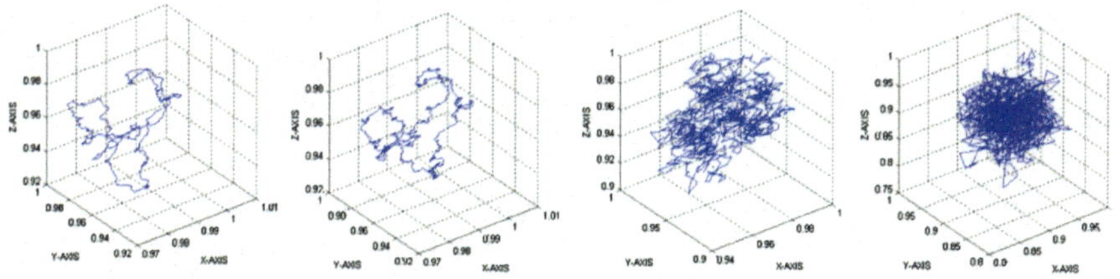

Fig. 7 Evolution of a three-dimensional parametric curve for (from left to right consecutively) $\alpha = 0.8$, $\alpha = 0.6$, $\alpha = 0.4$ and $\alpha = 0.2$ obtained using Eq. (18)

$$\begin{bmatrix} u_x(t) \\ u_y(t) \\ u_z(t) \end{bmatrix} = \frac{1}{\tau\Gamma(\alpha)t^{1-\alpha}} \otimes \begin{bmatrix} s_x(t) \\ s_y(t) \\ s_z(t) \end{bmatrix} \tag{18}$$

The Fourier space representation of this result is

$$\begin{bmatrix} U_x(\omega) \\ U_y(\omega) \\ U_z(\omega) \end{bmatrix} = \frac{1}{\tau(i\omega)^{\alpha}} \begin{bmatrix} S_x(\omega) \\ S_y(\omega) \\ S_z(\omega) \end{bmatrix}, \quad \omega > 0 \tag{19}$$

where the upper case functions of the angular frequency ω denote the Fourier transforms of the corresponding lower case function of time. It is then clear that the parametric curve is composed of elements that are characterised by the same value of α. Although the source functions are uncorrelated, their power spectral density functions are taken to be the same. The structure of the parametric curve is then determined by the value of α which, in turn, is a measure of the influence of the memory function in time. This is illustrated in Fig. 7 which shows parametric curves for various values of $\alpha \in (0, 1)$ illustrating that the complexity of the curve increases as the value of α decreases.

5.3 Discussion

If we can model the Covid-19 spike protein as a parametric curve with a known value α based on Eq. (18), then it may be possible to use this value in the search for other benign proteins that have a similar α value. Such proteins would then at least possess the same structural complexity which is an important factor in the development of any vaccine. One way to determine the value of α from protein models of the type given in Fig. 6 is to extract data associated with the functions $u_x(t)$, $u_y(t)$ and $u_z(t)$ (essentially the coordinate values of the structure obtained by moving along the protein strand), evaluate α in each case and compute the mean value.

6 Summary, Conclusions and Future Research

The material presented in this work has been developed to provide readers with an overview of the ways in which Eq. (2) can be used as a frame work for investigating epidemic and pandemic time series (and viral structures). In this context, a summary of the material presented is now given followed by some conclusions and directions for future research.

6.1 Summary

The evolution equation for a stochastic source given by Eq. (2) is a fundamental field equation of statistical mechanics. It is applicable in all topological dimensions and for any system composed of random interactions (elastic scattering). In the application of Eq. (2) to the evolution of an infectious disease, these interactions are taken to be the transmission of a pathogen from one person to another. In this regard, the focus of the work has been to develop time series models for the evolution of Covid-19 informed by the data that is currently available. For this purpose, and, using Eq. (4), a memory function has been considered—Eq. (10)—that yields a self-affine model for the time series. The reason for doing this is because it is known that biological and bio-medical time series are self-affine which is entirely compatible with the fractal geometry of nature [23]. Not surprisingly, therefore, this also appears to be the case for Covid-19 pandemic time series data.

Two time-only dependent equations have been derived, namely Eq. (7) and Eq. (8). The former equation is based on assuming the PDF in Eq. (2) is a delta function and corresponds to the case when $\tau << 1$. The latter equation is based on an asymptotic solution and is applicable for any PDF $p(\mathbf{r})$ which approaches zero as $r \to \infty$ and valid for all values of τ. However, through an analysis of the transfer functions for both equations as given in Sect. 4.2, it has been shown that the two equations have an equivalence in terms of the relationship between α for each equation as given by Eq. (14). This avoids having to resort to an iterative approach for solving Eq. (8). Moreover, it provides a method of determining the parameter α for Eq. (8) based on applying a recursion analysis using Eq. (7), i.e. given $u(t)$, compute α.

6.2 Conclusions

The application of stochastic models avoids the indeterminacy associated with implementing a deterministic model with many coefficients. On a global perspective, this approach assumes that there are no intrinsic correlations between the dynamics of the pandemic and its intervention and control. This is due to the multifaceted differences that are being introduced by different governments through different policies at different times in order to attempt to reduce the severity of the disease using 'solutions' that are not, as yet, fully proven (i.e. statistically significant), e.g. [25].

The models and results presented in this work are developments based exclusively on the evolution equation—Eq. (2). In this context, the time series model compounded in Eq. (11) is critically dependent on the memory function parameter α. From the example time series data given in Fig. 1, it is clear that the stochastic characteristics are non-ergodic (i.e. they changes significantly from one country to another) and that α changes from one country to another. Thus, the growth of the pandemic in each country is memory dependent. The distribution of α presented in Fig. 5 is informative but not yet statistically significant due to the lack of data that is currently available. Consequently, the results given in Fig. 5 need to be continually re-evaluated as the Covid-19 pandemic evolves.

The value of α provides a measure on the dissipation of the pandemic. It has a synergy with the reproduction number R associated with deterministic models which is a way of rating the ability for an infection to spread—the number of people (on average) that one infected person will pass the virus on to. To extinguish an infectious disease, we require that $R < 1$. To extinguish an infectious disease based on a self-affine evolutionary model based on Eq. (8), we require that $\alpha \rightarrow 0$. This is because $u(t)$ approaches zero due to the scaling of Equations (11) and (12) by $1/\Gamma(\alpha)$, i.e. $\Gamma(\alpha) \rightarrow \infty$ as $\alpha \rightarrow 0$. However, it is arguable that this is not physically possible, because it implies that the memory function is constant in time which in turn implies that the system is time-independent and that there is no time evolution of the density field.

On the basis of the evolution equation and the analysis used to derive a time-only-dependent representation for the density field $u(t)$, Equations (11) and (12) provide basic stochastic time series models which have an intrinsic relationship. If $\mid u(t) \mid$ is taken to be a model for the infections over a uniform period of time (e.g. each day), then the amplitude of this function is reduced as $\alpha \rightarrow 0$ and as $\tau \rightarrow \infty$. In terms of the dynamics of a global pandemic, this result implies that the longer the memory associated with a population maintaining a high value of τ is (giving a low infection rate), the greater the rate at which $\mid u(t) \mid$ reduces to zero, thereby extinguishing the pandemic.

In the same way that α is a gauge on viral infection rates, in the context of the Fig. 6 and the Bio-dynamics Hypothesis, it also relates to the self-affine structures that are prevalent in the spike protein. In both cases, the value of α determines the rate of infection and the structure of the protein that is causing the disease. The interesting question is whether there is a correlation between the two, i.e. the mean value of α that is characteristic of the infection rate in a global context and the value or α that is characteristic of the structural complexity of the spike protein.

The underlying principle is that the Covid-19 virus will fractionally diffuse in the early stages of the pandemic exhibiting self-affine characteristics, and, as time increases, the dynamics will become increasingly characterised by classical diffusion. This is a consequence of the Central Limit Theorem when $\gamma \rightarrow 2$ as $t \rightarrow \infty$. Further, as time increases, the value of α can be expected to approach zero for all countries thereby giving the appearance of the pandemic becoming extinct, the final density field then being given by Eq. (17) for $\gamma = 2$, i.e. the time-independent diffusion equation for a source.

In the context of this conceptual interpretation, the effect of attempting to control the infection rates will merely delay the transition from fractional to classical diffusion. Compared to the 1918 ‘Spanish flu’ pandemic, for example, which involved the H1N1 virus, taking a few years to be extinguished at the cost of many tens of millions lives [24], the current pandemic is likely to continue for a longer period of time but at the same final cost. This is not due to a difference in the dynamical behaviour of Covid-19 now compared to H1N1 in 1918, but the considerable difference in the moral imperatives of today compared to 100 years ago. In this regard, the failure of deterministic pandemic models is in part due to ‘interference’ of central governments and their time varying policies which alter the dynamics of the infection rate, one that is randomly inhomogeneous on a worldwide basis. Thus, a stochastic approach to modelling the pandemic is, in part, necessitated by the moral imperatives that modern governments are expect to adopt which injects randomness into the evolution of the disease when viewed on a global perspective [25]. On the basis of the models developed and the data analysed, this randomness appears to be self-affine. In this context, the models presented reflect the inconsistencies of implementing a lock-down and substantiates, on a theoretical level at least, the importance of evidence-based medicine rather than highly sensitive deterministic modelling based on assumptions and many unknowns [26] as briefly discussed in the introduction.

By way of an analogy, consider an ink drop which is introduced to the surface of some water that is contained in a vessel where it is assumed that the ink is the same density as the water and that the water is at a constant temperature and is homogeneous throughout the container. The ink will flow into the water producing complex patterns while spreading away from the point on the surface at which it has been introduced. These complex patterns represent the combined effects of each ink molecule undertaking a random walk. As time increases, the ink will diffuse into the water and eventually become equally distributed throughout, a process that is irreversible. A lock down is then analogous to draining the container by introducing a channel at the bottom of the vessel, for example, at the time the ink is first introduced in order to try and eradicate its presence. The effect of this is to drain some of the ink but at the expense of a falling water level. The difference between the initial and final water levels is then analogous to the difference between the economic prosperity of a country before and after lock down, especially in regard to the younger and more healthy component of the population who are inherently less vulnerable to the effects of infection. The economic effects of this may be destined to be significant [27]. In this context, the objective to suppress the pandemic through intermittent lock-downs, while waiting for an effective vaccine to be developed is, while laudable, not feasible and may lead to significant long-term damage, especially to those who are at the forefront of wealth creation in a society.

6.3 *Future Research*

Within the context of the material presented, example suggestions for future work include the following:

- Simulation of Covid-19 random walk fields using Eq. (12) for distributions in the values of the infection rate τ;
- evaluation of distributions for α using different data associated with the Covid-19 pandemic;
- evaluation of the time evolution of α as more data becomes available;
- evaluation of α using more advanced regression methods such as singular value decomposition which typically requires extensive data sets;
- simulation of spike proteins based on Eq. (18) when the value of α varies for each component of the parametric curve;
- computation of α for different continuous strands of proteins from which the spike protein is composed based on Eq. (18);
- analysis of solutions to Eq. (5) using time series data predicated on spatial locations, i.e. the geographical location of a country relative to a common origin such as Wuhan in China, for example (where the Covid-19 virus is considered to have emerged) and the location of isolated pockets of infections with each country as and when such data becomes available.

References

1. Han, et al.: Novel Coronavirus Pneumonia (COVID-19) progression course in 17 discharged patients: comparison of clinical and thin-section CT features during recovery. Clin. Infect. Dis. **71**(15), 723-731 (2020). https://doi.org/10.1093/cid/ciaa271
2. Bacaër, N.: McKendrick and Kermack on Epidemic Modelling (1926-1927). In: A Short History of Mathematical Population Dynamics, pp. 89–96. Springer, London (2011). https://doi.org/10.1007/978-0-85729-115-8_16
3. Jones, D., Helmreich, S.: A history of herd immunity, perspectives, the art of medicine. The Lancet **396** (2020). https://www.thelancet.com/journals/lancet/article/PIIS0140-67362031924-3/fulltext
4. Siettos, C.I., Russo, L.: Mathematical Modelling of iInfectious Disease Dynamics, vol. 4(4), pp. 295-306. Taylor & Francis, Virulence (2013). https://www.tandfonline.com/doi/pdf/10.4161/viru.24041
5. Cakan, S.: Dynamic analysis of a mathematical model with health care capacity for COVID-19 pandemic. Chaos, Solit. Fractals **139**, 110 033. Elsevier (2020)
6. Dayaratna, K.: Failures of an Influential COVID-19 Model Used to Justify Lockdowns. The Heritage Foundation. https://www.heritage.org/public-health/commentary/failures-influential-covid-19-model-used-justify-lockdowns. Accessed 21 Sept 2020
7. Crank, J.: The Mathematics of Diffusion. Clarendon Press, Oxford (1956)
8. Wyss, W.: The fractional diffusion equation. J . Math. Phys. **27**, 2782 (1986). https://doi.org/10.1063/1.527251
9. Blackledge, J.M., Barry, D.: Morphological analysis from images of hyphal growth using a fractional dynamic model. In: Carr, H., Grimstead, I. (eds) EG UK Theory and Practice of Computer Graphics (Warwick University), 17–24 (2011) https://doi.org/10.21427/3ssf-3335

10. Melin, P., Monica, J.C., Sanchez, D., Castillo, O.: Analysis of spatial spread relationships of Coronavirus (COVID-19) pandemic in the world using self organizing maps. Chaos, Solit. Fractals, Elsevier **138**, 109917–109918 (2020). https://doi.org/10.1016/j.chaos.2020.109917
11. Einstein, A.: On the motion of small particles suspended in liquids at rest required by the molecular-kinetic theory of heat. Annalen der Physik **17**, 549–560 (2016)
12. Samorodnitsky, G., Taqqu, M.S.: 1994. Stochastic Models with Infinite Variance, CRC Press, Stable Non-Gaussian Random Processes (1994)9780412051715
13. Kolmogorov, A.N.: On analytic methods in probability theory. In: Shiryaev, A. N. (ed) Selected Works of A. N. Kolmogorov, Volume II: Probability Theory and Mathematical Statistics1992, Kluwer, Dordrecht, 61-108 (1992). Based on the Original: Uber die Analytischen Methoden in der Wahrscheinlichkeitsrechnung, Math. Ann., **104**, 415-458 (1931)
14. Feller, W.: On boundaries and lateral conditions for the Kolmogorov differential equations. Ann. Math., Second Series **65**(3), 527–570 (1957)
15. Evans, G., Blackledge, J.M., Yardley, P.: Analytic Solutions to Partial Differential Equations, Springer Undergraduate Mathematics Series, Springer-Verlag. London (1999). https://doi.org/10.1007/978-1-4471-0379-0
16. Our World in Data, Coronavirus (COVID-19) Cases (2020). https://ourworldindata.org/coronavirus-data-explorer?Scale=log&zoomToSelection=true&casesMetric=true&interval=smoothed&aligned=true&smoothing=7&country. Accessed 21 Sept 2020
17. Papoulis, A.: Probability, pp. 427–442. Random Variables and Stochastic Processes, McGraw-Hill, New York (1991)0-07-048477-5
18. Turner, M.J., Blackledge, J.M., Andrews: Fractal Geometry in Digital Imaging, Academic Press, P. R. (1998)-10: 0127039708
19. Giesecke, J.: Why Lockdowns are the Wrong Policy, LockdownTV, Unherd.com/live ,17 April, 2020. https://www.youtube.com/watch?v=bfN2JWifLCY&feature=youtu.be. Accessed 20 Sept 2020
20. Neil A.: Interviews Anders Tegnell - A Second Wave and What Sweden Got Right | SpectatorTV, 18 Sep 2020. https://www.youtube.com/watch?v=6C99MtK4ogM. Accessed 21 Sept 2020
21. He, J.H.: Fatalness of virus depends upon its cell fractal geometry. Chaos, Solit. Fractals **38**, 1390–1393 (2008)
22. Scripps Research Institute, TSRI Scientists find Clues to Neutralizing Coronaviruses such as MERS, Public Release, 2 March, 2016. https://www.eurekalert.org/pub_releases/2016-03/sri-tsf022916.php. Last accessed 12 August, 2020
23. Mandelbrot, B.B.: The Fractal Geometry of Nature. W. H, Freeman and Co (1982)0-7167-1186-9
24. Center's for Disease Control and Prevention, 1918 Pandemic (H1N1 virus) (2020). https://www.cdc.gov/flu/pandemic-resources/1918-pandemic-h1n1.html. Last accessed 12 August 2020
25. Gandhi, M., Rutherford, G.: Facial Masking for Covid-19 - Potential for ‘ Variolation’ as we Await a Vaccine, *Perspective*, The New England Journal of Medicine, Massachusetts Medical Society, 1–3, September 8, (2020). https://doi.org/10.1056/NEJMp2026913
26. Kirkham, P. Yeadon, M., Thomas, B.: How Likely is a Second Waves, Lockdown Sceptics, 8 September (2020). https://lockdownsceptics.org/addressing-the-cv19-second-wave. Accessed 20 Sept 2020
27. Varoufakis, Y.: Something Remarkable just Happened this August: How the Pandemic has Sped up the Passage to Post-Capitalism, 25 August, 2020 https://diem25.org/something-remarkable-just-happened-this-august-how-the-pandemic-has-sped-the-passage-postcapitalism. Accessed 20 Sept 2020

Modelling the Dynamics of Fake News Spreading Transmission During Covid-19 Through Social Media

Saratha Sathasivam, Shehab Abdulhabib Alzaeemi, Teoh Poh Lin, and Woon Le Yu

Abstract On 12 January 2020, the World Health Organization (WHO) confirmed that a novel coronavirus was the cause of a respiratory illness in a cluster of people in Wuhan City, Hubei Province, China, which was reported to the WHO on 31 December 2019. The case fatality ratio for coronavirus disease 2019 (Covid-19) has been much lower than SARS of 2003, but the transmission has been significantly greater, with a significant total death toll. As of 20 May 2020, there are a total of 5,085,449 confirmed cases and 329,239 death cases in the world with more than 200 countries affected. Malaysia reported a total of 7,009 confirmed cases, 5,706 recoveries and 114 deaths. According to the Global Web Index (GWI), it can be seen that there is a significant increase in the usage of social media among global users for the past month, including Facebook, Instagram and WhatsApp. By going online, people can stay updated to the news more easily and information can be spread at a higher speed. However, it can also bring negative impact among the users when people misuse this platform to spread fake news, causing misconception, anxiety and fear as they become "viral". The spread of fake news can lead to several misconceptions among social media users, which can cause unnecessary fear and anxiety. For example, when Movement Control Order (MCO) was first announced in Malaysia on 16 March 2020, fake news about the shortage of food supply spread through the social media within hours, and this had led to more people rushing to the supermarkets to stock up their groceries. This paper discussed the transmission of fake news to understand the rate of spreading. Therefore, the objectives of this paper are to propose a mathematical model that can describe the dynamics of the spread of fake news through social media along the period of MCO through different social media platforms. This study also suggests some measures that can be taken by different parties, such as individuals, society and government to solve the issue of fake news transmission.

Keywords Covid-19 · Fake news · Social media · SIR model

S. Sathasivam (✉) · S. A. Alzaeemi · T. P. Lin · W. L. Yu
School of Mathematical Sciences, Universiti Sains Malaysia, 11800 USM Penang, Malaysia
e-mail: saratha@usm.my

P. Agarwal et al. (eds.), *Analysis of Infectious Disease Problems (Covid-19) and Their Global Impact*, Infosys Science Foundation Series,
https://doi.org/10.1007/978-981-16-2450-6_5

1 Introduction

Misinformation can amplify humanity's greatest challenges. A salient recent example of this is the Covid-19 pandemic, which has bred a multitude of falsehoods even as truth has increasingly become a matter of life and death [1]. The Covid-19 pandemic represents a substantial challenge to the maintenance of global human well-being. Unfortunately, misinformation about Covid-19 has proliferated on social media [2]. In the case of Covid-19, this misinformation comes in many forms—from conspiracy theories about the virus being created as a biological weapon in China to claims that coconut oil kills the virus [3]. At its worst, misinformation of this sort may cause people to turn to ineffective (and potentially directly harmful) remedies, as well as to either overreact (e.g. by hoarding goods) or, more dangerously, underreact (e.g. by deliberately engaging in risky behaviour and inadvertently spreading the virus) [4]. As an example, Cable News Network (CNN) has recently anticipated a rumour about the possible lockdown of Lombardy (a region in northern Italy) to prevent pandemics 3, publishing the news hours before the official communication from the Italian Prime Minister. As a result, people overcrowded trains and airports to escape from Lombardy towards the southern regions before the lockdown was in place, disrupting the government initiative aimed to contain the epidemics and potentially increasing contagion. Thus, an important research challenge is to determine how people seek or avoid information and how those decisions affect their behaviour [5], particularly when the news cycle dominated by the disintermediated diffusion of information alters the way information is consumed and reported on (GWI, 2020). Social media platforms such as YouTube and Twitter provide direct access to an unprecedented amount of content and may amplify rumours and questionable information [6, 7]. Some studies pointed out that fake news and inaccurate information may spread faster and wider than fact-based news [8].

In this work, a mathematical model is proposed called SIR model [9] that can describe the dynamics of the spread of fake news through social media along the period of MCO through different social media platforms.

2 Methodology/Proposal

2.1 SIR Model for Fake News Transmission

The Susceptible–Infected–Removed (SIR) model is used to compute the theoretical number of the flow of people between three states: the number of susceptible (S), the number of infectious (I) and the number of removed (R).

In this study, we will be using the SIR model to understand the transmission rate of fake news through social media. The assumptions to be made assume that the SIR model is homogeneous, and every social media user has identical touch to others within the population (social media user) that will be considered.

We assume that no one enters or leaves the community of the social media user and there is no contact outside the community. Each person is either susceptible, S (able to spread the fake news but still have not do so), infected, I (currently believe the fake news and still spreading the fake news) or removed, R (already get the correct source of the news and will not spread the fake news again). Thus, the total population for a specific social media platform is defined as [10]:

$$N(t) = S(t) + I(t) + R(t) \tag{1}$$

At the initial phase (which is at $t = 0$), every person is categorized as either S or I only. The time period for the model will be per day and will only discover the changes of S, I and R in 30 days. With some modifications from the simplest SIR model, the following shows the differential equations that will be using [11]:

$$\begin{aligned} \frac{dS}{dt} &= -\beta S(t)I(t) \\ \frac{dI}{dt} &= \beta S(t)I(t) - \gamma I(t) \\ \frac{dR}{dt} &= \gamma I(t) \end{aligned} \tag{2}$$

where $S(t)$ is the number of susceptible users in the community after time t., $I(t)$ is the number of infected users in the community after time t., $R(t)$ is the number of removed users in the community after time t., β is the transfer rate of the fake news around the social media platform or the transmission coefficient and γ is the removal rate of the fake news per day.

2.2 *Fake News Transmission Rate Through Different Social Media Platforms*

The social media platforms are Facebook [12], WhatsApp [6], Instagram [13, 14], Twitter [15] and Snapchat [16]. SIR model developed using MATLAB requires several variables and conditions.

Firstly, discover the initial number of susceptible users, S_0, and the initial number of infected users, I_0, for different social media platforms. Note that the initial number of removed users, R_0, is always zero as it takes some time for the people to realize that they had shared the wrong information or fake news around the social media community. Next, find the transmission coefficients, β. Suppose that each infected individual has k contact per day; that is, k users can receive the fake news per day when the infected user shares the fake news. Note that [17]:

Table 1 Initial number of susceptible users and the initial number of infected users for different social media platforms [6, 12, 15, 16, 18]

Social media	S_0(in billion)	I_0(in billion)	β
Facebook	$2.32 \times 0.90 = 2.088$	$2.32 \times 0.10 = 0.232$	$155 \times 0.001/2.32 = 0.06681$
WhatsApp	$1.6 \times 0.90 = 1.44$	$1.6 \times 0.10 = 0.16$	$145 \times 0.001/1.6 = 0.090625$
Instagram	$1 \times 0.90 = 0.90$	$1 \times 0.10 = 0.10$	$150 \times 0.001/1 = 0.15$
Twitter	$0.321 \times 0.90 = 0.2889$	$0.321 \times 0.10 = 0.0321$	$707 \times 0.001/0.321 = 2.202$
Snapchat	$0.36 \times 0.90 = 0.324$	$0.36 \times 0.10 = 0.036$	$34.1 \times 0.001/0.36 = 0.0947$

$$\beta = \frac{k}{N} \times \text{the transmission probability,}\tau. \tag{3}$$

Three assumptions are here:

1. Assume that 10% of the total monthly active users will be infected on the first day; that is, 10% of the total monthly active users will spread the fake news around the social media.
2. Assume that in each social media platform, there is around 0.1% of chance that a person reads and shares the fake news to others. Then, have $\tau = 0.001$.
3. Assume that it takes an average of 5 days for the people to realize that they had shared the wrong information on each social media platform. Then, have $\gamma = \frac{1}{5} = 0.2$.

Table 1 shows the initial number of susceptible users, S_0, the initial number of infected users, I_0, and β for different social media platforms.

2.3 *Fake News Transmission Rate Among Users of Different Age Groups*

This section investigates the fake news transmission rate among Facebook users of different age groups. There are a total of 2.32 billion in Facebook monthly active users. There are four age groups for SIR model use as in Table 2.

Table 2 Four age group targets in this study

Age group	Birth year	Current age (years)
Baby Boomers	1944–1964	56–76
Gen X	1965–1979	41–55
Millennials (Gen Y)	1980–1994	26–40
Gen Z	1995–2015	5–25

The following criteria are considered: 10% of the total monthly active users will be infected on the first day, 0.1% of chance that a person reads and shares the fake news to others, and it takes 5 days for the people to realize that they had shared the wrong information.

2.4 Fake News Transmission Rate Among Users of Facebook from Different Countries

Malaysia, USA and UK are been analysed. Table 4 shows the distribution of the Facebook users among different countries and their respective initial number of susceptible users, S_0, the initial number of infected users, I_0, and β [19].

3 Results, Interpretation and Discussion

In this section, the investigational outcome achieved is presented and discussed. In this study, the fake news dataset is used provided by Facebook, WhatsApp, Instagram, Twitter and Snapchat. The Optimization Toolbox in the MATLAB® software (MathWorks Inc.).

From Fig. 1, the number of susceptible Facebook users decreases over time as the number of removed users increases. This is because more and more users get to receive correct information about the news, and thus the number of shared posts starts to decrease. Besides, the figure can also observe that it takes roughly 10 days for the number of infected Facebook users to decrease to half of its initial number of infected users, $I(0) = 0.232$ billion. The transmission coefficient (β) of Facebook is considered small when compared to Twitter, mainly because Twitter users are used to sending tweets daily; thus, fake news spreads more faster; whereas Facebook has implemented the "flag" function to help remove misinformation on its platform, hence chances are less for users to spread the fake news.

The number of susceptible WhatsApp users decreases at a very low rate over time; this is probably due to the limit on messages forwarding through WhatsApp. The results of Fig. 2 can show that it takes around 26 days to reduce to 10% of the initial number of infected WhatsApp users, that is, from $I(0) = 0.16$ billion to $10\% \times I(0) = 0.016$ billion, which is roughly at $I(26) = 0.016986$ billion. The transmission coefficient of WhatsApp, $\beta = 0.090625$, is the second lowest among all five social media platforms. The limit on messages forwarding as well as its privacy usage on WhatsApp is believed to be the cause of its low transmission coefficient, which helps to reduce fake news transmission through its platform.

Figure 3 shows the SIR results from above figure are roughly similar to that of WhatsApp. It can be observed that after 30 days, the initial number of susceptible Instagram users, that is, $S(0) = 0.90$ billion, has decreased to only 83.35% of it,

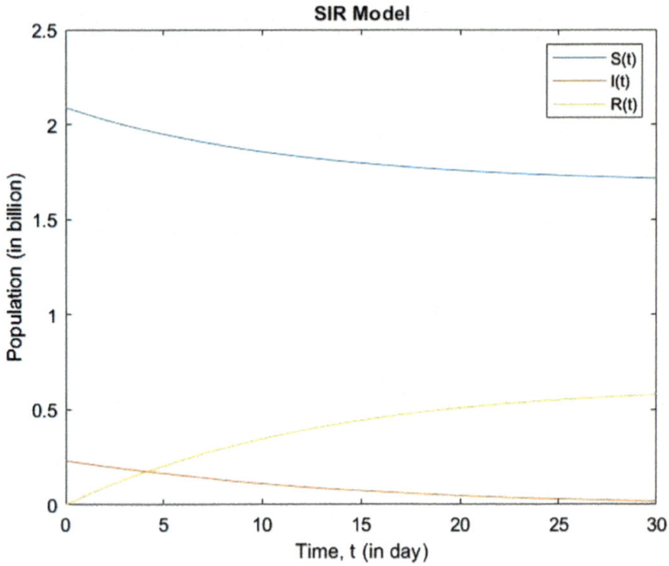

Fig. 1 SIR results for fake news transmission among Facebook users (population) over 30 days (time, t)

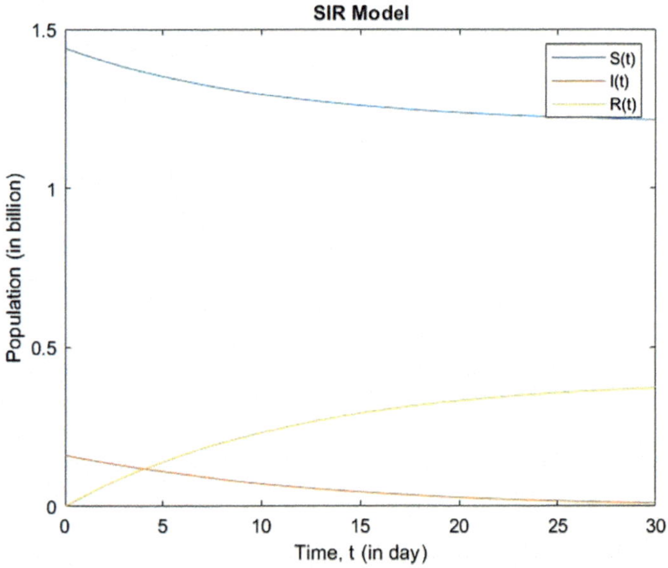

Fig. 2 SIR results for fake news transmission among WhatsApp users (population) over 30 days (time, t)

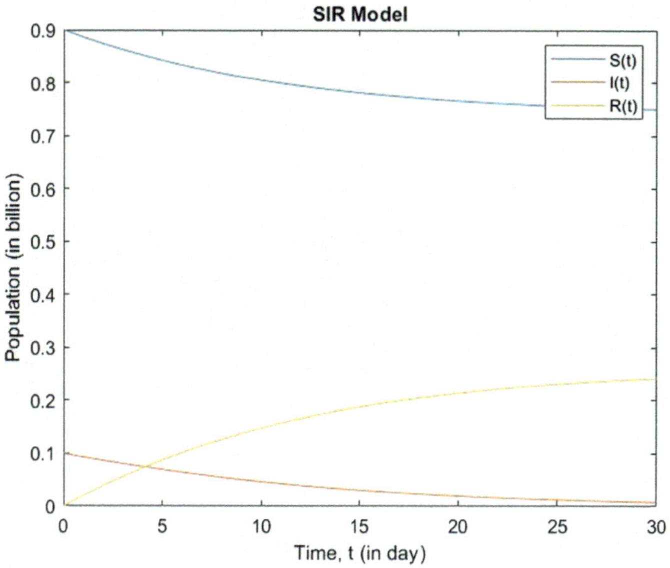

Fig. 3 SIR results for fake news transmission among Instagram users (population) over 30 days (time, t)

which is $S(30) = 0.75016$ billion. Also, notice from Table 1 that the transfer rate of fake news of Instagram, which is $\beta = 0.15$, is the second highest among all five social media platforms. The "discover" page allows Instagram users to see what is the current "hot" topic because the post with the most likes/comments/shares will be on top of the discover page, which leads users to read and share the post, which in turn increases the transfer rate.

Figure 4 clearly shows that the number of infected Twitter users increases the fastest among all five social media platforms. This is because the transfer rate of fake news through Twitter, that is, $\beta = 2.202$, is the highest as can be seen from Table 1. According to OmnicoreAgency.com, 71% of Twitter users say they use this platform to get their news, which is why it has a high transfer rate. Besides the results in the figure, we can also see that the number of infected Twitter users peaked at between days 5 and 10. At the same time, the number of susceptible Twitter users decreases significantly and only takes around 9 to 10 days to reduce to 10% of its initial susceptible users, that is, from $S(0) = 0.2889$ billion to $10\% \times S(0) = 0.0289$ billion, which lies between $S(9) = 0.03263$ billion and $S(10) = 0.024295$ billion. The reason is that there are roughly 500 million tweets sent per day, as seen from the statistics of OmnicoreAgency.com (2020); hence, a specific trendy news will be replaced by the other very soon.

Figure 5 shows us that the SIR of Snapchat is quite constant. According to OmnicoreAgency.com, the number of snaps created per day (including photographs and videos) is approximately 3 billion. However, users often use Snapchat to send photographs and videos related to their daily lives. Hence, fake news are less likely

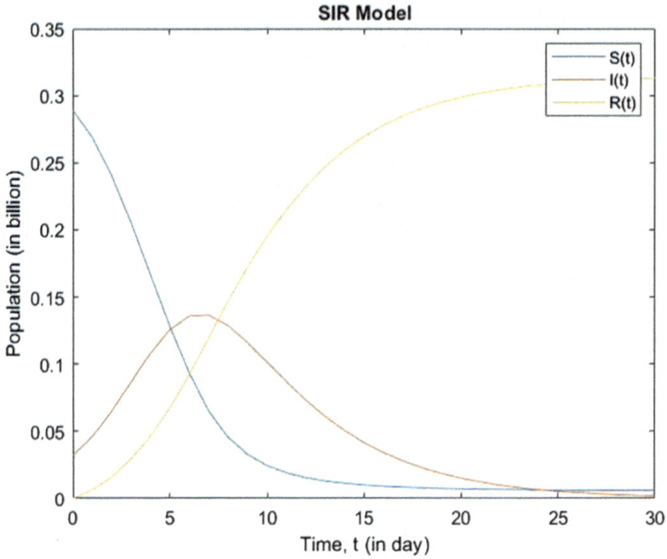

Fig. 4 SIR results for fake news transmission among Twitter users (population) over 30 days (time, t)

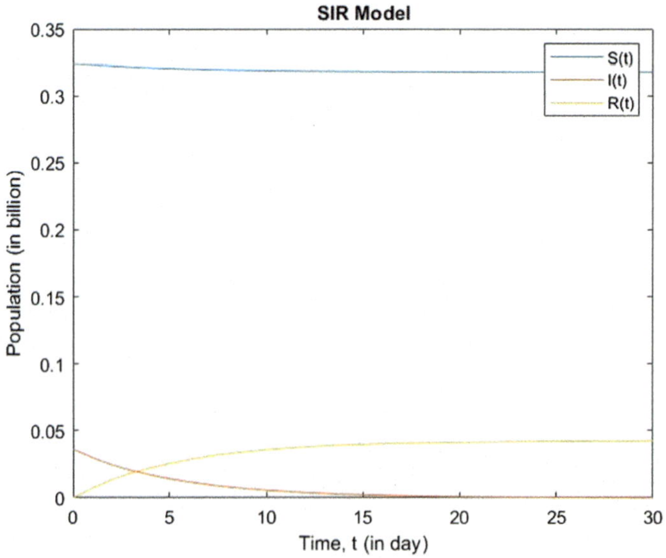

Fig. 5 SIR results for fake news transmission among Snapchat users (population) over 30 days (time, t)

Table 3 Age group users in Facebook [16]

Age groups	S_0(in billion)	I_0(in billion)	β
Baby Boomers	$2.32 \times 0.102 \times 0.90$ $= 0.212976$	$2.32 \times 0.102 \times 0.10$ $= 0.023664$	$115.5 \times 0.001/0.23664$ $= 0.48808$
Gen X	$2.32 \times 0.198 \times 0.90$ $= 0.413424$	$2.32 \times 0.198 \times 0.10$ $= 0.045936$	$248.5 \times 0.001/0.45936$ $= 0.54097$
Gen Y	$2.32 \times 0.404 \times 0.90$ $= 0.843552$	$2.32 \times 0.404 \times 0.10$ $= 0.093728$	$319 \times 0.001/0.93728$ $= 0.34035$
Gen Z	$2.32 \times 0.296 \times 0.90$ $= 0.618048$	$2.32 \times 0.296 \times 0.10$ $= 0.068672$	$507 \times 0.001/0.68672$ $= 0.73829$

to be spread through its platform and when it does, the users are less likely to be infected, which is why its infected number of users is able to decrease to 0.00376% of its initial infected number of users, $I(0) = \mathrm{I}(0) = 0.036$ billion after 30 days. With its low transfer rate, $\beta = 0.0947$, the S, I and R also have a significant small change daily, especially after day 15. Besides, we also can deduce that its low transfer rate is because it does not have the “share” function, meaning a user who receives a “snap” is unable to share or forward it.

Table 3 shows that the number of Facebook’s Baby Boomers users is the lowest among all 4 generations. This is clear because the users from this group are 56–76 years old today, and most of them are lagged from this technological world. Hence, the initial number of susceptible Baby Boomers users, $S(0)$, as well as the initial number of infected Baby Boomers users, $I(0)$, is low as well. Therefore, this study has less significant changes in the SIR as can be seen from Fig. 6.

The results from Fig. 7 tell us that the number of removed Facebook’s Gen X users, R, surpassed the number of infected Gen X users, I, on day 6, that is, $R(6) = 0.057403$ billion > 0.048712 billion $= I(6)$. This means most of the Gen X users will check on the correct sources of the fake news before spreading it. The Facebook users from this generation are mature and rational in handling fake news since their ages are between 41 and 55.

Table 3 shows us that the number of initial susceptible Facebook’s Gen Y users, S0, and the number of initial infected Gen Y users are the highest among all four generations. The users from this age group are currently 26 to 40 years old. As stated in Global Web Index [20], 50% of the Millennials said they are using Facebook for up-to-date news about Covid-19. That is why more active users will get exposed to fake news transmission. Figure 8 shows that on day 16, the number of removed Gen Y users, $R(16) = 0.4063$ billion, is close to the number of susceptible Gen Y users, $S(16) = 0.41597$ billion. It means that most of the Gen Y users take more than two weeks to realize that the fake news that has been spreading around is a misinformation.

Figure 9 clearly shows the significant SIR changes throughout 30 days. The transmission coefficient, $\beta = 0.73829$, is the highest within all age groups. The reason is

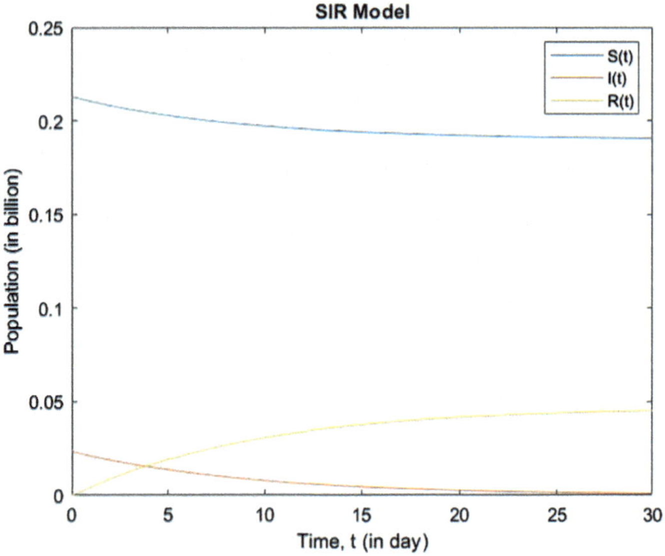

Fig. 6 SIR results for fake news transmission among Facebook's Baby Boomers users (population) over 30 days (time, t)

Table 4 Users on Facebook among various countries [19]

Countries	S_0(in billion)	I_0(in billion)	β
Malaysia	0.0231×0.90 $= 0.02079$	0.0231×0.10 $= 0.00231$	$223 \times 0.001/0.0231$ $= 9.65368$
USA	0.253×0.90 $= 0.2277$	0.253×0.10 $= 0.0253$	$338 \times 0.001/0.253$ $= 1.33597$
UK	0.04484×0.90 $= 0.040356$	0.04484×0.10 $= 0.004484$	$155 \times 0.001/0.04484$ $= 3.45674$

because these younger generation users are used to sharing trendy news, regardless of whether the information is correct or wrong. The number of infected Facebook's Gen Z users peaked at day 7 to day 9, which has reached 0.2 billion users. Then, the number significantly drops to $I(19) = 0.066497$ billion on day 19, which is less than its initial infected user, $I(0) = 0.068672$ billion. At the same time, the number of susceptible users drops significantly at day 7 to day 9 as most of them, S, have been converted to I. However, notice that S is still slightly higher than I after day 19, because the susceptible users who read the fake news still do not take any action after reading it, neither sharing nor correcting, whereas those who are infected, I, have already been converted to removed users, R, after receiving the correct sources of information.

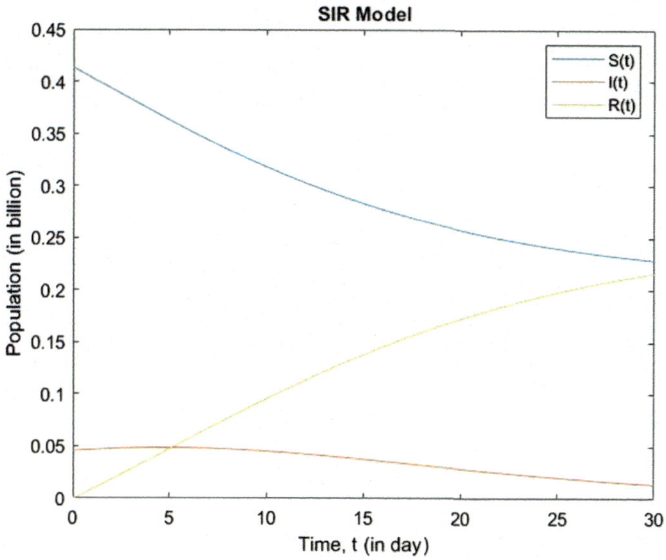

Fig. 7 SIR results for fake news transmission among Facebook's Gen X users (population) over 30 days (time, t)

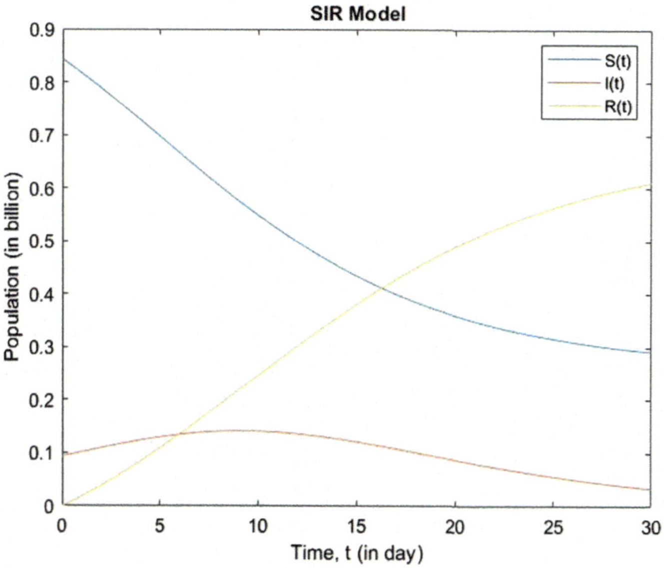

Fig. 8 SIR results for fake news transmission among Facebook's Millennials users (population) over 30 days (time, t)

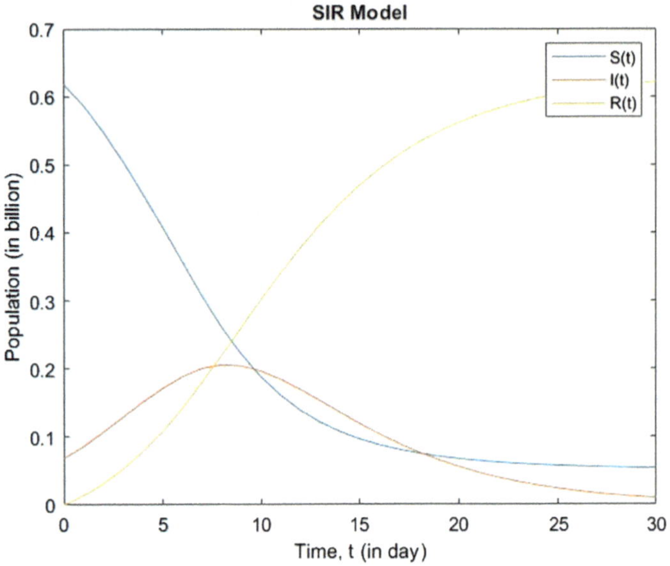

Fig. 9 SIR results for fake news transmission among Facebook's Gen Z users (population) over 30 days (time, t)

The Facebook users from different countries may have different usage activities on their social media platform since different countries have different implemented laws on controlling and filtering the fake news. In Fig. 10, we have divided the S, I and R of fake news transmission from different countries into three subplots. The figure shows an overview of the S, I and R of three different countries but as can notice, the results for Malaysia and UK are similar in the three subplots, not because they are constant, but because the scale used here is too big for the population of both the countries, since the population in USA is the largest among the three. Hence, to compare the results more clearly, we have divided them into their respective SIR model according to their countries.

Figure 11 shows that the number of infected Malaysia's Facebook users, I, intersects with the number of removed users approximately on day 5. This means the users realized that they received the fake news similar to our assumption made in Sect. 2.3, that is: "It takes 5 days for the people to realize that they had shared the wrong information". The total number of Malaysia's Facebook users is the lowest among the three countries, but the transmission coefficient, $\beta = 9.65368$, is the highest among all.

From Fig. 12, we can observe the significant changes of S, I and R among Facebook users from the USA. The population of Facebook users in the USA is the highest among the three countries. Also, we can see that the number of susceptible Facebook users intersects with the number of removed users on approximately day 15, where $S(15) = 0.10652$ billion and $R(15) = 0.11084$ billion. Besides, the number of infected Facebook users, I, peaked at approximately day 9, with $I(9) = 0.042037$

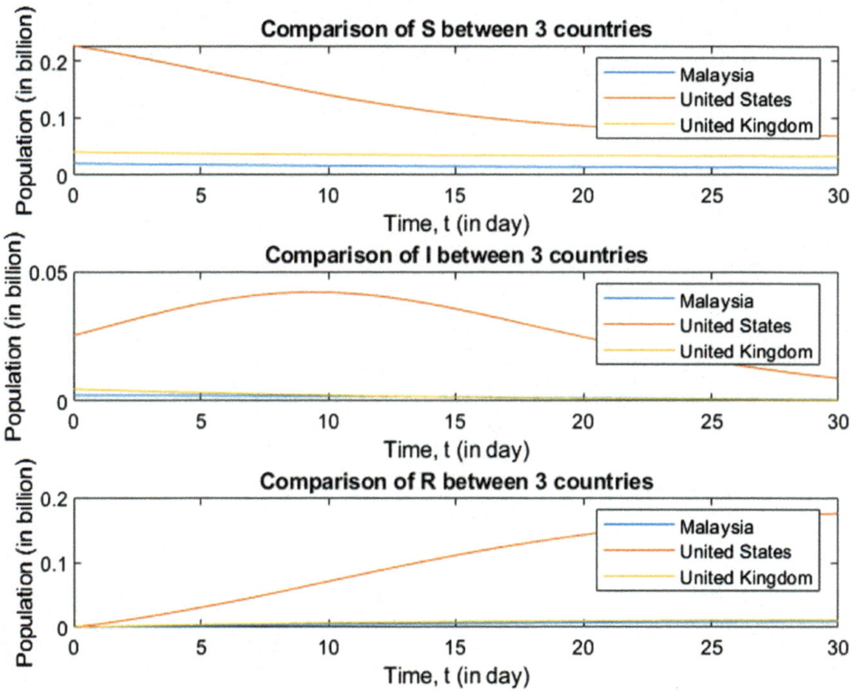

Fig. 10 Shows the *S*, *I* and *R* results for Facebook users from three different countries, which are Malaysia, USA and UK (population) over 30 days (time, t)

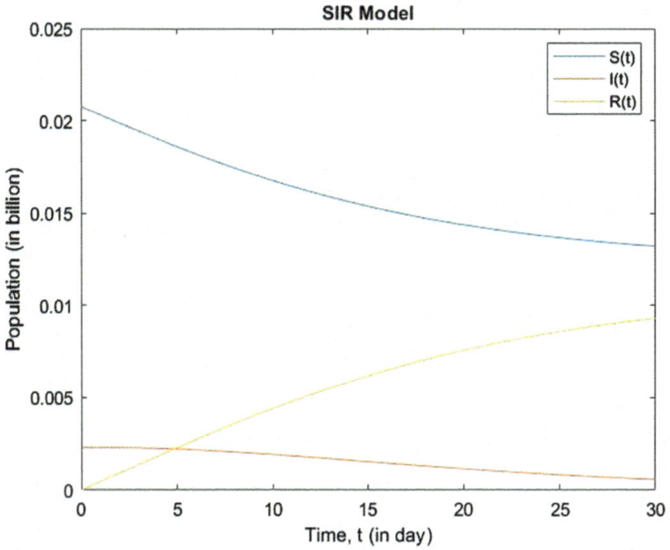

Fig. 11 SIR results for fake news transmission among Facebook users in Malaysia (population) over 30 days (time, t)

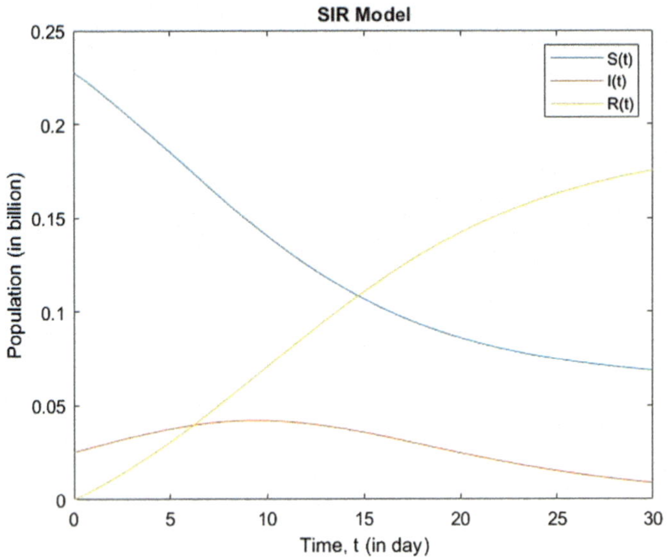

Fig. 12 SIR results for fake news transmission among Facebook users in the USA (population) over 30 days (time, t)

billion. And it takes roughly 27 days for the initial number of infected users, $I(0) = 0.0253$ billion, to drop to half of it, that is, $\frac{1}{2} \times I(0) = 0.01265$ billion, which is roughly at $I(27) = 0.012372$ billion.

From Fig. 13, we can observe the significant changes of S, I and R among Facebook users from the UK. The changes of SIR among Facebook users from UK are less significant over time. It takes around 4 days for the number of infected Facebook users, I, to intersect with the number of removed users, R, which is a good thing because it means that the users are less likely to spread the fake news, and most of them will check the validity of the information when they receive it, so the fake news are less likely to spread around its community. The number of susceptible users, S, does not decrease much even after 30 days, meaning the users usually read the news but they do not take any actions about it, which is important in controlling the widespread of fake news.

4 Conclusion

In this paper, fake news transmission through social media platforms from three different aspects has been investigated. We investigated the SIR trend of fake news transmission through different social media platforms. The results shown tell us that Twitter is the platform with the most dynamic SIR changes. Snapchat has the least SIR change over a month. We would say that the privacy function of Snapchat is

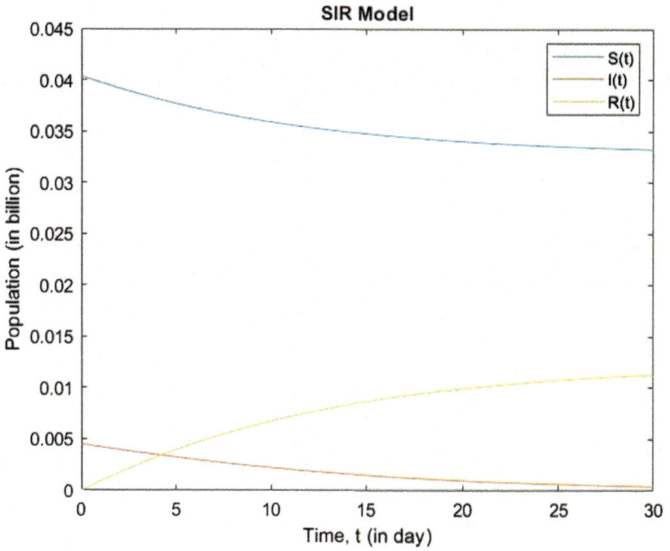

Fig. 13 SIR results for fake news transmission among Facebook users in the UK (population) over 30 days (time, t)

strong, whereas the "re-tweet" function in Twitter is the common reason why fake news can go viral so fast on its platform. The authorities and users are responsible for cutting down the transmission chain of fake news.

Acknowledgements This research was funded by Research University Grant (RUI)(1001/PMATHS/8011131) by Universiti Sains Malaysia.

References

1. Worldometers.: Coronavirus worldwide graphs. Retrieved from https://www.worldometers.info/coronavirus/worldwide-graphs/#total-cases (2020). Accessed 15 April 2020
2. Frenkel, S., Alba, D., Zhong, R.: Surge of Virus Misinformation Stumps Facebook and Twitter. New York Times. Retrieved from https://www.nytimes.com/2020/03/08/technology/coronavirus.misinformation-socialmedia.html (2020). Accessed on 2 April 2020
3. Pradhan, D., Biswasroy, P., Ghosh, G., Rath, G.: A review of current interventions for COVID-19 prevention. Archives Med. Res. (2020). Accessed 28 April 2020
4. Russonello, G.: Afraid of coronavirus? That might say something about your politics. New York Times. Retrieved from https://www.nytimes.com/2020/03/13/us/politics/coronavirus.trump-polling.html (2013). Accessed 5 April 2020
5. Sharot, T., Sunstein, C.R.: How people decide what they want to know. Nature Human Behav 1–6 (2020). Accessed 25 April 2020
6. Bovet, A., Makse, H.A.: Influence of fake news in twitter during the 2016 us presidential election. Nature commun. **10**(1), 1–14 (2019). Accessed on 25 March 2020

7. Smith., K : 60 Incredible and interesting twitter stats and statistics. Retrieved from https://www.brandwatch.com/blog/twitter-stats-and-statistics (2020). Accessed 10 April 2020
8. Vosoughi, S., Roy, D., Aral, S.: The spread of true and false news online. Science, **359**(6380) 1146–1151 (2018). Accessed 29 March 2020
9. Zakary, O., Rachik, M., Elmouki, I.: On the analysis of a multi-regions discrete SIR epidemic model: an optimal control approach. Int. J. Dyn. Control **5**(3), 917–930 (2017). Accessed 21 April 2020
10. Ledzewicz, U., Schättler, H.: On optimal singular controls for a general SIR-model with vaccination and treatment. In: Conference Publications, vol. 2011, No. Special, p. 981 (2011). Accessed 2 April 2020
11. Khurana, P., Kumar, D.: Sir model for fake news spreading through whatsapp. In Proceedings of 3rd International Conference on Internet of Things and Connected Technologies (ICIoTCT) pp. 26–27 (2018)
12. OmnicoreAgency.: Snapchat by the numbers: stats, demographics & fun facts. Retrieved from https://www.omnicoreagency.com/snapchat-statistics (2020). Accessed 25 April 2020
13. Hern, A. (2020). WhatsApp to impose new limit on forwarding to fight fake news. Retrieved from https://www.theguardian.com/technology/2020/apr/07/whatsapp-to-impose-new-limit-on-forwarding-to-fight-fake-news, 15 April 2020
14. Workmacro.: What your follower/ following ratio say about your instagram account. Retrieved from https://workmacro.com/instagram/follower-following-ratio-say-instagram-account/ (2018). Accessed 29 March 2020
15. Smith., K.: 60 Incredible and interesting twitter stats and statistics. Retrieved from https://www.brandwatch.com/blog/twitter-stats-and-statistics/ (2020). Accessed 10 April 2020
16. OmnicoreAgency.: Snapchat by the numbers: stats, demographics & fun facts. Retrieved from https://www.omnicoreagency.com/snapchat-statistics/ (2020). Accessed 10 April 2020
17. Ignatius, D.: Modeling the spread of information on twitter Doctoral dissertation, California State Polytechnic University, Pomona (2018). Accessed 2 April 2020
18. American Institute of Mathematical Sciences.: Data Policy. Instagram data policy. https://help.instagram.com/519522125107875 (2020). Accessed on 2, 5 April 2020
19. Statista.: Facebook users in the United Kingdom (UK) from september 2018 to March 2020. Retrieved from https://www.statista.com/statistics/1012080/uk-monthly-numbers-facebook-users/ (2020). Accessed 26 April 2020
20. Global Web Index.: Coronavirus Research: Media Consumption and Sport. Retrieved from https://www.globalwebindex.com/hubfs/1.%20Coronavirus%20Research%20PDFs/GWI%20coronavirus%20findings%20April%202020%20-%20Media%20Consumption%20(Release%204).pdf (2020). Accessed 28 April 2020

Generalized Logistic Equations in Covid-Related Epidemic Models

Daniele Ritelli

Abstract The logistic equation on population growth was proposed by Verhulst (Corresp Math Phys 10:113-126, 1838) [22], with the aim to provide a possible correction to the unrealistic exponential growth forecast by T. Malthus, (J Johnson, London, 1872) [13]. Population modeling became of particular interest in the 20th century to biologists urged by limited means of sustenance and increasing human populations. Verhulst's scheme was rediscovered by A. Lotka, (Elements of Mathematical Biology. Dover, New York, 1956) [12], as a simple model of a self-regulating population. Subsequently, the use of logistic dynamics spreads across a huge number of different frameworks, especially in diffusion phenomena. The logistic differential equation is a fundamental element in quantitative study of population dynamics, its use also extends to the field of epidemiology: both to describe the evolution of the infected population in deterministic models, and working in conditions of uncertainty it is the deterministic component of stochastic differential equations. This work brings a contribution to the foundational basic research on the logistic equation and its generalizations which hopefully have repercussions for epidemiologic applications.

Keywords Epidemiological models · Logistic Growth · Hypergeometric function · Periodic solutions

1 Introduction

If $x(t)$ is the population (which for us means single species in a closed ecosystem without migrations) at time t, the Verhulst model is ruled by the initial value problem:

D. Ritelli (✉)
Department of Statistics, University of Bologna, Bologna, Italy
e-mail: daniele.ritelli@unibo.it

P. Agarwal et al. (eds.), *Analysis of Infectious Disease Problems (Covid-19) and Their Global Impact*, Infosys Science Foundation Series,
https://doi.org/10.1007/978-981-16-2450-6_6

$$\begin{cases} \dot{x} = rx\left(1 - \dfrac{x}{K}\right) \\ x(0) = x_0 \end{cases} \tag{1}$$

where the dot means derivative with respect to time and the *intrinsic reproduction rate* r is a positive constant measuring the population average net growth reproduction. In the above equation, "any role of resources is subsumed in the idealized parameters r and K", [9]. In fact, being x^2 representative of the rate of pair interactions, then r/K will provide the rate of them acting as a decrease of population growth. The carrying capacity K, due to environmental pressures, stands for the saturation, or maximum sustainable value, of population; so that $r\,(1 - x(t)/K)$ means the *per capita birth rate* at epoch t. The carrying capacity utmost bound of a territory is not fixed: It can spread due external factors. So that all the growth models based on fixed K-values, are somewhat unrealistic. Therefore, in the above differential equation r and k have to be replaced by an exogenous functions $r(t),\ k(t)$: In such a way realism and complexity of the model are both increased. In fact both $r(t)$ and $K(t)$ can be any functions depending by the type of phenomenon studied. It is important to point out that Nkashama, [18, 19], proved that each Verhulst-type equation with positive non-autonomous bounded forcing coefficients has exactly one bounded solution that is positive, and that does not approach the zero-solution in the past and in the future.

The connection of the logistic model with epidemiology is well known. We begin with the simplest of the epidemic models, the SI (susceptible-infected) where every infected remains infected, like varicella-zoster virus. If $S(t)$ and $I(t)$ denote the number of susceptibles and infected at time t, the evolution of the disease is described by the system of differential equation

$$\begin{cases} \dot{S} = -\beta \dfrac{SI}{N} \\ \dot{I} = \beta \dfrac{SI}{N} \end{cases}$$

$N = S + I$ represents the total population, it follows that this model reduces to the logistic equation:

$$\dot{I} = \beta I\left(1 - \frac{I}{N}\right)$$

Similarly, the susceptible-infected-susceptible (SIS) model describes the spread of diseases with no permanent immunity, [3, 11] assuming that an individual starts being susceptible to a disease, at some point of time gets infected and then recovers after some other time interval, becoming susceptible again. If $S(t)$ and $I(t)$ denote again the number of susceptibles and infected at time t, respectively, then the differential equations describing the spread of the disease are

$$\begin{cases} \dot{S} = -\beta \dfrac{SI}{N} + \gamma I \\ \dot{I} = \beta \dfrac{SI}{N} - \gamma I \end{cases}$$

Again assuming $N = S + I$ to represent the total population the model reduces to the logistic equation:

$$\dot{I} = (\beta - \gamma) I - \frac{\beta}{N} I^2.$$

The introduction of stochastic elements allows to obtain more realistic and reliable models, and involves the introduction of variable coefficients in the logistic model. In epidemiology, two main kinds of stochasticity are relevant: demographic and environmental. Demographic stochasticity models the fact that, even if all individuals may be subject to the same possible events with the exact same probabilities, chance events may change the fates of individuals. When a phenomenon is the sum of a large number of small individual effects (as disease propagation in large population), the weak law of large numbers reduces the effects of demographic stochasticity and a deterministic model can be used. In contrast, when the population is small, random events cannot be neglected and a stochastic model is necessary. On the other side, environmental stochasticity deals with the situation where there is variation in the probability associated with an event. Therefore, some parameters in stochastic models may be uncertain and characterized by a probability distribution instead of a constant value. Fixing initial conditions, a deterministic model will produce a unique result, whereas a stochastic model will produce many different outputs, depending on the actual values the random variables take. For these reasons, we will study different occurrences and generalizations of the logistic equation, representing stochasticity using equations with variable coefficients.

For these reasons, in this chapter we present several modifications of the basic model, specifically we will deal with the following variants of the model:

(i) Model's coefficients are assumed to change logistically as exposed in [16]: We will provide explicit solutions using Gauss hypergeometric function ${}_2F_1$. Our computational results agree with the theoretical results established by Nkashama [18, 19].

(ii) We examine the situation of periodic coefficients to represent infections with seasonal effects. We confirm the important theoretical conclusions established by deMottoni and Schiaffino in [5, 6] in a particular situation then establishing an effective operational procedure for the implementation of the model.

(iii) The logistic model is upgraded introducing a periodic forcing term, following [17]: The relevant Riccati equation is solved in terms of Mathieu functions after linearization.

2 Logistic Coefficients Models

The use of variable coefficients in the logistic model, referring to its epidemiological occurrences, allows to analyze the effect of exogenous interventions, such as social distancing, hygiene measures, introduction of specific therapies, aimed at reducing the spread of infection. All this implies a variable carrying capacity: Here we refer to the contributions of [15, 16, 18], providing some extensions of the previous models. Write the general logistic differential equation with variable coefficient as:

$$\begin{cases} \dot{x} = a(t)x - b(t)x^2 \\ x(0) = x_0 > 0 \end{cases} \tag{2}$$

where we assume $a(t) > 0$ and $b(t) > 0$ are given continuous positive bounded functions of time. (2) is a Bernoulli equation that can be easily integrated:

$$x(t) = \frac{\exp\left(\int_0^t a(\tau)\mathrm{d}\tau\right)}{\frac{1}{x_0} + \int_0^t b(\tau)\exp\left(\int_0^\tau a(\xi)d\xi\right)\mathrm{d}\tau}. \tag{3}$$

The study of its asymptotic behavior is of great relevance and not helped by formula (3); moreover, the following remark is fundamental for the study of (2).

Remark 1 Since the zero function solves (2) on $\mathbb{R}$, by uniqueness any non-trivial solution of (2) must be either positive or negative on its interval of definition.

In the general case to variable, positive, bounded and continuous coefficients, we explicitly report the important, and relatively recent, contribution of Nkashama [18]: assume that

$$0 < \alpha \leq a(t) \leq A, \quad 0 < \beta \leq b(t) \leq B, \quad t \in \mathbb{R}, \tag{4}$$

for some positive constants α, β, A and B. In consequence of hypothesis (4), we can state the following Lemma which, in this particular situation, provides the existence of the horizontal asymptote for the solutions of (2).

Lemma 1 *If we assume, the existence of the limit*

$$\lim_{t\to\infty} \frac{a(t)}{b(t)} = \ell \in \mathbb{R}$$

then, solution of (2) is such that

$$\lim_{t\to\infty} x(t) = \ell$$

Proof The statement follows by de l'Hospital rule in formula (3). □

For completeness, we report three Theorems of Nkashama in view of their impact on the model we are going to present below.

Theorem 1 ([18]Theorem 2.1) *Suppose that (4) are fulfilled. Then equation (2) has exactly one bounded solution* $u : \mathbb{R} \to \mathbb{R}$ *that is positive, and that does not tend to zero as* $t \to \pm\infty$. *Actually,* u *satisfies the inequalities*

$$\frac{\alpha}{B} \leq u(t) \leq \frac{A}{\beta} \quad \textit{for all } t \in \mathbb{R}. \tag{5}$$

It turns out that the unique bounded solution $u(t)$ obtained in Theorem 1 is a forward attractor for all positive solutions (bounded and unbounded), and so is forward asymptotically stable. Also the zero-solution of (2) is a backward (exponential) attractor for all solutions $v(t)$ with $v(t_1) < u(t_1)$ for some $t_1 \in \mathbb{R}$, and so is backward exponentially stable. Thus, the zero-solution is a forward (exponential) repeller for all solutions that remain below the attractor. This is explained in the second and third Nkashama results.

Theorem 2 ([18] Theorem 3.1) *Suppose the conditions in (4) are met. Then, the bounded solution* $u(t)$ *given in Theorem 1 is an attractor for all positive solutions to (2). That is, if* $v(t)$ *is a positive solution to (2), then*

$$\lim_{t\to\infty} |u(t) - v(t)| = 0.$$

Theorem 3 ([18] Theorem 3.2) *Suppose the conditions in (4) are met. Then, the zero-solution exponentially repels all solutions* $v(t)$ *such that* $v(t_1) < u(t_1)$ *for some* $t_1 \in \mathbb{R}$. *That is, if* $v(t)$ *is a solution to (2) with* $v(t_1) < u(t_1)$ *for some* $t_1 \in \mathbb{R}$, *then*

$$\lim_{t\to-\infty} v(t) = 0$$

exponentially.

2.1 Computable Examples

Meyer and Ausubel, [15] introduce a variable carrying capacity, driven by a logistic law evolving sigmoidally between the initial value $\alpha > 0$ and the final value $\beta > 0$; the integration of the relevant equation is provided in [16]. After having recalled the integration in hypergeometric terms proposed in [16], we present two further integrations deriving from different representations of the two coefficients $a(t)$ and $b(t)$ that always produce solutions expressed through the Gaussian hypergeometric function. Consider equation (2) assuming:

$$a(t) = a_0 > 0, \qquad b(t) = \frac{a_0}{\alpha + (\alpha - \beta)\left(e^{-\gamma t} - 1\right)} \tag{6}$$

being $\gamma > 0$ a positive parameter that regulates the rate of change from the initial value α to the final asymptotic value β. We infer that solution of (2) when (6) holds verifies

$$\lim_{t \to \infty} x(t) = \beta.$$

To integrate equation (2) under assumption (6), we use the Gaussian ${}_2\mathrm{F}_1$ hypergeometric function. For completeness, we recall the properties we are going to use in the following; for further details we refer, for instance, to [1, 7] and [21]. ${}_2\mathrm{F}_1$ is defined by the power series, which converges for $|x| < 1$:

$${}_2\mathrm{F}_1\left(\begin{matrix} a,\, b \\ c \end{matrix} \middle| x\right) = \sum_{n=0}^{\infty} \frac{(a)_n\,(b)_n}{(c)_n} \frac{x^n}{n!},$$

$(a)_n$ stands for Pochhammer symbol, i.e., $(a)_n = a(a+1)\cdots(a+n-1)$. The integral representation theorem:

$${}_2\mathrm{F}_1\left(\begin{matrix} a,\, b \\ c \end{matrix} \middle| x\right) = \frac{\Gamma(c)}{\Gamma(c-a)\Gamma(a)} \int_0^1 \frac{t^{a-1}(1-t)^{c-a-1}}{(1-xt)^b}\,\mathrm{d}t,$$

where $\operatorname{Re} a > \operatorname{Re} c > 0$ ensures analytic continuation to the complex plane cut along the segment $[1, \infty)$. In what follows we will use a particular occurrence of ${}_2\mathrm{F}_1$, precisely:

$$\mathcal{F}(t) = {}_2\mathrm{F}_1\left(\begin{matrix} 1,\, 1 + \frac{a_0}{\beta\gamma} \\ 2 + \frac{a_0}{\beta\gamma} \end{matrix} \middle| t\right) \tag{7}$$

Theorem 4 *If conditions (6) hold and $\alpha \neq \beta$, formula (3) becomes*

$$x(t) = \frac{x_0(\alpha - \beta)(a_0 + \gamma)e^{a_0 t}}{(\alpha - \beta)(a_0 + \gamma) - a_0 x_0\left(\mathcal{F}\left(-\frac{\beta}{\alpha - \beta}\right) - e^{t(a_0+\gamma)}\,\mathcal{F}\left(-\frac{\beta}{\alpha - \beta}\,e^{t\gamma}\right)\right)}. \tag{8}$$

Proof From (3) we see that solution is obtained evaluating the integral

$$\boldsymbol{I}(t) = \int_0^t \frac{a_0 e^{a\tau}}{(\alpha - \beta)\left(e^{-\gamma\tau} - 1\right) + \alpha}\,\mathrm{d}\tau.$$

Using the change of variable $y = e^{\alpha\tau}$ we get:

$$\boldsymbol{I}(t) = \frac{a_0}{\gamma(\alpha - \beta)} \int_1^{e^{at}} \frac{u^{a_0/\gamma}}{1 + \frac{\beta}{\alpha - \beta}\,u}\,\mathrm{d}u \tag{9}$$

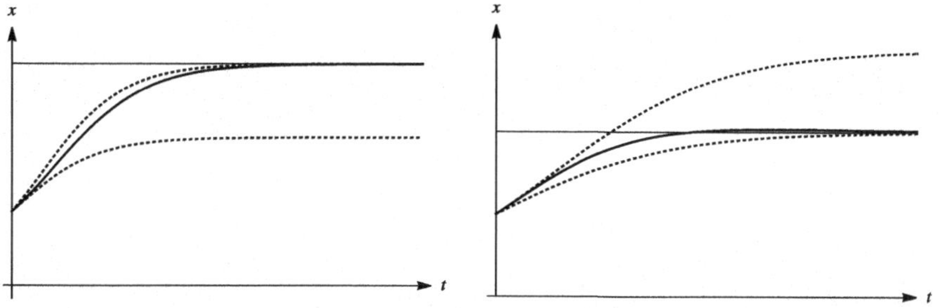

Fig. 1 Solutions for $\alpha < \beta$ and for $\alpha > \beta$

Write the integral in (9) as

$$\boldsymbol{I}(t) = \frac{a_0}{\gamma(\alpha-\beta)}\left(\int_0^{e^{a_0 t}} \frac{u^{a_0/\gamma}}{1+\frac{\beta}{\alpha-\beta}\,u}\,du - \int_0^1 \frac{u^{a_0/\gamma}}{1+\frac{\beta}{\alpha-\beta}\,u}\,du\right). \tag{10}$$

In the first integral in (10), we make the normalization $y = e^{\alpha t}\,u$, so that (8) follows by integral representation theorem for ${}_2F_1$. □

The explicit integration performed in Theorem 4 allows the complete description of the transient phase of demographic dynamics described in [15]. The following graphic representation, Fig. 1, is meaningful, since are represented the asymptotic level at which the system tends, with the dashed lines the logistic equations with constant coefficient with carrying capacities given by the two extreme values α and β both cases $\alpha < \beta$ and $\alpha > \beta$ the solution, represented with a continuous line of the equation (2) with coefficients given by (6) that governs Meyer–Ausubel's model.

The scenario in which, in the long term, the carrying capacity is reduced, i.e., $\alpha > \beta$, is, without doubt, the most interesting at epidemiological level, as it involves a significant reduction in the final number of the infected population. Moreover, for $\alpha > \beta$ solution of (2) under (6) is no longer monotonic, as shown in the right Fig. 1.

We remark that the asymptotic behavior detected is in full agreement with Nkashama's results: Theorems 1, 2 and 3.

Remark 2 Since there are many hypergeometric identities, it may happen, for particular configurations of the parameters, that the solutions can be represented through elementary functions. For instance, taking $\alpha = 3,\ \beta = 2\,\gamma = 1,\ a_0 = 1$ the identity, see http://functions.wolfram.com/07.23.03.3123.01, comes into play

$${}_2F_1\left(\begin{matrix}1,\ 3/2\\ 5/2\end{matrix}\,\middle|\, x\right) = \frac{3}{2x^{3/2}}\ln\frac{1+\sqrt{x}}{1-\sqrt{x}} - \frac{3}{x}.$$

Equations (2) with (6) assume the form of a elementary solvable initial value problem for a Bernoulli equation, namely:

$$\begin{cases} x' = x - \dfrac{x^2}{2+e^{-t}}, \\ x(0) = x_0. \end{cases}$$

Its solution is:

$$x(t) = \frac{4e^t x_0}{x_0\left(2e^t - 2 + \ln 3\right) - x_0 \ln\left(1 + 2e^t\right) + 4}.$$

In their possible practical applications, these specific situations are not indeed of great interest, given the very particular distribution of the parameters, whose estimation, on the contrary, allows, in light of the integration just carried out, to fully exploit the characteristics of the proposed model.
Now assume that the reproduction rate varies logistically, thus we consider (2) under condition

$$a(t) = \frac{a_0}{\alpha + (\alpha - \beta)\left(e^{-\gamma t} - 1\right)}, \qquad b(t) = a_0 \tag{11}$$

With this model, we try to represent the effect on the population dynamics regulated by the logistic equation (2) when the reproduction rate goes from an initial value to an asymptotic value: In this way we try thinking about possible epidemiological applications, to the effect of actions aimed at limiting, through exogenous interventions, the spread of an infection.

We skip the proof, since is similar to previous Theorem 4, of the following result, concerning the exact integration of logistic equation (2) under (11).

Theorem 5 *If conditions (11) hold and if $\alpha \neq \beta$ quadrature formula (3) becomes*

$$x(t) = \frac{x_0(\alpha - \beta)(a_0 + \beta\gamma)\left(\alpha + \beta\left(e^{\gamma t} - 1\right)\right)^{\frac{a_0}{\beta\gamma}}}{(\alpha - \beta)(a_0 + \beta\gamma)\alpha^{\frac{a_0}{\beta\gamma}} + a_0\beta x_0\, J(t)} \tag{12}$$

being

$$J(t) = \alpha^{\frac{a_0}{\beta\gamma}+1}\,\mathcal{F}\left(\frac{\alpha}{\alpha - \beta}\right) - \left(\alpha + \beta\left(e^{\gamma t} - 1\right)\right)^{\frac{a_0}{\beta\gamma}+1}\mathcal{F}\left(1 + \frac{\beta}{\alpha - \beta}\, e^{t\gamma}\right)$$

where, again, $\mathcal{F}$ is given by (7).

At this point, it is natural to consider the behavior of the logistic equation in which both functions $a(t)$ and $b(t)$ vary between an initial level and an asymptotic level. Indicated with α and β the two levels of the function $a(t)$ and with δ and ε those of the function $b(t)$, we treat the equation (2) assuming:

$$a(t) = \frac{a_0}{\alpha + (\alpha - \beta)\left(e^{-\gamma t} - 1\right)}, \qquad b(t) = \frac{a_0}{\delta + (\delta - \varepsilon)\left(e^{-\gamma t} - 1\right)} \tag{13}$$

Repeating, with the appropriate computational adjustments, the procedure applied in the theorem 4, we present in an explicit form the solution of the equation (2) under the condition (13).

Theorem 6 *If conditions (13) hold, and if* $\beta\delta - \alpha\varepsilon \neq 0$ *quadrature formula (3) becomes*

$$x(t) = \frac{x_0(a_0 + \beta\gamma)(\beta\delta - \alpha\varepsilon)\left(\alpha + \beta\left(e^{\gamma t} - 1\right)\right)^{\frac{a_0}{\beta\gamma}}}{(a_0 + \beta\gamma)\alpha^{\frac{a}{\beta\gamma}}(\beta\delta - \alpha\varepsilon) + b_0\beta x_0\, J_1(t)}. \tag{14}$$

being

$$J_1(t) = \left(\left(\alpha + \beta\left(e^{\gamma t} - 1\right)\right)^{\frac{a_0}{\beta\gamma}+1} \mathcal{F}\left(\frac{\left(\alpha + \left(e^{t\gamma} - 1\right)\beta\right)\varepsilon}{\alpha\varepsilon - \beta\delta}\right) - \alpha^{\frac{a_0}{\beta\gamma}+1} \mathcal{F}\left(\frac{\alpha\varepsilon}{\alpha\varepsilon - \beta\delta}\right)\right)$$

where $\mathcal{F}$ *is still given by* (7).

Remark 3 The explicit solutions found in Theorems 4, 5 and 6 exhibit the asymptotic behavior theoretically expected, reaching the level of the corresponding cases at constant coefficients. The possible employment of the obtained results regards the situations in which the functions $a(t)$ and $b(t)$ vary between two extreme values, assuming that such variation happens in a logistic-sigmoidal way. This last assumption can be seen as an approximation of convenience, since claiming, as we have done, that the variation between the two levels of the parameters occurs in a sigmoidal way allows the explicit integration of the differential equation thus obtained.

3 Carrying Capacity Periodically Variable

The idea of considering evolutions of population with periodically variable carrying capacity arises in a completely natural way, having in mind seasonal diseases and has, therefore, great interest from epidemiological applications. In this section, we recall the important theoretical results due to deMottoni and Schiaffino, [5], and then present a particular case, in which these theoretical evidences are reflected in the explicit calculation of the solution.

3.1 Existence of Periodic Solution

In [5], de Mottoni and Schiaffino consider this generalization of (1):

$$\dot{x} = x\, f(t, x) \tag{15}$$

and state the following result concerning existence of periodic solutions of (15).

Theorem 7 *Assume for $f : \mathbb{R} \times [0, +\infty) \to \mathbb{R}$ the following:*

(i) f is periodic in t (it does not go against the generality of the treatment to assume that the period is unitary)
(ii) f is continuous in t and C^1 in x
(iii) f is decreasing in x
(iv) xf_x is decreasing in x
(v) there exists $M_0 > 0$ such that $f(t, x) \le 0$ for $x \ge M_0 > 0$

Consider the mean μ of the function $f(t, 0)$ over one period, i.e.,

$$\mu = \int_0^1 f(t, 0)\,dt$$

then, if:

(a) $\mu \le 0$ there are no periodic non-negative non-trivial solutions of (15), moreover every solution such that $x(0) > 0$ tends for $t \to +\infty$ to the trivial solution.
(b) $\mu > 0$ there is a positive and periodic solution of (15), this solution is the sole periodic solution and it is globally stable, compared to all positive solutions. Henceforth, every solution such that $x(0) > 0$ tends for $t \to +\infty$ to the unique positive periodic solution of (15).

3.2 Cosinusoidal Carrying Capacity

Consider equation (1) assuming that K varies periodically with time ruled following a cosinusoidal rule:

$$K(t) = K_0\,(1 + \alpha \cos(\omega t))\,, \tag{16}$$

where we assume $K_0 > 0$ and $0 < \alpha < 1$. Using the notation of (15) we have

$$f(t, x) = r\left(1 - \frac{x}{K_0}\,(1 + \alpha \cos(\omega t))\right)$$

which immediately ensures for Theorem 7 existence of periodic solution of (1) when $K(t)$ is given by (16). In this particular situation, we are seeking for the explicit computation of the periodic solution theoretically individuated by Theorem 7.

Theorem 8 *Introduce, for $\alpha < 1$*

$$p = p(\alpha) = -\frac{1 - \sqrt{1 - \alpha^2}}{\alpha}, \tag{17}$$

and define

$$z(t) = \frac{1}{K_0}\left(\frac{1+p^2}{1-p^2}\right)\left\{1 + 2r\sum_{n=1}^{\infty}\left(\frac{r\cos(n\omega t) + n\omega\sin(n\omega t)}{r^2 + n^2\omega^2}\right)p^n\right\}. \tag{18}$$

Then $x(t) = 1/z(t)$ is periodic with period $T = 2\pi/\omega$ and solves equation

$$\dot{x} = r\,x\left(1 - \frac{x}{K_0\,(1+\alpha\cos(\omega\,t))}\right). \tag{19}$$

Proof The main ingredient for our proof is the Poisson kernel identity, entry 1.447.3 page 40 of [8], i.e.:

$$\frac{1-p^2}{1-2p\cos(\omega\,\tau)+p^2} = 1 + 2\sum_{n=1}^{\infty}p^n\,\cos(n\omega\,\tau), \qquad |p|<1. \tag{20}$$

Using standard substitution $z = 1/x$ equation (19) is linearized:

$$\dot{z} = -rz + \frac{r}{K_0}\,(1+\alpha\cos(\omega t))\,, \tag{19L}$$

We underline that here we are not working on the general solution nor on the solution of an initial value problem, but we are trying to represent explicitly the periodic solution theoretically identified by deMottoni and Schiaffino in Theorem 7. This computational approach has great importance in applications, because it allows to estimate the value of the periodic limiting solution, theoretically foreseen and, therefore, to calculate it according to the usual procedure of the initial value problems. At this aim, integrating, starting at $-\infty$ we get the particular solution of $(19L)$

$$z(t) = \frac{r\,e^{-r\,t}}{K_0}\int_{-\infty}^{t}\frac{e^{r\tau}}{1+\alpha\cos(\omega\tau)}\mathrm{d}\tau. \tag{21}$$

The integral appearing in (21) can be computed using (20). We need to find $|p|<1$ in order to express the denominator of the integrand as $1 - 2p\cos(\omega\,\tau) + p^2$. For the purpose, multiply and divide for $\beta > 0$ (we will choose the appropriate value later) in (21) getting:

$$z(t) = \frac{r\beta}{K_0}e^{-rt}\int_{-\infty}^{t}\frac{e^{r\tau}}{\beta + \alpha\beta\cos(\omega\tau)}d\tau. \tag{21'}$$

Thus, β must be such that $\beta = 1 + p^2$ and $\alpha\beta = -2p$, hence β is easily detected:

$$\beta^2 - \frac{4}{\alpha^2}\beta + \frac{4}{\alpha^2} = 0 \implies \beta = \frac{2}{\alpha^2}\left(1 - \sqrt{1-\alpha^2}\right)$$

where the smallest root has been selected so that $|p|<1$. And, then (17) follows. For this choice of $p = p(\alpha)$, we represent solution of $(19L)$ as:

$$z(t) = \frac{r\beta}{K_0} e^{-rt} \int_{-\infty}^{t} \frac{e^{r\tau}}{1 - 2p\cos(\omega\tau) + p^2}\, d\tau. \tag{22}$$

Inserting (20) into (22), we arrive at:

$$z(t) = \frac{r\beta}{K_0} \frac{1}{1-p^2} e^{-rt} \left\{ \int_{-\infty}^{t} e^{r\tau} d\tau + 2\sum_{n=1}^{\infty} p^n \int_{-\infty}^{t} e^{r\tau} \cos(k\omega\,\tau)\, d\tau \right\}, \tag{23}$$

where the integration and summation have been interchanged due to the uniform convergence. The second integral in the right-hand side of (23) is elementary, one can see [8] entry 2.663.3 p.196. Canceling e^{-rt}, we arrive at, recalling that $\beta = 1 + p^2$, at (18), which ends our proof. □

Remark 4 Form the proof of theorem 8, we can observe that:

(i) For $\alpha = 0$, and then, $p = 0$, one has simply $x(t) = K_0$, corresponding to the equilibrium solution for the constant coefficients case.
(ii) Series (18) converges fastly being $-1 < p < 0$.

As stated by Theorem 7, when considering any initial value problem associated with the equation (19), the relevant solution will not be in general periodic, but is asymptotic to the periodic solution individuated in Theorem 7 and computed in Theorem 8 for the particular cosinusoidal case. The initial value at $t = 0$ of the periodic solution is given by the infinite series

$$x(0) = K_0 \left(\frac{1-p^2}{1+p^2}\right) \left(1 + 2r \sum_{n=1}^{\infty} \frac{rp^n}{n^2\omega^2 + r^2}\right)^{-1}. \tag{24}$$

Series obtained in (24) can, in fact, be calculated in closed form, however the expression we get comes from an identity, verifiable via Mathematica®, of the form:

$$\sum_{n=0}^{\infty} \frac{p^n}{a\,n^2 + b} = \frac{1}{2b} \left({}_2F_1\left(\left. \begin{matrix} 1,\ -i\sqrt{\frac{b}{a}} \\ 1 - i\sqrt{\frac{b}{a}} \end{matrix} \right| p \right) + {}_2F_1\left(\left. \begin{matrix} 1,\ i\sqrt{\frac{b}{a}} \\ 1 + i\sqrt{\frac{b}{a}} \end{matrix} \right| p \right) \right) \tag{25}$$

which, in view of the fact that in applications we need a numerical evaluation of the initial condition associated only with the periodic solution of the equation (19), does not seem useful to us, given the transcendence of the expression obtained in (25).

In Fig. 2, we compare, in a time span of 30, for the set of particular values given by $r = .1,\ \alpha = .5,\ K_0 = 1,\ \omega = 2\pi$ the periodic solution, corresponding, following (24), at the initial value

$$\frac{1}{x(0)} = \frac{2}{5\sqrt{3}} \left(\sum_{n=1}^{\infty} \frac{\left(\sqrt{3}-2\right)^n}{10\left(4\pi^2 n^2 + \frac{1}{100}\right)} + 5 \right) \simeq 1.15455$$

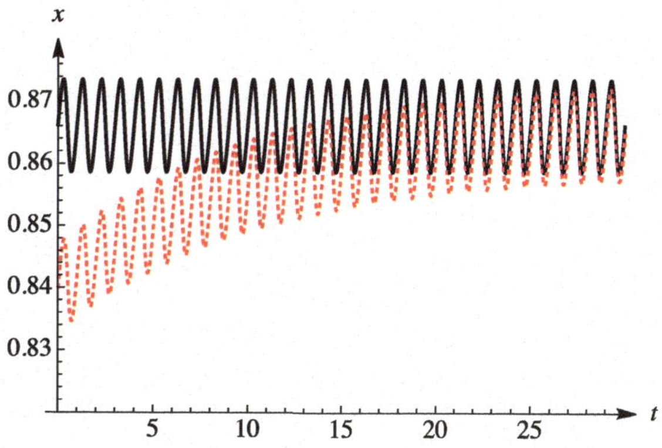

Fig. 2 Illustrating Theorems 7 and 8

thus $x(0) \simeq 0.84$ being here the period equal to 1.

4 Periodic Harvesting

The logistic constant coefficient equation with constant harvesting, $a,\ b,\ h > 0$ is:

$$\begin{cases} \dot{x}(t) = a\,x(t) - b\,x^2(t) - h, \\ x(0) = x_0, \end{cases} \tag{26}$$

(26) is an elementary Riccati equation, it is treated in [2] Chap. 2, Sects. 2.7.2 and 2.7.2. By the way in this case, equation (26) can be solved using the fact that a stationary solution, putting $\Delta = a^2 - 4bh$, assuming $\Delta > 0$, is given by:

$$x_0(t) = \frac{a + \sqrt{\Delta}}{2b}$$

hence, with standard methods, we see that solution $x(t)$ of (26) is given by

$$x(t) = \frac{a + \sqrt{\Delta}}{2b} + \frac{1}{ce^{\sqrt{\Delta}t} - \frac{b}{\sqrt{\Delta}}}$$

Moreover, if $\Delta < 0$ the integration of (26) is obtained using trigonometric functions, generated by the inversion of the algebraic integral:

$$\int_{x_0}^{x} \frac{\mathrm{d}s}{-h + as - bs^2} = t.$$

That said, we will study the initial value problem:

$$\begin{cases} \dot{x}(t) = a\,x(t) - b\,x^2(t) + c\,\cos(\omega\,t) - h\,, \\ x(0) = x_0 > 0. \end{cases} \tag{27}$$

Throughout the cycle of the exogenous, time-dependent, periodic forcing term $f(t) = c\,\cos(\omega t) - h,\ c > 0$, the population is unceasingly lowered by a constant harvesting of rate $h > 0$, plus a periodic unbalance $c\,\cos(\omega t)$. The birth parameter a is not under control, but the overcrowding and harvesting parameters b and c, as well as the harvesting/restocking parameters h and ω, present an avenue for exogenous control. We will integrate the Riccati equation (27) through its standard transformation into a second order linear (Mathieu) equation (see [4, 14]). Moreover, we establish (Theorem 9) the analytical relationship among the coefficients a, b, c, h, while ω remains not involved, and the initial condition x_0, sufficient to ensure that (27) has a defined, bounded and positive solution $x(t)$ for any $t > 0$, namely $|x(t)| \le K$ for a suitable positive number $K > 0$ for any $t \ge 0$. The proposed model aims to represent situations in which seasonal conditions occur that lead to the spread of a viral infection.

4.1 Global Features of the Solution

We transform (27) with the usual change of variable

$$u(t) = \exp\left(b \int_0^t x(\tau)\,d\tau\right) \Leftrightarrow x(t) = \frac{1}{b}\frac{\dot{u}(t)}{u(t)}, \tag{28}$$

obtaining:

$$\begin{cases} \ddot{u} - a\,\dot{u} - b\,c\,\cos(\omega t)\,u - b\,h\,u = 0, \\ u(0) = 1,\ \dot{u}(0) = b\,x(0) = b\,x_0 > 0. \end{cases} \tag{29}$$

Notice that (29) is a *damped* Mathieu equation, by the way the term $-a\dot{u}(t)$, is removed using a second (standard) change of variable, see, for instance, [20, chapter 1, Sect. 3, pp. 7–8], namely $v(t) = e^{-(a/2)t}u(t)$ which provides the normal form equation

$$\begin{cases} \ddot{v} - \left(\dfrac{a^2}{4} - b\,h + b\,c\,\cos(\omega t)\right)\,v = 0, \\ v(0) = 1,\ \dot{v}(0) = bx_0 - \dfrac{1}{2}a. \end{cases} \tag{30}$$

Equation (30) will be integrated using Mathieu functions later. Let us first provide relationships ensuring that (27) has a bounded solution. Recall that (27) is solved by:

$$x(t) = \frac{a}{2b} + \frac{1}{b}\frac{\dot{v}(t)}{v(t)}. \tag{31}$$

Therefore, we need to prove that the logarithmic derivative of the solution of (30) is bounded. Write for simplicity (30) as:

$$\ddot{v} - A(t)v = 0, \text{with} A(t) = a^2/4 - b\,h + b\,c\,\cos(\omega t). \tag{32}$$

We require the boundedness for the logarithmic derivative of solution of (32). First notice that if v is solution of (32), then its logarithmic derivative solves the first-order Riccati equation:

$$\dot{y} = A(t) - y^2. \tag{33}$$

We will use standard results on differential inequalities, provided in [10], in order to deduce the boundedness of $y(t)$ depending on $A(t)$. To this end, let us prove the following Lemma, which holds for any bounded real function $A(t)$.

Lemma 2 *Consider differential equation* (33) *assuming $A(t)$ bounded, and let y the solution of* (33) *such that $y(0) = y_0$.*

(i) If $0 < m^2 = \inf_{t\in\mathbb{R}} A(t) < M^2 = \sup_{t\in\mathbb{R}} A(t)$ and $|y_0| < |m|$, then y is bounded, while for $|y_0| > |M|$ y is unbounded.
(ii) If $-m^2 = \inf_{t\in\mathbb{R}} A(t) < -M^2 = \sup_{t\in\mathbb{R}} A(t) < 0$, then $y(t)$ is unbounded.
(iii) If $-m^2 = \inf_{t\in\mathbb{R}} A(t) < 0 < M^2 = \sup_{t\in\mathbb{R}} A(t)$, then neither the boundedness, nor the unboundedness of y can be inferred.

Proof We begin with (i). Using a standard argument, see for instance Corollary 4.2 page 27 of [10], we find that $y_m(t) \le y(t) \le y_M(t)$ where y_m and y_M are the solutions of the two initial value problems:

$$\begin{cases} \dot{y}_m = m^2 - y_m^2, \\ y_m(0) = y_0, \end{cases} \qquad \begin{cases} \dot{y}_M = M^2 - y_M^2, \\ y_M(0) = y_0, \end{cases}$$

namely:

$$y_m(t) = m\frac{m\sinh(mt) + y_0\cosh(mt)}{m\cosh(mt) + y_0\sinh(mt)}, \; y_M(t) = M\frac{M\sinh(Mt) + y_0\cosh(Mt)}{M\cosh(Mt) + y_0\sinh(Mt)}.$$

Such functions are both bounded if $|y_0| < m$, and then solution of (33) is also bounded. Similarly, if $|y_0| > M$ the functions $y_m(t)$, $y_M(t)$ are unbounded, and then y is unbounded too. The proof of (ii) is similar; in this case we have:

$$-m^2 = \inf_{t\in\mathbb{R}} A(t) < -M^2 = \sup_{t\in\mathbb{R}} A(t) < 0.$$

Thus, once again, we find $y_m \le y \le y_M$, but now y_m and y_M are solutions of the initial value problems:

$$\begin{cases} \dot{y}_m = -m^2 - y_m^2, \\ y_m(0) = y_0, \end{cases} \qquad \begin{cases} \dot{y}_M = -M^2 - y_M^2, \\ y_M(0) = y_0, \end{cases}$$

namely:

$$y_m(t) = m \tan\left(-mt + \arctan \frac{y_0}{m}\right), \quad y_M(t) = M \tan\left(-Mt + \arctan \frac{y_0}{M}\right),$$

that are both unbounded, and not globally defined, imposing the same behavior upon y. Finally, in the case of (iii), we can deduce only an upper bound for y but not a lower bound. □

By the above Lemma 2, we can establish the following sufficient condition for the boundedness of the solutions of (27).

Theorem 9 *Consider the initial value problem* (27). *If the following inequalities hold:*

$$4b\,(h+c) < a^2, \quad |2bx_0 - a| < \sqrt{a^2 - 4b\,(h+c)}\,, \tag{34}$$

the solution of (27) *is bounded.*

Remark 5 It is easy to evaluate the mean value $\bar{x}(t)$ in $[0, t]$ of the solution of (27); for recalling (31), we have:

$$\bar{x}(t) = \frac{1}{t}\int_0^t x(\tau)d\tau = \frac{a}{2b} + \frac{1}{bt}\ln\left|\frac{v(t)}{v(0)}\right|, \tag{35}$$

where v solves (30).

4.2 Closed-Form Integration and Examples

The Mathieu equation is a linear second-order equation of the form:

$$y'' + (\lambda - 2q\cos(2t))\,y = 0 \tag{36}$$

A fundamental system of solutions of (36) is given by the elliptic sine $\mathrm{Se}(\lambda, q, t)$ which is such that $\mathrm{Se}(\lambda, q, 0) = 0$ and is in odd function and the elliptic cosine $\mathrm{Ce}(\lambda, q, t)$, which is such that $\mathrm{Ce}(\lambda, q, 0) = 1$ and is even. For further details one can see [4, 14, 23]. Rewrite (30) as:

$$\begin{cases} \ddot{v} - (\Lambda + \Omega\cos(\omega t))\,v = 0, \\ v(0) = 1, \ \dot{v}(0) = X, \end{cases} \tag{30b}$$

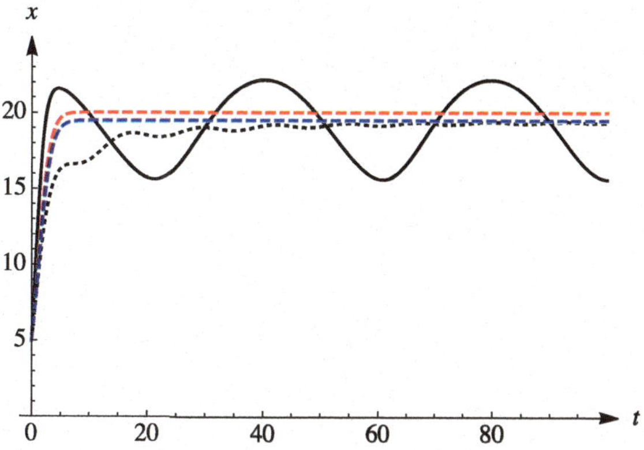

Fig. 3 The stable case: the population is bounded but oscillating at any time

where: $\Lambda = \Lambda(a, b, h) = a^2/2 - bh$, $\Omega = \Omega(b, c) = bc$ and $X = X(a, b, x_0) = bx_0 - (1/2)a$. Solution of v of (30b) is then:

$$v(t) = \frac{N_1 \operatorname{Se}\left(\frac{-4\,\Lambda}{\omega^2}, \frac{2\,\Omega}{\omega^2}, \frac{\omega}{2}t\right) + N_2 \operatorname{Ce}\left(\frac{-4\,\Lambda}{\omega^2}, \frac{2\,\Omega}{\omega^2}, \frac{\omega}{2}t\right)}{\omega\,(D_1 - D_2)}, \tag{37}$$

where:

$$\begin{aligned} N_1 &= \omega \operatorname{Ce}'\left(\frac{-4\,\Lambda}{\omega^2}, \frac{2\,\Omega}{\omega^2}, 0\right) - 2\,X \operatorname{Ce}\left(\frac{-4\,\Lambda}{\omega^2}, \frac{2\,\Omega}{\omega^2}, 0\right), \\ N_2 &= 2\,X \operatorname{Se}\left(\frac{-4\,\Lambda}{\omega^2}, \frac{2\,\Omega}{\omega^2}, 0\right) - \omega \operatorname{Se}'\left(\frac{-4\,\Lambda}{\omega^2}, \frac{2\,\Omega}{\omega^2}, 0\right), \\ D_1 &= \operatorname{Ce}'\left(\frac{-4\,\Lambda}{\omega^2}, \frac{2\,\Omega}{\omega^2}, 0\right) \operatorname{Se}\left(\frac{-4\,\Lambda}{\omega^2}, \frac{2\,\Omega}{\omega^2}, 0\right), \\ D_2 &= \operatorname{Ce}\left(\frac{-4\,\Lambda}{\omega^2}, \frac{2\,\Omega}{\omega^2}, 0\right) \operatorname{Se}'\left(\frac{-4\,\Lambda}{\omega^2}, \frac{2\,B}{\omega^2}, 0\right), \end{aligned}$$

and the primes $'$ denote derivatives with respect to t. To express the solution of (27), we have to insert (37) into (31).

4.3 A Sample Problem

To illustrate the concrete effects of the introduction of a periodic term in the logistics model, we present a simulation in the case providing bounded solution, therefore using data meeting condition (34) of Theorem 9. Let $a = 1$, $b = 1/20$, $c = 3$, $h = 1/2$, $\omega = 1/(2\pi)$, $x_0 = 5$.

Exact solution implementation

```
In[ ]:= exs[t_, a_, α_, β_, γ_, ξ_] := (ⅇ^(a t) (α - β) (a + γ) ξ) /
   (Factor[a α - a β + α γ - β γ] + Factor[-a ξ Hypergeometric2F1[1, (a + γ)/γ, 2 + a/γ, -β/(α - β)] +
      a ⅇ^(t (a+γ)) ξ Hypergeometric2F1[1, (a + γ)/γ, 2 + a/γ, -(ⅇ^(t γ) β)/(α - β)]]);
```

Numerical solution implementation

```
In[ ]:= eq[a_, α_, β_, γ_, ξ_] := {x'[t] == a x[t] - a/(α + (α - β) (E^(-γ t) - 1)) x[t]^2, x[0] == ξ};
nus[a_, α_, β_, γ_, ξ_] := NDSolveValue[eq[a, α, β, γ, ξ], x, {t, 0, 100}]
```

Choose a set of parameters and overlap the solutions

```
In[ ]:= s1 = nus[.1, 2, 3, .1, 1];
Max[Table[Abs[exs[t, .1, 2, 3, .1, 1] - s1[t]], {t, 0, 30, .05}]]
Out[ ]= 2.42031 × 10^-7
```

Fig. 4 Solution comparison from Sect. 2

In Fig. 3, the continuous black line indicates the solution of the initial value problem (27), expressed explicitly in terms of Mathieu's functions, the dotted black line is $\bar{x}(t)$, i.e., the mean value of the solution as computed in (35), the red dashed line represents the unperturbed solution of the constant coefficient logistic equation, corresponding to $c = 0$ and $h = 0$ in our notations, eventually the blue dashed line represents the logistic equation perturbed only by the harvesting effect, corresponding to $c = 0$ and $h > 0$ in our notations. The fact that the harvesting solution is dominated by the logistics solution with constant coefficients is, as expected, found. Moreover, the mean value $\bar{x}(t)$ goes asymptotically to the asymptotic value reached by eliminating the periodic effect: This is also a reasonable behavior confirmed by the computational evidence. The most interesting aspect is, certainly, the fact that the influence of the periodic term accentuates the oscillations of the solution, reproducing the effects of epidemic waves brought by seasonal viral infections, like the coronaviruses.

Explicit solutions and Mathematica®

In Sects. 2 and 4, we have obtained explicit solutions in closed form of the logistic differential equations used for the description of epidemiological models. Although the formulas obtained in the respective integration processes are structurally complicated, given that, thanks to the current computer algebra resources, they can still be implemented and, therefore, can be used operationally. Moreover, as the following two examples, one related to Sect. 2, see Fig. 4 and the second to Sect. 4, Fig. 5, show

Exact solution implementation

```
In[ ]:= exs[t_, a_, b_, c_, h_, ω_, ξ_] :=
  (ω (a MathieuC[-(a^2 - 4 b h)/ω^2, (2 b c)/ω^2, (t ω)/2] + ω MathieuCPrime[-(a^2 - 4 b h)/ω^2, (2 b c)/ω^2, (t ω)/2])
     MathieuSPrime[-(a^2 - 4 b h)/ω^2, (2 b c)/ω^2, 0] -
    (a - 2 b ξ) MathieuC[-(a^2 - 4 b h)/ω^2, (2 b c)/ω^2, 0] (a MathieuS[-(a^2 - 4 b h)/ω^2, (2 b c)/ω^2, (t ω)/2] +
      ω MathieuSPrime[-(a^2 - 4 b h)/ω^2, (2 b c)/ω^2, (t ω)/2]))/
  (2 b (-(a - 2 b ξ) MathieuC[-(a^2 - 4 b h)/ω^2, (2 b c)/ω^2, 0] MathieuS[-(a^2 - 4 b h)/ω^2, (2 b c)/ω^2, (t ω)/2] +
      ω MathieuC[-(a^2 - 4 b h)/ω^2, (2 b c)/ω^2, (t ω)/2] MathieuSPrime[-(a^2 - 4 b h)/ω^2, (2 b c)/ω^2, 0]));
```

Numerical solution implementation

```
In[ ]:= eq[a_, b_, c_, h_, ω_, ξ_] := {x'[t] == a x[t] - b x[t]^2 + c Cos[ω t] - h, x[0] == ξ};
nus[a_, b_, c_, h_, ω_, ξ_] := NDSolveValue[eq[a, b, c, h, ω, ξ], x, {t, 0, 200}]
```

Choose a set of parameters and overlap the solutions

```
In[ ]:= s1 = nus[1, 1/20, 1/5, 1/2, 1/(2 π), 5];
Max[Table[Abs[exs[t, 1, 1/20, 1/5, 1/2, 1/(2 π), 5] - s1[t]], {t, 0, 30, .05}]]

Out[ ]= 1.41356 × 10^-6
```

Fig. 5 Solution comparision from Sect. 4

a remarkable numerical precision in the Mathematica® libraries. Below we show the comparison, obtained by discretizing the maximum difference between numerical solution and solution obtained in closed form in two sample problems.

Conclusion

In this chapter, we have set out three different generalizations of the logistic equation, providing models more suitable to represent real cases, also and especially in the field of epidemiology. In the first two models, we considered two particular occurrences of the logistic equation with non-constant coefficients, which confirmed the theoretical analyses conducted by Nkashama [18, 19] and deMottoni and Schiaffino [5] in two particular cases, but significant in the concrete implementation. The last model instead deals with a periodic perturbation of a logistic equation with constant coefficients. All models presented allow explicit and concrete calculations, illustrated in detail by the use of Mathematica®.

The spirit of our contribution is that of fundamental research, aimed at offering new possible future instruments of investigation to scholars of phenomena in real situations.

Acknowledgements The model presented in Sect. 3 dates back to a collaboration started with Professor Stefano Alliney, which could not materialize due to the worsening of his health, which led to his premature death. This work is dedicated to his memory.

References

1. Andrews, G.E., Askey, R., Roy, R.: Special Functions. Cambridge University Press, Cambridge (1999)
2. Banks, R.B.: Growth and diffusion phenomena: Mathematical frameworks and applications. Springer, New York (2013)
3. Brauer, F., van der Driesche, P., Wu, J.: Lecture notes in mathematical epidemiology. Springer, New York (2008)
4. Campbell, R.: Théorie générale de l'équation de Mathieu et de quelques autres équations différentielles de la mécanique. Masson, Paris (1955)
5. de Mottoni, P., Schiaffino, A.: On logistic equations with time periodic coefficients. Istituto per le Applicazioni del Calcolo Mauro Picone **1–17** (1979)
6. de Mottoni, P., Schiaffino, A.: Competition systems with periodic coefficients: a geometric approach. J. Math. Biol. **11**, 1–17 (1981)
7. Duren, P.: Invitation to Classical Analysis. American Mathematical Society, Providence (2012).
8. Gradshteyn, I.S., Ryzhik, J.M.: Table of Integrals, Series and Products, 6th edn. Academic Press, New York (2000)
9. Grover, J.P.: Resource Competition. Springer, New York (1997)
10. Hartman, P.: Differential Equations, 2nd edn. SIAM, Philadelphia (1982)
11. Hethcote, H.W., Yorke, J.A.: Gonorrhea transmission dynamics and control. Springer, New York (2014)
12. Lotka, A.J.: Elements of mathematical biology. Dover, New York (1956)
13. Malthus, T.R.: An Essay on the Principle of Population. J. Johnson, London (1872)
14. McLachlan, N.W.: Theory and application of Mathieu functions. Oxford University Press, Oxford (1951)
15. Meyer, P.S., Ausubel, J.H.: Carrying capacity: a model with logistically varying limits. Technol. Forecast. Soc. Change. 61(3), 209–214 (1999).
16. Mingari Scarpello, G., Palestini, A., Ritelli, D.: Closed form solutions to generalized logistic-type nonautonomous systems. Appl. Sci. **12**, 134–145 (2010)
17. Mingari Scarpello, G., Ritelli, D.: Closed form solution of a periodically forced logistic model. Ann. Univ. Ferrara Sez. VII Sci. Mat. **54**(1), 85–94 (2008)
18. Nkashama, M.N.: Dynamics of logistic equations with non-autonomous bounded coefficients. Electr. J. Differ. Equ. **2000**(2), 1–8 (2000)
19. Nkashama, M.N.: Bounded and almost-periodic solutions of nonlocal perturbations of nonautonomous logistic-type equations. Acta Appl. Math. **65**, 283–293 (2001)
20. Rainville, E.D.: Intermediate differential equations, 2nd edn. Mcmillian, New York (1964)
21. Seaborn, J.B.: Hypergeometric functions and their applications. Springer, New York (1991)
22. Verhulst, P.F.: Notice sur la loi que la population suit dans son accroissement. Corresp. Math. Phys. 10, 113–126 (1838).
23. Wang, Z.X., Ren Guo, D.: Special functions. World Scientific, Singapore (1989)

A Transition of Shared Mobility in Metro Cities—A Challenge Post-Lockdown Covid-19

Mohd Aman and Bushra Miftah

Abstract This chapter is written for the welfare of the society, to question and enlighten on effects of the increment or decrement in the percentage of quality of air causing pollution due to the rise in the traffic post-lockdown due to Covid-19 in metro cities, specifically in Delhi. In this chapter, we address the question about people's preference of moving in the shared taxis to their workplaces or their reluctance travelling in shared vehicle because of the fear of getting infected. The sensitivity of the situation will compel the people to move in a single-occupied vehicle (SOV). The rise in the number of vehicles on the roads will result in traffic jams, and different kinds of pollutions where people battling with the pandemic will inevitably get exposed to other health-related issues. We use a Bureau of Public Roads (BPR) model to combat this issue endangering the environment and public health. We exploit the BPR function to relate average travel time to the estimated number of commuters travelling by car. We collect mode share data from the NITI Ayog, the State Resource Centre and other authentic sources, which gives unique figures of the impact of shared mobility in India and how, in its absence, various sectors will get affected. Using the given data and the BPR, we evaluate increased vehicle volumes on the road if different portions of transit and carpool users switch to single-occupancy vehicles and its effect on multiple other factors. Based on the study of densely populated city, Delhi, we predict that cities with significant transit ridership are at risk for extreme traffic and pollution unless transit systems can resume safe with effective protocols.

Keywords Covid-19 · Commute · Mobility practice · Low carbon travel · Transport sector

M. Aman (✉)
Department of Mathematics, University Institute of Sciences, Chandigarh University, Mohali 140413, India

B. Miftah
Department of English, Faculty of Arts, Aligarh Muslim University, 202002 Aligarh, India

P. Agarwal et al. (eds.), *Analysis of Infectious Disease Problems (Covid-19) and Their Global Impact*, Infosys Science Foundation Series,
https://doi.org/10.1007/978-981-16-2450-6_7

1 Introduction

The twenty-first century saw the emergence of a newly found coronavirus, also known as the Severe Acute Respiratory Syndrome (SARS) COV–2 in the Wuhan city of China. Unaware of the cause of transmission to the human body, the deadly virus which had been declared Public Health Emergency of International Concern by WHO earlier this year has been contracted by more than one crore population across the globe causing more than 1 lakh fatalities bringing the entire world to a standstill.

India, which holds a population of more than 130 crores, has been severely affected by the newly found virus. However, to curb the same, India went under what is known as the strictest lockdown on March 22, 2020. The stay-at-home orders had a drastic effect on the life of every common person. It caused a direct impact on the usage of the transport system. As the stay-at-home order took effect, ridership data show steep decline in both transit ridership and vehicular traffic.

According to the data collected in from NITI Ayog [1, 2], a State-Resource-Centre of Government of India established with the aim to achieve sustainable development goals in the economic policy-making process; there was an usurp growth in the vehicle ownership and transportation in the last few years which led to overcrowding and unsorted situation that resulted in the loss of 1.42 lakh crore INR annually alone in the cities of Delhi, Mumbai, Kolkata and Bangalore. It has had severe and adverse implications on the health and environment. The increment in the number of vehicles had severely affected India's energy consumption, energy security and economy, pollution, congestion, health and safety. The graphs in Figs. 1 and 2 depict a more detailed picture of the congestion and its cost across metro cities.

The transportation sector in India accounts for 18% of commercial energy consumption and is highly dependent on oil imports. India imported 80% of its oil at the cost of Rs. 4.2 lakh crore in recent years. Additionally, private vehicle use has significant implications on land requirement for parking: In Delhi, for example, parking accounts for 8–10% of the available land pool.

There is a direct effect of ridesharing practice on space. The Fig. 3 gives the idea of estimated space that could be saved by switching to rideshare from private vehicles in big cities in 2017.

Weighing the seriousness of the situation, it is deducted that with the complete unlocking of the lockdown, there will be a drastic mode shift of transportation to single-occupied vehicles (SOV).

Definitely, there will be a massive change in the traffic volume caused due to a sudden drop in transit usage and its impact on the commute time on the road. With the collected data from verified sources, we estimate the number of cars on the road if certain proportions of commuters switch from transit and carpool modes to single occupancy vehicle (SOV), thus increasing the total number of vehicles on the road and the average travel time. The total traffic volume is therefore taken as the number of vehicles commuting from this mode. This data when applied on the BPR model [3–6] to calculate the traffic volume and average traffic time give us an idea of the

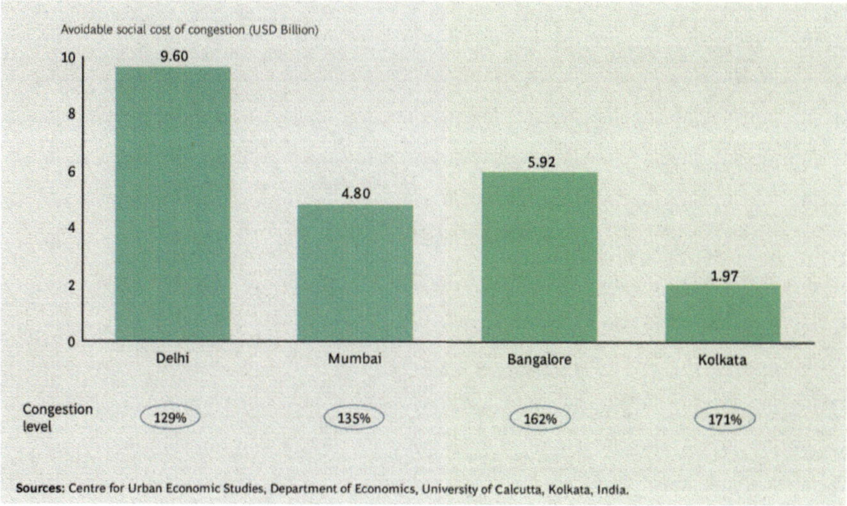

Fig. 1 Cost of congestion across cities (2017) in USD Billion

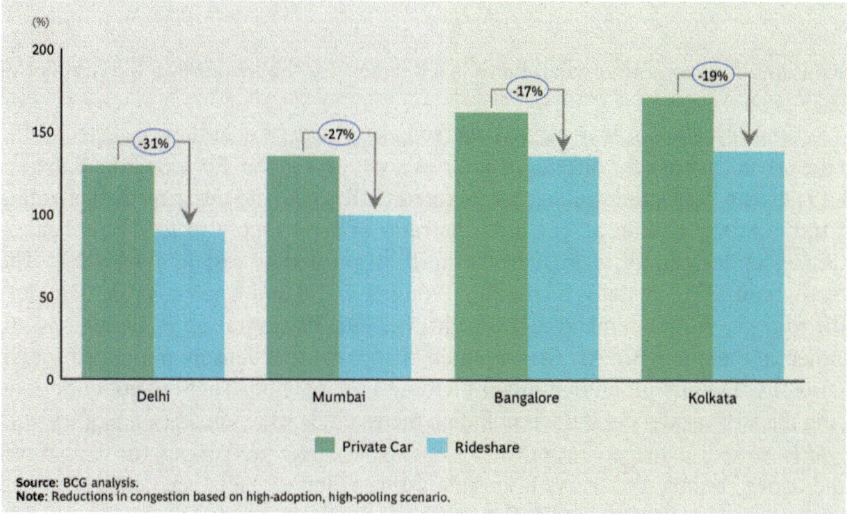

Fig. 2 Road congestion during peak hours before vs. after rideshare (2017)

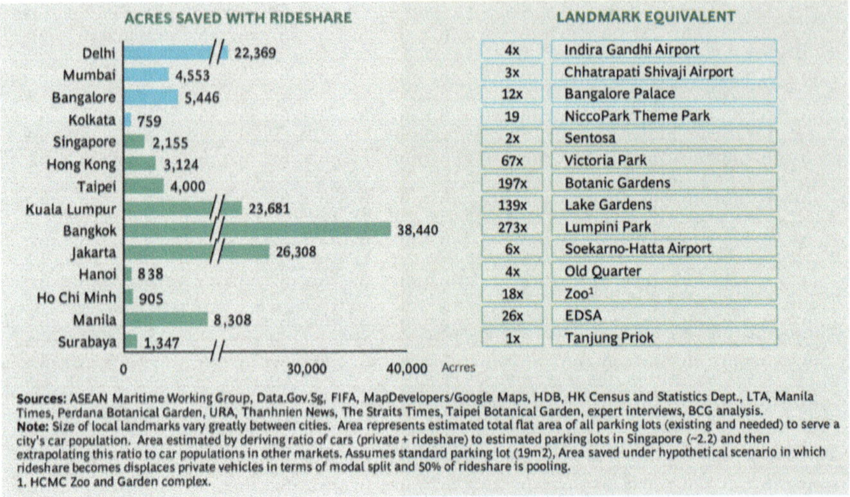

Fig. 3 Estimated space that can be saved by adopting rideshare assuming rideshare substitutes for private cars (2017)

travel time in a condition when there is a decrease or the increase in the number of vehicles on the road.

Several researchers have carried out studies trying to model the congested traffic in the urban network for different countries across the globe. For example, Saberi et al. [7] used a susceptible-infected-recovered (SIR) model to describe the spreading of traffic jam. Colak et al. [8] used the ratio of road supply to travel demand as a dimensionless factor to explain the percentage of time lost in congestion. The macroscopic BPR model is studied by Wong et al. [9] and Kucharski and Drabicki [10] to relate traffic demand and travel time. One or several cities or regions are studied in the above works. Our research is specific to a densely populated Indian metro city, Delhi with an exorbitant increase in the traffic. There is no work done using the BPR analytical model on Indian metro cities which makes an inquiry with regards to road management in Indian cities and make predictions for their travel time under various scenarios of possible traffic volume. India accounts for top 15 most polluted cities in the world. Figure 4 gives the average travel time of four highly congested metro cities in India in 2018.

The major finding on the collected data throws light on the greater risk of high transit cities of increased traffic so that system can resume safely without any complications.

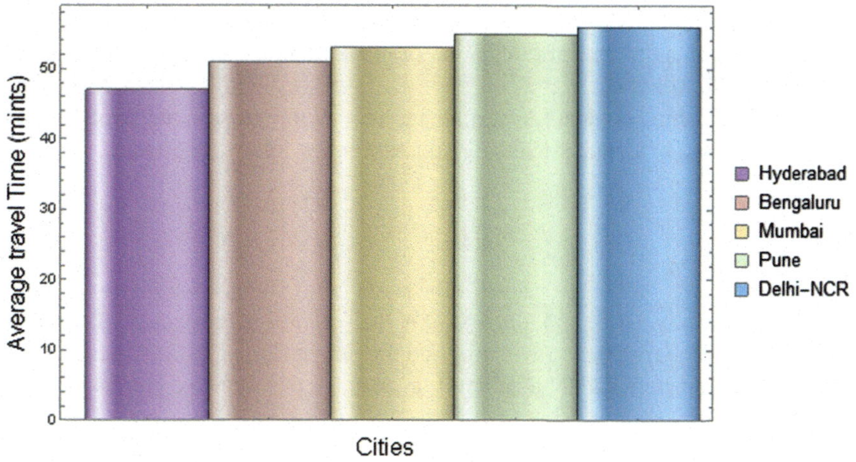

Fig. 4 Travel time of congested metro cities of India (2018)

The high-transit metro cities are at a higher risk with potentially 4–30 min additional commute travel time in a one-way trip. This unusual rise in road transport which will result in a sudden increment in the number of vehicles will cause serious health and environmental issues. This can be curbed, and the transit ridership can be brought to normalcy with returns in trips by car, thereby bringing down the traffic.

The rest of the chapter deals with the introduction of the formulation of BPR model and the introduction of data on traffic in metro cities of India and show the forecast result of traffic in different reopening scenarios.

Our main finding is that the high–transit cities are at greater risk for increased traffic volume unless their transit systems can resume safe, high throughput operations quickly.

2 BPR Model

A widely used impedance calculation model, the Bureau of Public Roads (BPR) model [3–6] states that traffic flow affects the traffic speed. The Bureau of Public Roads is a federal agency created in 1918. Lodged in the US Department, it has taken up much responsibility of building roads in national parks and forests, assisted states with road construction, helped beautify highways, and conducted various transportation studies.

The Bureau of Public Roads (BPR) function [3, 4] is a model that relates the volume of traffic on the road to the travel time to traverse it. It has a great deal of usage in transportation management [11, 12] and network traffic stimulation [13]. According to recent studies, apart from being applied on single–road traffic [9, 10], it also has applicability on urban scale transportation analysis. A BPR function thus provides us with a theoretical foundation of predicting metro area travel congestion based on traffic volume.

The relationship between travel time and the volume (total number of vehicles) can be expressed by the classical BPR function in the following ways:

$$\mathcal{T} = \mathcal{T}_0 \left[1 + a \left(\frac{N}{C} \right)^b \right], \tag{1}$$

where, $\mathcal{T}$ is the travel time as a function of N the volume on the roadway. The parameters $\mathcal{T}_0$, C are the free-flow travel time and the practical road capacity, respectively. The shape parameters a and b can be fit or assumed to follow a common choice of $a = 0.15$ and $b = 4$.

In order to apply the function at the scale of a city, we interpret the BPR model as a function that takes the total number of road users in a city N as a proxy for volume and returns the average commute travel time $\mathcal{T}$ in the city. In this interpretation, the capacity C should be viewed as the total number of road users that can be accommodated in the city before average travel time begins to increase. The average travel time is overall users at all time of the day.

Rewriting (1), we have

$$\mathcal{T} = \mathcal{T}_0 \left[1 + 0.15 \left(\frac{N}{C} \right)^b \right], \tag{2}$$

or

$$\mathcal{T} = \mathcal{T}_0 \, \mu + N. \tag{3}$$

The above equation clearly shows that the travel time $\mathcal{T}$ and the traffic volume N have a linear relationship. The model parameters in (1) can be estimated using linear regression. With the historic data from NITI Ayog and other sources [1, 2, 14–16], we conduct a linear regression on the data from 2012–2018 to find the coefficients $\mathcal{T}_0$ and μ. This allows us to estimate the free-flow travel time $\mathcal{T}_0$ and the practical road capacity

$$c = \left(\frac{0.15\,\mathcal{T}}{\mu} \right), \tag{4}$$

for the metro city Delhi deriving from (2).

3 Data Analysis & Implementation

3.1 Data Description

The data used in the given equation has been derived mainly from NITI Ayog which is a State-of-Art Resource Centre with in-demand knowledge and some other sources as well [1, 2, 14–16]. Using the data, we can answer the following questions:

```
How many cars are on the road in each city?

What is the average travel time experienced by commuters in
each city?
```

The data records means of transportation to work by selected characteristics. For Delhi, annual statistics of a given time (2012–2018) is recorded including the total number of road users for each commute mode (shared vehicles including public transit, single-occupancy vehicles (SOV)), as well as the average commute time (Fig. 5).

The road commute metrics are calculated with the help of raw data. The average travel time of the four-wheelers is taken. The total number of vehicles is computed by converting cars, jeeps, shared vehicles and buses into equivalent vehicles on the road.

We have estimated the resulting vehicles on the road when 25%, 50%, 75% and 100% of commuters using shared vehicles switch to SOV.

We use the latest statistics from the 2018 data to estimate the number of vehicles on the road. The data from 2018 to present can be considered in an extension and

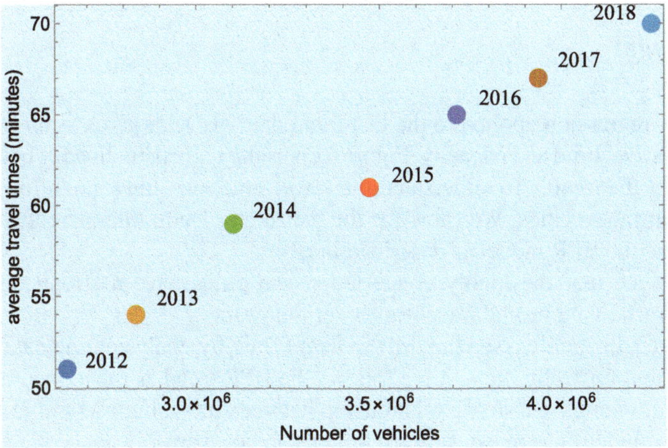

Fig. 5 Observed data of number of vehicles and average one-way tavel time (Delhi) from 2012–2018

Table 1 Exploitation of historical data[a] & Data computed using BPR function (Delhi)

Year	No. of Vehicles	Avg. Travel Time	Trave Time Ratio Capacity Ratio
2012	2644520	51	1.007 0.807
2013	2831460	54	1.067 0.864
2014	3102442	59	1.165 0.946
2015	3470526	61	1.205 1.059
2016	3711060	65	1.284 1.132
2017	3937104	67	1.324 1.201
2018	4245760	70	1.383 1.295

[a] Historical data collected from NITI Ayog & other reliable sources

is not taken into account in this analysis. We also note that the mode share data for taxis and ride-hailing is mixed in with motorcycles, bike and others, and we omit the influence of taxis (not OLA, UBER, etc.) in this study and do not count taxis in the total number of vehicles. Table 1 gives the historical commute data of Delhi from 2012 to 2018.

3.2 *Model Application & Results*

BPR Model

The linear regression applied to the historical data of Delhi gives us an estimate of free-flow travel time and capacity. Figure 6 gives the regression line for better understanding of the trend. To understand the travel time, we study the traffic scenarios in different metro cities. We show for the metro city Delhi, the increment in travel time follow the BPR model as described in (2).

We deduce that the highly congested metro cities have a strong relationship between traffic volume and travel time over the years.

For better insight, we see the drift in travel time by analysing the data of Delhi. We show that for Delhi, travel time follows the BPR trend as mentioned in (2). The cities that do not have a strong relationship between the volume of traffic and travel time are excluded. The reasons for excluding can be an error in data collection or the traffic volume not being the main factor for increase in travel time. We exclude these cities in analysis as the traffic volume does not facilitate in predicting the commute

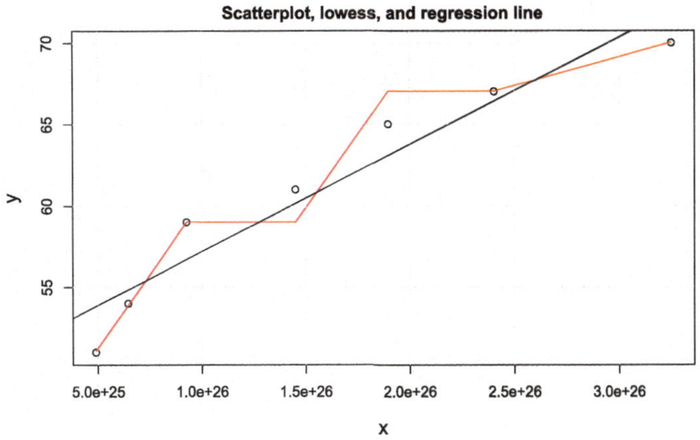

Fig. 6 Regression line and scatter plot for the data of Delhi from 2012–2018

time. The exclusion is done based on some statistical analysis. We measure the linear correlation between travel time T and the fourth order of traffic volume N^4 and calculate their Pearson's correlation coefficient and two-tailed p value. We filter out the metro areas where Pearson's correlation coefficient is larger than 0.5, and p value is smaller than 0.1. On the basis of threshold, we predict that the analysis is applicable to the cities including Delhi, Bangalore, Mumbai and Kolkata and some other that are not included in the further analysis. The BPR model is then applied to Delhi and other metro cities. We see that in Delhi travel time increases with the increase in the number of vehicles, nicely following the BPR function.

We can observe a similar trend in the other mentioned metro cities using the BPR model, which gives us the estimated free-flow time and practical road capacity. Using the estimated free-flow travel time and road capacity, we calculate two important metrics for mentioned metro area:

- Travel time ratio: the ratio of actual travel time versus free-flow travel time. A travel time ratio of 1.1 means the current travel time is 1.1 time (or 10% higher) than the empty road travel time.
- Capacity ratio: the ratio of traffic volume versus road capacity. A capacity ratio of 1.1 means there are 10% more cars than the road capacity.

Travel time ratio and capacity ratio allows us to standardize each city, accounting for the fact that larger cities tend to have larger capacities and longer commutes, even when the roads are empty.

Figure 7 shows the standardized relationship of travel time ratio and capacity ratio of Delhi (Blue dots are historical data and yellow dots are prediction for 25%, 50%, 75% and 100% switch to SOV). We see that the city follows the same growing curve when there is a decrease in the number of shared vehicles on the road. Essentially, what we are doing in the standardization is looking at the rate travel time ratio increases with capacity ratio, then estimate where the city sits on the BPR curve. For

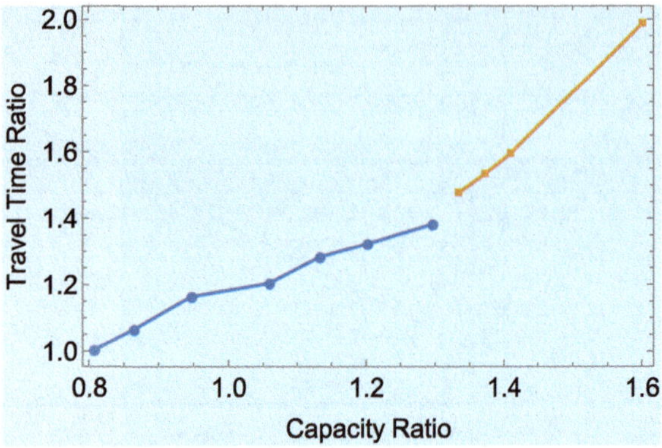

Fig. 7 Travel time ratio vs. capacity ratio for Delhi under different scenarios

Delhi, there is an increase in travel time ratio with an increase in capacity ratio. This indicates that the traffic volume of Delhi is way above road capacity. The same can be observed in Fig. 7.

3.3 Prediction of Traffic Scenarios Post-Lockdown

For decades now, there has been a massive amount of pollutants in the atmosphere, which is a cause of major concern. The air quality has however enormously improved from hazardous to moderate during the lockdown imposed due to Covid-19.

A massive rise of pollutants is expected post-lockdown with increasing number of vehicles on roads with commuters switching to SOV. A sudden drift in the number of vehicles will cause an adverse effect on the traffic system. However, a massive decrement in the amount of pollutants in the atmosphere has been observed, which was a cause of major concern pre-lockdown. It has been successfully reduced, improving the air quality from hazardous to moderate.

According to the Air Quality Index, the unprecedented growth in the pollutants in the atmosphere has caused not only environmental and health issues but a heavy impact on the economy.

If we focus on the situation on the road traffic before lockdown, we see a high level of congestion in four megacities in India, namely Delhi, Mumbai, Bangalore and Kolkata, where total congestion cost was estimated to be more than USD 22 billion per year. We can thus estimate the potential positive impact on ridesharing in each city.

Delhi and Mumbai have been two mega urban centres with relatively more developed modern public transport system. The congestion levels remained high during the pre-lockdown era due to high level of private vehicles in the city. With the burgeoning population and the growing prosperity of Delhi and Mumbai, the reliance on cars has increased, adding more pressure to the road network.

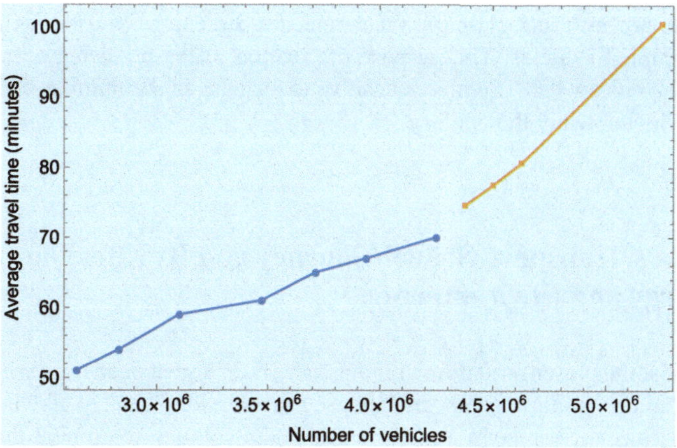

Fig. 8 Example of BPR travel time prediction for Delhi. The blue points are the observed data, and the yellow points are the predictions when 25%, 50%, 75% and 100% of the carpool and transit commuters switch to SOV

Bangalore and Kolkata have a relatively smaller population; these two cities have been more dependent on motorbikes and cars adding to huge ownership of private vehicles causing intense congestion.

Government has urged the cities to maintain control over vehicle growth and encourages the use of public transport as key objectives for going forward. A combination of infrastructure improvement, addition of more mass transit, as well as efficient alternatives to vehicle ownership, will facilitate in curbing congestion.

It can be easily predicted that if commuters quickly return to road, the transit users are more likely to switch to SOV. We have considered three scenarios, namely when 25%, 50%, 75% and 100% of the carpool and transit users switch to SOV. The assumed scenarios are created to show a range of possibilities of the mode shift to SOV, which is highly likely post-lockdown in the country. It does not necessarily predict the actual mode shift.

The predictions for Delhi under each of the four scenarios is shown in Fig. 8. The data plotted using the BPR model can be seen to be easily fitted along the curve. We can determine from Fig. 8 that cities having more cars than the network can handle (e.g., Delhi here) are sensitive to the changes in the number of vehicles on the road. A few minutes of increment in average travel time can make a huge impact on the traffic network if multiplied by the number of road users in the city, and this can result in thousands of additional hours time spent in traffic each day. However, the rate of actual mode shift of transit and carpool users that will shift to personal vehicles or SOV depends on a multitude of factors. They may be specific of each traveller and each city, such as unemployment, cost of maintaining SOV, remote work.

We are, however, not claiming that a specific percentage of users will switch to single-occupied vehicles. The purpose of creation of the predicted scenarios is to identify the cities which are more sensitive to changes in the number of cars on the road post-lockdown in the country.

4 India's Transport Growth Journey and Its Effect on Energy and Environment

If we look at the present situation in India, there is an urgent need to conserve energy and land, control pollution and "greenhouse gas emissions", and to alleviate poverty.

Urban transport has been a major cause and a solution to combat these issues. The need of the hour is planned urban mobility solutions where all categories of road users are facing problems in commuting.

If we look at the scenario before the pandemic brought the world to a standstill the increment in the number of vehicles on the road has caused problems to everybody, the pedestrians do not get a safe, conflict-free and obstruction-free path to walk. The cyclists have to fight for the space to cycle with fast moving motorized modes of transport, many a time risking their lives. This is due to overcrowding of vehicles reducing the area of parking, compelling people to park their vehicles out of the allotted area.

The users of shared vehicles face long waiting periods, uncertainty in travel time and difficult conditions of travel. The movement of personal motorized modes of transport is slowed down by the slow-moving passenger and goods traffic and face significant delays at traffic signals and road junctions. Road users get restless leading to road rage, rash driving and accidents.

The use of desirable modes, walk, bicycle and PT, is declining and the use of undesirable modes, i.e. car and two-wheelers, is growing. As a result, congestion is increasing, urban mobility as well as road safety are declining, and pollution and use of fossil fuel and accidents are rising everyday.

4.1 Transport and Environment

The second largest consumer of energy in India is the transport sector. The unprecedented and haphazard growth of the transport has been a major cause of concern, for it has not only increased pressure on the limited non-renewable energy resources but has considerably increased environmental pollution.

Increasing car dependency in India, especially in the urban areas, is most visible in vehicular emissions which cause air pollution, noise pollution and corresponding health effects. Increasing energy consumption, pollution, land intrusion and congestion are some of the areas that need urgent attention.

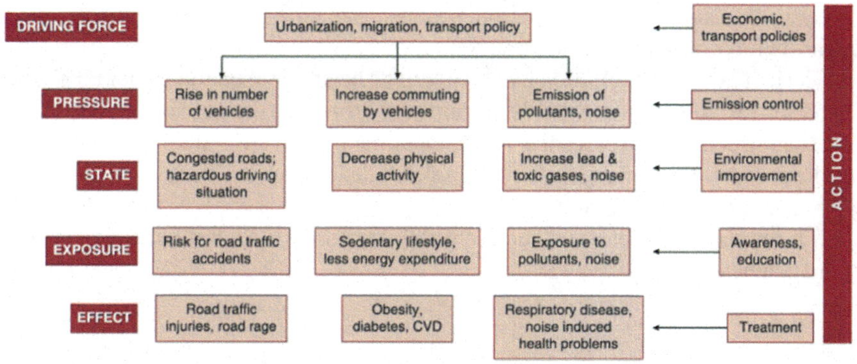

Fig. 9 Effects of Road Transport on Growth. Source: ncbi.nlm.nih.gov/pmc/articles/PMC4746948/

Transport planning is intrinsically linked to land use planning and both need to be developed together in a manner that serves the entire population and yet minimizes travel needs. An integrated master plan needs to internalize the features of sustainable urban transport.

Rapid motorization of Indian cities has led to a public health crisis in the form of increased traffic injuries and fatalities, exposure to air and noise pollution and decreased physical activity among many other adverse health and environmental impacts (Fig. 9).

4.2 *Health and Social Issues*

Adverse effects of increasingly car-based urban transport systems in India and other emerging economies are most visible on the local level. Vehicle emissions such as particulate matter, NO_x or SO_x pollute the atmosphere. Traffic noise act as a hindrance in conversation and disturbs the sleep. Road accidents pose further risk to the citizens' health, affecting especially vulnerable groups such as pedestrians, cyclists or children.

The transport sector has contributed significantly to the emissions of toxic substances into the atmosphere. High demand for used automobiles might have sufficed and catered the need of the people, but it has made the situation worse for their health. Every vehicle on the road adds to the harmful substance in the atmosphere.

Many surveys reveal that 45% of the respondents claimed that they have transport-related diseases in the city. It is pertinent to note that 50% of the respondents who claim that they have transport-related health challenges have eye problems, approximately 16% has asthma and the same percentage has skin-burn diseases. In addition, 8% and 5% of the patients claim that they have upper respiratory tract infections and hypertension, respectively. Only 2% of respondents indicated that they have hearing impairment resulting from unpleasant sounds emanating from indiscriminate use of horns by motorists and record players.

The increase in air pollution has very serious health implications. Poor air quality increases respiratory ailments like asthma and bronchitis, heightens the risk of life-threatening conditions like cancer and burdens our health care system with substantial medical costs. Particulate matter is singlehandedly responsible for up to 30, 000 premature deaths each year.

It is impossible to reduce all environmental exposures to a level at which the risk to human health is zero.

4.3 Personal Vehicles and Their Impact

Use of personal motorized vehicles and its significant contribution to air pollution, greenhouse gas emissions and fossil fuel consumption are well accepted. The main reason for the increasing use of personal vehicles is the reluctance of the people to travel in public transports (PTs) for the inefficiency in maintaining the quality of the transport. Not until this situation was tackled that Covid-19 hit the country, making the situation even worse where even a greater population will now switch to a personal mode of commute, turning the whole situation gross.

Simultaneously, there is an urgent need to put a restraint on the use of personal vehicles. Government of India is already supporting measures such as traffic-calmed areas, pedestrianized areas, car limited zones, congestion pricing zones, no-emission zones, high parking charges, park & ride facility and other economic instruments to control the indiscriminate use of personal motorized modes. However, these may not suffice in the current panic-like situation.

Increase in the number of PT would not suffice in such a situation of crisis. The pandemic is more likely to force people to choose private vehicle ownership for the fear of infection, reducing their dependency on PTs.

AQI calculates the air pollutants and particulate matter, nitrogen oxide, sulphur dioxide, ozone, carbon monoxide, etc. The ones that are of most concern is particulate matter with a diameter of 2.5 and 10 microns. The PT of these sizes cannot be removed and filtered from the body.

It is obvious that low levels of air pollution reached during the lockdown have considerably reduced the particulate matter in the atmosphere, thus reducing the deaths to approximately six lakhs. Due to the restricted activities during the period of lockdown, the particulate matter was reduced by 52% nationwide.

According to the Central Government's System of Air Quality and Weather Forecasting and Research, all the sources of pollution have decreased during the lockdown period to a considerably lower level which has not been seen in the past four decades.

These changes are however temporary, and once the lockdown is brought to closure, the vehicles will increase at an alarming rate due to a sudden switch to SOV or personal vehicles. A measure to save oneself from one deadly disease, i.e. Covid-19, would push them to the risk of another.

This situation needs dire and urgent attention to the public transport in India is not very developed and walkable and cycling environment needs to be promoted at a larger scale. With lakhs of travel trips a day, cities without adequate measures to tackle the situation will lock in an enormous amount of pollution and carbon.

There is a rise of 7–14 time more pollutants contributed by car or two-wheelers than by buses in Delhi in every trip. There is a constant decline in the usage of the buses in Delhi which is expected to witness even a steeper decline post-lockdown.

4.4 Measures to Curb the Traffic Upsurge

With the unlocking of the cities, there will be steep inclination in the people switching to private mode of transport. The spread of the infectious disease can be easily contracted in close proximity of the infected person; therefore, people will keep off from enclosed spaces especially the shared mode of transport.

Confined and crowded environment result in easy contraction of the disease which might result in an outbreak. The restarting of the public transport with reduced crowding is an issue of paramount importance.

The safety measures should be incorporated in such a manner to protect commuters and on-board staff. Proper and regular sanitization of public transport with proper distancing might serve as a boon.

Several other ways are being discussed by the government keeping in view the welfare of the society.

Conclusion

After performing the experiment with the help of the given data, it is observed that the increase in the average travel time is only by few minutes. This may appear as a minimal change, but the delay takes place in each trip. To understand the actual time-lapse if it is multiplied by the total number of travellers in the city, even a minute of change will result in thousands of additional hours in the traffic.

The data on road commute mode and travel time in different cities has been accumulated from the verified sources such as State Resource Centre, NITI Aayog and Transport Sector of India.

A BPR model is further used to establish a relation between the average travel time to the estimated number of commuters travelling by car. The resulting travel time is thus deduced using the BPR model by estimating the number of cars on the road wherein the transit and carpool users switch to single-occupancy vehicles.

Therefore, it can be concluded that

- When the number of vehicles is more than the capacity of the road. The increasing cars are inimical to everyone's commute. This is calculated and analysed using the BPR model.
- Covid-19 brought serious implication in the mode shift of traffic. The imposition of lockdown throughout the country resulted in deserted roads thereby decreasing the pollution. With the reopening, traffic will eventually spring back. If transit ridership does not return, travel time will increase, sometimes dramatically.
- A possible increase in travel time per trip is of 5–20 minutes in high-transit cities, which add up to several hundreds of thousands of hours of travel time each day.
- These discordant and erratic increases are avoidable if transit ridership resumes in accordance with car traffic.

Acknowledgements The authors are thankful to the Government of India and their respective bodies for putting up important data related to urban transport which was the main source of data for the analysis.

References

1. *Transforming India's Mobility–a Perspective.* NITI Aayog and Boston Consulting Group (BCG). 2018
2. Bhandari, A., Juyal, S., Maini, H., Saxena, A., Srivastava, A.: Moving forward together-enabling shared mobility in India. NITI Aayog, Global Mobility Submit (2018)
3. Bureau of Public Roads. Traffic assignment manual. U.S. Department of Commerce, Urban Planning Division. Washington DC. (1964)
4. Bureau of Public Roads. Traffic Assignment Manual for Application With a Large, High Speed Computer. U.S. Department of Commerce, Bureau of Public Roads, Office of Planning, Urban Planning Division, Washington, DC (1964)
5. Daskin, M.S.: Urban transportation networks: Equilibrium analysis with mathematical programming methods. JSTOR (1985)
6. Hu, Y., Barbour, W., Samaranayake, S., Work, D.: Impacts of Covid–19 mode shift on road traffic. arXiv:2005.01610v1 [physics.soc-ph]. 4 May, 2020
7. Saberi, M., Hamedmoghadam, H., Ashfaq, M., Hosseini, S.A., Gu, Z., Shafiei, S., Nair, D.J., Dixit, V., Gardner, L., Waller, S.T., et al.: A simple contagion process describes spreading of traffic jams in urban networks. Nat. Commun. **11**(1), 1–9 (2020)
8. Çolak, S., Lima, A., Gonzáalez, M.C.: Understanding congested travel in urban areas. Nat. Commun. **7**(1), 1–8 (2016)
9. Wong, W., Wong, S.C.: Network topological effects on the macroscopic bureau of public roads function. Transportmetrica A: Transp. Sci. **12**(3), 272–296 (2016)
10. Kucharski, R., Drabicki, A.: Estimating macroscopic volume delay functions with the traffic density derived from measured speeds and flows. J. Adv. Transp. (2017)
11. Highway Capacity Manual. Highway capacity manual. Washington DC. 2 (2000)
12. Dowling, R.G., Singh, R., Cheng, W.W.: Accuracy and performance of improved speed-flow curves. Transp. Res. Rec. **1646**(1), 9–17 (1998)
13. Florian, M., Nguyen, S.: Recent experience with equilibrium methods for the study of a congested urban area. In: Traffic Equilibrium Methods, pp. 382–395. Springer (1976)

14. Bandyopadhyay, K.: Life in transit is easy in Kolkata, shows study. The Times Of India. November 2, 2018
15. Shaikh, Z.: Census data: Most Mumbai commuters travel less than 10 km, says report. The Indian Express. Novermber 16, 2015
16. Chin, V., Jaafar, M., Subudhi, S., Shelomentsev., N., Do, D., Prawiradinata, I.: Unlocking cities: The impact of ridesharing across India. Boston Consulting Group (2018)

Analysis of Covid-19 Virus Spreading Statistics by the Use of a New Modified Weibull Distribution

Abdelmajid Belafhal, Salma Chib, and Talha Usman

Abstract Since the World Health Organization has declared Coronavirus a pandemic, researchers have given several interpretations on how this virus is spreads. In the present work, in anticipation of substantial fatal effects on health of people following this human-to-human spread, we aim to propose a new six parameter-modified Weibull distribution to analyze the spread of Covid-19 virus. We apply this model to study the cumulative cases infected in some countries, we give a global analysis of the statistical data of the pandemic, and we prove that our new distribution efficiently generalizes some existing models and fits correctly some data registered from February to June 2020. We use these results to assess the potential for human-to-human spread to occur around the globe.

Keywords Covid-19 virus · Modified Weibull distribution · Moments · Reliability function · Statistical properties

1 Introduction and Preliminaries

In December 2019, Covid-19, as a new coronavirus declared as a global pandemic by the World Health Organization, is spreading quickly in more than 214 countries. A large cases reported by June 30, 2020, became infected in the world by this novel virus which caused in the world 10435321 cases and 508844 deaths. These numbers are distributed as: 396674 cases and 52699 deaths in Africa, 5318248 cases and 251324 deaths in America, 2272566 cases and 56207 deaths in Asia and 2437636 cases and 191255 deaths in Europe [1]. The basic issue to be addressed is to give

A. Belafhal · S. Chib
LPNAMME, Laser Physics Group, Department of Physics, Faculty of Sciences, Chouaïb Doukkali University, P. B 20, 24000 El Jadida, Morocco

T. Usman (✉)
Department of Mathematics, School of Basic and Applied Sciences, Lingaya's Vidyapeeth, Faridabad 121002, Haryana, India

P. Agarwal et al. (eds.), *Analysis of Infectious Disease Problems (Covid-19) and Their Global Impact*, Infosys Science Foundation Series,
https://doi.org/10.1007/978-981-16-2450-6_8

an analysis of the Covid-19 virus spreading statistics on a lot of cases from some countries.

For this problematic, we have studied different published models used in the past to model some distributions, because we have need to promote the use of statistical analyses that provide guidance for the evolution of the virus. Until now, many researches have been developed to study the development, propagation law and prediction of Covid-19 [2–13].

In the past and for modeling lifetime data, many distributions are proposed. The most popular ne is the Weibull distribution introduced in 1951 by Weibull [14] and applied by Bailly and Bell [15] in forestry and in other fields [16]. Many works have been investigated about modified forms of the Weibull distribution with two [17–19], three [20–24] four [25–31] and five parameters [32–39].

In this work, we propose a modified Weibull distribution, referred as NMW_B, with six parameters for given a generalization of some previous distributions. To our knowledge, no study has proposed with this form and with this number of parameters. The present investigation, based on the results of Refs. [31, 36], is used to analyze the Covid-19 virus spreading statistics by taking different countries as examples.

For the present investigation, we recall in the following some theoretical notions.

1.1 The New Model NMW_B Distribution

We introduce our new modified Weibull distribution by proposing the following cumulative distribution function (CDF)

$$F(x) = \left[1 - e^{-\left(\alpha x^{\theta} + \beta x^{\gamma} e^{\chi x}\right)}\right]\left[1 + \lambda e^{-\left(\alpha x^{\theta} + \beta x^{\gamma} e^{\chi x}\right)}\right],\ x \geq 0. \tag{1}$$

In this expression, the five parameters $\alpha,\ \beta,\ \theta,\ \gamma$ and χ are shape parameters and λ, called the transmuted parameter, is defined by $-1 \leq \lambda \leq 1$. α is a non-negative scale parameter representing the characteristic life and χ is the acceleration parameter. From Eq. (1), and by deriving the CDF, one can determine the failure probability density function (PDF) of our model as

$$f(x) = \left[\alpha\theta x^{\theta-1} + \beta\left(\gamma + \chi x\right) x^{\gamma-1} e^{\chi x}\right] e^{-\left(\alpha x^{\theta} + \beta x^{\gamma} e^{\chi x}\right)}\left[1 - \lambda + 2\lambda e^{-\left(\alpha x^{\theta} + \beta x^{\gamma} e^{\chi x}\right)}\right]. \tag{2}$$

This PDF can be also expressed in terms of survival and hazard functions S_w and h_w of the Weibull and modified Weibull distributions S_{MW} and h_{MW} as

$$f(x) = [h_W(x, \alpha, \theta) + h_{MW}(x, \beta, \gamma, \chi)]S_W(x, \alpha, \theta)S_{MW}(x, \beta, \gamma, \chi)[1 - \lambda + 2\lambda S_W S_{MW}]. \tag{3}$$

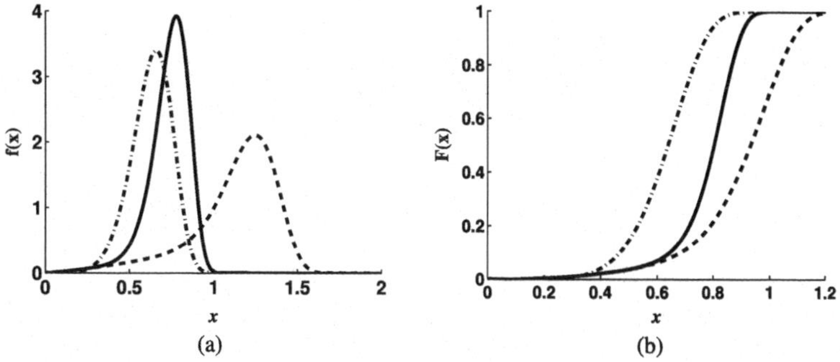

Fig. 1 (a) Probability Density Function and (b) Cumulative Distribution Function for the NMW_B distribution with the following parameters: Solid curve ($\alpha = 0.087, \beta = 4, \gamma = 6.03, \theta = 2.3, \chi = 0.01, \lambda = 1$), Dotdash curve ($\alpha = 5, \beta = 0.8, \gamma = 9, \theta = 6.3, \chi = 0.01, \lambda = 1$) and Dashed curve ($\alpha = 0.087, \beta = 0.05, \gamma = 6.03, \theta = 2.3, \chi = 0.01, \lambda = 1$)

By taking values of the six parameters, one obtains the NMW_B distribution behavior described by the corresponding PDF. We illustrate in Fig. 1 the comportment of the PDF and the CDF for some special packets of parameters interesting in the description of the propagation analysis of the Covid-19. In Fig. 1, and based on a preliminary analysis of the evolution of the pandemic, we observe that the PDF of our new model has the same shape of the propagation of Covid-19 in some countries.

1.2 The Reliability Function

This function is defined as [31, 40]

$$R(x) = 1 - F(x), \tag{4}$$

which gives the hazard function h by the relation

$$h(x) = \frac{f(x)}{1 - F(x)} = \frac{f(x)}{R(x)}. \tag{5}$$

Also, we can evaluate the cumulative hazard function by the expression

$$H(x) = -\ln|F(x)|. \tag{6}$$

For our model, these functions are given, respectively by

$$R(x) = e^{-\left(\alpha x^{\theta} + \beta x^{\gamma} e^{\chi x}\right)} \left[(1 - \lambda) + \lambda e^{-\left(\alpha x^{\theta} + \beta x^{\gamma} e^{\chi x}\right)}\right], \tag{7}$$

$$h(x) = \frac{\left[\alpha\theta x^{\theta-1} + \beta(\gamma + \chi x) x^{\gamma-1} e^{\chi x}\right]\left[1 - \lambda + 2\lambda e^{-\left(\alpha x^{\theta} + \beta x^{\gamma} e^{\chi x}\right)}\right]}{\left[(1-\lambda) + \lambda e^{-\left(\alpha x^{\theta} + \beta x^{\gamma} e^{\chi x}\right)}\right]}, \tag{8}$$

and

$$H(x) = \ln\left|\frac{1}{1 + \lambda e^{-\left(\alpha x^{\theta} + \beta x^{\gamma} e^{\chi x}\right)}}\right| - \ln\left|1 - e^{-\left(\alpha x^{\theta} + \beta x^{\gamma} e^{\chi x}\right)}\right|. \tag{9}$$

Figure 2 shows the patterns of these functions in terms of the variable x with different choices of our six parameters.

1.3 Moments of the Distribution

The kth moments of random variable X with the PDF $f(x)$ or the CDF $F(x)$ is defined by [30, 31]

$$\mu_k = E(X) = \int_0^{\infty} x^k f(x)\,dx = \int_0^{\infty} x^k dF(x). \tag{10}$$

From this definition, one can evaluate other coefficients of the proposed distribution as

$$CV = \sqrt{\frac{\mu_2}{\mu_1^2} - 1}, \tag{11}$$

$$CS = \frac{\mu_3 - 3\mu_1\mu_2 + 2\mu_1^3}{\left(\mu_2 - \mu_1^2\right)^{3/2}}, \tag{12}$$

and

$$CK = \frac{\mu_4 - 4\mu_1\mu_3 + 6\mu_1^2\mu_2 - 3\mu_1^4}{\left(\mu_2 - \mu_1^2\right)^2}. \tag{13}$$

These coefficients are called: the coefficient of Variation, coefficient of Skewness and coefficient of Kurtosis, respectively. We illustrate in Fig. 3 the behavior of these coefficients in terms of the parameter γ for different values of λ. The other parameters are chosen as follows: $\alpha = 5$, $\beta = 0.8$, $\theta = 6.3$ and $\chi = 0.01$.

From Fig. 3, we can clearly see that the three coefficients keep a similar shape profile for the three values of the parameter λ. It is also observed from these plots that the CV decreases with the increment of γ, the CS first decreases and reaches its

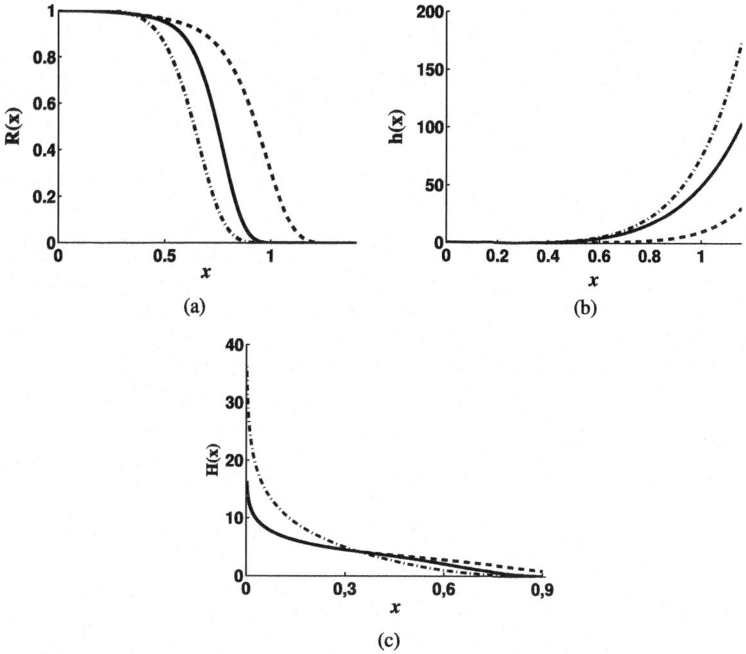

Fig. 2 Representation of (a) the reliability function (b) the hazard function and (c) the cumulative hazard function for the NMW_B distribution with the following parameters: solid curve ($\alpha = 0.087$, $\beta = 4$,$\gamma = 6.03$, $\theta = 2.3$, $\chi = 0.01$, $\lambda = 1$), dotdash curve ($\alpha = 5$, $\beta = 0.8$, $\gamma = 9$, $\theta = 6.3$, $\chi = 0.01$, $\lambda = 1$) and dashed curve ($\alpha = 0.087$, $\beta = 0.05$, $\gamma = 6.03$, $\theta = 2.3$, $\chi = 0.01$,$\lambda = 1$)

minimum at $\gamma = 2.0$ and its maximum around $\gamma = 4.5$. However, the CK takes its maximum around $\gamma = 3.6$.

Note that, for the case of $\lambda = 0$ corresponding to the distribution of Almalki and Yuan [36] and by setting $\chi = 0$ and $\theta = 1$, we obtain the different coefficients of the distribution of Khan and King [31].

Another important moment of the distribution is the moment generating function (MGF), which is obtained from the measure of the central tendency and of the dispersion. This function is defined as

$$M_X(t) = \int_0^\infty e^{xt} f(x)\, dx. \tag{14}$$

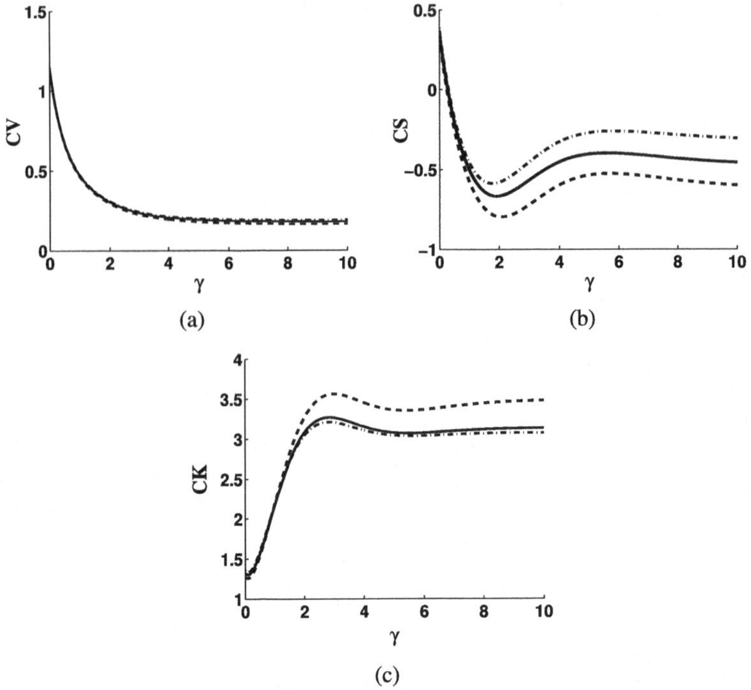

Fig. 3 Illustration in terms of the parameter γ of (a): the coefficient of variation, (b): coefficient of skewness and (c): coefficient of kurtosis, respectively, for the NMW_B distribution with the three values of λ dashed curve: $\lambda = -0.4$, solid curve: $\lambda = 0$ and dotdash curve $\lambda = 0.6$

1.4 Order Statistics

The PDF of the rth order statistic $X_{(r)}$ $(1 \leq r \leq n)$ from the continuous distribution of a random sample $(X_{1:n} \leq \ldots \leq X_{n:n})$ is defined by [40]

$$f_{r:n}(x) = \frac{F(x)^{r-1}(1 - F(x))^{n-r} f(x)}{B(r, n - r + 1)}, \tag{15}$$

where B is the beta function given by

$$B(r, n - r + 1) = \frac{1}{C_{r:n}} = \frac{(r-1)!\,(n-r)!}{n!}. \tag{16}$$

We define also the joint PDF of $X_{r:n}$ and $X_{s:n}$ $(1 \leq r \leq s \leq n)$ by

$$f_{r:s:n}(x, u) = C_{r:s:n}[F(x)]^{r-1}[F(u) - F(x)]^{s-r-1}[1 - F(x)]^{n-s} f(x) f(u), \tag{17}$$

where

$$C_{r:s:n} = \frac{n!}{(r-1)!\,(s-r-1)!\,(n-s)!} \text{ and } 0 \leq x \leq u \leq \infty. \tag{18}$$

1.5 Parameter Estimation

We consider a random sample $x_1, \ldots, x_n$ with n observations from the NMW_B distribution with six parameters $(\alpha, \beta, \theta, \gamma, \chi, \lambda)$ and we use the approach to estimate the parameters called the maximum likelihood. We define the likelihood function of the model by [40]

$$L\left(x_1, \ldots, x_n, \alpha, \beta, \theta, \gamma, \chi, \lambda\right) = \prod_{i=1}^{n} f\left(x_i\right). \tag{19}$$

So, the log-likelihood function of this expression is given by

$$\mathcal{L} = \ln\left(L\right) = \sum_{i=1}^{n} \ln f\left(x_i\right). \tag{20}$$

The estimating equations are obtained by differentiating this last expression with respect to each parameter then equating it to zero.

1.6 Relationship with Weibull-Related Results

We give in Table 1 a list of models that are generalized by NMW_B distribution with their CDF and parameters.

2 Main Results

2.1 Statistical Properties

Here, we announce some theorems to evaluate the above expressions of the proposed distribution NMW_B as the kth moment

Theorem 1 *The kth moment of the NMW_B is given as follows*

$$\mu_k = \frac{1}{\alpha^{k/\theta}} \left(\frac{k}{\theta}\right)! \left[\frac{\lambda}{2^{k/\theta}} R_k^{\theta,\gamma}\left(x_2, y_2\right) - \left(\lambda - 1\right) R_k^{\theta,\gamma}\left(x_1, y_1\right)\right], \tag{21}$$

Table 1 CDF and special parameters of sub-models of NMW_B distribution

Distribution	$F(x)$	Parameters	Reference
NMW_B	$[1-e^{-(\alpha x^{\theta}+\beta x^{\gamma}e^{\chi x})}][1+\lambda e^{-(\alpha x^{\theta}+\beta x^{\gamma}e^{\chi x})}]$	$(\alpha, \beta, \theta, \gamma, \chi, \lambda)$	Present work
TMW_A	$[1-e^{-(\alpha x^{\theta}+\beta x^{\gamma}e^{\chi x})}]$	$(\alpha, \beta, \theta, \gamma, \lambda, 0)$	[36]
TMW_K	$[1-e^{-(\alpha x+\beta x^{\gamma})}][1+\lambda e^{-(\alpha x+\beta x^{\gamma})}]$	$(\alpha, \eta, 1, \beta, 0, \lambda)$	[31]
TME	$[1-e^{-(\alpha x+\beta x)}][1+\lambda e^{-(\alpha x+\beta x)}]$	$(\alpha, \beta, 1, 1, 0, \lambda)$	[31]
TMR	$[1-e^{-(\alpha x+\beta x^2)}][1+\lambda e^{-(\alpha x+\beta x^2)}]$	$(\alpha, \beta, 1, 2, 0, \lambda)$	[31]
MW	$[1-e^{-(\alpha x+\beta x^{\gamma})}]$	$(\alpha, \beta, 1, \gamma, 0, 0)$	[31]
MR	$[1-e^{-(\alpha x+\beta x^2)}]$	$(\alpha, \beta, 1, 2, 0, 0)$	[31]
ME	$[1-e^{-(\alpha x+\beta x)}]$	$(\alpha, \beta, 1, 1, 0, 0)$	[31]
TW	$(1-e^{-\beta x^{\gamma}})(1+\lambda e^{-\beta x^{\gamma}})$	$(0, \beta, 0, \gamma, 0, \lambda)$	[31]
TR	$(1-e^{-\beta x^2})(1+\lambda e^{-\beta x^2})$	$(0, \beta, 0, 2, 0, \lambda)$	[31]
TE	$(1-e^{-\beta x})(1+\lambda e^{-\beta x})$	$(0, \beta, 0, 1, 0, \lambda)$	[31]
W	$(1-e^{-\beta x^{\gamma}})$	$(0, \beta, 0, \gamma, 0, 0)$	[14]
R	$(1-e^{-\beta x^2})$	$(0, \beta, 0, 2, 0, 0)$	[19]
E	$(1-e^{-\beta x})$	$(0, \beta, 0, 1, 0, 0)$	[19]

where the function $R_k^{\theta,\gamma}$ *is defined by*

$$R_k^{\theta,\gamma}(x, y) = \sum_{m,n=0}^{\infty} \left(\frac{k}{\theta}\right)_{\frac{m\gamma+n}{\theta}} \frac{x^m}{m!} \frac{(my)^n}{n!}, \tag{22}$$

with

$$x_1 = -\frac{\beta}{\alpha^{\gamma/\theta}},\ x_2 = -\frac{2\beta}{(2\alpha)^{\gamma/\theta}}, \tag{23}$$

$$y_1 = \frac{\chi}{\alpha^{1/\theta}},\ y_2 = \frac{\chi}{(2\alpha)^{1/\theta}} \text{ and } (\alpha)_p = \frac{\Gamma(\alpha+p)}{\Gamma(\alpha)}. \tag{24}$$

Proof By substituting Eq. (1), which can be written as

$$F(x) = 1 + (\lambda - 1)\, e^{-(\alpha x^{\theta}+\beta x^{\gamma}e^{\chi x})} - \lambda e^{-2(\alpha x^{\theta}+\beta x^{\gamma}e^{\chi x})}, \tag{25}$$

into Eq. (10), one obtains

$$\mu_k = \lambda k I^{(2)} - (\lambda - 1)\, k I^{(1)}, \tag{26}$$

where

$$I^{(a)} = \int_0^{\infty} x^{k-1} e^{-a\left(\alpha x^{\theta} + \beta x^{\gamma} e^{\chi x}\right)} dx, \tag{27}$$

with $a = 1$ or 2.
To evaluate the integral $I^{(a)}$, we use the Taylor expansion of exponential function twice. So, Eq. (27) can be written as

$$I^{(a)} = \sum_{m,n=0}^{\infty} \frac{(-a\beta)^m}{m!} \frac{(m\chi)^n}{n!} \int_0^{\infty} x^{k-1} x^{m\gamma+n} e^{-a\alpha x^{\theta}} dx. \tag{28}$$

The integral in this last equation can be evaluated by the help of the following identity [41]

$$\int_0^{\infty} x^{\nu-1} e^{-\mu x^p} dx = \frac{\Gamma\left({}^{\nu}/_{p}\right)}{p\mu^{\nu/p}}, \tag{29}$$

with $\mathrm{Re}\,(\mu) = \mathrm{Re}\,(a\alpha) > 0$, $\mathrm{Re}\,(\nu) = \mathrm{Re}\,(m\gamma + n + k) > 0$ and $p = \theta > 0$.
Then, $I^{(a)}$ becomes

$$I^{(a)} = \sum_{m,n=0}^{\infty} \frac{(-a\beta)^m}{m!} \frac{(m\chi)^n}{n!} \frac{1}{\theta (a\alpha)^{\frac{m\gamma+n+k}{\theta}}} \Gamma\left(\frac{m\gamma + n + k}{\theta}\right). \tag{30}$$

We use the function given by Eq. (22), and $I^{(a)}$ can be rearranged as

$$I^{(a)} = \frac{1}{\theta} \frac{1}{(a\alpha)^{k/\theta}} \Gamma\left(\frac{k}{\theta}\right) R_k^{\theta,\gamma}\left(x_a, y_a\right). \tag{31}$$

Finally, by inserting $I^{(1)}$ and $I^{(2)}$ in Eq. (26), one obtains

$$\mu_k = \frac{\lambda k}{\theta} \frac{1}{(2\alpha)^{k/\theta}} \Gamma\left(\frac{k}{\theta}\right) R_k^{\theta,\gamma}\left(x_2, y_2\right) - (\lambda - 1) \frac{k}{\theta} \frac{1}{\alpha^{k/\theta}} \Gamma\left(\frac{k}{\theta}\right) R_k^{\theta,\gamma}\left(x_1, y_1\right), \tag{32}$$

with x_1, x_2, y_1 and y_2 are given by Eqs. (23) and (24).
So, we get the required result. This completes the proof. □

Corollary 1 *If $\lambda = 0$ and $\chi = \lambda$, the kth moment of the NMW_B distribution is given as follows*

$$\begin{aligned} \mu_{k_A} &= \frac{1}{\alpha^{k/\theta}} \left(\frac{k}{\theta}\right)! R_k^{\theta,\gamma}\left(-\frac{\beta}{\alpha^{\gamma/\theta}}, \frac{\lambda}{\alpha^{1/\theta}}\right) \\ &= \frac{k}{\theta} \sum_{n,m=0}^{\infty} \frac{(-\beta)^n}{n!} \frac{(n\lambda)^m}{m!} \alpha^{-\left(\frac{n\gamma+m+k}{\theta}\right)} \Gamma\left(\frac{n\gamma + m + k}{\theta}\right), \end{aligned} \tag{33}$$

This result is the same as the kth moment found by Almalki and Yuan [36].

Corollary 2 *If $\theta = 1$, $\beta = \eta$, $\gamma = \beta$, $\chi = 0$ and $\lambda \neq 0$, one finds the kth moment corresponding to TMW_K distribution*

$$\mu_{k_K} = (1-\lambda)\sum_{m=0}^{\infty}\frac{k\Gamma(k+m\beta)}{\alpha^{m\beta+k}}\frac{(-\eta)^m}{m!} + \lambda\sum_{m=0}^{\infty}\frac{k\Gamma(k+m\beta)}{(2\alpha)^{m\beta+k}}\frac{(-2\eta)^m}{m!}. \tag{34}$$

Theorem 2 *If X has NMW_B distribution, then its moment generating function is given by*

$$M_X(t) = \sum_{l=0}^{\infty}\frac{t^l}{l!}\mu_l, \tag{35a}$$

and

$$M_X(t) = \sum_{l=0}^{\infty}\frac{\left({}^t/_{\alpha^\theta}\right)^l}{l!}\left(\frac{l}{\theta}\right)!\left[\frac{\lambda}{2^{l/\theta}}R_l^{\theta,\gamma}(x_2, y_2) - (\lambda-1)R_l^{\theta,\gamma}(x_1, y_1)\right], \tag{35b}$$

where the function $R_l^{\theta,\gamma}$ is given by Eq. (22) and the other variables are defined by Eqs. (23) and (24).

Proof Starting from Eq. (14) and by applying the Taylor expansion of e^{tx} , one obtains for M_X

$$M_X(t) = \sum_{l=0}^{\infty}\frac{t^l}{l!}\int_0^{\infty}x^l f(x)dx. \tag{36}$$

The integral of this expression is the lth moment μ_l, so

$$M_X(t) = \sum_{l=0}^{\infty}\frac{t^l}{l!}\mu_l. \tag{37}$$

By using Theorem 1, Eq. (35-b) is proved, and this completes the proof. □

Corollary 3 *If $\lambda = 0$,*

$$M_X^A(t) = \sum_{l=0}^{\infty}\frac{\left({}^t/_{\alpha^\theta}\right)^l}{l!}\left(\frac{l}{\theta}\right)!R_l^{\theta,\gamma}(x_1, y_1). \tag{38}$$

Proof It is easy to prove this corollary. So, by using the expression of R given by Eq. (22), this last equation becomes

$$M_X^A(t) = \sum_{l,m,n=0}^{\infty} (1)_{l/\theta} \left(\frac{l}{\theta}\right)_{\frac{m\gamma+n}{\theta}} \frac{x^l}{l!} \frac{y^m}{m!} \frac{(mz)^n}{n!}, \tag{39}$$

where

$$x = \frac{t}{\alpha\theta},\ y = -\frac{2\beta}{(2\alpha)^{\gamma/\theta}} \text{ and } z = \frac{\chi}{(2\alpha)^{1/\theta}}. \tag{40a}$$

□

Corollary 4 *If* $\theta = 1,\ \beta = \eta,\ \gamma = \beta,\ \chi = 0$ *and* $\lambda \neq 0$

$$M_X^K(t) = \sum_{l=0}^{\infty} t^l \left[\frac{\lambda}{2^l} R_l^{1,\beta}(x_2, y_2) - (\lambda - 1) R_l^{1,\beta}(x_1, y_1)\right], \tag{41}$$

where $x_1 = -\frac{2\eta}{(2\alpha)^\beta},\ x_2 = \frac{1}{2^{(\beta-1)}},\ y_1 = 0$ *and* $y_2 = \frac{1}{2}$.

Proof For the proof of this identity, we use the expression of the function $R_l^{1,\beta}$ given by

$$R_l^{1,\beta}(x_1, y_1) = \sum_{m=0}^{\infty} (l)_{m\beta} \frac{x_1^m}{m!}, \tag{41a}$$

and

$$R_l^{1,\beta}(x_2, y_2) = \sum_{m,n=0}^{\infty} (l)_{(m\beta+n)} \frac{x_2^m}{m!} \frac{(my_2)^n}{n!}, \tag{41b}$$

and the expression of the moment generating function is

$$\begin{aligned} M_X^S(t) = \lambda \sum_{l,m,n=0}^{\infty} (1)_l (l)_{(m\beta+n)} \frac{\left(\frac{t}{2}\right)^l}{l!} \frac{\left({}^1/_{2^{\beta-1}}\right)^m}{m!} \frac{\left({}^m/_2\right)^n}{n!} \\ + (1-\lambda) \sum_{l,m=0}^{\infty} (1)_l (l)_{m\beta} \frac{(t)^l}{l!} \frac{\left({}^{-2\eta}/_{(2\alpha)^\beta}\right)^m}{m!}. \end{aligned} \tag{42}$$

□

Table 2 Quantile of particular distributions

Distribution	Parameters $(\alpha, \beta, \theta, \gamma, \chi, \lambda)$	The qth quantile of the distribution
TMW_K	$(\alpha, \eta, 1, \beta, 0, \lambda)$	See Eq. (8) of Ref. [31]
TR	$(0, \beta, 0, 2, 0, \lambda)$	$\sqrt{-\frac{A}{\beta}}$
$TLFRD$	$(\alpha, \beta, 0, 2, 0, \lambda)$	$\frac{-\alpha+\sqrt{\alpha^2-4\beta A}}{2\beta}$
TE	$(0, \beta, 0, 1, 0, \lambda)$	$\frac{-A}{\beta}$
TW	$(0, \beta, 0, \gamma, 0, \lambda)$	$\left(\frac{-A}{\beta}\right)^{1/\gamma}$
TME	$(\alpha, \beta, 1, 1, 0, \lambda)$	$\frac{-(\alpha+A)}{\beta}$
TMR	$(\alpha, \beta, 1, 2, 0, \lambda)$	$\left[\frac{-(\alpha+A)}{\beta}\right]^{1/2}$
TWD	$(0, \beta, 0, \gamma, 0, \lambda)$	$\left(-\frac{\ln A}{\beta}\right)^{1/\gamma}$

Theorem 3 *The quantile t_q of NMW_B distribution is given as the real solution of the following equation*

$$\beta t_q^{\gamma} e^{\chi t_q} + \alpha t_q^{\theta} + \ln\left[1 - \frac{(1+\lambda) - \sqrt{(1+\lambda)^2 - 4\lambda q}}{2\lambda}\right] = 0. \tag{43}$$

Proof For this reason, we get that $a = \alpha t_q^{\theta} + \beta t_q^{\theta} e^{\chi t_q}$ and it easy to find the solution of the equation $F(x) = t_q$ with $x = e^{-a}$, which can be written as

$$x = e^{-a} = 1 - \frac{(1+\lambda) - \sqrt{(1+\lambda)^2 - 4\lambda q}}{2\lambda}. \tag{44}$$

After some algebraic manipulations, one finds Eq. (43). This completes the proof. □

From Theorem 3, one can deduce the median of NMW_B distribution by taking $q = \frac{1}{2}$. We put $t_{1/2} = t_m$ which is the solution of the following equation

$$\beta t_m^{\gamma} e^{\chi t_m} + \alpha t_m^{\theta} + B = 0, \tag{45}$$

with

$$B = \ln\left(\frac{\lambda - 1 + \sqrt{\lambda^2 + 1}}{2\lambda}\right).$$

From Eq. (44), we can deduce some special cases which are listed in Table 2 for $\beta = 0$, t_q is given by $t_q = \left(\frac{-A}{\alpha}\right)^{1/\theta}$ with $A = \ln\left[1 - \frac{(1+\lambda)-\sqrt{(1+\lambda)^2-4\lambda q}}{2\lambda}\right]$.

2.2 Least Square Estimates (LSES)

LSES are evaluated by minimizing the following quantity

$$Q = \sum_{i=1}^{n} \{F\,(t_i) - E\,[F\,(t_i)]\}^2, \tag{46}$$

where t_i $(1 \leq i \leq n)$ is the ordered sample and $E\,[F\,(t_i)] = E_i$ is given (for three methods for estimating F by graphical procedure) as [42]

$$-\ for\ the\ mean\ rank:\ E_i = \frac{i}{(n+1)}, \tag{47a}$$

$$-\ for\ the\ median\ rank:\ E_i = \frac{i-0.3}{n+0.4}\ and \tag{47b}$$

$$-\ for\ the\ symmetrical\ rank\ CDF:\ E_i = \frac{i-0.5}{n}. \tag{47c}$$

Theorem 4 *The estimators of NMW_B distribution are governed by*

- *for $p = \lambda$*

$$\sum_{i=1}^{n} [(1 - f\,(t_i))\,(1 + \lambda f\,(t_i)) - E_i]\,(1 - f\,(t_i))\,f\,(t_i) = 0, \tag{48}$$

- *and for $p \neq \lambda$*

$$\sum_{i=1}^{n} [(1 - f\,(t_i))\,(1 + \lambda f\,(t_i)) - E_i]\,(\lambda - 1 - 2\lambda f\,(t_i))\,\frac{\partial f\,(t_i)}{\partial p} = 0, \tag{49}$$

with $p = \alpha, \beta, \theta, \gamma$ or χ.

Proof For our proposal distribution, Eq. (46) is expressed as follows

$$Q = \sum_{i=1}^{n} [(1 - g(t_i))(1 + \lambda g(t_i)) - E_i]^2, \tag{50}$$

where

$$g\,(t_i) = e^{-\left(\alpha t_i^{\theta} + \beta t_i^{\gamma} e^{\chi t_i}\right)}. \tag{51}$$

Note that the expression of Q depends on six parameters and in the following, we give the corresponding equations deduced by minimizing Eq. (48) with respect first

to the parameter λ and second to the parameter $p = \alpha, \beta, \theta, \gamma$ or χ.
So, Theorem 4 is proved. □

By using the following expressions

$$\frac{\partial f(t_i)}{\partial \alpha} = -t_i^{\theta} f(t_i), \tag{52a}$$

$$\frac{\partial f(t_i)}{\partial \beta} = -t_i^{\gamma} e^{\chi t_i} f(t_i), \tag{52b}$$

$$\frac{\partial f(t_i)}{\partial \theta} = -\alpha t_i^{\theta} f(t_i) \, ln(t_i), \tag{52c}$$

$$\frac{\partial f(t_i)}{\partial \gamma} = -\beta t_i^{\gamma} e^{\chi t_i} f(t_i) \, ln(t_i), \tag{52d}$$

and

$$\frac{\partial f(t_i)}{\partial \chi} = -\beta t_i^{\gamma+1} e^{\chi t_i} f(t_i), \tag{52e}$$

and Eqs. (48) and (49) because it is difficult to obtain a closed-form solution. One can deduce, by using an adequate numerical technique, the estimated parameters $\lambda, \alpha, \beta, \theta, \gamma$ and χ from the following equations

a- for λ

$$\sum_{i=1}^{n} u_{\lambda}(t_i) \, w(t_i) = 0, \tag{53a}$$

b- for α

$$\sum_{i=1}^{n} t_i^{\theta} u_{\lambda}(t_i) \, v_{\lambda}(t_i) = 0, \tag{53b}$$

c- for β

$$\sum_{i=1}^{n} t_i^{\gamma} e^{\chi t_i} u_{\lambda}(t_i) \, v_{\lambda}(t_i) = 0, \tag{53c}$$

d- for θ

$$\sum_{i=1}^{n} \alpha t_i^{\theta} \ln(t_i) \, u_{\lambda}(t_i) \, v_{\lambda}(t_i) = 0, \tag{53d}$$

e- for γ

$$\sum_{i=1}^{n} \beta t_i^{\gamma} e^{\chi t_i} \ln(t_i) \, u_{\lambda}(t_i) \, v_{\lambda}(t_i) = 0, \tag{53e}$$

f- and for χ

$$\sum_{i=1}^{n} \beta t_i^{\gamma+1} e^{\chi t_i} u_\lambda (t_i)\, v_\lambda (t_i) = 0, \tag{53f}$$

where

$$u_\lambda (t_i) = \left[1 - e^{-\left(\alpha t_i^\theta + \beta t_i^\gamma e^{\chi t_i}\right)}\right]\left[1 + \lambda e^{-\left(\alpha t_i^\theta + \beta t_i^\gamma e^{\chi t_i}\right)}\right], \tag{53g}$$

$$v_\lambda (t_i) = \left[\lambda - 1 - 2\lambda e^{-\left(\alpha t_i^\theta + \beta t_i^\gamma e^{\chi t_i}\right)}\right] e^{-\left(\alpha t_i^\theta + \beta t_i^\gamma e^{\chi t_i}\right)}, \tag{53h}$$

and

$$w (t_i) = \left[1 - e^{-\left(\alpha t_i^\theta + \beta t_i^\gamma e^{\chi t_i}\right)}\right] e^{-\left(\alpha t_i^\theta + \beta t_i^\gamma e^{\chi t_i}\right)}. \tag{53i}$$

2.3 Order Statistics

In this subsection, we present the formulae about the PDF of the rth order statistic and the joint PDF for NMW_B distribution.

Theorem 5 *The PDF of the rth order statistic for NMW_B distribution is given by*

$$f_{r:n} (x) = n \binom{n-1}{r-1} \sum_{l,m=0}^{r-1} \sum_{k=0}^{n-r} \binom{r-1}{l} \binom{r-1}{m} \binom{n-r}{k} \lambda^{(m+n-r-k)} \times (1-\lambda)^k \frac{(-1)^l}{\varepsilon_{lmk}} f\left(x, \alpha', \beta', \theta, \gamma, \chi, \lambda\right), \tag{54}$$

where

$$f\left(x, \alpha', \beta', \theta, \gamma, \chi, \lambda\right) = \left[\alpha' \theta x^{\theta-1} + \beta' (\gamma + \chi x) x^{\gamma-1} e^{\chi x}\right]\left[1 - \lambda + 2\lambda e^{S(x)}\right] e^{\varepsilon_{lmk} S(x)}, \tag{55a}$$

$$\alpha' = \varepsilon_{lmk} \alpha, \tag{55b}$$

$$\beta' = \varepsilon_{lmk} \beta, \tag{55c}$$

with

$$\varepsilon_{lmk} = l + m + 2n - 2r - k + 1,$$

and

$$S (x) = -\left(\alpha x^\theta + \beta x^\gamma e^{\chi x}\right). \tag{55e}$$

Proof By using the Taylor expansion of e^x and the identity $(x+y)^n = \sum_{k=0}^{n} \binom{n}{k} x^{n-k} y^k$, one obtains for each term of Eq. (15) the following expressions

$$F(x) = \left[1 - e^{S(x)}\right]\left[1 + \lambda e^{S(x)}\right], \tag{56}$$

$$\begin{aligned} [F(x)]^{r-1} &= \left[1 - e^{S(x)}\right]^{r-1}\left[1 + \lambda e^{S(x)}\right]^{r-1} \\ &= \sum_{l,m=0}^{r-1} \binom{r-1}{l}\binom{r-1}{m} (-1)^l \lambda^m e^{(l+m)S(x)}, \end{aligned} \tag{57}$$

$$[1 - F(x)] = \lambda e^{2S(x)} + (1-\lambda)\, e^{S(x)}, \tag{58}$$

$$[1 - F(x)]^{n-r} = e^{(n-r)S(x)} \sum_{k=0}^{n-r} \binom{n-r}{k} \lambda^{(n-r-k)} e^{(n-r-k)S(x)} (1-\lambda)^k, \tag{59}$$

and

$$f(x) = \left[\alpha\theta x^{\theta-1} + \beta(\gamma + \chi x)\, x^{\gamma-1} e^{\chi x}\right] e^{S(x)} \left[1 - \lambda + 2\lambda e^{S(x)}\right]. \tag{60}$$

So, Eq. (15) can be rearranged as

$$\begin{aligned} f_{r:n}(x) &= n \binom{n-1}{r-1} \sum_{l,m=0}^{r-1} \binom{r-1}{l}\binom{r-1}{m} (-1)^l \lambda^m e^{(l+m)S(x)} e^{(n-r)S(x)} \\ &\times \sum_{k=0}^{n-r} \binom{n-r}{k} \lambda^{(n-r-k)} e^{(n-r-k)S(x)} (1-\lambda)^k \\ &\times \left[\alpha\theta x^{\theta-1} + \beta(\gamma + \chi x)\, x^{\gamma-1} e^{\chi x}\right]\left[1 - \lambda + 2\lambda e^{S(x)}\right] e^{S(x)}. \end{aligned} \tag{61}$$

After some algebraic manipulations, one finds Eq. (54). This completes the proof. □

From Theorem 5 and by taking $r = 1$ and $r = n$, one can deduce the first order and nth order probability density functions. So, it is easy to establish the following corollaries.

Corollary 5 *The first order and nth order probability density functions for NMW_B distribution are given by*

$$f_{1:n}(x) = nS'(x) \sum_{k=0}^{n-1} \binom{n-1}{k} \lambda^{(n-k-1)} (1-\lambda)^k e^{(2n-k-1)S(x)}, \tag{62}$$

and

$$f_{n:n}(x) = n\binom{n-1}{r-1} S'(x) \sum_{l,m=0}^{n-1} \sum_{k=0}^{n-1} \binom{n-1}{l}\binom{n-1}{m}\binom{n-1}{k} \lambda^{m-k}(1-\lambda)^k \times (-1)^l e^{(l+m-k+1)S(x)}, \tag{63}$$

where

$$S'(x) = \left[\alpha\theta x^{\theta-1} + \beta(\gamma+\chi x) x^{\gamma-1} e^{\chi x}\right]\left[1-\lambda+2\lambda e^{S(x)}\right]. \tag{64}$$

Proof It is easy to prove Eqs. (62) and (63) by setting $r = 1$ and n into Eq. (61), respectively. □

Corollary 6 *The joint distribution of rth order statistic X_r and sth order statistic X_s is expressed as*

$$\begin{aligned} g(x_1, x_n) &= n(n-1)\left[F(x_n) - F(x_1)\right]^{n-2} f(x_1) f(x_n) \\ &= n(n-1)(\lambda-1)^{n-2} e^{(n-2)S(x_n)} \sum_{p,q=0}^{n-2} \sum_{v=0}^{q} \binom{n-2}{p}\binom{n-2}{q}\binom{q}{v}(-1)^{p+q}\left(\frac{\lambda}{\lambda-1}\right)^q \\ &\times e^{qS(x_n)} e^{(p+v)[S(x_1)-S(x_n)]} S'(x_1) S'(x_n) e^{[S(x1)+S(x_n)]}. \end{aligned} \tag{65}$$

Proof It is evident to prove Eq. (65) by using the definition of g and Eqs. (59) and (60). □

Theorem 6 *The joint PDF of $X_{r:n}$ and $X_{s:n}$ $(1 \le r \le s \le n)$ is expressed as*

$$\begin{aligned} f_{r:s:n}(x,u) &= \frac{n!}{(r-1)!(s-r-1)!(n-s)!} \frac{\lambda^n}{(\lambda-1)^{r+1}} \left(\frac{\lambda-1}{\lambda}\right)^s S'(x) \\ &\times S'(u) e^{(s-r)S(u)} e^{[2(n-s)+1]S(x)} \sum_{k=0}^{n-s} \binom{n-s}{k}\left(\frac{1-\lambda}{\lambda}\right)^k e^{-kS(x)} \\ &\times \sum_{m,l=0}^{r-1} \sum_{p,q=0}^{s-r-1} \sum_{v=0}^{q} \binom{r-1}{m}\binom{r-1}{l}\binom{s-r-1}{p}\binom{s-r-1}{q}\binom{q}{v} \\ &\times (-1)^{l+p+q} \lambda^m \left(\frac{\lambda}{\lambda-1}\right)^q e^{(l+m+p+v)S(x)+(q-p-v)S(u)}. \end{aligned} \tag{66}$$

Proof We start by evaluating each term of Eq. (17). So, we give the expressions of these terms as follows

$$[F(x)]^{r-1} = \sum_{l,m=0}^{r-1} \binom{r-1}{l}\binom{r-1}{m} (-1)^l \lambda^m e^{(l+m)S(x)}, \tag{67a}$$

$$[F(u)-F(x)]^{s-r-1}=(\lambda-1)^{(s-r-1)}e^{(s-r-1)S(u)}$$
$$\times\sum_{p,q=0}^{s-r-1}\sum_{v=0}^{q}\binom{s-r-1}{p}\binom{s-r-1}{q}\binom{q}{v}(-1)^{p+q}\left(\frac{\lambda}{\lambda-1}\right)^{q}e^{(q-p-v)S(u)}e^{(p+v)S(x)}, \tag{67b}$$

$$[1-F(x)]^{n-s}=e^{(n-s)S(x)}\sum_{k=0}^{n-s}\binom{n-s}{k}\lambda^{(n-s-k)}e^{(n-s-k)S(x)}(1-\lambda)^{k}, \tag{67c}$$

$$F(x)=1+(\lambda-1)e^{S(x)}-\lambda e^{2S(x)}, \tag{67d}$$

and

$$F(u)=1+(\lambda-1)e^{S(u)}-\lambda e^{2S(u)}. \tag{67e}$$

By substituting these last equations into Eq. (17), one finds Eq. (66). This completes the proof. □

2.4 Parameter Estimation

2.4.1 Maximum Likelihood Estimators

The usual estimation method of parameters is by maximum likelihood. For that we consider a random sample $x_1, \ldots, x_n$ consisting of n observations from the NMW_B distribution. We know that the likelihood function of our failure probability density function of six parameters given by Eq. (2) is expressed as

$$\begin{aligned}L(x_1,\ldots,x_n,\alpha,\beta,\theta,\gamma,\chi,\lambda)&=\prod_{i=1}^{n}f(x_i)\\&=\prod_{i=1}^{n}\left[\alpha\theta x_i^{\theta-1}+\beta(\gamma+\chi x_i)x_i^{\gamma-1}e^{\chi x_i}\right]e^{-\left(\alpha x_i^{\theta}+\beta x_i^{\gamma}e^{\chi x_i}\right)}\\&\times\left[1-\lambda+2\lambda e^{-\left(\alpha x_i^{\theta}+\beta x_i^{\gamma}e^{\chi x_i}\right)}\right].\end{aligned} \tag{68}$$

So, the log-likelihood function can be expressed according to the following relation

$$\begin{aligned}\mathcal{L}=\ln(L)&=\sum_{i=1}^{n}\ln\left[\alpha\theta x_i^{\theta-1}+\beta(\gamma+\chi x_i)x_i^{\gamma-1}e^{\chi x_i}\right]\\&-\alpha\sum_{i=1}^{n}x_i^{\theta}-\beta\sum_{i=1}^{n}x_i^{\gamma}e^{\chi x_i}+\sum_{i=1}^{n}\ln\left[1-\lambda+2\lambda e^{-\left(\alpha x_i^{\theta}+\beta x_i^{\gamma}e^{\chi x_i}\right)}\right].\end{aligned} \tag{69}$$

Differentiating this last equation with respect to parameters $(\alpha, \beta, \theta, \gamma, \chi, \lambda)$ and by equating it to zero, one obtains the following estimating equations

$$\sum_{i=1}^{n} \frac{\theta x_i^{\theta-1}}{D_i^{(1)}} - \sum_{i=1}^{n} x_i^{\theta} - 2\lambda \sum_{i=1}^{n} \frac{x_i^{\theta} N_i}{D_i^{(2)}} = 0, \tag{70a}$$

$$\sum_{i=1}^{n} \frac{(\gamma + \chi x_i)\, x_i^{\gamma-1} e^{\chi x_i}}{D_i^{(1)}} - \sum_{i=1}^{n} x_i^{\gamma} e^{\chi x_i} - 2\lambda \sum_{i=1}^{n} \frac{x_i^{\gamma} e^{\chi x_i} N_i}{D_i^{(2)}} = 0, \tag{70b}$$

$$\sum_{i=1}^{n} \frac{x_i^{\theta-1} (1 + \theta \ln x_i)}{D_i^{(1)}} - \sum_{i=1}^{n} x_i^{\theta} \ln x_i - 2\lambda \sum_{i=1}^{n} \frac{x_i^{\theta} N_i \ln x_i}{D_i^{(2)}} = 0, \tag{70c}$$

$$\sum_{i=1}^{n} \frac{x_i^{\gamma-1} e^{\chi x_i} \left[1 + (\gamma + \chi x_i) \ln x_i\right]}{D_i^{(1)}} - \sum_{i=1}^{n} x_i^{\gamma} e^{\chi x_i} \ln x_i - 2\lambda \sum_{i=1}^{n} \frac{x_i^{\gamma} e^{\chi x_i} \ln x_i N_i}{D_i^{(2)}} = 0, \tag{70d}$$

$$\sum_{i=1}^{n} \frac{x_i^{\gamma} (1 + \gamma + \chi x_i) e^{\chi x_i}}{D_i^{(1)}} - \sum_{i=1}^{n} x_i^{\gamma+1} e^{\chi x_i} - 2\lambda \sum_{i=1}^{n} \frac{x_i^{\gamma+1} e^{\chi x_i} N_i}{D_i^{(2)}} = 0, \tag{70e}$$

and

$$\sum_{i=1}^{n} \frac{(2N_i - 1)}{(1 - \lambda + 2\lambda N_i)} = 0, \tag{70f}$$

where

$$N_i = e^{-\left(\alpha x_i^{\theta} + \beta x_i^{\gamma} e^{\chi x_i}\right)}, \tag{71a}$$

$$D_i^{(1)} = \alpha \theta x_i^{\theta-1} + \beta (\gamma + \chi x_i) x_i^{\gamma-1} e^{\chi x_i}, \tag{71b}$$

and

$$D_i^{(2)} = 1 - \lambda + 2\lambda N_i. \tag{71c}$$

Finally, one can deduce, by solving the nonlinear equations (70) numerically for $\alpha, \beta, \theta, \gamma, \chi$ and λ, the maximum likelihood estimators $\hat{\alpha}, \hat{\beta}, \hat{\theta}, \hat{\gamma}, \hat{\chi}$ and $\hat{\lambda}$. As $\frac{\partial \mathcal{L}}{\partial p}$ $(p = \alpha, \beta, \theta, \gamma, \chi \text{ or } \lambda)$ is a continuous function, so this quantity is differentiable and $\frac{\partial^2 \mathcal{L}}{\partial p \partial p'}$ exist.

We give in Appendix all the second partial derivatives of the log-likelihood function $\mathcal{L}$ for the construction of the observed information matrix of the six parameters. This 6×6 Fisher information matrix [43], given in terms of the second partial derivatives of the log-likelihood function $\mathcal{L}$ as [44]

$$I = -\begin{pmatrix} \frac{\partial^2 \mathcal{L}}{\partial \alpha^2} & \cdots & \frac{\partial^2 \mathcal{L}}{\partial \alpha \partial \lambda} \\ \cdots & \cdots & \cdots \\ \frac{\partial^2 \mathcal{L}}{\partial \lambda \partial \alpha} & \cdots & \frac{\partial^2 \mathcal{L}}{\partial \lambda^2} \end{pmatrix}. \tag{72}$$

This matrix yields also the approximate variance–covariance matrix

$$V = \begin{pmatrix} V_{11} & \cdots & V_{16} \\ \cdots & \cdots & \cdots \\ V_{61} & \cdots & V_{66} \end{pmatrix} = \begin{pmatrix} \text{var}\left(\hat{\alpha}\right) & \ldots & \text{cov}\left(\hat{\alpha}, \hat{\lambda}\right) \\ \vdots & \ddots & \vdots \\ \text{cov}\left(\hat{\lambda}, \hat{\alpha}\right) & \cdots & \text{var}\left(\hat{\lambda}\right) \end{pmatrix} = I^{-1} \tag{73}$$

Approximately, $100\,(1-\varepsilon)\,\%$ confidence intervals for the six parameters can be evaluated as $\hat{\alpha} \pm Z_{\varepsilon/2}\sqrt{\text{var}\left(\hat{\alpha}\right)}$, $\hat{\beta} \pm Z_{\varepsilon/2}\sqrt{\text{var}\left(\hat{\beta}\right)}$, $\hat{\theta} \pm Z_{\varepsilon/2}\sqrt{\text{var}\left(\hat{\theta}\right)}$, $\hat{\gamma} \pm Z_{\varepsilon/2}\sqrt{\text{var}\left(\hat{\gamma}\right)}$, $\hat{\chi} \pm Z_{\varepsilon/2}\sqrt{\text{var}\left(\hat{\chi}\right)}$ and $\hat{\lambda} \pm Z_{\varepsilon/2}\sqrt{\text{var}\left(\hat{\lambda}\right)}$, with $Z_{\varepsilon/2}$ is the upper εth percent of the standard normal distribution and $\varepsilon > 0$.

3 Applications

In this section, we present a data analysis in order to show the efficacy of our new model to describe the propagation of the novel virus Covid-19 in some countries. The data represents the daily infected by this kind of virus in each country treated which is registered from February to June 2020.

In Fig. 4, we fit the PDF of our new modified Weibull distribution expressed in Eq. (2) to the data of the daily cases infected by Covid-19. As shown in the below figure, our model has agreed with the propagation of this novel virus and describe its behavior.

The table below presents the MLEs of the parameters of the NMW_B distribution for the data registered (Table 3).

Table 3 MLEs of parameters for daily cases infected by Covid-19 in six treated countries

Countries	$\hat{\alpha}$	$\hat{\beta}$	$\hat{\theta}$	$\hat{\gamma}$	$\hat{\chi}$	$\hat{\lambda}$
Canada	0.01	0.5	2.3	6.03	1.1	1
India	2.10^{-5}	0.0257	6	6	0	10^{-3}
Iraq	9.10^{-5}	0.02004	10	6	1.1	−1
Qatar	2.10^{-7}	0.15	0.65	6.8	0.018	0.5
Mexico	2.10^{-6}	0.02001	1.5	5	0.15	1
Oman	5.10^{-5}	0.02025	0.75	5	1	−0.45

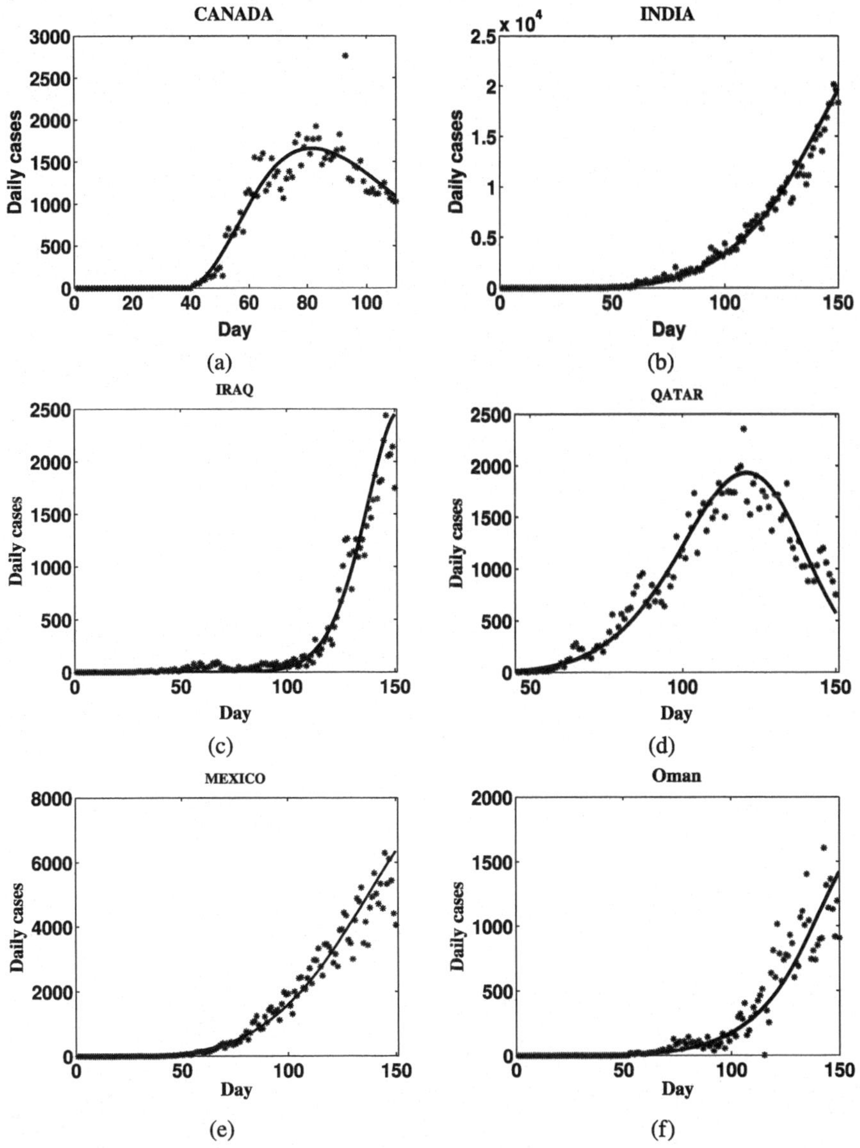

Fig. 4 Fitted PDF of daily cases infected by Covid-19 in (a) Canada (b) India (c) Iraq (d) Qatar (e) Mexico and (f) Oman with (*)is the data registered and solid curve is the NMW_B distribution

Finally, we give the approximate 95% confidence intervals for $(\alpha, \beta, \theta, \gamma, \chi, \lambda)$ respectively, for the current data:

- Canada:

$$\alpha \in [0, 5.63], \ \beta \in [0.492, 0.508], \ \theta \in [2.25, 2.34],$$
$$\gamma \in [5.88, 6.18] \ \chi \in [0.01, 2.19] \ \text{and} \ \lambda \in [0.59, 1].$$

- India:

$$\alpha \in [0, 0.00146], \ \beta \in [0.025695, 0.025706], \ \theta \in [5.999, 6.001],$$
$$\gamma \in [5.848, 6.152], \ \chi \in [-0.04782, 0.04782] \ \text{and} \ \lambda \in [-0.190, 0.192].$$

- Iraq:

$$\alpha \in [0, 0.00149], \ \beta \in [0.020035, 0.020045], \ \theta \in [9.999, 10.001],$$
$$\gamma \in [5.85, 6.15], \ \chi \in [1.05, 1.15] \ \text{and} \ \lambda \in [-1, -0.81].$$

- Qatar:

$$\alpha \in [0, 5.7 \times 10^{-7}], \ \beta \in [0.149, 0.151], \ \theta \in [0.619, 0.681],$$
$$\gamma = [6.78, 6.82], \ \chi \in [0.0167, 0.0193] \ \text{and} \ \lambda \in [0.2, 0.8].$$

- Mexico:

$$\alpha \in [0, 0.03005], \ \beta \in [0.01482, 0.02520], \ \theta \in [0.05, 2.96],$$
$$\gamma \in [4.93, 5.08], \ \chi = [-0.27, 0.57] \ \text{and} \ \lambda \in [0.61, 1].$$

- Oman:

$$\alpha \in [0, 0.0986], \ \beta \in [0.0183, 0.0222], \ \theta \in [-0.32, 1.82],$$
$$\gamma \in [4.96, 5.04], \ \chi \in [0.28, 1.72] \ \text{and} \ \lambda \in [-0.57, -0.33].$$

4 Conclusion

The proposal new Weibull distribution with six parameters is studied. We have derived various structural properties of this distribution as moments, moment generating function, relationship with previous Weibull distributions, parameter estimation, statistical properties, the qth quantile, estimators and order statistics.

As application, we analyzed the Covid-19 virus spreading statistics by our extended distribution to fit the cases infected in some countries. We proved that our new distribution generalizes some existing models and gives the correct fits of some data.

Our hope is that our new distribution will attract wider applications and replace other models which are valid for modeling real data in several fields.

Appendix

All the second partial derivatives of the log-likelihood function are obtained in this appendix as follows

$$\mathcal{L}_{\alpha\alpha} = -\sum_{i=1}^{n} \frac{h_{\alpha}^{2}}{h^{2}} + 2\lambda \sum_{i=1}^{n} t_i^{2\theta} h_{S\lambda}, \tag{74}$$

$$\mathcal{L}_{\beta\beta} = -\sum_{i=1}^{n} \frac{h_{\beta}^{2}}{h^{2}} + 2\lambda \sum_{i=1}^{n} t_i^{2\gamma} e^{2\chi t_i} h_{S\lambda}, \tag{75}$$

$$\mathcal{L}_{\theta\theta} = \sum_{i=1}^{n} \frac{\left(h_{\theta\theta} h - \alpha^{2} h_{\alpha\theta}^{2}\right)}{h^{2}} - \alpha \sum_{i=1}^{n} t_i^{\theta} \ln^{2}(t_i) - 2\alpha\lambda \sum_{i=1}^{n} t_i^{\theta} h_{S\lambda}^{\alpha} \ln(t_i), \tag{76}$$

$$\mathcal{L}_{\gamma\gamma} = \sum_{i=1}^{n} \frac{\left(h_{\gamma\gamma} h - \beta^{2} h_{\beta\gamma}^{2}\right)}{h^{2}} - \beta \sum_{i=1}^{n} t_i^{\gamma} e^{\chi t_i} \ln^{2}(t_i) - 2\beta\lambda \sum_{i=1}^{n} t_i^{\gamma} e^{\chi t_i} h_{S\lambda}^{\beta\chi} \ln^{2}(t_i), \tag{77}$$

$$\mathcal{L}_{\chi\chi} = \sum_{i=1}^{n} \frac{\left(h_{\chi\chi} h - h_{\beta\chi}^{2}\right)}{h^{2}} - \beta \sum_{i=1}^{n} t_i^{\gamma+2} e^{\chi t_i} - 2\beta\lambda \sum_{i=1}^{n} t_i^{\gamma+2} e^{\chi t_i} h_{S\lambda}^{\beta\chi}, \tag{78}$$

$$\mathcal{L}_{\lambda\lambda} = -\sum_{i=1}^{n} h_{\lambda}^{2}, \tag{79}$$

$$\mathcal{L}_{\theta\alpha} = \sum_{i=1}^{n} \frac{\left(h_{\alpha\theta} h - \alpha h_{\alpha\theta} h_{\alpha}\right)}{h^{2}} - \sum_{i=1}^{n} t_i^{\theta} \ln(t_i) - 2\lambda \sum_{i=1}^{n} t_i^{\theta} h_{S\lambda}^{\alpha}, \tag{80}$$

$$\mathcal{L}_{\beta\alpha} = -\sum_{i=1}^{n} \frac{h_{\alpha} h_{\beta}}{h^{2}} + 2\lambda \sum_{i=1}^{n} t_i^{\theta+\gamma} e^{\chi t_i} h_{S\lambda}, \tag{81}$$

$$\mathcal{L}_{\gamma\alpha} = -\beta \sum_{i=1}^{n} \frac{h_{\alpha} h_{\beta\gamma}}{h^{2}} + 2\beta\lambda \sum_{i=1}^{n} t_i^{\theta+\gamma} e^{\chi t_i} h_{S\lambda} \ln(t_i), \tag{82}$$

$$\mathcal{L}_{\chi\alpha} = -\sum_{i=1}^{n} \frac{h_{\alpha} h_{\beta\chi}}{h^{2}} + 2\beta\lambda \sum_{i=1}^{n} t_i^{\theta+\gamma+1} e^{\chi t_i} h_{S\lambda}, \tag{83}$$

$$\mathcal{L}_{\lambda\alpha} = -2\sum_{i=1}^{n} t_i^{\theta} \frac{e^S}{S_\lambda^2}, \tag{84}$$

$$\mathcal{L}_{\theta\beta} = -\alpha\sum_{i=1}^{n} \frac{h_{\alpha\theta}h_\beta}{h^2} + 2\alpha\lambda\sum_{i=1}^{n} t_i^{\theta+\gamma} e^{\chi t_i} h_{S\lambda} \ln(t_i), \tag{85}$$

$$\mathcal{L}_{\gamma\theta} = -\alpha\beta\sum_{i=1}^{n} \frac{h_{\alpha\theta}h_{\beta\gamma}}{h^2} + 2\alpha\beta\lambda\sum_{i=1}^{n} t_i^{\theta+\gamma} e^{\chi t_i} h_{S\lambda} \ln^2(t_i), \tag{86}$$

$$\mathcal{L}_{\chi\theta} = -\alpha\sum_{i=1}^{n} \frac{h_{\alpha\theta}h_{\beta\chi}}{h^2} + 2\alpha\beta\lambda\sum_{i=1}^{n} t_i^{\theta+\gamma+1} e^{\chi t_i} h_{S\lambda} \ln(t_i), \tag{87}$$

$$\mathcal{L}_{\lambda\theta} = -2\alpha\sum_{i=1}^{n} t_i^{\theta} \frac{e^S}{S_\lambda^2} \ln(t_i), \tag{88}$$

$$\mathcal{L}_{\gamma\beta} = \sum_{i=1}^{n} h_{\beta\gamma} \frac{\left(h - \beta h_\beta\right)}{h^2} - \sum_{i=1}^{n} t_i^{\gamma} e^{\chi t_i} \ln(t_i) - 2\lambda\sum_{i=1}^{n} t_i^{\gamma} e^{\chi t_i} h_{S\lambda}^{\beta\chi} \ln(t_i), \tag{89}$$

$$\mathcal{L}_{\chi\beta} = \sum_{i=1}^{n} \frac{\left(h_{\chi\gamma}h - h_{\beta\chi}h_\beta\right)}{h^2} - \sum_{i=1}^{n} t_i^{\gamma+1} e^{\chi t_i} - 2\lambda\sum_{i=1}^{n} t_i^{\gamma+1} e^{\chi t_i} h_{S\lambda}^{\beta\chi}, \tag{90}$$

$$\mathcal{L}_{\lambda\beta} = -2\sum_{i=1}^{n} t_i^{\gamma} e^{\chi t_i} h_S^{\lambda}, \tag{91}$$

$$\begin{aligned}\mathcal{L}_{\chi\gamma} = {} & \beta\sum_{i=1}^{n} \frac{\left(h_{\beta\gamma}^{\chi}h - h_{\beta\chi}h_{\beta\gamma}\right)}{h^2} - \beta\sum_{i=1}^{n} t_i^{\gamma+1} e^{\chi t_i} \ln(t_i) \\ & - 2\beta\lambda\sum_{i=1}^{n} t_i^{\gamma+1} e^{\chi t_i} h_{S\lambda}^{\beta\chi} \ln(t_i),\end{aligned} \tag{92}$$

$$\mathcal{L}_{\lambda\gamma} = -2\beta\sum_{i=1}^{n} t_i^{\gamma} e^{\chi t_i} h_S^{\lambda} \ln(t_i), \tag{93}$$

and

$$\mathcal{L}_{\lambda\chi} = 2\beta\lambda\sum_{i=1}^{n} t_i^{\gamma+1} e^{\chi t_i} \frac{e^S}{S_\lambda^2}, \tag{94}$$

where

$$h_{\alpha} = \theta t_i^{\theta-1}, \tag{95}$$

$$h_{S\lambda} = \frac{\left(S_{\lambda} - 2\lambda e^{S}\right) e^{S}}{S_{\lambda}^{2}}, \tag{96}$$

$$h_{\beta} = (\gamma + \chi t_i)\, t_i^{\gamma-1} e^{\chi t_i}, \tag{97}$$

$$h_{\beta\gamma} = e^{\chi t_i} t_i^{\gamma-1} \left[1 + (\gamma + \chi t_i) \ln (t_i)\right], \tag{98}$$

$$h_{\chi\chi} = \beta t_i^{\gamma+1} e^{\chi t_i} (2 + \gamma + \chi t_i), \tag{99}$$

$$h_{\gamma\gamma} = \beta e^{\chi t_i} t_i^{\gamma-1} \left[2 + (\gamma + \chi t_i) \ln (t_i)\right] \ln (t_i), \tag{100}$$

$$h_{\alpha\theta} = t_i^{\theta-1} (1 + \theta \ln (t_i)), \tag{101}$$

$$h_{\theta\theta} = \alpha t_i^{\theta-1} (2 + \theta \ln (t_i)) \ln (t_i), \tag{102}$$

$$h_{S\lambda}^{p\chi} = \frac{\left[S_{\lambda} - p t_i^{\gamma} e^{\chi t_i} \left(S_{\lambda} - 2\lambda e^{S}\right)\right] e^{S}}{S_{\lambda}^{2}}, \tag{103}$$

$$h_{S\lambda}^{p} = \frac{\left[S_{\lambda} - p t_i^{\theta} \left(S_{\lambda} - 2\lambda e^{S}\right)\right] e^{S} \ln (t_i)}{S_{\lambda}^{2}}, \tag{104}$$

$$h_{\beta\chi} = \beta t_i^{\gamma} e^{\chi t_i} (1 + \gamma + \chi t_i), \tag{105}$$

$$h_{\chi\gamma} = t_i^{\gamma} e^{\chi t_i} \left[1 + (\gamma + \chi t_i)\right], \tag{106}$$

$$h_{\lambda} = \frac{(S_{\lambda} - 1)}{\lambda S_{\lambda}}, \tag{107}$$

$$h_{S} = \frac{\left(2e^{S} - 1\right) e^{S}}{S_{\lambda}^{2}}, \tag{108}$$

$$h_{S}^{\lambda} = \frac{\left[S_{\lambda} - \lambda \left(2e^{S} - 1\right)\right] e^{S}}{S_{\lambda}^{2}} \tag{109}$$

and

$$h_{\beta\gamma}^{\chi} = t_i^{\gamma} e^{\chi t_i} \left[1 + \ln (t_i) + (\gamma + \chi t_i) \ln (t_i)\right]. \tag{110}$$

References

1. http://www.sehhty.com/
2. Gondauri, D., Mikautadze, E., Batiashvili, M.: Research on COVID-19 Virus spreading statistics based on the examples of the cases from different countries. Electron. J. Gen. Med. **17**, 1–4 (2020)
3. Li, L., Yang, Z., Dang, Z., Meng, C., Huang, J., Meng, H., Wang, D., Chen, G., Zhang, J., Peng, H., Shao, Y.: Propagation analysis and prediction of the COVID-19. Infect. Dis. Model. **5**, 282–292 (2020)
4. Corman, V.M., Landt, O., Kaiser, M., et al.: Detection of 2019 novel coronavirus (2019-nCoV) by real-time RT-PCR. Euro Surveill. **25**(3), 2000045 (2020)
5. Hui, D.S., Azhar, E.I., Madani, T.A., et al.: The continuing 2019-nCoV epidemic threat of novel coronaviruses to global health-the latest 2019 novel coronavirus outbreak in Wuhan. China. Int. J. of Infect. Dis. **91**, 264–266 (2020)
6. Mizumoto, K., Chowell, G.: Transmission potential of the novel coronavirus (COVID-19) onboard the diamond Princess Cruises Ship. Infect. Dis. Model. **5**, 264–270 (2020)
7. Riou, J., Althauss, C.L.: Pattern of early human-to-human transmission of Wuhan 2019 novel coronavirus (2019-nCoV), December 2019 to January 2020. Euro Surveill. **25**(4), 2000058 (2020)
8. Shao, Y., Wu, J.: IDM editorial statement on the 2019-nCoV. Infect. Dis. Model. **5**, 233–234 (2020)
9. Zhu, N., Zhang, D., Wang, W., et al.: A Novel Coronavirus from Patients with Pneumonia in China, 2019. N. Engl. J. Med. **382**, 727–733 (2020)
10. Wu, J.T., Leung, G.M.: Nowcasting and forecasting the potential domestic and international spread of the 2019-nCoV outbreak originating in Wuhan, China: a modelling study. Lancet **395**, 689–697 (2020)
11. He, F., Deng, Y., Li, W.: Coronavirus Discasc 2019 (COVID-2019): What we know? J. Med. Virol. **92**, 719–725 (2020)
12. Lu, R., Zhao, X., Wang, Li. J, et al.: Grnomic characterisation and epidemiology of 2019 novel coronavirus: implications for virus origins and receptor binding. Lancet. **395**, 565–574 (2020)
13. Zhou, P., Yang, X.L., Wang, X.G., et al.: A pneumonia outbreak associated with a new coronovirus of probable bat origin. Nature **579**, 270–273 (2020)
14. Weibull, W.A.: Statistical distribution function of wide applicability. J. App. Mech. **18**, 293–296 (1951)
15. Bailey, R.L., Dell, T.R.: Quantifying diameter distributions with the Weibul function. For. Sci. **19**, 97–104 (1973)
16. Murthy, D.N.P., Xie, M., Jiang. R.: Weibull Models. Wiley, New York (2013)
17. Bebbingtom, M.S., Lai, C.D., Zitikis, R.: A flexible Weibull extension. Reliab. Eng. Sys. Safe. **92**, 719–726 (2007)
18. Zhang, T., Xie, M., Zitikis, R.: On the upper truncated Weibull distribution and its reliability implications. Reliab. Eng. Sys. Safe. **92**, 194–200 (2011)
19. Bain, L.J.: Analysis for the linear feailure-rate life-testing distribution. Technometrics. **42**, 299–302 (1993)
20. Mudholkar, G.S., Srivastava. D.K.: Exponentiated Weibull family for analysing bathtub failure rate data. IEEE T. Reliab. **42**, 299–302 (1993)
21. Marshall, A.W., Olkin. I.: A new method for adding a parameter to a family of distributions with application to the exponential and Weibull families. Biometrika. **84**, 641–652 (1997)
22. Remolls, K., Geary, D.N., Rollinson, T.J.D.: Characterizing diameter distributions by the use of the Weibull distribution. Foresty. **58**, 57–66 (1985)
23. Maltamo, M.: Comparing basal area diameter distributions estimated by tree species and for the entire growing stock in a mixed stand. Silva Fenn. **31**, 53–65 (1996)
24. Xie, M., Tang, Y., Goh, T.N.: A modified Weibull extension with bathtub-shaped failure rate function. Reliab. Eng. Sys. Safe. **76**, 279–285 (2002)

25. Xie, M., Lai, C.D.: Reliability analysis using an additive Weibull model with bathtub-shaped failure ratefunction. Reliab. Eng. Sys. Safe. **52**, 87–93 (1995)
26. Sarhan, A.M., Zaindin, M.: Modified Weibull distribution. Appl. Sci. **11**, 123–136 (2009)
27. Famoye, F., Lee, C., Olumolade, O.: The beta-Weibull distribution. JSTA **4**, 121–136 (2005)
28. Shahbaz, M.Q., Shahbaz, S., Butt, N.S.: The Kumaraswamy-inverse weibull distribution. PAK. J. Sta. Oper. Res. **8**, 479–489 (2012)
29. Ahmad, Z., Iqbal, B.: Generalized flexible Weibull extension distribution. Circ. Comput. Sci. **2**, 68–75 (2017)
30. Ahmad, Z., Hussain, Z.: New extended weibull distribution. Circ. Comput. Sci. **2**, 14–19 (2017)
31. Khan, M.S., King, R.: Transmuted modified Weibull distribution: a generalization of the modified Weibull probability distribution. Eur. J. Pure appl. Math. **6**, 66–88 (2013)
32. Phani, K.K.: A new modified Weibull distribution function. J. Am. Ceram. Soc. **70**, 182–184 (1987)
33. Silva, G.O., Ortega, E.M., Cordeiro, G.M.: The beta modified Weibull distribution. Lifetime Data Anal. **16**, 409–430 (2010)
34. Singla, N., Jain, K., Kumar, Sharma S.: The beta generalized Weibull distribution: properties and applications. Reliab. Eng. Sys. Safe. **102**, 5–15 (2012)
35. Exponentiated generalized linea exponential distribution: Sarhan, A. M., Abd EL-Baset, A A., Alasbahi, I. A. Appl. Math. Model. **37**, 2838–2849 (2013)
36. Almalki, S.J., Yuan, J.: A new modified Weibull distribution. Reliab. Eng. Sys. Safe. **111**, 164–170 (2013)
37. Abd EL-Baset, A.A., Ghazal, M.G.M.: Exponentiated additive Weibull distribution. Reliab. Eng. Sys. Safe. **193**, 106663 (2020)
38. He, B., Cui, W., Du, X.: An additive modified Weibull distribution. Reliab. Eng. Sys. Safe. **145**, 28–37 (2016)
39. Ashour, S.K., Eltehiwy, M.A.: Transmuted exponentiated modified Weibull distribution. IJBAS **2**, 258–269 (2013)
40. Arnold, B.C., Balakrishnan, N., Nagaraja, H.N.: A first course in order statistics. Society for Industrial and Applied Mathematics (2008)
41. Gradshteyn, I.S., Ryzhik, I.M.: Table of Integrals, Series, and Products, 5th edn. Academic Press, New York (1994)
42. Al-Fawzan, M.A.: Methods for estimating the parameters of the Weibull distribution. (2000) (Unpublish) King Abdulaziz City for Science and Technology, Saudi Arabia
43. Fisher, R.A.: On the mathematical foundations of theoretical statistics. Philos. Trans. R. Soc. A **222**, 309–368 (1922)
44. Lawless, J.F.: Statistical Models and Methods for Lifetime Data, vol. 20, pp. 1108–1113. John Wiley and Sons, New York (2003)

Lifting Lockdown Control Measure Assessment: From Finite-to Infinite-Dimensional Epidemic Models for Covid-19

Redouane Qesmi and Aayah Hammoumi

Abstract The main focus of this chapter is on public health control strategies which are currently the main way to mitigate Covid-19 pandemic. We introduce and compare compartmental models of increasing complexity for Covid-19 transmission to describe dynamics of the disease spread. We begin by considering an SEAIR model including basic characteristics related to Covid-19. Next, we shall pay attention to age-structured modeling to emphasis the role of age-group individuals on the disease spread. A model with constant delay is also formulated to show the impact of the latency period on the severity of Covid-19. Since there is evidence that for Covid-19 disease, important relationships exist between what is happening in the host and what is occurring at the population level, we shall link the basic model to in-host dynamics through the so-called threshold-type delay models. Finally, we will include demographic effects to the most complex models, and we will conduct rigorous bifurcation analysis to quantify possible factors responsible for disease progression.

Keywords Covid-19: Spreading statistics · Modified Weibull distribution · Mean · Variance · Standard deviation · Moments

1 Introduction

The SARS-CoV-2, designated as Severe Acute Respiratory Syndrome CoronaVirus-2, is a causative agent of Covid-19 disease that first emerged in China on December 2019 [28]. Up to date, 213 countries and territories are affected by the disease, with nearly 19 million confirmed cases and more than 700,000 deaths. Unfortunately, there are no current effective therapeutic agents or vaccines for treatment of Covid-

R. Qesmi (✉)
Superior School of Technology, Sidi Mohamed Ben Abdellah University, Fez 30000, Morocco
e-mail: redouane.qesmi@usmba.ac.ma

A. Hammoumi
Department of Biology, Cadi Ayyad University, Semlalia, Marrakech 40000, Morocco
e-mail: a.hammoumi@uca.ma

P. Agarwal et al. (eds.), *Analysis of Infectious Disease Problems (Covid-19) and Their Global Impact*, Infosys Science Foundation Series,
https://doi.org/10.1007/978-981-16-2450-6_9

19 and, consequently, public health control strategies that diminish contact between infectious and susceptible individuals are actually the main way to contain and mitigate the pandemic [36]. Examples of such a control include the personal protective measures (e.g., hand hygiene, cough or sneeze etiquette and face coverings), social distancing measures (e.g., increasing physical distance from other people, avoiding social gathering and stay at home) and environmental surface cleaning [12]. However, despite health control interventions seem to be successful in reducing the spread of the pandemic, they are also responsible of global economic crisis. It is estimated that Covid-19 could cost the global economy more than $10 trillion [1, 21]. Millions of individuals throughout the world have been forced to reduce their working hours or have lost their jobs and around 900 million students are affected by national school closures [30, 33]. Furthermore, because of the isolation and the increase of social class inequalities, the lockdown is badly lived by the majority of children and adults who have developed mental health disorders and familial problems [1, 8, 21]. Although many information related to Covid-19, such as its potential to reoccur, remain unclear, lifting lockdown measure became an urgent need to avoid the worsening of the global crisis caused by Covid-19 [22]. Governments around the world encountered serious difficulties to adopt the best lockdown lifting strategy balancing between economy recovery and health protection of citizens.

Fortunately, since the beginning of the outbreak of Covid-19, mathematical modeling proved to be an effective tool to predict the course as well as the severity of the epidemic and to help decision-makers to evaluate the effectiveness of health control measures (See [4, 13, 15, 20, 32] and references therein). Generally, at the beginning of an emergent epidemic, the novel pathogenic agent lacks detailed knowledge. Mathematicians begin by using simplest compartmental models to estimate the key epidemiological parameters (such as the basic reproduction number R_0, peak time, peak size, latency period, infectious period) which are necessary to set up public health strategies and monitor the disease progression [3]. Most such models consider individuals in a closed population that are classified according to their disease status: susceptible (S), latent or exposed (E), infectious (I) and recovered (R). These basic models have the great advantage of being easy to investigate but, on the other hand, often oversimplify the existing complexity of disease processes which underestimate or overestimate the magnitude of the disease spread. However, more complex models can be considered in case the scientists provide more epidemiological evidences leading to detailed knowledge of Sars-Cov-2 pathogenic mechanism and its mode of transmission. Even if they are more difficult to analyze and need more detailed data, these models could be more realistic since they take into account more realistic epidemiological properties such as the heterogeneity of disease transmission, age-subgroups, latent periods and so on. The purpose of this chapter is to consider and compare different deterministic compartmental models of increasing complexity that will be useful to clarify how Sars-CoV-2 spread within individuals while considering the relaxation of the compulsory lockdown to prevent dissemination of the Covid-19 disease.

The main contribution of this chapter is organized as follows. In Sect. 3, we will consider and investigate an extended basic SEAIR model which is widely used for Covid-19 disease. Indeed, this model takes into account the standard epidemiological states such as the exposed individuals to the Sars-CoV-2 virus which are infected but can not transmit the virus to others. In Sect. 4, we consider an extension of the previous model with particular focus on an identified route of Covid-19 transmission from children to adults and vice versa. In other words, we present a discrete age-structured model, by separating the population into two different age-subgroups with different contact rates, to look at the heterogeneity of Covid-19 transmission within a population. Indeed, it is proved that children are less affected by Sars-Cov-2 than adults and play a minor role in disease transmission [2, 17]. Seniors and person with existing chronic medical conditions develop more severe form of disease and are more likely to die [34]. Furthermore, individuals with different ages may also have different behaviors and behavioral changes which are crucial in the assessment of control scenarios targeted at particular groups, such as reopening schools or relaunch of economic activities. The impact of the latent period on disease transmission is also evaluated in Sect. 5 by incorporating a time delay to the basic SAIR model instead of considering the latent stage as a model component. In Sect. 6, we examine a threshold-type delay model by incorporating a series of smaller Sars-CoV-2 viral loads, due to close contact with infectious individuals, into the within-host virus dynamics. This type of model can be used for example to study the impact of Covid-19 exposure to health care workers who are daily in close contacts with Covid-19 patients, visitors or co-workers in a population and are more likely to be infected [7]. In Sect. 7, we include vital dynamics to the constant and threshold-type delay models by assuming that the Covid-19 disease could persist for a long period. Indeed, with the evidence of sensibility of Sars-CoV-2 to climatic factors such as temperature and humidity, scientists think that the Covid-19 allows a seasonal cycle and could reduce with climate change. But, even with the arrival of the warm weather, the disease still evolved and could persist for several months or years. This demonstrates that the climate change is not the main parameter which influences the disease transmission but also, the people's behavior, the low immunity of individuals to a novel coronavirus and the immunity period (the amount of time that people remain immune after infection) [9, 11]. We will then conduct rigorous qualitative analysis including bifurcation investigation of both models with demographic effect to quantify possible factors responsible for disease progression and highlight long-term qualitative behavior of Covid-19 spread. Next, in order to help scientists to avoid major blunders and generate models that fit the data reasonably accurately, we compare in Sect. 8 the proposed models to identify which one best fits the reported data and provide a better prediction for Covid-19. Results of our models will help to tackle health concerns that are of great importance and will draw of the hospitals research and surveillance data to create, optimize and parameterize disease models, focusing on Covid-19.

2 Data Collection

The data of reported symptomatic infectious cases is collected each day at 11 pm from the official Coronavirus Portal of Morocco [27]. Data information covers the cumulative number of reported cases from March $2nd$ to June $10th$, 2020. The data from March $2nd$ to March 20 (first day of lockdown measure) are used to estimate the basic reproduction number and adjust the investigated models to become closer to reality, while data from March $21st$ to June $10th$ (last day of lockdown measure) are used to adjust the models and estimate the lockdown rate during this period of lockdown.

3 Basic Covid-19 Model

The population, with size N, considered in this basic model is stratified into seven disease status. Individuals are classified as susceptible (S), exposed noninfectious (E) , asymptomatic infectious (A), unreported symptomatic infectious (I_u), reported symptomatic infectious or hospitalized (H), recovered (R) and dead (D). We formulate the model to describe the course of Covid-19 epidemic under the assumptions:

1. Reported symptomatic infectious individuals are hospitalized and can not contact susceptibles anymore.
2. As confirmed by Rothe et al. [24], asymptomatic individuals can infect susceptible individuals.
3. Confined asymptomatic and confined unreported individuals can still spread the virus to their families.
4. Exposed infected individuals cannot immediately spread the virus to other individuals.
5. As proved by MacIntyre in [18], asymptomatic and symptomatic infectious individuals share the same infection probability.

Taking account of the previous assumptions, the dynamics of Covid-19 can be described as follows: Individuals are confined at rate p. Unconfined (resp. confined) susceptibles $(1-p)S$ (resp. (pS)) contacted with either unreported symptomatic (I_u) or asymptomatic infectious individuals (A) are infected with infection probability, β_N (resp. β_c), and move to the exposed infected class (E). Exposed individuals then become asymptomatic infectious at rate k. After an average period $1/\delta$ days the asymptomatic infectious individuals (A) become symptomatic and proceed either to the unreported symptomatic infectious (I_u), at rate δ_1, or to the reported symptomatic infectious (H) at rate δ_2 with $\delta = \delta_1 + \delta_2$. Once becoming symptomatic, individuals of class I_u and H remain symptomatic for $1/\mu$ days on average before they are recovered or dead at rate d. The parameter γ corresponds to the lifting rate while parameter θ corresponds to the contact reduction, due to wearing masks, washing hands and social distancing practices of unconfined individuals. The general basic model equations including parameters control are given as follows

$$
\begin{cases}
\frac{dS}{dt} &= -\left((1-\gamma)\, p\beta_c + (1-\theta)\,(1-(1-\gamma)\,p)\,\beta_N\right) S(t)\,(A(t)+I_u(t))\,/N, \\
\frac{dE}{dt} &= \left((1-\gamma)\, p\beta_c + (1-\theta)\,(1-(1-\gamma)\,p)\,\beta_N\right) S(t)\,(A(t)+I_u(t))\,/N - kE, \\
\frac{dA}{dt} &= kE - \delta A(t), \\
\frac{dI_u}{dt} &= \delta_1 A(t) - \mu I_u(t) - d I_u(t), \\
\frac{dH}{dt} &= \delta_2 A(t) - \mu H - dH, \\
\frac{dR}{dt} &= \mu(H + I_u), \\
\frac{dD}{dt} &= d(H + I_u).
\end{cases}
\tag{1}
$$

3.1 Reproduction Numbers

The basic reproduction number, R_0, is the average number of secondary infections produced when one infectious individual is introduced into a host susceptible population. This quantity determines whether a given disease may spread, or die out in a population. To compute this number, we assume that $p = \theta = \gamma = 0$ and we apply the next generation matrix method in [31]. We obtain

$$
R_0 = \frac{(a+k)\,(a+\delta)\,(a+\mu+d)}{k\,(\delta_1 + a + \mu + d)} \left(\frac{1}{\delta} + \frac{\delta_1}{\delta\mu}\right) \tag{2}
$$

where a is an estimated constant given in Sect. 3.2. Here, R_0 can be explained as follows: Assume that one asymptomatic infectious individual is introduced into the susceptible population. This asymptomatic individual produces, on average, $\beta_N S_0 \frac{1}{\delta}$ asymptomatic individuals during his average lifespan $1/\delta$. These asymptomatic individuals then become unreported symptomatic infectious individuals over their lifespan $1/\delta$ at a rate δ_1 and then each infectious symptomatic produces, on average, $\beta_N S_0 \frac{1}{\mu}$ asymptomatic individuals during his lifespan $1/\mu$.

Let us show the formula of R_0. The linearized system related to infectious individuals , around $(S_0, 0, 0, 0)$, of system (1) is given by

$$
\begin{cases}
\frac{dE}{dt} &= -kE(t) + \beta_N S_0 A(t) + \beta_N S_0 I_u(t) \\
\frac{dA}{dt} &= kE(t) - \delta A(t), \\
\frac{dI_u}{dt} &= \delta_1 A(t) - (\mu + d)\, I_u(t),
\end{cases}
$$

and the associated Jacobian matrix is given by $M = F - E$ where

$$F = \begin{pmatrix} 0 & \beta_N S_0 & \beta_N S_0 \\ k & 0 & 0 \\ 0 & \delta_1 & 0 \end{pmatrix} \text{ and } E = \begin{pmatrix} k & 0 & 0 \\ 0 & \delta & 0 \\ 0 & 0 & \mu + d \end{pmatrix}.$$

Therefore, $FE^{-1} = \begin{pmatrix} 0 & \beta_N S_0/\delta & \beta_N S_0/(\mu + d) \\ 1 & 0 & 0 \\ 0 & \delta_1/\delta & 0 \end{pmatrix}$ and R_0 is its spectral radius. Using the formula of β_N in (9), we obtain the formula given in (2).

The control reproduction number, R_c, is an important value, used to determine whether a control policy, such as lockdown, lifting, behavioral practices, etc., will be efficient to decrease the number of secondary infections to be less than one. Computation method of R_c is similar to the one of R_0 and leads to the following formula

$$R_c = ((1 - \gamma)\, p\beta_c + (1 - \theta)\,(1 - (1 - \gamma)\, p)\, \beta_N) \left(\frac{1}{\delta} + \frac{\delta_1}{\delta\mu} \right).$$

3.2 Parameter and Initial Data Estimation

To estimate the model parameters, we will consider two different stages. The first stage is between the beginning of the Covid-19 epidemic and the first time of containment control (i.e., $p = 0$ and $\theta = 0$) for which we will estimate the initial data of the model, the parameters related to infection and the basic reproduction number. The second stage will be during the lockdown period ($\gamma = 0$ and $\theta = 0$) for which we will estimate the lockdown rate.

Since the first and the only symptomatic infectious individual is reported on March $2nd$, 2020, which corresponds to $t = 0$, then $H(0) = 1$, $R(0) = 0$ and $D(0) = 0$. For the estimation of β_N, $E(0)$, $A(0)$ and $I_u(0)$ we will use the data of cumulative reported cases collected from March 2nd to March 20 (before the start of lockdown) and we follow the procedure by [15]. The cumulative reported infectious population is given, for $t \geq 0$, by $F(t) = \delta_2 \int_0^t A(s)ds + 1$. It is obvious that cumulative reported infectious population increases slowly and then accelerates rapidly with time. Hence, we will use exponential regression with 95% of confidence level to find an exponential function that best fits the data, from March $2nd$ to June $10th$. Using SPSS software (Statistical Package for the Social Sciences), we found that exponential model given by be^{at} with $a = 0.263$ with confidence interval CI $(0.229 - 0.297)$ and $b = 0.507$

with CI (0.3444 – 0.7475) fits well the data with a correlation coefficient given by $R = 0.97$. It follows from $F(t) = \delta_2 \int_0^t A(s)ds + 1 = be^{at}$ that

$$A(t) = \frac{ba}{\delta_2} e^{at}. \tag{3}$$

Since the initial susceptible population is not dramatically affected in the early phase of the epidemic, we will assume that $S(t) \approx S(0)$. Let $S_0 := S(0)$, $E(0) := E_0$, $A(0) := A_0$ and $I_u(0) := I_0$. From the second and the third equations of system (1) and using (3) we obtain

$$\left(\left(\frac{a+\delta}{k} \right) + (a+\delta) \right) A(t) = \beta_N S(0) \left(A(t) + I_u(t) \right), \tag{4}$$

$$E(t) = E_0 e^{at} \text{ and } I_u(t) = I_0 e^{at}, \tag{5}$$

where

$$E_0 = \frac{a+\delta}{k} \frac{ba}{\delta_2} \text{ and } I_0 = \frac{ba \left(\left(\frac{a+\delta}{k} \right) + (a+\delta) - \beta_N S(0) \right)}{\delta_2 \beta_N S_0}. \tag{6}$$

Now, using formulas (5) and the third equation of system (1), we obtain after simplification

$$aE_0 = \beta_N S_0 (A_0 + I_0) - kE_0 \tag{7}$$

and

$$aI_0 = \delta_1 A_0 - (\mu + d) I_0. \tag{8}$$

Solving Eqs. (6), (7) and (8) for β_N and I_0 lead to

$$\beta_N = \frac{(a+k)(a+\delta)(a+\mu+d)}{k(\delta_1 + a + \mu + d)} \text{ and } I_0 = \frac{\delta_1}{a+\mu+d} A_0. \tag{9}$$

To estimate the transmission rate, β_c, and the lockdown rate, p during the lockdown period, we assume that $\gamma = 0$ and $\theta = 0$ and we use the nonlinear least squares solver "lsqcurvefit" in MATLAB R2019b software. The values of the estimated parameters are summarized in Table 1.

Define the sum of squared residuals (SSR) as

$$SSR = \sqrt{\frac{1}{n} \sum_{i=1}^{n} (\delta_2 A(t) - \text{Newcase}(i))^2}$$

where Newcase(i) is the number of new reported cases on the day i and n is the number of collected new cases. This number measures the discrepancy between the data and the estimation model of new reported cases per day and will serve us to

Table 1 Parameter definitions and values of model (1)

Symbol	Definition	Parameter value	Confidence interval	Reference
$S(0)$	Initial susceptible population	35865191		[5]
$E(0)$	Initial exposed noninfecious population	0.3175	00.8 – 1.37	Estimated
$A(0)$	Initial asymptomatic population	11.9921	9.42 – 15.03	Estimated
$I_u(0)$	Initial unreported symptomatic population	0.8414	0.592 – 1.3	Estimated
$H(0)$	Initial reported symptomatic population	1		See text
$R(0)$	Initial recovered population	0		See text
$D(0)$	Initial dead population	0		See text
β_{N}	Infection rate for unconfined population	2.87	0.5 – 4.2	Estimated
β_{C}	Infection rate for confined population	0.57	0.1 – 0.84	Estimated
$1/\delta$	Asymptomatic duration	6 days		[27]
k	Exposed noninfectious rate	3	2 – 4	See text
δ_1	Asymptomatic unreported rate	0.017 per day		Assumed
δ_2	Symptomatic reported rate	0.15 per day		Assumed
$1/\mu$	Symptomatic duration	14 days		[35]
p	Proportion of lockdown	0.7	0.5 – 0.76	Estimated
R_0	Basic reproduction number	2.88	2.55 – 2.99	Estimated

compare the suggested models of this chapter. A small SSR indicates a better fit of the model to the data. A computation of this measure for model (1) leads to $SSR_{basic} = 93.4$.

4 Discrete Age-Structured Covid-19 Model

Basic discrete age-structured compartmental models seem to be more appropriate for Covid-19 disease since it is claimed that adults have a greater risk of transmitting SARS-CoV-2 virus than children do toward susceptibles (See Sect. 1). This suggests that in order to give more appropriate description of Covid-19 transmission, it is important to separate the population into two different age-subgroups.

The population considered in this section is stratified into two age categories and ten disease status. Individuals are classified as susceptible children (T), susceptible adult (S), exposed noninfectious (E_T), exposed noninfectious adult (E_s), asymptomatic infectious adult (A), asymptomatic infectious children (B), unreported symptomatic infectious (I_u), hospitalized symptomatic infectious (H), recovered individuals (R) and dead individuals (D). We assume that infected children do not show symptoms and can still transmit the disease. Covid-19 disease dynamics can be described as follows: Let β^{χ} be the transmission rate from infectious individuals to confined susceptible individuals and β^{N} be the transmission rate from infectious individuals to unconfined susceptible individuals. Then, for $i \in \{\chi, N\}$, susceptibles adults (S) (resp. susceptible children (T)) are infected through contact with infectious adults ($A + I_u$) at a transmission rate β^i_{aa} (resp. β^i_{ca}) or through contact with infectious children (B) at a transmission rate β^i_{ac} (resp. β^i_{cc}) and move to the exposed noninfectious adult class (E_s) (resp. the exposed noninfectious children class (E_T)). Adult exposed individuals (resp. children exposed individuals) then become asymptomatic infectious at rate k_s (resp. k_T). After an average period $1/\delta$ days the asymptomatic infectious individuals (A) become symptomatic and proceed either to the unreported symptomatic infectious (I_u), at rate δ_1, or to the hospitalized individual (H) at rate δ_2 with $\delta = \delta_1 + \delta_2$. Once becoming symptomatic, individuals of class I_u and H either remain asymptomatic for $1/\mu$ days on average before they are recovered or remain asymptomatic for $1/d$ days on average before they are dead. Asymptomatic children can either be recovered without being hospitalized at rate δ or detected and hospitalized at rate σ. The control parameters are as defined in Sect. 3. The subscripts c and a, respectively, characterize children and adults. The model will be given by the following equations

$$
\begin{cases}
\dfrac{dT}{dt} &= -\left(1-\gamma_c\right)p_c\left(\beta^{\chi}_{ac}T(t)\left(A(t)+I_u(t)\right)+\beta^{\chi}_{cc}T(t)B(t)\right)\\
&\quad -\left(1-\theta_c\right)\left(1-\left(1-\gamma_c\right)p_c\right)\left(\beta^{N}_{ac}T(t)\left(A(t)+I_u(t)\right)+\beta^{N}_{cc}T(t)B(t)\right),\\
\dfrac{dE_T}{dt} &= \left(1-\gamma_c\right)p_c\left(\beta^{\chi}_{ac}T(t)\left(A(t)+I_u(t)\right)+\beta^{\chi}_{cc}T(t)B(t)\right)\\
&\quad +\left(1-\theta_c\right)\left(1-\left(1-\gamma_c\right)p_c\right)\left(\beta^{N}_{ac}T(t)\left(A(t)+I_u(t)\right)+\beta^{N}_{cc}T(t)B(t)\right)-k_T E_T,\\
\dfrac{dB}{dt} &= k_T E_T-(\sigma+\delta)B(t),\\
\dfrac{dS}{dt} &= -\left(1-\gamma_a\right)p_a\left(\beta^{\chi}_{aa}S(t)\left(A(t)+I_u(t)\right)+\beta^{\chi}_{ca}S(t)B(t)\right)\\
&\quad -\left(1-\theta_a\right)\left(1-\left(1-\gamma_a\right)p_a\right)\left(\beta^{N}_{aa}S(t)\left(A(t)+I_u(t)\right)+\beta^{N}_{ca}S(t)B(t)\right),\\
\dfrac{dE_s}{dt} &= \left(1-\gamma_a\right)p_a\left(\beta^{\chi}_{aa}S(t)\left(A(t)+I_u(t)\right)+\beta^{\chi}_{ca}S(t)B(t)\right)\\
&\quad +\left(1-\theta_a\right)\left(1-\left(1-\gamma_a\right)p_a\right)\left(\beta^{N}_{aa}S(t)\left(A(t)+I_u(t)\right)+\beta^{N}_{ca}S(t)B(t)\right)-k_s E_s,\\
\dfrac{dA}{dt} &= k_s E_s-\delta A(t),\\
\dfrac{dI_u}{dt} &= \delta_1 A(t)-\mu I_u(t)-d I_u(t),\\
\dfrac{dH}{dt} &= \delta_2 A(t)+\sigma B(t)-\mu H-dH,\\
\dfrac{dR}{dt} &= \delta B(t)+\mu(H+I_u),\\
\dfrac{dD}{dt} &= d(H+I_u).
\end{cases}
\tag{10}
$$

4.1 Reproduction Numbers

Here, the basic and control reproduction numbers will be given by

$$
R_0=\frac{\beta^{N}_{cc}T(0)/N}{\sigma+\delta}+\frac{\beta^{N}_{aa}S(0)/N}{\delta}+\frac{\delta_1\beta^{N}_{aa}S(0)/N}{\delta\left(\mu+d\right)}
\tag{11}
$$

and

$$
\begin{aligned}
R_c=&\frac{\left(\left(1-\gamma_c\right)p_c\beta^{\chi}_{cc}+\left(1-\theta_c\right)\left(1-\left(1-\gamma_c\right)p_c\right)\beta^{N}_{cc}\right)T(0)/N}{\sigma+\delta}\\
&+\frac{\left(\delta_1+\mu+d\right)\left(\left(1-\gamma_a\right)p_a\beta^{\chi}_{aa}+\left(1-\theta_a\right)\left(1-\left(1-\gamma_a\right)p_a\right)\beta^{N}_{aa}\right)S(0)/N}{\delta\left(\mu+d\right)}.
\end{aligned}
\tag{12}
$$

Let us show the formula of $R_{0.}$ By setting $\gamma=\theta=0$, the linearized system related to infectious individuals, around $(T(0), 0, 0, S_0, 0, 0, 0)$, of system (3) is given b

$$\begin{cases} \dfrac{dE_T}{dt} &= -k_T E_T + \beta_{cc}^N T(0)B(t)/N + \beta_{ac}^N T(0)A(t)/N + \beta_{ac}^N T(0)I_u(t)/N \\ \dfrac{dB}{dt} &= k_T E_T - (\sigma + \delta)B(t), \\ \dfrac{dE_S}{dt} &= \beta_{ca}^N S(0)B(t)/N - k_s E_S + \beta_{aa}^N S(0)A(t)/N + \beta_{aa}^N S(0)I_u(t)/N \\ \dfrac{dA}{dt} &= k_s E_s - \delta A(t), \\ \dfrac{dI_u}{dt} &= \delta_1 A(t) - (\mu + d)\, I_u(t). \end{cases}$$

Moreover, the associated Jacobian matrix will be given by $M = F - E$ where

$$F = \begin{pmatrix} 0 & \beta_{cc}^N T(0)/N & 0 & \beta_{ac}^N T(0)/N & \beta_{ac}^N T(0)/N \\ k_T & 0 & 0 & 0 & 0 \\ 0 & \beta_{ca}^N S(0)/N & 0 & \beta_{aa}^N S(0)/N & \beta_{aa}^N S(0)/N \\ 0 & 0 & k_s & 0 & 0 \\ 0 & 0 & 0 & \delta_1 & 0 \end{pmatrix} \text{ and } E = \begin{pmatrix} k_T & 0 & 0 & 0 & 0 \\ 0 & \sigma+\delta & 0 & 0 & 0 \\ 0 & 0 & k_s & 0 & 0 \\ 0 & 0 & 0 & \delta & 0 \\ 0 & 0 & 0 & 0 & \mu+d \end{pmatrix}.$$

Therefore,

$$FE^{-1} = \frac{1}{N} \begin{pmatrix} \dfrac{\beta_{cc}^N T(0)}{\delta+\sigma} & \dfrac{\alpha_c \beta_{cc} T(0)}{\delta+\sigma} & \dfrac{(d+\mu+\delta_1)\,\beta_{ac}^N T(0)}{\delta(d+\mu)} & \dfrac{(d+\mu+\delta_1)\,\beta_{ac}^N T(0)}{\delta(d+\mu)} & \dfrac{\beta_{ac}^N T(0)}{d+\mu} \\ 0 & 0 & 0 & 0 & 0 \\ \dfrac{\beta_{ca}^N S(0)}{\delta+\sigma} & \dfrac{\beta_{ca}^N S(0)}{\delta+\sigma} & \dfrac{(d+\mu+\delta_1)\,\beta_{aa}^N S(0)}{\delta(d+\mu)} & \dfrac{(d+\mu+\delta_1)\,\beta_{aa}^N S(0)}{\delta\,(d+\mu)} & \dfrac{\beta_{aa}^N S(0)}{d+\mu} \\ 0 & 0 & 0 & 0 & 0 \\ 0 & 0 & 0 & 0 & 0 \end{pmatrix}$$

and R_0 is its spectral radius which is given by formula (11). Moreover, assuming that $\gamma\theta_c\theta_a \neq 0$ and following the same process above, the control reproduction number will be given by formula (12).

4.2 Parameter and Initial Data Estimation

Note that the first infected child was reported 22 days since the beginning of the epidemic. Furthermore, the maximum asymptomatic duration including the exposure period is about 14 days. Consequently, there were neither exposed nor asymptomatic infected children under 15 years old at $t = 0$. Thus, the initial data values related to infected adult individuals are the same as those in system (3). Furthermore, $E_0 = B_0 = 0$, $T_0 = 9683602$ and $S_0 = 26181589$. As mentioned in Sect. 1, we assume that $\beta_{ac}^i = \beta_{aa}^i$, $\beta_{ca}^i = \beta_{cc}^i$ where $i \in \{\chi, N\}$. Using the same fitting solver as in Sect. 3.2, we obtain the parameter values shown in Table 2. The SSR related to this model is estimated to be $SSR_{age} = 98.76$.

Table 2 Parameter definitions and values of model (10)

Symbol	Definition	Parameter value	Confidence interval	Reference
$\beta_{aa}^N, \beta_{ac}^N$	Infection rate from infectious adults to unconfined population	0.41	$0.1 - 0.63$	Estimated
$\beta_{ca}^N, \beta_{cc}^N$	Infection rate from infectious children to unconfined population	0.2	$0.05 - 0.31$	Estimated
$\beta_{aa}^X, \beta_{ac}^X$	Infection rate from infectious adults to confined population	0.1	$0.007 - 0.15$	Estimated
$\beta_{ca}^X, \beta_{cc}^X$	Infection rate from infectious children to confined population	0.014	$0.002 - 0.16$	Estimated
p	Proportion of lockdown	0.65	$0.57 - 0.86$	Estimated
k	Exposed noninfectious individuals	3	$2 - 4$	See text
R_0	Basic reproduction number	2.06	$0.5 - 3.19$	Estimated

5 Covid-19 Model with Constant Delay

In order to enable the study of the effect of the period time, in which infected individuals are asymptomatic and noninfectious, on the Covid-19 dynamics, we will incorporate the time delay (latency period) in the basic model instead of considering the noninfectious latent state as a model component. Let η denotes the death rate of noninfectious exposed individuals. Once infected through contact with infectious individuals at rate β, the susceptible individuals that survive with probability $e^{-\eta\tau}$ become infectious (able to transmit the infection) when the time since exposure exceeds an exposure period time τ. The dynamics of the model are described by the following system of differential equation with delay

$$\begin{cases} \frac{dS}{dt} &= -\alpha e^{-\eta\tau} S(t)\left(A(t)+I_u(t)\right)/N, \\ \frac{dA}{dt} &= \alpha e^{-\eta_a\tau} S(t-\tau)\left(A(t-\tau)+I_u(t-\tau)\right)-\delta A(t), \\ \frac{dI_u}{dt} &= \delta_1 A(t)-\mu I_u(t)-dI_u(t), \\ \frac{dH}{dt} &= \delta_2 A(t)-\mu H-dH, \\ \frac{dR}{dt} &= \mu(H+I_u), \\ \frac{dD}{dt} &= d(H+I_u) \end{cases} \tag{13}$$

where $\alpha = (1-\gamma)\,p\beta_c + (1-\theta)\,(1-(1-\gamma)\,p)\,\beta_N$ and all the model parameters, except η and τ, are described similarly to those in Sect. 3.

5.1 Reproduction Numbers

The control and basic reproduction numbers for system (13) are successively given by

$$R_c = \frac{\alpha S_0 e^{-\eta\tau}}{N}\left(\frac{1}{\delta}+\frac{\delta_1}{\delta\,(\mu+d)}\right) \text{ and } R_0 = \frac{\beta_N S_0 e^{-\eta\tau}}{N}\left(\frac{1}{\delta}+\frac{\delta_1}{\delta\,(\mu+d)}\right).$$

To compute the basic reproduction number, we apply the survival function approach described by Heffernan, Smith, and Wahl [6]. Let R_{01} (respectively, R_{02}) be the average number of secondary infections produced when one asymptomatic infected (respectively, symptomatic unreported infected) individual is introduced into the host virgin population. Following the work in [6], we have $R_{01} = \int_0^\infty F(s)ds$ where $F(s)$ is the probability that a newly asymptomatic infected individual has been produced by an existing asymptomatic infectious individual and lives for at least time s. The probability function $F(s)$ can be expressed as $F(s) = \displaystyle\int_0^s P_1(t)P_2(s,t)dt$, where $P_1(t)$ is the probability that an asymptomatic infected individual of age t infects a susceptible individual and is given by $\dfrac{\beta_N S_0}{N}$ and $P_2\,(s,t)$ is the probability that exposed infected individual lives to age $s-t$ and is given by $e^{-\eta\tau}e^{-\delta(s-t)}$ before becoming infectious. Consequently, $R_{01} = \frac{\beta_N S_0}{N}e^{-\eta\tau}\int_0^\infty\int_0^s e^{-\delta(s-t)}dtds$ which can be reduced to $R_{01} = \frac{\beta_N S_0 e^{-\eta\tau}}{N\delta}$. Since asymptomatic individuals can become unreported symptomatic infectious individuals over their lifespan $1/\delta$ at a rate δ_1 and each infectious symptomatic individual produces, on average, $\beta_N S_0 \dfrac{1}{\mu+d}$ asymptomatic individuals during his lifespan $1/(\mu+d)$ then, similarly, we can express R_{02} as

$R_{02}=\frac{\beta_N S_0 e^{-\eta\tau}}{N}\frac{\delta_1}{\delta(\mu+d)}$. Thus, the basic reproduction number R_0 will be given by

$$R_0=\frac{\beta_N S_0 e^{-\eta\tau}}{N}\left(\frac{1}{\delta}+\frac{\delta_1}{\delta\,(\mu+d)}\right).$$

Similarly, we can obtain the control reproduction number for system (13).

5.2 Parameter and Initial Data Estimation

Since the parameters δ, δ_1,δ_2, μ and d are not affected by the age then their values are the same as those in Sect. 3.2. Note that since there were no death of exposed individuals then it is meaningful to assume that $\eta = 0$. To estimate the initial data, we will use the same process as in Sect. 3.2 so that $A(t)$ will be given by (3) for t close to 0. Thus, using the second and the third equations of system (13) we obtain, for t close to 0,

$$aA(t) = \beta_N S(0)\,(A(t-\tau) + I_u(t-\tau))\,/N - \delta A(t), \tag{14}$$

and

$$I_u(t+0) = I_0\,(\theta)\,e^{at}, \tag{15}$$

where

$$I_0(\theta) = \frac{\delta_1}{a+\mu+d}\frac{ba}{\delta_2}e^{a\theta}. \tag{16}$$

Now, using Eqs. (14) and (15) and the third equation of system (13), we obtain after simplification

$$aA_0 = \beta_N S_0\left(A_0 + \frac{\delta_1}{a+\mu+d}A_0\right)e^{-a\tau}/N - \delta A_0 \tag{17}$$

and

$$aI_0 = \delta_1 A_0 - \mu I_0 - dI_0. \tag{18}$$

Solving Eqs. (16), (17) and (18) for β_N and A_0 lead to

$$\beta_N = \frac{(a+\delta)\,(a+\mu+d)}{a+\mu+d+\delta_1}e^{a\tau} \text{ and } I_0 = \frac{\delta_1}{a+\mu+d}A_0. \tag{19}$$

Table 3 Parameter definitions and values of model (13)

Symbol	Definition	Parameter value	Confidence Interval (95%)	Reference
β_N	Infection rate for unconfined population	0.4596	0.4492 – 0.48	Estimated
β_c	Infection rate for confined population	0.091	0.089 – 0.096	Estimated
τ	latency period	0.33	0.25 – 0.5	See text
R_0	Basic reproduction number	3.03	2.96 – 3.174	Estimated
p	Proportion of lockdown	0.75	0.53 – 0.82	Estimated

Furthermore, the initial data $A_0(\theta)$ and $I_0(\theta)$ are given for $\theta \in [-\tau, 0]$ by $A_0(\theta) = \frac{ba}{\delta_2}e^{a\theta}$ and $I_0(\theta) = \frac{\delta_1}{a+\mu+d}A_0(\theta)$. We will assume, as in Sect. 3, that the latency duration varies between 6 and 12 h. Consequently, β_N is estimated to be between 0.4492 and 0.48 with an average of 0.4596. In this case, the basic reproduction number varies between 2.96 and 3.174 with 3.03 in average. Finally, by repeating the same above process between the first and last day of lockdown we can estimate the parameters β_c and p (See Table 3). Here, the sum of squared residuals is estimated to be $SSR_{dde} = 92.63$. When considering 6 and 12 h as latency periods, then their SSR are given respectively by $SSR_{\tau=0.25} = 93.23$ and $SSR_{\tau=0.5} = 95.55$.

6 Covid-19 Model with Threshold-Type Delay

Threshold delay equations (TDEs) ensue in a natural way in compartmental models for which the time in residence in a particular compartment is determined by the stipulation that a fixed threshold load of an entity is racked up during the time spent in that compartment. A susceptible individual that is first exposed to a pathogen at time $t-\sigma$ will become infectious at time t provided the individual receives a sufficient load of the virus during the time from $t-\sigma$ to t. We will assume that an individual is exposed to an infectious quantum, c, which is the unit of SARS-CoV-2 viral load needed to produce an infection. Therefore, we will assume that the infectious SARS-CoV-2 viral load will grow, overcoming the nonspecific immune response. When the pathogen load has increased to a threshold Q, or equivalently, when the age since exposure is greater than the latency period τ, we then consider the individual to be infectious. We assume, as mentioned in [7], that the repeated exposures to smaller viral loads increase the pathogen load in-host. Furthermore, since transmission occurs from infected individuals, the pathogen load due to an exposure will depend on the infected population.

Let r be the internal growth rate of the SARS-CoV-2 virus, b is the number of effective contacts between an exposed and infectious individuals, k is an adjustable parameter which measures how soon saturation occurs. Following the modeling approach in [23], the threshold condition is governed by the following formula

$$\Psi(t) := ce^{r\tau(A_t+I_{u,t})} + \int_{-\tau(A_t+I_{u,t})}^{0} e^{-vr} G(A(t+v) + I_u(t+v))dv - Q = 0 \quad (20)$$

where $A_t + I_{u,t}$ are the history functions of the infectious individuals defined for $\xi \in [-\tau^{\infty} := -\max_{\phi\in C} \tau(\phi), 0]$ by

$$A_t(\xi) + I_{u,t}(\xi) = A(t+\xi) + I_u(t+\xi)$$

and $\tau : C \mapsto \mathbb{R}^+$ is a decreasing and continuously differential map on the space of continuous functions,$C := C\left([-\tau^{\infty}, 0], \mathbb{R}^+\right)$, satisfying $\tau(0) = \frac{1}{r}\ln\left(\frac{Q}{c}\right)$. Furthermore, F is the additive SARS-CoV-2 viral load in the exposed individual due to multiple exposures to infectious individuals which is given, for $x \geq 0$, by the following Holling functional response-type 2

$$G(x) = \frac{bcx}{kx+1}.$$

The Covid-19 model will then be given by the following threshold-type delay system

$$\begin{cases} \frac{dS}{dt} &= -\alpha S(t)\left(A(t) + I_u(t)\right)/N, \\ \frac{dA}{dt} &= \alpha e^{-\eta\tau(A_t+I_{u,t})} S\left(t - \tau\left(A_t + I_{u,t}\right)\right)\left(A\left(t - \tau\left(A_t + I_{u,t}\right)\right) + I_u\left(t - \tau\left(A_t + I_{u,t}\right)\right)\right) \\ & -\delta A(t), \\ \frac{dI_u}{dt} &= \delta_1 A(t) - \mu I_u(t) - dI_u(t), \\ \frac{dH}{dt} &= \delta_2 A(t) - \mu H - dH, \\ \frac{dR}{dt} &= \delta B(t) + \mu(H + I_u), \\ \frac{dD}{dt} &= d(H + I_u), \\ \Psi(t) &= 0 \end{cases} \quad (21)$$

where τ, A and I_u satisfy the threshold condition (20).

Applying the survival function approach described by Heffernan, Smith, and Wahl [6] as done in Sect. 5.1, the control and basic reproduction numbers are given by

Table 4 Parameter definitions and values of model (21)

Symbol	Definition	Parameter value	Confidence Interval (95%)	Reference
β_N	Infection rate for unconfined population	0.4596	0.4492 – 0.48	Estimated
β_c	Infection rate for confined population	0.091	0.089 – 0.096	Estimated
r	Internal growth rate	1.02		Adjusted
b	Effective contact number	20		Adjusted
k	Adjustable parameter	10^{-5}		Adjusted
c	Viral load per contact	49, 79	18.31 – 135.33	Estimated
$\tau(0)$	Maximal latency duration	0.33 days	0.25 – 0.25	See text
R_0	Basic reproduction number	3.03	2.96 – 3.174	Estimated
p	Proportion of lockdown	0.73	0.51 – 0.78	Estimated

$$R_c = \frac{\alpha S_0 e^{-\eta\tau(0)}(\mu+d+\delta_1)}{\delta N(\mu+d)} \text{ and } R_0 = \frac{\beta_N S_0 e^{-\eta\tau(0)}(\mu+d+\delta_1)}{\delta N(\mu+d)}.$$

In order to estimate the model parameters and simulate its dynamics we use MATLAB ddesd solver [25] for state-dependent delay differential equations to compute the solutions of (21) numerically. However, we should note that simulating the behavior of solutions of system (21) for the general state-dependent delay τ is a challenging task. To overcome this difficulty, we will estimate the parameters and perform our simulations using constant initial data. Let $\tilde{C} = \{\phi \in C : \phi(s) = \phi(0) \text{ for all } s \in [-\tau^\infty, 0]\}$ be the space of constant initial data. Thus, for $\phi \in \tilde{C}$, the equation $\Psi(\tau(\phi), \phi) = 0$ given by (20) is equivalent to

$$ce^{r\tau(\phi)} + \int_{-\tau(\phi)}^{0} e^{-rs} G(\phi(0))dv - Q = 0.$$

Solving this equation for $\tau(\phi)$, we obtain

$$\tau(\phi) = \frac{1}{r} \ln\left(\frac{rQ + G(\phi(0))}{cr + G(\phi(0))}\right). \tag{22}$$

It is experimentally shown that the minimal viral load needed for the infection to occur in hamsters is 1000 particles (See [10] more details). Thus, we assume that $Q = 1000$. Furthermore, since the maximal latency duration $\tau(0)$ varies between 6 and 12 hours then, from formula (22) the viral load, c, per each contact will vary between $Qe^{-r/2}$ and $Qe^{-r/4}$ with an average of $Qe^{-r/3}$. However, another difficulty we encounter for this model is that the parameters b, r and k related to Covid-19 disease are still unknown and we are compelled to fairly adjust them to fit the reported cases (see Table 4). In this case, we will be able to follow the same process as the one in Sect. 5.2 to obtain the remaining model parameters (See Table 4). Furthermore, we obtain $SSR_{sde} = 94.3$.

7 Models with Demographic Effects

In the previous section, we have omitted births and deaths in our description of models because it was believed that the time scale of of Covid-19 epidemic is much shorter than the demographic time scale. Indeed, we have used a time scale on which the number of births and deaths in unit time is negligible. However, as mentioned in Sect. 1, there is a possibility that the Covid-19 may not go away after a short time and could stay for years. Thus, we need to think on a longer time scale and include a birth rate parameter, π_S and a death rate parameter d_S. In what follows, we will reconsider models (13) and (21) including demographic effects and we shall give a rigorous mathematical analysis to the both models. The reason for which we select these models is that model (13) is shown to be the best one to fit well the data while model (21), as we will see in Subsection 7.2, generates more complicated behavior then the three other models.

7.1 *Covid-19 Model with Constant Delay*

Let us analyze the following constant-delay Covid-19 model

$$\begin{cases} \frac{dS}{dt} &= \pi_S - \alpha e^{-\eta\tau} S(t)\left(A(t) + I_u(t)\right)/N - d_S S(t), \\ \frac{dA}{dt} &= \alpha e^{-\eta_a\tau} S(t-\tau)\left(A(t-\tau) + I_u(t-\tau)\right) - \delta A(t) - -d_S A(t), \\ \frac{dI_u}{dt} &= \delta_1 A(t) - \mu I_u(t) - d I_u(t) - d_S I_u(t), \\ \frac{dH}{dt} &= \delta_2 A(t) - \mu H(t) - d H(t) - d_S H(t), \\ \frac{dR}{dt} &= \mu\left(H(t) + I_u(t)\right) - d_S R(t), \\ \frac{dD}{dt} &= d\left(H(t) + I_u(t)\right) \end{cases} \tag{23}$$

where

$$\alpha = ((1-\gamma)\, p\beta_c + (1-\theta)\,(1-(1-\gamma)\, p)\, \beta_N)\,.$$

Since the three last components H, R and D do not appear in the three first equations of model (23), then we will focus our local stability study on the three first equations.

7.1.1 Equilibria

Computing the equilibria of system (23), we see that a positive steady state $\left(\tilde{S}, \tilde{A}, \tilde{I}_u\right)$ must satisfy

$$\begin{cases} \pi_S - \alpha e^{-\eta\tau}\tilde{S}\left(\tilde{A}+\tilde{I}_u\right)/N - d_S\tilde{S} & = 0, \\ \alpha e^{-\eta\tau}\tilde{S}\left(\tilde{A}+\tilde{I}_u\right)/N - (\delta + d_S)\,\tilde{A} & = 0, \\ \delta_1\tilde{A} - (\mu + d + d_S)\,\tilde{I}_u & = 0. \end{cases}$$

A straightforward calculation of the above system leads to the following result.

Proposition 1 *The model (23) has a disease-free equilibrium (DFE) given by* $\overline{E} = (\frac{\pi_S}{d_S}, 0, 0)$ *in which there is no disease. Furthermore, the DFE is unique when* $R_c \leq 1$ *and a unique endemic equilibrium of (23) appears when* $R_c > 1$.

Moreover, the endemic equilibrium, $E^* = \left(\tilde{S}, \tilde{A}, \tilde{I}_u\right)$, *satisfies*

$$\tilde{S} = \frac{\delta}{\alpha e^{-\eta\tau}\left(1+\frac{\delta_1}{\mu+d+d_S}\right)/N},\ \tilde{A} = \delta\left(\pi_S - d_S\tilde{S}\right)/N \text{ and } \tilde{I}_u = \frac{\delta_1}{\mu+d+d_S}\tilde{A}, \tag{24}$$

7.1.2 Control Thresholds

Following the work done in Sect. 5.1 we can easily obtain the basic reproduction number related to model (23) as follows

$$R_0 = \frac{\pi_S\beta_N e^{-\eta\tau}}{d_S N}\left(\frac{1}{\delta+d_S} + \frac{\delta_1}{(\delta+d_S)\,(\mu+d+d_S)}\right).$$

The control reproduction number is given by

$$R_c = \frac{\pi_S\alpha e^{-\eta\tau}}{d_S N}\left(\frac{1}{\delta+d_S} + \frac{\delta_1}{(\delta+d_S)\,(\mu+d+d_S)}\right).$$

7.1.3 Bifurcation Analysis

In the following, we shall prove that system (23) produces a forward transcritical bifurcation. The linearization of system (23) around any steady state $\mathrm{E} = \left(S^e, A^e, I_u^e\right)$ characteristic equation

$$\Delta(\lambda) = (\lambda + \delta + d_S)\left(\lambda + \alpha e^{-\eta\tau}\left(A^e + I_u^e\right)/N + d_S\right)(\lambda + \mu + d + d_S) \tag{25}$$
$$-\alpha e^{-\eta\tau} S^e (\lambda + \mu + d + \delta_1 + d_S)(\lambda + d_S) e^{-\lambda\tau}/N.$$

The local behavior of the DFE of system (23) is given by the following theorem.

Theorem 1 *The boundary steady state $\overline{E}$ of system (23) is unstable when $R_c > 1$ and locally asymptotically stable when $R_c < 1$.*

Proof The characteristic equation associated with the DFE is given by

$$\Delta(\lambda) = (\lambda + d_S)\left((\lambda + \delta + d_S)(\lambda + \mu + d + d_S) - \alpha e^{-\eta\tau}\overline{S}(\lambda + \mu + d + \delta_1 + d_S) e^{-\lambda\tau}/N\right).$$

Then the associated eigenvalues are given by $\lambda = -d_S$ and the roots of

$$\tilde{\delta}(\lambda) = (\lambda + \delta + d_S)(\lambda + \mu + d + d_S) - \alpha e^{-\eta\tau}\overline{S}(\lambda + \mu + d + \delta_1 + d_S) e^{-\lambda\tau}/N. \tag{26}$$

Let λ be any eigenvalue associated with Eq. (26) with nonnegative real part (i.e. $\Re e(\lambda) \geq 0$) and assume that $R_c < 1$. Then $e^{-\Re e(\lambda)\tau} \leq 1$ and

$$\frac{|\lambda + \delta + d_S||\lambda + \mu + d + d_S|}{|\lambda + \mu + d + \delta_1 + d_S|} \leq \alpha e^{-\eta\tau}\overline{S}/N.$$

On the other hand, it follows from $R_c < 1$ that

$$\alpha e^{-\eta\tau}\overline{S}/N < \frac{(\delta + d_S)(\mu + d + d_S)}{\mu + d + \delta_1 + d_S}.$$

This is a contradiction since the map $\lambda \mapsto \dfrac{|\lambda + \delta + d_S||\lambda + \mu + d + d_S|}{|\lambda + \mu + d + \delta_1 + d_S|}$ is increasing. Consequently, the DFE is locally asymptotically stable. On the other hand if $R_c > 1$ then

$$\tilde{\delta}(0) = \delta(\mu + d + d_S)(1 - R_c) < 0.$$

Then $\tilde{\delta}$ has one positive root and the DFE is unstable. □

The forward transcritical bifurcation of the endemic equilibrium as R_c moves through 1 is stated as follows.

Theorem 2 *When $R_c < 1$, the endemic equilibrium of system (23) is locally asymptotically stable while the DFE is unstable, and for $R_c > 1$ the DFE is unique and* *locally asymptotically stable. That is, forward transcritical bifurcation occurs at* $R_c = 1$.

Proof The characteristic equation associated with the endemic equilibrium is given by

$$\Delta(\lambda) = \frac{(\lambda+\delta+d_S)\left(\lambda+\alpha e^{-\eta\tau}\left(\tilde{A}+\tilde{I}_u\right)/N+d_S\right)(\lambda+\mu+d+d_S)}{(\lambda+\mu+d+\delta_1+d_S)(\lambda+d_S)} - \alpha e^{-\eta_a\tau}\tilde{S}/Ne^{-\lambda\tau}.$$

Let λ be any eigenvalue associated with Eq. (26) with nonnegative real part. Then

$$\begin{aligned}\frac{|\lambda+\delta+d_S||\lambda+\mu+d+d_S|}{|\lambda+\mu+d+\delta_1+d_S|} &\leq \frac{|\lambda+\delta+d_S||\lambda+\alpha e^{-\eta\tau}\left(\tilde{A}+\tilde{I}_u\right)/N+d_S||\lambda+\mu+d+d_S|}{|\lambda+\mu+d+\delta_1+d_S||\lambda+d_S|}\\ &= \alpha e^{-\eta\tau}\tilde{S}\,|e^{-\lambda\tau}|/N\\ &\leq \frac{(\mu+d+d_S)\,\delta}{\mu+d+\delta_1+d_S}\end{aligned}$$

However, $\lambda \mapsto \dfrac{|\lambda+\delta+d_S||\lambda+\mu+d+d_S|}{|\lambda+\mu+d+\delta_1+d_S|}$ is increasing which is a contradiction. It follows that all characteristic roots of Δ are negative. Thus, the local asymptotic stability of the positive steady state immediately follows. Furthermore, from Theorem 1 we deduce the local behavior of the DFE. This completes the proof. □

7.2 Covid-19 Model with Threshold-Type Delay

In this section, we will perform qualitative analysis of the following threshold-type delay Covid-19 model. We shall prove that system (23) produces two potential cases of bifurcation depending on the chosen parameter values.

$$\begin{cases}\frac{dS}{dt} &= \pi_S - \alpha S(t)\left(A(t)+I_u(t)\right)/N - d_S S,\\ \frac{dA}{dt} &= \alpha e^{-\eta\tau(A(t)+I_u(t))}S(t-\sigma(t))\left(A(t-\sigma(t))+I_u(t-\sigma(t))\right)\\ &\quad -(\delta+d_S)A(t),\\ \frac{dI_u}{dt} &= \delta_1 A(t) - \mu I_u(t) - (d+d_S)I_u(t),\\ \frac{dH}{dt} &= \delta_2 A(t) - \mu H - (d+d_S)H,\\ \frac{d\tilde{R}}{dt} &= \delta B(t) + \mu(H+I_u),\\ \frac{dD}{dt} &= d(H+I_u)\end{cases} \tag{27}$$

where $\sigma(t) = \tau\left(A(t)+I_u(t)\right)$.

7.2.1 Equilibria

As mentioned in Sect. 7.1, we will focus our study only on the three first equations. Computing the equilibria of the system (27), we see that an endemic equilibrium $\left(\tilde{S}, \tilde{A}, \tilde{I}_u\right)$ must satisfy

$$\begin{cases} \pi_S - \alpha \tilde{S}\left(\tilde{A} + \tilde{I}_u\right)/N - d_S \tilde{S} & = 0, \\ \alpha e^{-\eta\tau(\tilde{A}+\tilde{I}_u)} \tilde{S}\left(\tilde{A} + \tilde{I}_u\right)/N - (\delta + d_S)\tilde{A} & = 0, \\ \delta_1 \tilde{A} - (\mu + d + d_S)\tilde{I}_u & = 0. \end{cases}$$

Let, for $y > 0$, $\nu(y) = \tau\left(\left(\frac{\mu + d + \delta_1 + d_S}{\mu + d + d_S}\right) y\right)$,

$$W(y) = \eta\nu'(y)\left(\alpha\left(\frac{\mu + d + \delta_1 + d_S}{\mu + d + d_S}\right) y/N + d_S\right) + \alpha\left(\frac{\mu + d + \delta_1 + d_S}{\mu + d + d_S}\right)/N$$

and

$$\chi(y) = \frac{\pi_S \alpha e^{-\eta\nu(y)}(\mu + d + \delta_1 + d_S)}{\alpha\left(\frac{\mu + d + \delta_1 + d_S}{\mu + d + d_S}\right) y/N + d_S}.$$

A straightforward calculation of the above system leads to the following result.

Proposition 2 *The model (27) has a disease-free equilibrium (DFE) given by,*

$$\overline{E} = \left(\frac{\pi_S}{d_S}, 0, 0\right)$$

in which there is no disease. Furthermore,

(i) if $R_c \le 1$ and $W\left(\tilde{A}\right) > 0$ then there is no endemic equilibria,

(ii) if $R_c > 1$ and $W\left(\tilde{A}\right) > 0$ then there exists only one endemic equilibrium,

(iii) if $R_c < 1$ and there exist $A^* > 0$ such that $\chi(A^*) > \delta N(\mu + d)$, then there exist at least two endemic equilibria,

(vi) if $R_c \le 1$ and, for all $y > 0$, $\chi(y) < \delta N(\mu + d)$, then there is no endemic equilibria.

Moreover, the endemic equilibrium, $E^* = \left(\tilde{S}, \tilde{A}, \tilde{I}_u\right)$, satisfies

$$\tilde{S} = \frac{\pi_S}{\alpha\left(\frac{\mu + d + \delta_1 + d_S}{\mu + d + d_S}\right)\tilde{A}/N + d_S}, \quad \tilde{I}_u = \frac{\delta_1}{\mu + d + d_S}\tilde{A} \text{ and } \chi\left(\tilde{A}\right) = \delta N(\mu + d + d_S). \tag{28}$$

Proof After few calculations, we obtain

$$\chi(0) = \frac{\pi_S \alpha e^{-\eta\nu(0)}(\mu + d + \delta_1 + d_S)}{d_S} = R_c \delta N(\mu + d + d_S),$$

$\lim_{y\to\infty} \chi(y) = 0$ and

$$\chi'\left(\tilde{A}\right) = -\frac{\pi_S \alpha (\mu + d + \delta_1 + d_S) e^{-\eta\nu(\tilde{A})}}{\left(\alpha\left(\frac{\mu + d + \delta_1 + d_S}{\mu + d + d_S}\right)\tilde{A}/N + d_S\right)^2} W\left(\tilde{A}\right).$$

This proves all the assertions of the proposition. □

7.2.2 Control Thresholds

Similarly to the proof in Sect. 5.1, the basic and control reproduction numbers for system (27) are successively given by
vspace*-8pt

$$R_0 = \frac{\pi_S \beta_N e^{-\eta\nu(0)}(\mu + d + \delta_1 + d_S)}{\delta N(\mu + d + d_S) d_S} \text{ and } R_c = \frac{\pi_S \alpha e^{-\eta\nu(0)}}{N d_S}\left(\frac{1}{\delta + d_S} + \frac{\delta_1}{(\delta + d_S)(\mu + d + d_S)}\right).$$

7.2.3 Bifurcations

Here we focus on local asymptotic stability and bifurcation analysis of equilibria of system (27) .

Theorem 3 *The DFE* $\overline{E} = \left(\overline{S}, 0, 0\right)$ *of (27) is unstable when* $R_c > 1$*, and locally asymptotically stable when* $R_c < 1$*.*

Proof The characteristic equation associated with the DFE is given by

$$\begin{aligned}\Delta(\lambda) &= (\lambda + \delta + d_S)(\lambda + \mu + d + d_S) - \alpha e^{-\eta\nu(0)}\overline{S}e^{-\lambda\nu(0)}(\lambda + \mu + d + \delta_1 + d_S)/N \\ &= \lambda^2 + \left(\mu + d + \delta + d_S - \alpha\overline{S}/N\right)\lambda - \alpha e^{-\eta\nu(0)}\overline{S}/N(\lambda + \mu + d + \delta_1 + d_S)e^{-\lambda\nu(0)} \\ &\quad + (\delta + d_S)(\mu + d + d_S).\end{aligned}$$

When $\nu = 0$ then $\Delta(\lambda) = \lambda^2 + \left(\mu + d + \delta + d_S - \alpha\overline{S}/N\right)\lambda + \delta(\mu + d + d_S)$ $(1 - R_c)$. Furthermore, we have

$$\begin{aligned}\mu + d + \delta + d_S - \overline{S}\alpha/N &= \frac{(\delta + d_S)(\mu + d + d_S)}{\mu + d + \delta_1 + d_S}\frac{(\mu + d + \delta + d_S)(\mu + d + \delta_1 + d_S)}{(\delta + d_S)(\mu + d + d_S)} \\ &> \frac{(\delta + d_S)(\mu + d + d_S)}{\mu + d + \delta_1 + d_S}(1 - R_c).\end{aligned}$$

Thus, the DFE is stable when $\nu = 0$ and $R_c < 1$. Assume that $\nu > 0$ and let $\omega > 0$. Separating real and imaginary parts, equality $\Delta(i\omega) = 0$ is equivalent to

$$\omega^4 + \left((\mu + d + d_S)^2 + (\delta + d_S)^2 - \left(\alpha e^{-\eta\nu(0)}\overline{S}/N\right)^2\right)\omega^2 + (\delta + d_S)^2 (\mu + d + d_S)^2 - \left(\alpha e^{-\eta\nu(0)}\overline{S}/N\,(\mu + d + \delta_1 + d_S)\right)^2 = 0.$$

A simple calculation of the discriminant $\tilde{\delta}$ leads to

$$\tilde{\delta} = \left((\mu + d + d_S)^2 - (\delta + d_S)^2 - \left(\alpha e^{-\eta\nu(0)}\overline{S}/N\right)^2\right)^2 + 4\,(\delta + d_S)^2 \left(\alpha e^{-\eta\nu(0)}\overline{S}/N\right)^2 + 4\left(\alpha e^{-\eta\nu(0)}\tilde{S}/N\,(\mu + d + \delta_1 + d_S)\right)^2$$

which is positive. It follows that $i\omega$ is not a root of Δ and, consequently, the DFE is LAS for all $\nu > 0$ such that $R_c < 1$. On the other hand, if $R_c > 1$ then

$$\begin{aligned}\Delta(0) &= \delta\,(\mu + d + d_S)\left(1 - \frac{\alpha e^{-\eta\nu(0)}\pi_S\,(\mu + d + \delta_1 + d_S)/N}{d_S\delta\,(\mu + d + d_S)}\right)\\ &= (\delta + d_S)\,(\mu + d + d_S)\,(1 - R_c)\end{aligned}$$

which is negative. It follows that Δ has a positive root and the DFE is unstable. □

Theorem 4 *When $R_c = 1$ and $W\left(\tilde{A}\right) > 0$, the endemic equilibrium undergoes a forward transcritical bifurcation, that is for $R_c > 1$, R_c close to 1, the endemic equilibrium is locally asymptotically stable, whereas the DFE is unstable, and for $R_c < 1$ the DFE is locally asymptotically stable and is the only steady state of (27).*

Proof The characteristic equation is given by

$$\Delta(\lambda) = (\lambda + \delta + d_S)\,(\lambda + \mu + d + d_S) - \alpha\tilde{S}e^{-\eta\nu\left(\tilde{A}\right)}e^{-\lambda\nu\left(\tilde{A}\right)}\,(\lambda + \mu + d + \delta_1 + d_S)/N + Q(\lambda)$$

where

$$Q(\lambda) = \alpha e^{-\eta\nu\left(\tilde{A}\right)}\left(\tilde{A} + \tilde{I}_u\right)\tilde{S}\,(\lambda + \mu + d + \delta_1 + d_S)\left(\frac{e^{-\lambda\nu\left(\tilde{A}\right)}\alpha/N}{\lambda + \alpha\left(\tilde{A} + \tilde{I}_u\right)/N + d_S} + \eta\nu'\left(\tilde{A}\right)\right)/N.$$

Then

$$\begin{aligned}\Delta(0) &= \delta\,(\mu + d + d_S) - \alpha e^{-\eta\nu\left(\tilde{A}\right)}\tilde{S}\,(\mu + d + \delta_1 + d_S)/N\\ &\quad + \alpha e^{-\eta\nu\left(\tilde{A}\right)}\left(\tilde{A} + \tilde{I}_u\right)\tilde{S}\,(\mu + d + d_S)\left(\frac{\alpha\left(\frac{\mu+d+\delta_1}{\mu+d}\right)/N}{\alpha\left(\tilde{A} + \tilde{I}_u\right)/N + d_S} + \eta\nu'\left(\tilde{A}\right)\right)/N.\end{aligned}$$

On the other hand, from the equilibrium Eq. (28), we have

$$\alpha e^{-\eta_a \nu(\tilde{A})} \tilde{S} \left(\mu + d + \delta_1 + d_S\right) / N - \left(\delta + d_S\right) \left(\mu + d + d_S\right) = 0.$$

Then

$$\Delta (0) = \alpha e^{-\eta \nu\left(\tilde{A}\right)} \left(\tilde{A} + \tilde{I}_u\right) \tilde{S} \left(\mu + d + d_S\right) \left(\frac{\alpha \left(\dfrac{\mu + d + \delta_1 + d_S}{\mu + d + d_S} \right) / N}{\alpha \left(\tilde{A} + \tilde{I}_u\right) / N + d_S} + \eta \nu' \left(\tilde{A}\right) \right) / N.$$

It follows from condition (ii) in Proposition 2 that $\Delta(0) > 0$. This proves that $\lambda = 0$ is not a root of $\Delta(\lambda) = 0$.

Now, let λ be a root of $\Delta(.)$ with nonnegative real part and $Z = \mid \lambda + \mu + d + \delta_1 + d_S \mid \alpha e^{-\eta \nu(\tilde{A})} \tilde{S} / N$. Thus, $\mid e^{-\lambda \nu(\tilde{A})} \mid \leq 1$ and

$$\begin{aligned} \mid Q(\lambda) \mid &\leq Z \left(\frac{\alpha \left(\tilde{A} + \tilde{I}_u\right) / N}{\mid \lambda + \alpha \left(\tilde{A} + \tilde{I}_u\right) / N + d_S \mid} \right) \\ &< Z. \end{aligned}$$

Set $X = \frac{(\delta + d_S)(\mu + d + d_S)}{\mu + d + \delta_1 + d_S} - \alpha \tilde{S} e^{-\eta \nu(\tilde{A})} e^{-\lambda \nu(\tilde{A})} / N$ and $Y = \alpha e^{-\eta_a \nu(\tilde{A})} \tilde{S} / N - \alpha$ $\tilde{S} e^{-\eta \nu(\tilde{A})} e^{-\lambda \nu(\tilde{A})} / N$. Then, using formula (28), we have $X = Y$ and

$$\begin{aligned} \mid (\lambda + \delta + d_S)(\lambda + \mu + d + d_S) - \alpha \tilde{S} e^{-\eta \nu\left(\tilde{A}\right)} e^{-\lambda \nu\left(\tilde{A}\right)} / N \mid &\geq \mid \lambda + \mu + d + \delta_1 + d_S \mid\mid Y \mid \\ &= Z \mid 1 - e^{-\lambda \nu\left(\tilde{A}\right)} \mid . \end{aligned}$$

Therefore, $\mid 1 - e^{-\lambda \nu(\tilde{A})} \mid < 1$ which is a contradiction since $\Re e(\lambda) \geq 0$. Consequently, the endemic equilibrium is LAS. □

Theorem 5 *Assume that case (iii) in Proposition 2 holds true. When $R_c = 1$, the system (27) undergoes a backward bifurcation. That is, for $R_c > 1$, R_c close to 1, the endemic equilibrium is the unique equilibrium which is locally asymptotically stable; and for $R_c < 1$ R_c close to 1, the DFE together with an endemic equilibria is locally asymptotically stable, whereas a second endemic equilibrium exists and is unstable.*

Proof When case (iii) hold, then there exist at least two positive steady states, $E_m = \left(S^m, A^m, I_u^m\right)$ and $E_M = \left(S^M, A^M, I_u^M\right)$. The selected equilibria E_m and E_M we will use are the first two solutions A^m and A^M of equation $\chi(y) = \delta N (\mu + d)$such that $\chi'(A^M) < 0$ and $\chi'(A^m) > 0$. Thus, the proof of the LAS of equilibrium E^M is similar to the one of Theorem 4.

The characteristic equation associated with E_m satisfies

$$\Delta(0) = \alpha e^{-\eta\nu(A_m(\zeta))} (A_m(\zeta) + I_m(\zeta)) S_m(\zeta) (\mu + d + d_S) \chi'(A^m)/N.$$

Consequently $\Delta(0) < 0$ and, since $\lim_{\lambda\to\infty} \Delta(\lambda) = +\infty$, then there exists $\lambda^* > 0$ such that $\Delta(\lambda^*) = 0$. This concludes the proof of the theorem. □

The existence of a backward bifurcation is an interesting artifact since this means that repeated exposures of susceptibles to the SARS-CoV-2 virus can cause bistability dynamics and, subsequently, infection persistence even when the control reproduction number R_c is less than unity. An interesting query that emanates from the backward bifurcation is "What is the maximum effective contact number, b, or viral load per each contact, c, below which the Covid-19 disappear one we reduce R_c below one?". Note that, as mentioned and proved in [23], in the case of single exposure model (27) is a system of constant-delay differential equations which is equivalent to system (23). Moreover, no backward bifurcation occurs. Generally, there is a threshold b^* below which the backward bifurcation disappear (The proof is similar to the one in [23]). This result could have a significant biological interpretation since, as stated in [10], minimization of exposure to SARS-COV-2 is key to reducing the chance of infection and developing disease.

8 Discussion

Since the beginning of Covid-19 pandemic, numerous mathematical models with increasing complexity are developed worldwide to understand the course of Covid-19 disease. The modeling results have shown a wide large of variations, especially in the basic reproduction numbers. This leads to ask some questions such as: Why these variations exist between models? Which model is the most realistic for the Covid-19 disease? WHO had reported that the basic reproduction number is estimated to be between 1.4 and 2.5 [26] while other interesting contributions reported that the Covid-19 is more transmissible than what WHO mentioned. In [16], the authors estimated, through a comparison study of 12 different results, that the median value of R_0 for Covid-19 is expected to be around $2-3$. However, only 6 among these studies have used mathematical models leading to a higher variation of R_0 $(1.5-6.49)$, with an average of 4.2. Another systematic review in [14] screened 75 mathematical and statistical models published between December $1st$ 2019 and February $21st$ 2020 and concluded that the median of R_0 for Covid-19 was 3.77 (Fig. 1). In this chapter, we developed, fitted and compared four mathematical models with increasing complexity, that incorporate lifting lockdown strategy, to check out which one among them provides the best prediction for Covid-19 disease. We considered a progressive relaxation of the compulsory lockdown performed in two stages and supported by a reduction of 60% of the contact rate. In the first stage, 30 % of the total confined population lifted the lockdown on June 10th, while in the second stage another 30%

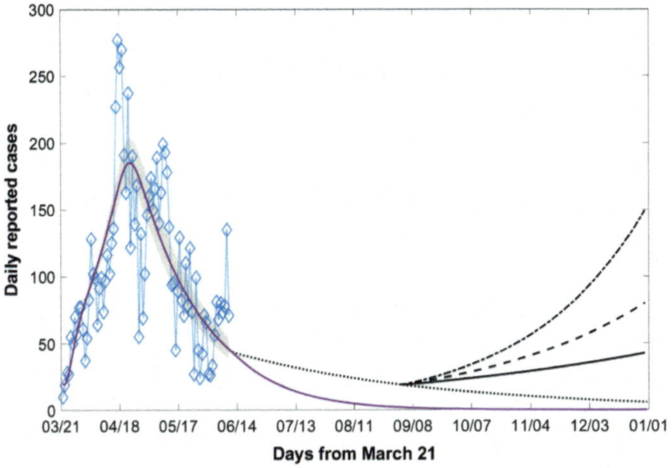

Fig. 1 Time series plot for model (1), starting from March 21, 2020, of the numbers of reported individuals change using different lifting rates at different times as follows: 30% of the total population is lifted on June 10 (dot line) and a fraction γ of the remaining confined individuals ($\gamma = 0.3$, $\gamma = 0.4$, and $\gamma = 0.5$, solid line, dashed line and dot-dashed line respectively) is lifted on September $1st$

lifted the lockdown on September 1st. Our investigation of the proposed models showed a small variation of R_0 ranging from 2.06 to 3.03, and according to the SSR measure (see Sect. 3), the best fit of reported data is achieved for the model with constant delay (13) with $SSR = 92.63$. Consequently, our results show that model (13) is the most reliable to estimate the value of R_0 ($R_0 = 3.03$), which is higher than those estimated by models (1), (10) and (21) (Fig. 2). Although it is believed that the discrete age-structured model (10) is more realistic, our investigations show that this model is the least accurate of any of the models used to estimate the basic reproduction number R_0 since its SSR is the highest one with $SSR = 98.76$. This leads us to think to extend the proposed models by gathering both age and constant-delay factors at once. On the other hand, using our proposed models, the examination of the lockdown lifting scenario shows a prominent difference between disease predictions. Furthermore, no eradication of Covid-19 disease is observed before the end of the year when relaxing the compulsory lockdown on September 1st. The discrete age-structured model (10), which have estimate the lowest R_0 value, predict a less severe disease persistence when comparing with the other models. Lifting 30% of the total confined population on June 10th will lead to a slight second wave of infection followed by a rapid decrease till the eradication of the disease before the end of the year (Fig. 3). However, if this strategy is accompanied with a second lockdown lifting of at least 30% of the total confined population (11.5% of adults and 80% of children under 15 years old) on September 1st then the extinction of the virus cannot happen (Fig. 2) and a third wave could arise. However, it is obvious that the reopening of primary and junior high schools does not lead to an important wave of

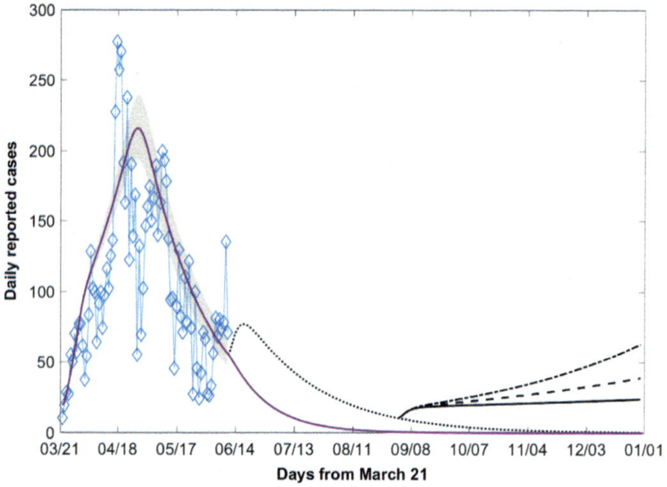

Fig. 2 Time series plot for model (10), starting from March 21, 2020, of the numbers of reported individuals change using different lifting rates at different times as follows: 30% of children and 30% of adults are lifted on June 10 (dot line) and a fraction γ of the remaining confined individuals $((\gamma_a = 0.115, \gamma_c = 0.8)$, $(\gamma_a = 0.25, \gamma_c = 0.8)$, and $(\gamma_a = 0.39, \gamma_c = 0.8)$, solid line, dashed line, dot-dashed line respectively) is lifted on September $1st$

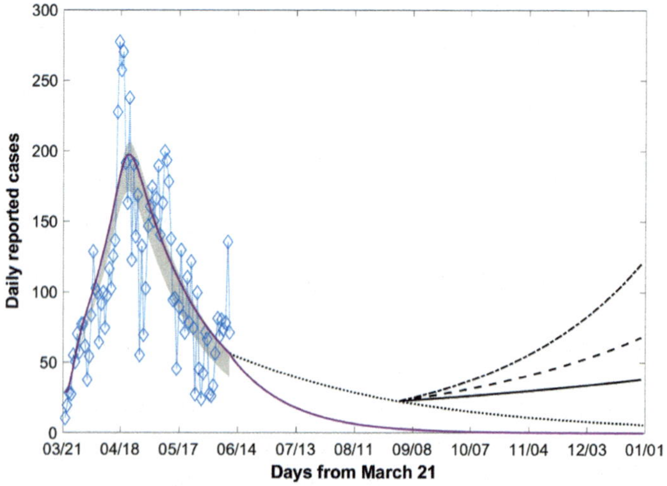

Fig. 3 Time series plot for model (13), starting from March 21, 2020, of the numbers of reported individuals change using different lifting rates at different times as follows: 30% of the total population is lifted on June 10 (dot line) and a fraction γ of the remaining confined individuals ($\gamma = 0.3$, $\gamma = 0.4$, and $\gamma = 0.5$, solid line, dashed line, dot-dashed line respectively) is lifted on September $1st$

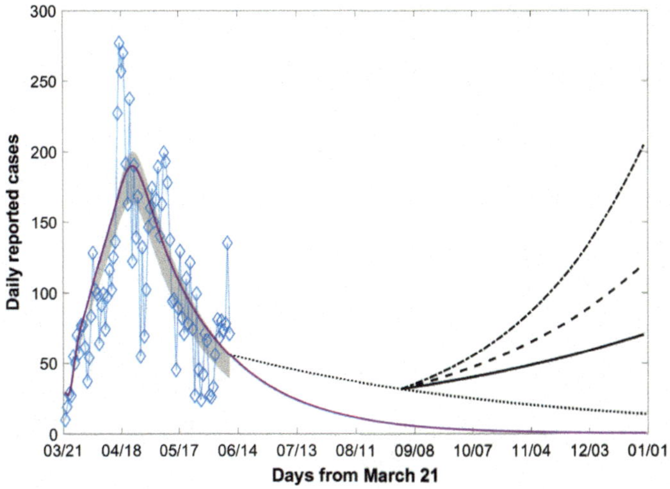

Fig. 4 Time series plot for model (21), starting from March 21, 2020, of the numbers of reported individuals change using different lifting rates at different times as follows: 30% of the total population is lifted on June 10 (dot line) and a fraction γ of the remaining confined individuals ($\gamma = 0.3$, $\gamma = 0.4$, and $\gamma = 0.5$, solid line, dashed line, dot-dashed line respectively) is lifted on September $1st$

infection, when comparing with models (1), (13) and (21). Figures 1, 3 and 4 show, however, that no second wave will reoccur but a longer lasting persistence of the infection occurs when 30% of the population lifted on June 10th. However, when comparing with the both basic model (1) and constant-delay model (13), threshold-type delay model (21) show a higher size of reported cases as well as an important second wave when a second stage of lifting lockdown strategy occurs on September 1st. Furthermore, it seems that the latency period influences the model fitting to data. Figure 5 and the SSR measure ($SSR_{\tau=0.33} = 92.63$), related to the delay model (13), shows that the constant-delay model with latency period of 8 h is the best fit to data and, thus, this period gives a better prediction than 6 or 12 h of latency.

In summary, there are no mathematical models able to correctly capture all complexity of Covid-19 disease in general. Each model, either simple or complex, has its own advantages and disadvantages. Besides the availability of data, the choice of model depends on the goal sought by scientists to answer a question of interest. Furthermore, the use of complex models does not necessarily provide the most precise answers than the simplest. Indeed, since many biological and epidemiological issues related to SARS-CoV-2 remain to be clarified, parameters considered in the proposed model can be underestimated or overestimated and, consequently, can lead to wrong results. An unsuccessful evaluation of the disease behavior could cost serious damage because it leads to an incorrect estimate of the control health measures that are necessary to contain the disease transmission. However, although a lot of issues

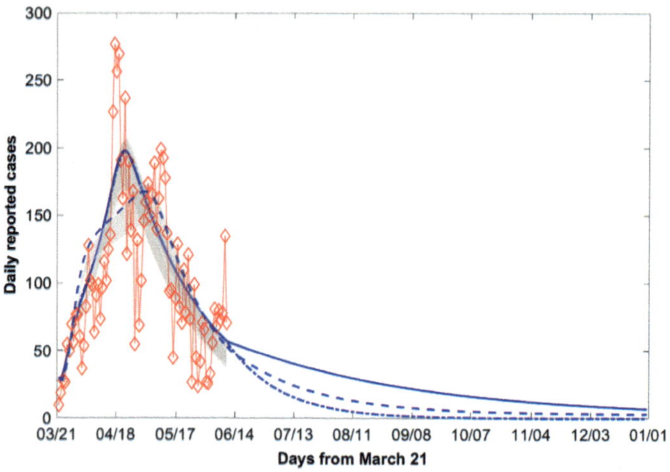

Fig. 5 Time series plot for model (13), starting from March 21, 2020, of the numbers of reported individuals change using different latent periods ($\tau = 0.25$, $\tau = 0.33$, and $\tau = 0.5$, dashed line, solid line, dot-dashed line respectively) with 30% of the total population is lifted on June 10

must be considered to provide the built model a maximum of realism, mathematical modeling remains a crucial tool to understand and control the behavior of Covid-19 disease.

Acknowledgements The authors are grateful to the anonymous referees for their valuable and helpful comments that improved this chapter.

References

1. Ahmed, F., Ahmed, N., Pissarides, C., Stiglitz, J.: Why inequality could spread COVID-19. The Lancet Regional Health **5**(5), E240 (2020). https://doi.org/10.1016/S2468-2667(20)30085-2
2. Benjamin, L., William V.R.: Pediatrics August, 146 (2) e2020004879; doi: https://doi.org/10.1542/peds.2020-004879 (2020)
3. Britton, T., Tomba, G.S.: Estimation in emerging epidemics: biases and remedies. J. R. Soc. Interface **16**(150), 20180670 (2019)
4. Hammoumi, A., Qesmi, R.: Impact assessment of containment measure against COVID-19 spread in Morocco. Chaos Solit. Fractals **140** (110231). https://doi.org/10.1016/j.chaos.2020.110231 (2020)
5. HCP of Morocco, https://www.hcp.ma/Population_r143.html (2020)
6. Heffernan J.M., Smith R.J., Wahl L.M.: Perspectives on the basic reproductive ratio, J.R. Soc. Interf. (2) 281 (2005)
7. Heneghan, C., Brassey J., Jefferson, T.: SARS-CoV-2 viral load and the severity of COVID-19. 26 March, 2020; https://www.cebm.net/covid-19/sars-cov-2-viral-load-and-the-severity-of-covid-19/ (2020)
8. Jakovljevic, M., Bjedov, S., Jaksic, N., Jakovljevic, I.: Covid-19 pandemia and public and global mental health from the perspective of global health securit. Psychiatr. Danub. Spring. **32**(1), 6–14 (2020). https://doi.org/10.24869/psyd.2020.6

9. Kanzawa, M., Spindler, H., Anglemyer, A., Rutherford, W.: Will coronavirus disease 2019 become seasonal? J. Infect. Dis. **22**(5), 719–721 (2020)
10. Karimzadeh, S., Bhopal, R., Nguyen Tien, H.: Review of viral dynamics, exposure, infective dose, and outcome of COVID-19 caused by the SARS-CoV-2 Virus: Comparison with Other Respiratory Viruses. Preprints **2020070613** (2020)
11. Kissler, S.M., Tedijanto, C., Goldstein, E., Grad, Y.H., Lipsitch, M.: Projecting the transmission dynamics of SARS-CoV-2 through the postpandemic period. Science **368**(6493), 860–868 (2020)
12. Lasry, A., Kidder, D., Hast, M., Poovey, J., Sunshine, G., Winglee, K., Zviedrite, N., Ahmed, F., Ethier, K.A.: Timing of community mitigation and changes in reported COVID-19 and community mobility- four U.S. metropolitan areas, February 26-April 1, 2020. MMWR Morb. Mortal. Wkly. Rep. **69**(15), 451–457 (2020)
13. Leung, K., Wu, J.T.: The gradual release exit strategy after lockdown against COVID-19. The Lancet Regional Health-Western Pacific (2020). https://doi.org/10.1016/j.lanwpc.2020.100008
14. Lin, Y.-F., Duan, Q., Zhou, Y., Yuan, T., Li, P., et al.: Spread and impact of COVID-19 in China: a systematic review and synthesis of predictions from transmission-dynamic models. Front. Med. (2020). https://doi.org/10.3389/fmed.2020.00321
15. Liu, Z., Magal, P., Seydi, O., Webb, G.: Understanding unreported cases in the 2019-nCov epidemic outbreak in Wuhan. China, and the importance of major public health interventions, MPDI Biology **9**(3), 50 (2020)
16. Liu, Y., et al.: The reproductive number of COVID-19 is higher compared to SARS coronavirus. J. Travel Med., 27 (2) (2020)
17. Macartney, K., Quinn, H.E., Pillsbury, A.J., Koirala, A., Deng, L., Winkler, N., Katelaris, A.L., O'Sullivan, M.V.N., Dalton, C., Wood, N. and the NSW COVID-19 schools study team: transmission of SARS-CoV-2 in Australian educational settings: a prospective cohort study. Lancet Child. Adolesc. Health. doi: https://doi.org/10.1016/S2352-4642(20)30251-0 (2020)
18. MacIntyre, C.R.: Global spread of COVID-19 and pandemic potential. Global Biosecur. **1**(3),(2020)
19. Martinez, M.E.: The calendar of epidemics: seasonal cycles of infectious diseases. PLOS Pathogens **14**(11), e1007327 (2018)
20. Ndariou, F., Area, I., Nieto, J.J., Torres, D.F.: Mathematical modeling of COVID-19 transmission dynamics with a case study of Wuhan. Chaos Solit. Fractals (2020). https://doi.org/10.1016/j.chaos.2020.109846
21. Nicola, M., Alsafi, Z., Sohrabi, C., Kerwan, A., Al-Jabir, A., Losifidis, C., Agha, M., Agha, R.: The socio-economic implications of the coronavirus pandemic (COVID-19): a review. Int. J. Surg. **78**, 185–193 (2020)
22. Prem, K., Liu, Y., Russell, T.W, Kucharski, A.J., Eggo, R.M., Davies, N., Jit, M., Klepac, P.: The effect of control strategies to reduce social mixing on outcomes of the COVID-19 epidemic in Wuhan, China: a modelling study. Lancet Public Health. doi.org./10.1016/s2468-2667(20)30072-4 (2020)
23. Qesmi, R., Heffernan, J., Wu, J.: An immuno-epidemiological model with threshold delay: a study of the effects of multiple exposures to a pathogen. J. Math. Biol. **70**, 343–366 (2015)
24. Rothe, C., et al.: Transmission of 2019-nCoV infection from an asymptomatic contact in Germany. N. Engl. J. Med. **382**, 970–971 (2020)
25. Shampine, L.F.: Solving ODEs and DDEs with residual control. Appl. Numer. Math. **52**, 113–127 (2005)
26. Statement on the meeting of the International Health Regulations: Emergency Committee regarding the outbreak of novel coronavirus 2019 (n-CoV) on 23 January 2020. (2005)
27. The Ministry of Health of Morocco, The Official Coronavirus Portal of Morocco. www.covidmaroc.ma (2020)
28. Ye, Z-W. Yuan, S., Yuen, K-S., Fung, S-Y., Chan, C-P., Jin, D-Y,: Zoonotic origins of human coronavirus. Int. J. Biol. Sci. **16**(10): 1686–1697 (2020)

29. Zhang, Y., Geng, X., Tan, Y., Qiang, L., Can, X., Jianglong, X., Liangchao, H., Zhaomu, Z., Xianpu, L., Fulin, L., Wong, H.: New understanding of the damage of SARS-CoV-2 infection outside the respiratory system. Biomed. Pharmacother. J. **127**, 110195 (2020)
30. UNESCO Educational disruption and response. https://plus.google.com/+UNESCO COVID-19 (2020)
31. Van den Driessche, P., Watmough, J.: Reproduction numbers and subthreshold endemic equilibria for compartmental models of disease transmission. Math. Biosci. **180**, 29–48 (2002)
32. Vespignani, A., Tian, H., Dye, C., et al.: Modelling COVID-19. Nat. Rev. Phys. **2**, 279–281 (2020). https://doi.org/10.1038/s42254-020-0178-4
33. Viner, R.M., Russel, S.J., Croker, H., Packer, J., Ward, J., Stansfield, C., et al.: School closure and management practices during coronavirus outbreaks including COVID-19: a rapid systematic review. Lancet Child Adolesc. Health **4**(5), 397–404 (2020)
34. WHO Modes of transmission of virus causing COVID-19: implications for ICP precaution recommendations (2020)
35. WHO, News briefing on 24th February 2020; [updated, : 24; cited 2020 February 24]. (2020 February)
36. Wilder-Smith, A., Freedman, D.O.: Isolation, quarantine, social distancing and community containment: pivotal role for old-style public health measures in the novel coronavirus (2019-nCoV) outbreak. J. Travel Med., 27(2) (2020)

Introduction to the Grey Systems Theory and Its Application in Mathematical Modeling and Pandemic Prediction of Covid-19

Hoang Anh Ngo, Thai Nam Hoang, and Mehmet Dik

Abstract Firstly, this chapter is devoted to present the scientific background for the appearance of Grey Systems in the 1980s. Then, the history of astonishing development, along with the main components and fundamental principles of the Grey Systems, is also introduced. Currently, Grey Systems is an emerging research area with strong possibilities to transect across and apply to a wide range of scientific areas, including industry, agriculture, geology, ecology, medicine, education, etc. However, most applications of the Systems are from Chinese-speaking researchers, while the theory itself is still uncommon in Uncertainty Mathematics. Finally, the representative models with high accuracy are put into practice by predicting and handling the outbreak of Covid-19 pandemic. Not only can the Systems predict the total number of positive cases, but it can also be applied in various other medical practices, including telecare and data management. Their performances are also compared with other uncertainty models, including Machine Learning, which has proven that Grey System models have the ability to perform equally well, or even better, especially in the context of limited data.

Keywords Mathematical modeling · SEAIR model · MATLAB

1 A Brief Introduction to the Grey Systems Theory

Grey method was proposed by Deng Ju-Long in March, 1982 [12]. In Grey system theory [12, 29], considered the degree of information, a white system is a system in which all information is known, while a black system is a system that contains all

H. A. Ngo
École Polytechnique, Institut Polytechnique de Paris, 91128 Palaiseau, France
e-mail: hoang-anh.ngo@polytechnique.edu

T. N. Hoang · M. Dik (✉)
Department of Mathematics and Computer Science, Beloit College, Beloit, WI 53511, USA
e-mail: dikm@beloit.edu

T. N. Hoang
e-mail: hoangnt@beloit.edu

P. Agarwal et al. (eds.), *Analysis of Infectious Disease Problems (Covid-19) and Their Global Impact*, Infosys Science Foundation Series,
https://doi.org/10.1007/978-981-16-2450-6_10

unknown parts. Additionally, a system which consists of both known and unknown information is called a Grey system [12]. According to Guo, R. [14], the Grey system outperforms other methods with just a limited number of discrete data, to achieve an insignificant margin of error of prediction versus real value. The system of total Covid-19 infected cases can be treated as a Grey system due to its constraint of data.

Mathematically, the traditional Grey predicting model is based on the least square reduction and the first-order linear ordinary differential equation. For instance, traditional GM(1, 1) can be taken into account [25, 63] to solve this problem. Notably, to reinforce the predicting accuracy, some researchers have studied and combined to create hybrid Grey models, such as Grey-Markov [25, 62], Grey-Fourier [46], Grey-Taguchi [13]. Some more hybrid models such as Grey rolling mechanism [1, 4, 27] or Nonlinear Grey Bernoulli method [5, 31, 50, 54] can also be taken into consideration.

Those alternatives of original Grey models aforementioned can be applied to a variety of topics, including Grey Relational Analysis [10, 21, 23] and Grey prediction [39, 47]. Grey Relational Analysis has an important role in fields of data analysis to make assumptions based on two or more Relational data. Taking the relationship between a country's energy consumption and its GDP, Grey Relational Analysis can scrutinize how energy resources like oil and renewable energy have major impacts on Turkey's GDP. This method yields a potential result, compared to other econometric models [23]. While Grey Relational Analysis can delineate the relationship of different topics, Grey prediction can make future assumptions based on given data. Due to the dynamics of system evolution, the biological limitations of the human sensing organs, and the constraints of relevant economic conditions and technological availability, most nowadays problems can be regarded as time-series problems, or in other words, prediction problems. Using Grey prediction, Wang et al. applied Grey systems theory to a comprehensive index to represent the condition of food security to predict the changing trend of the constructed index in the future and judge the condition of food security risk [47].

As an unascertained system, Grey method comprises many fundamental characteristics to solve uncertainty problems. The first and foremost characteristic is the incompleteness in the information. The situation of incomplete information is often seen in our social, economic, and scientific research activities. For instance, in agricultural productions, even if we know all the exact information regarding the areas of plantation, seeds, fertilizers, irrigations, due to the uncertainties in areas like labor quality, natural environments, weather conditions, the commodity markets, etc., it is still extremely difficult to precisely predict the production output and the consequent economic values. For biological prevention systems, even if we clearly know the relationship between insects and their natural enemies, it is still very difficult for us to achieve the expected prevention effects due to our ignorance with the knowledge on the relationships between the insects and the baits, their natural enemies and the baits, and a specific kind of natural enemy with another kind of natural enemy. Another fundamental characteristic is the inaccuracy of data. Both incompleteness and inaccuracy in data are roughly the same, as glancing through. However, inaccuracy triggers the insightful of Grey method: data fluctuation can affect the outcome [30].

Within the first parts of this chapter, univariate Grey models (both linear and non-linear) will be introduced, along with different methods/mechanisms of optimization. Then, some models that have been proposed and applied in predicting the number of Covid-19 cases will be investigated, showing that Grey models have the ability to return excellent results compared to various other traditional or modern statistical methods.

2 Description of the Traditional Linear and Nonlinear Univariate Grey Models GM(1, 1) and NGBM(1, 1)

A very brief introduction of the mathematical modeling of two traditional Grey models: GM(1, 1) and Nonlinear Grey Bernoulli Model NGBM(1, 1) is presented in this section.

2.1 Building the Traditional Grey Model GM(1, 1)

Assume that $x^{(0)}$ is a non-negative original historical time series of data with m entries

$$x^{(0)} = \{x^{(0)}(1), x^{(0)}(2), ..., x^{(0)}(k), ..., x^{(0)}(m)\} \tag{1}$$

According to Nguyen et al., the initial data has to be tested using the following conditions to check if it is consistent with the prediction model. Then, $\sigma^{(0)}(k)$ is called class ration when the initial value has $m \geq 4, x^{(0)} \in \mathbb{R}$, and $k = 2, 3, \cdots, n$ [35].

$$\frac{x^{(0)}(k-1)}{x^{(0)}k} = \sigma^{(0)}(k) \in \left(e^{-\frac{2}{m+1}}, e^{\frac{2}{m+1}}\right) \tag{2}$$

Next, defining $x^{(1)}$ using one-time accumulated generating operation (1 - AGO) as

$$x^{(1)} = \{x^{(1)}(1), x^{(1)}(2), ..., x^{(1)}(k), ..., x^{(1)}(m)\} \tag{3}$$

where

$$\begin{cases} x^{(1)}(1) = x^{(0)}(1) \\ x^{(1)}(k) = \sum_{i=1}^{k} x^{(0)}(i), k = 2, 3, ..., m \end{cases} \tag{4}$$

As $x^{(1)}$ is a monotonic increasing sequence—same as the solution of a first-order linear differential equation, one can assume that the solution of the following differential equation will be

$$\frac{d\hat{x}^{(1)}}{dt} + a\hat{x}^{(1)} = b \tag{5}$$

representing the Grey predicted value complement to the initial condition $\hat{x}^{(1)}(1) = x^{(0)}(1)$ and parameters a and b.

By definition, $\frac{d\hat{x}}{dt}$ can be written as

$$\frac{d\hat{x}^{(1)}}{dt} = \lim_{\Delta t \to 0} \frac{\hat{x}^{(1)}(t + \Delta t) - \hat{x}^{(1)}(t)}{\Delta t} \tag{6}$$

However, to discretize the differential equation, Δt can be set to be equal to 1, which makes (5) to be rewritten as

$$\frac{d\hat{x}^{(1)}}{dt} = \hat{x}^{(1)}(t+1) - \hat{x}^{(1)}(t) = x^{(1)}(t+1) - x^{(1)}(t) = x^{(0)}(t+1) \tag{7}$$

The Grey predicted value is now defined as

$$\hat{x}^{(1)}(t) \approx Px^{(1)}(k) + (1-P)x^{(1)}(k+1) = z^{(1)}(k+1), k = 1, 2, 3, \ldots, m \tag{8}$$

with P usually set as $\frac{1}{2}$ in the traditional models.

The differential equation can now be discretized as

$$x^{(0)}(k) + az^{(1)}(k) = b \tag{9}$$

By the least-squared method, the coefficients a and b can be determined by

$$\begin{bmatrix} a \\ b \end{bmatrix} = \left(B^T B\right)^{-1} B^T Y \tag{10}$$

with

$$B = \begin{bmatrix} -z^{(1)}(2) & 1 \\ -z^{(1)}(3) & 1 \\ \ldots & \\ -z^{(1)}(m) & 1 \end{bmatrix}, Y = \begin{bmatrix} x^{(0)}(2) \\ x^{(0)}(3) \\ \ldots \\ x^{(0)}(m) \end{bmatrix} \tag{11}$$

The particular solution of Eq. (4) with the initial condition is

$$\hat{x}^{(1)}(k+1) = \left(x^{(0)}(1) - \frac{b}{a}\right)e^{-ak} + \frac{b}{a}, k = 1, 2, 3, \ldots, m-1 \tag{12}$$

The prediction of the historical time series of data at point $k+1$ can now be deduced by

$$\hat{x}^{(0)}(k+1) = \hat{x}^{(1)}(k+1) - \hat{x}^{(1)}(k) = \left(1 - e^{-a}\right)\left(x^{(0)}(1) - \frac{b}{a}\right)e^{-ak} \tag{13}$$

with

$$\begin{cases} \hat{x}^{(0)}(k) = x^{(0)}(k), k = 1, 2, ..., m \text{ fitted values,} \\ \hat{x}^{(0)}(m+1), \hat{x}^{(0)}(m+2), ..., x^{(0)}(m+h) \text{ predicted values} \end{cases} \tag{14}$$

2.2 The Nonlinear Grey Bernoulli Model NGBM(1, 1)

In order to obtain higher accuracy in predicting comparing to the original GM(1,) model, Professor Chen [5] had proposed the Nonlinear Bernoulli Grey Model NBGM(1, 1) as follows.

Similarly to the traditional Grey model GM(1, 1), assume that $x^{(0)}$ is the non-negative original historical time series of data with m entries

$$x^{(0)} = \{x^{(0)}(1), x^{(0)}(2), ..., x^{(0)}(k), ..., x^{(0)}(m)\} \tag{15}$$

Next, we define $x^{(1)}$ using one-time accumulated generating operation (1 - AGO), which is as

$$x^{(1)} = \{x^{(1)}(1), x^{(1)}(2), ..., x^{(1)}(k), ..., x^{(1)}(m)\} \tag{16}$$

where

$$\begin{cases} x^{(1)}(1) = x^{(0)}(1) \\ x^{(1)}(k) = \sum_{i=1}^{k} x^{(0)}(k), k = 2, 3, ..., m \end{cases} \tag{17}$$

As indicated previously, Eq. (4) is a linear differential equation. A similar form of this equation, which is nonlinear and has the form of

$$\frac{d\hat{x}^{(1)}}{dt} + a\hat{x}^{(1)} = b\left[\hat{x}^{(1)}\right]^n \tag{18}$$

where $n \in \mathbb{R}$ any real number is called a Bernoulli equation, or the with then differential equation of the NGBM(1, 1) model.

The background value is now also defined as

$$z^{(1)}(k+1) = (1-P)x^{(1)}(k) + Px^{(1)}(k+1) \tag{19}$$

with $P = \frac{1}{2}$ for the traditional model. Then, discretizing the ODE, one obtains

$$x^{(0)}(k) + az^{(1)}(k) = b\left[x^{(1)}(k)\right]^n \tag{20}$$

which is called the basic Grey differential equation of the NGBM(1, 1) model. It can easily be recognized that for $n = 0$, this equation turns to equation (4), which is the traditional GM(1, 1) model; for $n = 2$, the equation turns to the Grey - Verhulst equation.

By the least square method, the parameters a and b can be determined by

$$\begin{bmatrix} a \\ b \end{bmatrix} = \left(B^T B\right)^{-1} B^T Y \tag{21}$$

with

$$B = \begin{bmatrix} -z^{(1)}(2) & \left[z^{(1)}(2)\right]^n \\ -z^{(1)}(3) & \left[z^{(1)}(3)\right]^n \\ \cdots & \\ -z^{(1)}(m) & \left[z^{(1)}(m)\right]^n \end{bmatrix}, Y = \begin{bmatrix} x^{(0)}(2) \\ x^{(0)}(3) \\ \cdots \\ x^{(0)}(m) \end{bmatrix} \tag{22}$$

The particular solution of Eq. (17), or the discrete time function, with the initial condition is

$$\hat{x}^{(1)}(k) = \left[\left(x^{(0)}(1)^{(1-n)} - \frac{b}{a}\right) e^{-a(1-n)(k-1)} + \frac{b}{a}\right]^{\frac{1}{1-n}}, k = 1, 2, 3, ..., m \tag{23}$$

The prediction of the historical time series of data at point k can now be deduced by

$$\hat{x}^{(0)}(k) = \hat{x}^{(1)}(k) - \hat{x}^{(1)}(k-1) \tag{24}$$

3 Optimization of the Univariate Grey Models

3.1 *Optimization of Hyper-parameters*

Optimization of hyper-parameters in Grey models includes optimizing the exponential value (in non-linear models) and of the background value estimation.

Previously, based on the basic principle of the overlapping information of the Grey systems and approximation of the integral, Wang et al. (2009) [48] and Tan (2000) [40] has proposed different formula in determining the optimal value of the parameter P in the background value and the exponential parameter n. However, NGO and HOANG (2020) [34] has investigated that, with the existence of modern programming languages, the formula yield the problem of inflexibility and ineffectiveness compared to the method of iterating on the pre-defined range with the maximum likelihood of optimality

- (0, 1) for the background value P
- $[-1, 1)$ for the exponential parameter n

Similar to the Fractional Order r in multivariate Grey models (Sect. 6.4), the two hyper-parameters can also be simultaneously optimized by applying evolutionary algorithms independently without spending enormous resources on iterating with small steps.

3.2 Rolling Mechanism

In case when a prediction series has a substantial number of data points, a rolling mechanism for a short data sequence is preferred. The purpose of the rolling mechanism is that, in each rolling step, the next forecasting data points are derived based on the most recent data (including data that has recently been predicted). The standard algorithm that is widely applied in various newly proposed models can be found at [27].

3.3 Optimization of the Initial Condition

In traditional univariate Grey models, the initial condition is set as $x^{(0)}(1)$. However, using the principle of new information prior choosing, Dang (2004) [9] has confirmed that $x^{(1)}(m)$ can be used to increase the accuracy of the model. This can be further developed by adding a correction term as $x^{(1)}(m) + c$ to form a new initial condition, minimizing the following function (proposed by Lu et al. (2016) [31])

$$f(c) = \sum_{k=1}^{m} \left\{ \left[\hat{x}^{(1)}(k)\right]^{1-n} - \left[x^{(1)}(k)\right]^{1-n} \right\}^2 \tag{25}$$

By setting

$$\begin{cases} E(k) = e^{-a(1-n)(k-m)} \\ A(k) = \left[x^{(1)}(k)\right]^{1-n} - \frac{b}{a}(1 - E(k)) \end{cases} \tag{26}$$

the new initial condition with correction term can be written as

$$x^{(1)}(m) + c = \left[\frac{\sum_{k=1}^{m} A(k)E(k)}{\sum_{i=1}^{n} E(k)^2} \right]^{1-n} \tag{27}$$

4 Applications of Univariate Grey Models in Predicting Total Covid-19 Infected Cases

Due to the current situation of limited data available for Covid-19 related research, especially to pandemic modeling and prediction, univariate models are currently more preferred in terms of feasibility and practicality. With its advantage in dealing with limited available information and data sequences, Grey models have the potential to return excellent result compared to other epidemiological or machine learning models, both short-term and long-term. However, there are still very limited research papers using Grey models as a prediction tool, as follows

- Forecasting the cumulative number of confirmed cases of Covid-19 in Italy, UK and USA using Fractional nonlinear Grey Bernoulli model by Sahin, U. and Sahin, T (2010). [38]. This paper uses three traditional models: GM(1, 1), NGBM(1, 1) and Fractional NGBM(1, 1), along with optimizing hyper-parameters of the models (γ—power index value and r—Fractional Order value) by a generative algorithm. The Fractional NGBM(1, 1) performed significantly better compared to other models, with MAPE of $\leq 4.895\%$ and R-squared values of ≥ 0.999 for all three countries.
- Prediction of the Number of Patients Infected with Covid-19 Based on Rolling Grey-Verhulst Models by Zhao et al. (2020) [61]. At the time of research, the pandemic curve in China is increasing in an S-shaped trend, which is suitable for the strong prediction capacity of Grey-Verhulst models. Six models, along with the rolling mechanism on 7-, 8- and 9-day data sequences are built to predict the number of cumulative cases from January 20th to February 20th, with the training set depending on the length of the rolling sequence. The minimum and maximum MAPE in each stage is presented in Table 1, which shows that the proposed model showed a significantly high level of robustness and accuracy.
- A Rolling Optimized Nonlinear Grey Bernoulli model and application in predicting total Covid-19 infected cases by NGO and HOANG (2020) [34]. In this paper, the authors proposed a novel model by optimizing two hyper-parameters simultaneously (the background value P and the power index value n), while applying a rolling mechanism to take advantage of newly generated data points. The model is first tested on predicting Vietnam's GDP from 2004 to 2018 and the compared with modern machine learning models (ANN and LSTM) in predicting total Covid-19 cases in China from January 28th to February 18th, 2020. The novel model outperformed any other models compared in the paper. The authors do not consider saturating factors in the model due to the epidemiological suggestions and confirmation that China is still in its initial stage of containing the virus until February 20th, 2020 [8].

From the three research papers shown above, univariate Grey models have shown their massive advantage in handling limited data situations with consistently strong performance (Figs. 1 and 2).

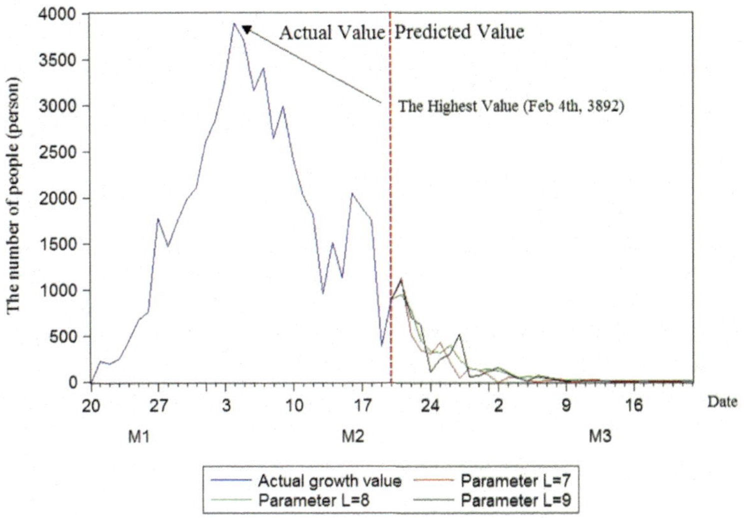

Fig. 1 Prediction of rolling Grey–Verhulst models with 7-, 8- and 9-day data sequence, Zhao et al. (2020)

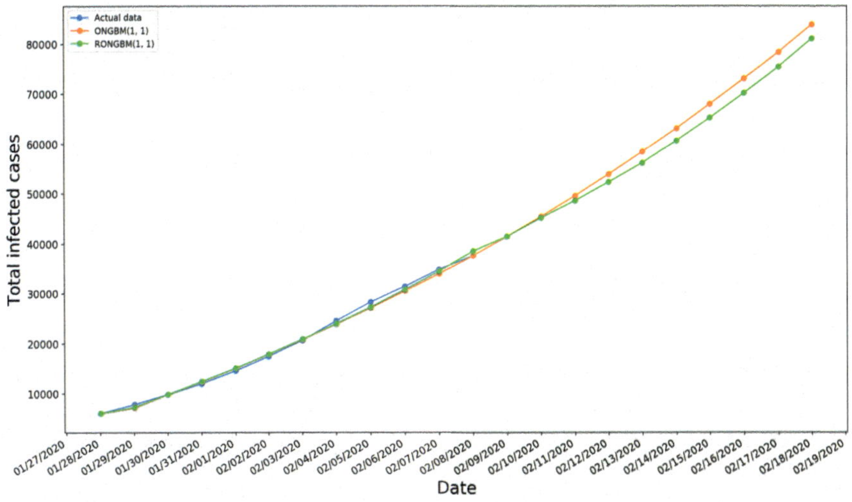

Fig. 2 Prediction of total Covid-19 infected cases predicted using Grey models (2020-01-28 - 2020-02-08), NGO and HOANG (2020)

Table 1 Prediction results (MAPE) of rolling Grey-Verhulst models proposed by Zhao et al. (2020)

	Training stage (%)	Testing stage (%)
Minimum MAPE	1.80	1.65
Maximum MAPE	4.74	4.72

The next sections are devoted to elaborating on the series of multivariate Grey models. Due to the limited data sources available, there has been little to no applications of these models in predicting Covid-19 related figures. When data are becoming more and more available, these models will have a greater impact in making predictions; for example, the daily number of confirmed Covid-19 cases can be predicted based on various variables such as

- Number of tests conducted within the previous days
- Number of imported/local cases; Number of active clusters
- Number of quarantined patients due to close contact with previous positive cases
- Number of available staffed / ICU beds available for Covid-19 patients, etc.

5 Description of the Existing GM(1, N) and GMC(1, N) Models

5.1 The Traditional GM(1, N) Model

Assume that there exist pairs of observations $X^{(0)} = \left(X_1^{(0)}, X_2^{(0)}, \ldots, X_n^{(0)}\right)$ available at equispaced intervals of time with $n - 1$ inputs $\left(X_2^{(0)}, X_3^{(0)}, \ldots, X_n^{(0)}\right)$ and an output $X_1^{(0)}$ from a certain dynamic system.

Let

- r be the number of data points (number of time intervals) used in building the model
- rp be the delay period
- rf be the number of data points to be forecasted

Then, the original data points would be

$$X_i^{(0)} = \left\{X_i^{(0)}(1), X_i^{(0)}(2), \ldots, X_i^{(0)}(r)\right\}, i = 2, 3, \ldots, n \tag{28}$$

while the predicted series (series that need prediction) would be

$$X_1^{(0)} = \left\{X_1^{(0)}(rp+1), X_1^{(0)}(rp+2), \ldots, X_1^{(0)}(rp+r)\right\} \tag{29}$$

The first order accumulated generating operation (1-AGO) data for

$$\begin{cases} X_i^{(1)} = \left\{X_i^{(1)}(1), X_i^{(1)}(2), \ldots, X_i^{(1)}(r)\right\}, i = 2, 3, \ldots, n \\ X_1^{(1)} = \left\{X_1^{(1)}(rp+1), X_1^{(1)}(rp+2), \ldots, X_i^{(1)}(rp+r)\right\} \end{cases} \tag{30}$$

are given as follows

$$\begin{cases} X_i^{(1)}(k) = \sum_{j=1}^{k} X_i^{(0)}(j) \\ X_1^{(1)}(rp+k) = \sum_{j=1}^{k} X_1^{(0)}(rp+j) \end{cases}, k = 1, 2, \ldots, r \tag{31}$$

Deng (1989) [11] suggests that the discrete systems of GM(1, n) model can be described by the following Grey differential equation

$$\frac{dx_1^{(1)}(rp+t)}{dt} + b_1 X_1^{(1)}(rp+t) = \sum_{i=2}^{n} b_i X_i^{(1)}(t); t = 1, 2, \ldots, r \tag{32}$$

The Grey derivative for the 1-AGO representation, for $\Delta t \to 1$ is described as

$$\begin{aligned} \frac{dx_1^{(1)}(rp+t)}{dt} &= \lim_{\Delta t \to 1} \frac{X_1^{(1)}(rp+t+\Delta t) - X_1^{(1)}(rp+t)}{\Delta t} \\ &= X_1^{(1)}(rp+t+1) - X_1^{(1)}(rp+t) \\ &= X_1^{(0)}(rp+t) \end{aligned} \tag{33}$$

The background value of the Grey derivative $\frac{dX^{(1)}(rp+t)}{dt}$ is taken as

$$z_1^{(1)}(rp+t) = \frac{1}{2}\left(X_1^{(1)}(rp+t) + X_1^{(1)}(rp+t-1)\right) \tag{34}$$

while those of the series $X_i^{(1)}(t)$ would be

$$z_i^{(1)}(t) = \frac{1}{2}\left(X_i^{(1)}(t) + X_i^{(1)}(t-1)\right) \tag{35}$$

The least-square solution for the model parameters can be determined by

$$\left[b_1\ b_2\ \ldots\ b_n\right]^T = \left(B^T B\right)^{-1} B^T Y_R \tag{36}$$

with

$$B = \begin{bmatrix} -\frac{1}{2}\left(X_1^{(1)}(rp+1) + X_1^{(1)}(rp+2)\right) & X_2^{(1)}(2)\ X_3^{(1)}(2)\ \ldots\ X_n^{(1)}(2) \\ -\frac{1}{2}\left(X_1^{(1)}(rp+2) + X_1^{(1)}(rp+3)\right) & X_2^{(1)}(3)\ X_3^{(1)}(3)\ \ldots\ X_n^{(1)}(3) \\ \vdots & \vdots\ \vdots\ \ldots\ \vdots \\ -\frac{1}{2}\left(X_1^{(1)}(rp+r-1) + X_1^{(1)}(rp+r)\right) & X_2^{(1)}(r)\ X_3^{(1)}(r)\ \ldots\ X_n^{(1)}(r) \end{bmatrix} \tag{37}$$

and

$$Y_R = \left[X_1^{(0)}(rp+2)\ X_1^{(0)}(rp+3)\ \ldots\ X_1^{(0)}(rp+r)\right] \tag{38}$$

The particular solution of the Grey differential equation (32), or the 1-AGO modeling values of the series, according to Tien (2012) [44] is

$$\hat{X}_1^{(1)}(rp+t) = \left[X_1^{(0)}(rp+1) - \frac{1}{b_1}\sum_{i=2}^{n} b_i X_i^{(1)}(t)\right] \times e^{-b_1(t-1)} + \frac{1}{b_1}\sum_{i=2}^{n} b_i X_i^{(1)}(t)$$
$$(t = 2, 3, \ldots, r + rf) \tag{39}$$

From 1-IAGO, the predicted values of the model can be derived as

$$\begin{cases} \hat{X}_1^{(0)}(rp+1) = \hat{X}_1^{(1)}(rp+1) = X_1^{(0)}(rp+1) \\ \hat{X}_1^{(0)}(rp+t) = \hat{X}_1^{(1)}(rp+t) - \hat{X}_1^{(1)}(rp+t-1) \end{cases}, t = 2, 3, \ldots, r + rf \tag{40}$$

5.2 The Grey Model with Convolution Integral GMC(1, N)

The model GMC(1, n) is a new model, as an improvement to the existing GM(1, 1) with a so-called Grey control parameter u introduced. This means that the representation for GMC(1, 1) becomes a linear differential equation, as follows

$$\frac{dx_1^{(1)}(rp+t)}{dt} + b_1 X_1^{(1)}(rp+t) = \sum_{i=2}^{n} b_i X_i^{(1)}(t) + u; t = 1, 2, \ldots, r + rf \tag{41}$$

Similarly to the GM(1, n) model, by the least-square method, the model parameters of GMC(1, n) can be estimated by

$$\left[b_1\ b_2\ \ldots\ b_n\ u\right]^T = \left(B^T B\right)^{-1} B^T Y_R \tag{42}$$

with

$$B = \begin{bmatrix} -z_1^{(1)}(rp+2) & z_2^{(1)}(2) & z_3^{(1)}(2) & \dots & z_n^{(1)}(2) \\ -z_1^{(1)}(rp+3) & z_2^{(1)}(3) & z_3^{(1)}(3) & \dots & z_n^{(1)}(3) \\ \vdots & \vdots & \vdots & \dots & \vdots \\ -z_1^{(1)}(rp+r) & z_2^{(1)}(r) & z_3^{(1)}(r) & \dots & z_n^{(1)}(r) \end{bmatrix} \tag{43}$$

and

$$Y_R = \left[X_1^{(0)}(rp+2)\ X_1^{(0)}(rp+3)\ \dots\ X_1^{(0)}(rp+r)\right] \tag{44}$$

If we set the right hand side of (41) to be a discrete function $f(t)$ as

$$f(t) = b_2 X_2^{(1)}(t) + b_3 X_3^{(1)}(t) + \dots + b_n X_n^{(1)}(t) + u, t = 1, 2, \dots, rf \tag{45}$$

The particular solution of the equation (41) can be derived as

$$\hat{X}_1^{(1)}(rp+t) = X_1^{(1)}(rp+1)e^{-b_1(t-1)} + \int_1^t e^{-b_1(t-\tau)} f(\tau) d\tau \tag{46}$$

which can be approximated by

$$\hat{X}_1^{(1)}(rp+t) \approx X_1^{(0)}(rp+1)e^{-b_1(t-1)} + u(t-2) \times \left\{ \sum_{k=2}^{t} e^{-b_1\left(t-k+\frac{1}{2}\right)} \cdot \frac{1}{2}\left[f(t) + f(t-1)\right] \right\} \tag{47}$$

with $u(t-2)$ being the unit step function.

The predicted values of the model can be derived similarly with the traditional GM(1, n) model, using the first-order inverse accumulative generating operation (1-IAGO).

5.3 *Variations of the Current GMC(1, N) and GMC(1, N) Models*

5.3.1 A New Multivariable Grey Prediction Model with Structure Compatibility NMGM(1, N)

Assume all initial conditions exactly identical to previous settings. Then,

$$X_1^{(1)}(rp+t) = \sum_{i=2}^{n} b_i X_i^{(1)}(t) + \beta_1 X_1^{(1)}(t-1) + \beta_2(t-1) + \beta_3 \tag{48}$$

is referred to as the New Multivariable Grey prediction Model with structure compatibility, or usually abbreviated as NMGM(1, n) [60].

With

$$B = \begin{bmatrix} X_2^{(1)}(2) \; X_3^{(1)}(2) \; ... \; X_n^{(1)}(2) & X_1^{(1)}(1) & 1 & 1 \\ X_2^{(1)}(3) \; X_3^{(1)}(3) \; ... \; X_n^{(1)}(3) & X_1^{(1)}(2) & 2 & 1 \\ \vdots \quad \vdots \quad ... \quad \vdots & \vdots & \vdots & \vdots \\ X_2^{(1)}(r) \; X_3^{(1)}(r) \; ... \; X_n^{(1)}(r) & X_1^{(1)}(r-1) & r-1 & 1 \end{bmatrix} \tag{49}$$

and

$$Y_R = \left[X_1^{(0)}(rp+2) \; X_1^{(0)}(rp+3) \; ... \; X_1^{(0)}(rp+r)\right] \tag{50}$$

the least square solution for the model parameters $\left[b_2, b_3, ..., b_n, \beta_1, \beta_2, \beta_3\right]$ can be derived as

1. If $r = n + 3$ and $|B| \neq 0$, $\left[b_2, b_3, ..., b_n, \beta_1, \beta_2, \beta_3\right] = B^{-1}Y_R$.
2. If $r > n + 3$ and $\left|B^T B\right| \neq 0$, $\left[b_2, b_3, ..., b_n, \beta_1, \beta_2, \beta_3\right] = \left(B^T B\right)^{-1} B^T Y_R$.
3. If $r > n + 3$ and $\left|B B^T\right| \neq 0$, $\left[b_2, b_3, ..., b_n, \beta_1, \beta_2, \beta_3\right] = B^T \left(B B^T\right)^{-1} Y_R$.

For the NMGM(1, n) model, the time-response function, or the particular solution for the 1-AGO modeling values of Eq. (48), is given by Zeng (2019) [60] as

$$\begin{aligned} \hat{X}^{(1)}(rp+t) = & \sum_{u=1}^{t-1}\left[\sum_{i=2}^{n} \beta_1^{u-1} b_i X_i^{(1)}(t-u+1)\right] + \beta_1^{(t-1} X_1^{(1)}(1) \\ & + \sum_{v=0}^{t-2} \beta_1^{v} \left[(t-v-1\beta_2+\beta_3\right] \end{aligned} \tag{51}$$

In Grey System theory, there are various univariate and multivariate models in different forms and formats. Applying these models improperly will lead to poor, or even misleading, predicted results. Due to the wide range of available models with different complexity, the compatibility (or generalization ability) of a model is at utmost importance. The following proposition will prove the compatibility of NMGM(1, n) with the other commonly used Grey models.

Proposition 1 *1. When $n = 1$ and $\beta_1\beta_2\beta_3 \neq 0$, the proposed model NMGM(1, n) model is equivalent to the model NHGM(1, 1, k).*

2. *When $n = 1$, $\beta_2 = 0$ and $\beta_1\beta_3 \neq 0$, the proposed model NMGM(1, n) becomes the traditional GM(1, 1) model.*
3. *When $n > 1$, $\beta_1 \neq 0$ and $\beta_2 = \beta_3 = 0$, the proposed model NMGM(1, n) is equal to the traditional multivariate GM(1, n) model.*

5.4 Representation of the Nonlinear Grey Model with Convolution Integral NGMC(1, N)

To apply GMC(1, n) for nonlinear data series, Wang (2014) [49] proposed an improved version of the model, namely NGMC(1, n). The Grey differential equation of this model now becomes

$$\frac{dx_1^{(1)}(rp+t)}{dt}+b_1X_1^{(1)}(rp+t)=\sum_{i=2}^{n}b_i\left[X_i^{(1)}(t)\right]^{\beta_i}+u;t=1,2,...,r \tag{52}$$

where $b_1, b_2, ..., b_n; u, \beta_2, \beta_3, ..., \beta_n$ are parameters that need estimating. $\beta_2, \beta_3, ..., \beta_n$ are introduced into the model as power exponents of the predicted variables, reflecting the behavior of nonlinear systems. Note that when $n = 1$ or $\beta_2 = \beta_3 = ... = \beta_n = 0$, (52) becomes the traditional GM(1, 1) model.

To evaluate all parameters in the model, the exponential parameters $\beta_2, \beta_3, ..., \beta_n$ are assumed to be known. Using the same least-square method as that of GMC(1, n), the estimates of $b_1, b_2, ..., b_n, u$ are made. After deriving the particular solution and applying 1-IAGO to obtain the predicted values of the model $\hat{X}_1^{(0)}$, the optimization algorithm is applied to obtain the values of $\beta_2, \beta_3, ..., \beta_n$.

6 Grey System Models with Fractional Order Accumulation

6.1 *Definition of the Fractional Order Accumulation*

Let $x^{(0)} = \left\{x^{(0)}(1), x^{(0)}(2), ..., x^{(0)}(n)\right\}$ be the original time-series data sequence. If the first - order accumulated generating operator (1-AGO) is applied r times on $x^{(0)}$, we obtain

$$x^{(r)} = \left\{x^{(r)}(1), x^{(r)}(2), ..., x^{(0)}(n)\right\} \tag{53}$$

By mathematical induction, setting $\binom{\frac{p}{q}-1}{0} = 1$ and $\binom{k-1}{k} = 0$, Wu et al. (2013) [52] has proven that its r-order Fractional accumulation (r-FOA) is

$$x^{(r)}(k)=\sum_{i=1}^{k}\binom{k-i+r-1}{k-i}x^{(0)}(i), k=1,2,...,n \tag{54}$$

where

$$\binom{k-i+t-1}{k-i}=\frac{(r+k-i-1)(r+k-i-2)...(r+1)r}{(k-i)!} \tag{55}$$

It is worth noting that the larger the value of r, the larger the weight of old data points in the time-series sequence would be; the lower the value of r, the smaller the weight of the old data would be.

The r-order inverse Fractional accumulation (r-IFOA) is also defined as

$$x^{(r)}(k) = \sum_{i=1}^{k} \binom{k-i-r-1}{k-i} x^{(0)}(i), k = 1, 2, ..., n \tag{56}$$

which means that the definition of the r-FOA and r-IFOA share basically the same formulation, with the only difference at the sign of r. From (54) and (56), we have the following relationship [32]

$$\left(x^{(r)}(k)\right)^{(-r)} = \sum_{i=1}^{k} \binom{k-i-r-1}{k-i} x^{(r)}(i) = x^{(0)}(k) \tag{57}$$

6.2 The Fractional $GM^{\frac{p}{q}}$(1, 1) Model

In line with the traditional model GM(1, 1) introduced previously, the Grey differential equation of $GM^{\frac{p}{q}}(1, 1)$ model can be expressed as

$$x^{\left(\frac{p}{q}\right)}(k) - x^{\left(\frac{p}{q}\right)}(k-1) + az^{\frac{p}{q}}(k) = b \tag{58}$$

with

$$z^{\frac{p}{q}}(k) = \frac{1}{2}\left(x^{\left(\frac{p}{q}\right)}(k) + x^{\left(\frac{p}{q}\right)}(k-1)\right), k = 2, 3, ..., n \tag{59}$$

Using the least-squares method, the coefficients a and b of the Eq. (58) can be determined by

$$\begin{bmatrix} a \\ b \end{bmatrix} = \left(B^T B\right)^{-1} B^T Y \tag{60}$$

where

$$B = \begin{bmatrix} -z^{\frac{p}{q}}(2) & 1 \\ -z^{\frac{p}{q}}(3) & 1 \\ \cdots \\ -z^{\frac{p}{q}}(n) & 1 \end{bmatrix}, Y = \begin{bmatrix} x^{\left(\frac{p}{q}\right)}(2) - x^{\left(\frac{p}{q}\right)}(1) \\ x^{\left(\frac{p}{q}\right)}(3) - x^{\left(\frac{p}{q}\right)}(2) \\ \cdots \\ x^{\left(\frac{p}{q}\right)}(n) - x^{\left(\frac{p}{q}\right)}(n-1) \end{bmatrix} \tag{61}$$

Similar to the GM(1, 1) model, the particular solution for the whitenization differential Eq. $\frac{dx^{\frac{p}{q}(t)}}{dt} + ax^{\left(\frac{p}{q}\right)}(t) = b$ is

$$x^{\left(\frac{p}{q}\right)}(k+1) = \left[x^{(0)}(1) - \frac{b}{a}\right]e^{-ak} + \frac{b}{a} \tag{62}$$

In order to optimize the effects of the model parameters in the particular solution, we can assume that

$$x^{\left(\frac{p}{q}\right)}(k+1) = ce^{-ak} + d \tag{63}$$

Applying again the least squares method for parameters c and d, we obtain

$$\begin{bmatrix} c \\ d \end{bmatrix} = \left(B^T B\right)^{-1} B^T Y \tag{64}$$

with

$$B = \begin{bmatrix} e^{-a} & 1 \\ e^{-2a} & 1 \\ \cdots & \\ e^{-(n-1)a} & 1 \end{bmatrix}, Y = \begin{bmatrix} x^{\left(\frac{p}{q}\right)}(2) \\ x^{\left(\frac{p}{q}\right)}(3) \\ \cdots \\ x^{\left(\frac{p}{q}\right)}(n) \end{bmatrix} \tag{65}$$

Thus, the final solution for equation (58), which is a 3-parametric exponential expression, would be

$$x^{\left(\frac{p}{q}\right)}(k+1) = ce^{-ak} + d, k = 1, 2, ..., n-1 \tag{66}$$

If we replace the constant b on the right-hand side of equation (58) with a polynomial function with respect to k, the new form of the model would be

$$x^{\left(\frac{p}{q}\right)}(k) - x^{\left(\frac{p}{q}\right)}(k-1) + az^{\frac{p}{q}}(k) = \beta_1 \sum_{i=1}^{k} i^1 + \beta_2 \sum_{i=1}^{k} i + \beta_3 \tag{67}$$

This model is named the Time - Delayed Polynomial Grey System Model with the Fractional Order Accumulation (TDPFOGM(1, 1)) [6].

6.3 *The Fractional Multivariate Grey Model with Convolutional Integral GMC $^{\frac{p}{q}}$(1, N)*

Let $X_i^{(r)}(i = 1, 2, ..., rp + n)$ be the r-order Fractional accumulation of the original series $X_i^{(0)}$, with rp beign the time delay factor. The Fractional multivariate Grey model with convolutional integral GMC$^{\frac{p}{q}}$(1, n) can be represented by the following Grey differential equation

$$\frac{d_1^{(r)}(rp+t)}{dt} + b_1 X_1^{(r)}(t) = \sum_{i=2}^{n} b_i X_i^{(r)}(t) + u \tag{68}$$

Applying the trapezoid formula for each of the intervals $[k-1, k]$, the differential equation can be discretized as

$$\left(X_1^{(r)}(rp+k) - X_1^{(r)}(rp+k-1)\right) + b_1 Z_1^{(r)}(k) = \sum_{i=2}^{n} b_i Z_i^{(r)}(k) + u \quad (69)$$

where $Z_i^{(r)}(i = 1, 2, ..., rp+n)$ are called background values,

$$Z_i^{(r)}(k) = \frac{1}{2}\left(X_i^{(r)}(k) + X_i^{(r)}(k-1)\right) \quad (70)$$

Similar to the traditional GMC(1, 1) model, the parameters $b_1, b_2, ..., b_n$ and u can be estimated using least-squares method, as follows

$$\left[b_1\ b_2\ ...\ b_n\ u\right]^T = \left(B^T B\right)^{-1} B^T Y \quad (71)$$

where

$$B = \begin{bmatrix} -Z_1^{(r)}(2) & -Z_2^{(r)}(2) & ... & -Z_n^{(r)}(2) & 1 \\ -Z_1^{(r)}(3) & -Z_2^{(r)}(3) & ... & -Z_n^{(r)}(3) & 1 \\ \vdots & \vdots & ... & \vdots & \vdots \\ -Z_1^{(r)}(n) & -Z_2^{(r)}(n) & ... & -Z_n^{(r)}(n) & 1 \end{bmatrix}, Y = \begin{bmatrix} X_1^{(r)}(rp+2) - X_1^{(r)}(rp+1) \\ X_1^{(r)}(rp+3) - X_1^{(r)}(rp+2) \\ \vdots \\ X_1^{(r)}(rp+n) - X_1^{(r)}(rp+n-1) \end{bmatrix} \quad (72)$$

The continuous response function for (68) can be estimated using the discrete function $f(t)$ and estimation methodology previously mentioned

$$X_1^{(r)}(rp+t) = X_1^{(0)} e^{-b_1(t-1)} + \sum_{k=2}^{t} \left\{ e^{-b_1\left(t-k+\frac{1}{2}\right)} \cdot \frac{1}{2}\left[f(k) + f(k-1)\right] \right\} \quad (73)$$

From $X^{(r)}$, the predicted value of the original sequence can be calculated using the 1-IFOA Eq. (57).

6.4 Optimization of the Fractional Order r

Considering all the previously proposed model, the Fractional Order r has been assumed to be given before running the model. However, selecting the optimal value of r is also of significant importance in improving the accuracy of the final model. Once again, to evaluate the accuracy, we will use the mean absolute percentage error (MAPE).

Table 2 Prediction results of $GM^{\frac{p}{q}}(1, 1)$ with different values of Fractional Order r

	$GM^{1.1}(1, 1)$	$GM^{1}(1, 1)$	$GM^{0.3}(1, 1)$	$GM^{0.2}(1, 1)$	$GM^{0.1}(1, 1)$	$GM^{0}(1, 1)$
MAPE (2001–2006)	2.55	1.13	1.27	1.17	**1.07**	1.18
MAPE (2007–2009)	28.37	6.54	3.83	2.31	**1.49**	2.23

Table 3 Prediction results of the optimal FDGM(1, n) comparing with different multivariate Grey models

Year	FDGM $r = -1.24234$	FGMC $r = -0.41939$	GMC_G	GMC_T	NGMC
Fitting ARPE	**0.0002**	0.7664	6.2579	10.7512	1.4752
Prediction ARPE	**13.0452**	103.6555	2118.5894	985.1529	17.5114

There has been a lot of well-known evolutionary algorithms that have been used to optimize hyper-parameters of Grey models (background value, power coefficient and now, the Fractional Order), including Particle Swarm Optimization (PSO), Genetic Algorithm (GA), Ant Colony Optimization (ACO), Evolution Strategy (ES), Population-based Incremental Learning [32] and Adaptive Dynamic Cat Swarm Algorithm (ADCSA) [26]. Ma et al. (2019) [32] also suggested using Grey Wolf Optimizer, one of the most intelligent optimizers proposed in 2014, to solve the nonlinear programming problem for the Fractional Order r. However, most of the optimizers proposed only concern non-constrained optimization, which means that we have to validate the constrains for every iteration of the optimizer.

In terms of empirical results, Wu et al. (2012) [52] confirmed that different values of Fractional Order r returns significantly different results of ARPE (Table 2). Besides, application of Grey Wolf Model by Ma (2019) (Table 3) also received significantly better results compared to other existing models, especially upon comparing with the traditional Grey model with convolutional integral.

The final parts of this chapter introduces another important part of Grey systems: Grey Relational Analysis (GRA). While Grey models handle prediction and regression tasks, Grey Relational Analysis resolves the relationship between factors when experimental methods can not be carried out properly, or when data becomes ambiguous, overcoming the disadvantages of traditional statistical methods.

7 Introduction to the Grey Relational Analysis

7.1 Data Preprocessing

Data preprocessing is a process in which the data get transformed, or modified, to a more comparable series. For this purpose, all variables are normalised to be within the range [0, 1].

There are various approaches in normalising the original sequence, including

1. If the target value of the sequence is infinite ($\pm\infty$) and has the characteristic of "the higher, the better," the sequence can be minimized as

$$x_i^*(k) = \frac{x_i^0(k) - \min x_i^0(k)}{\max x_i^0(k) - \min x_i^0(k)} \tag{74}$$

2. If the target value of the sequence is expected to be "the lower, the better," in this case, the original sequence should be normalized as

$$x_i^*(k) = \frac{\max x_i^0(k) - x_i^0(k)}{\max x_i^0(k) - \min x_i^0(k)} \tag{75}$$

3. If there is a finite target values for the sequence to reach, the original sequence shall be normalized by

$$x_i^*(k) = 1 - \frac{\left|x_i^0(k) - x^0\right|}{\max x_i^0(k) - x^0} \tag{76}$$

   with x^0 being the desired/preferred output value of the sequence.
4. Most simply, the sequence can be normalized based on its first value

$$x_i^*(k) = \frac{x_i^0(k)}{x_i^0(1)} \tag{77}$$

7.2 Grey Relational Coefficient and Grey Relational Grade

Grey Relational Coefficient is meant to express the relationship between the idea (desired) and actual normalized results. This coefficient, according to Yang (2006) [57], can be calculated as follows

$$\xi_i(k) = \frac{\Delta_{\min} + \xi \cdot \Delta_{\max}}{\Delta_{0i}(k) + \xi \cdot \Delta_{\max}} \tag{78}$$

where

- $\Delta_{0i}(k)$ is the deviation sequence of the reference sequence and the comparability sequence, namely

$$\Delta_{0i}(k) = \left\| x_0^*(k) - x_i^*(k) \right\| \tag{79}$$

- ξ is the distinguishing or identification coefficient, $\xi \in [0, 1]$. Normally, $\xi = 0.5$ is commonly used.
- Δ_{max} and Δ_{min} is the maximum and minimum deviation of the reference sequence from the comparability sequence, which is described as

$$\Delta_{max} = \max_{\forall j \in i} \max_{\forall k} \left\| x_0^*(k) - x_j^*(k) \right\| \tag{80}$$

$$\Delta_{min} = \min_{\forall j \in i} \min_{\forall k} \left\| x_0^*(k) - x_j^*(k) \right\| \tag{81}$$

After all the Grey Relational Coefficients are calculated, the Grey Relational Grade is obtained simply by taking the mean of all the Grey Relational Coefficients, as follows

$$\gamma_i = \frac{1}{n} \sum_{i=1}^{n} \xi_i(k) \tag{82}$$

However, since the effects of each variable (factor) on the output sequence is not the same, the Grey Relational Grade formula (82) can be modified as

$$\gamma_i = \sum_{k=1}^{n} \omega_k \cdot \xi_i(k), \sum_{k=1}^{n} \omega_k = 1 \tag{83}$$

with ω_k beign the normalized weighting value of factor k.

In the Grey Relational Analysis, Grey Relational Grade represents the relationship among sequences or variables. If the two sequence are identical, the Grey Relational Grade will be equal to 1. If a particular comparability sequence has more impact than another comparability sequence, the Grey Relational Grade for that particular sequence will also be higher than the other [58].

8 Applications of Grey Relational Analysis In medicine

8.1 General Applications of Grey Relational Analysis in Medical Data Analysis

With advantages in handling limited data sequence, Grey Relational Analysis has more applications compared to traditional statistical methods in multi-variable analysis. Grey Relational Analysis can be used in verification of medical theory [7, 18] or results of empirical research [42, 43]. Besides, with the assistance of Grey Relational Analysis, either evaluation of the curative effect on a single variable can be evaluated without the usage of placebo control or all side effects can be evaluated in overall in multi-variable model judgement environment [28].

Grey Relational Analysis has also been applied to generate clustering algorithms, namely

- Hierarchical Grey relation clustering algorithm with application to the geographic information system of hospitals in Taiwan [53].
- Grey Relational pattern analysis approach for data clustering and comparison with well-known existing algorithms, including fuzzy c-means and hard c-means methods [3, 19].

8.2 Application in Telecare

8.2.1 The Role and Development of Telecare in Covid-19 Pandemic

Remote healthcare is easier to access in this era than ever, thanks to the constant improvement of technology. The term 'telecare' or 'telehealth' is the care offered to patients remotely via live video, or remote patient monitoring. Telecare is often used to expand patient access to care, help patients manage recovery and well-being at home, and remotely monitor risks or early warning signs of health conditions. The care could be handled through a range of technology—from telephones to online virtual visits to remote patient monitoring centers [45].

In this Covid-19 situation, the advantage of telecare is radically utilized. Patients can receive immediate feedback on their environment, health, or situation, which can alleviate memory issues and help the person to maintain their dignity and independence [45], also doctors can keep distance to patients to minimize the chance of being exposed to coronavirus. Electronic intensive care unit (e-ICU) monitoring programs, which allow nurses and physicians to remotely monitor the status of 60 to 100 patients in ICUs in multiple hospitals are ideal for monitoring sicker patients. Technological and staffing complexities make it impossible to create such a program on short notice, but rapid deployment of the two-tablet approach can reduce health care workers' contact with infected patients in the ICU.

Telehealth has had a positive impact on a number of pandemic diseases similar to Covid-19 in the past. During the years 2014–2016, when Africa was dealing with the Ebola crisis, there was a challenge of how to interrupt the ongoing transmission of the Ebola virus to others. In this situation, an approach was used to combat the disease using a mobile app named Ebola Contact Tracing (ECT), which helped remotely monitor and contact trace confirmed cases of Ebola virus disease. Data gathered by the ECT app were faster, secure, and complete as compared with a paper-based form and it could accurately monitor a large number of contacts [22, 37].

Disasters and pandemics pose unique challenges to health care delivery. Though telehealth will not solve them all, it's well suited for scenarios in which infrastructure remains intact and clinicians are available to see patients. Payment and regulatory structures, state licensing, credentialing across hospitals, and program implementation all take time to work through, but health systems that have already invested in telemedicine are well-positioned to ensure that patients with Covid-19 receive the care they need. In this instance, it may be a virtually perfect solution [16].

In general, the mentioned applications of telecommunications in past and current crises demonstrate the potential of remote teleconsultation in the management of viral pandemics. The important issue is that many developing countries are not ready to take advantage of telehealth, especially for their remote and rural areas despite the significant growth of technology, such as increased penetration of smartphones and the expansion of 3G and 4G internet networks [22].

8.2.2 Previous Application of Grey Relational Analysis in Telecare

Huang (2011) [17] conducted a survey on 76 adult users of age 55 or above about their perception of the telecare services. There are 7 factors that are used to measure effects of using telecare on Quality of Life, including health promotion, safety, accessibility of medical care services, overall living quality, financial burden, social relationship, and acquisition of information. This study adopted Grey system theory to propose an effective method of data analysis, which is different from most of the traditional statistical methods.

Based on users' preference for the influence of telecare on the quality of life, the results showed that the overall living quality has the greatest effect on the effect generated by telecare on the quality of life (0.808). It is followed by the acquisition of information (0.785), accessibility of medical care services (0.748), and safety (0.741) (Fig. 3). This research also suggests that the Grey system theory (in general), or the Grey rational analysis (in particular), is an effective method for data analysis. The results and methodology of this research can be considered as a reference for later studies, especially when telecare is playing a more and more important role in increasing the treatment effect on Covid-19 patients.

8.3 Grey Data Management in Medicine

Handling data is indeed a crucial part of Covid-19 pandemic response in every country. Medical history, information about movements, and interactions are of equal importance as quarantine or social lockdown in dealing with this pandemic. For certain regions, for example, the US and European Union, these types of data are also very sensitive and concern a lot of privacy measures. There have been numerous applications of data analysis into Covid-19 research, some of which have reached early success, including contact tracing, resource optimization, aiding at-risk populations,

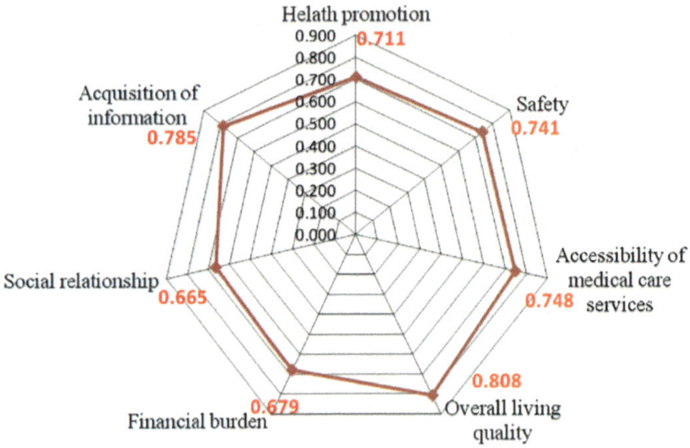

Fig. 3 Grey Relational Grade of each quality of life (Huang, 2011)

and demand planning [36]. Medical data are considered minor in this experimental context as information is divided into small-sized samples against the proposition information field of the whole human body [55].

The Grey data management, in general, refers to the first step of Grey data analysis, including data collection, data imputation, data storage, and management.

1. **Data collection**: In most cases, data collection starts with an incomplete data requirement, which means that the incompleteness will be shown right from the beginning. Each sample will be considered as a Grey dataset, with Grey number as a representation of its incompleteness.
2. **Data imputation, data storage, and management**: Within this step, a data format and storage management plan has to be come up with to keep not only the information available but also all the details of its Greyness. Instead of converting or guessing unknown value to a more reliable existing value (mean, median, or mode), Grey data imputation focuses on reducing the degree of Greyness rather than completely removing all uncertainty.

Due to the minor data and uncertain characteristics of medical data (similar to Grey systems), combined with mathematical modeling and quantification of medical information, Tan et al. (2007) [41] proposed some of the most basic concepts of Grey medicine, including Grey medical cognition mode, Grey Relational Coefficient, Grey polarity besides the previously defined terms, Grey Relational Analysis or Grey Relational Grade.

Conclusion

Although the research on Covid-19 has been continuously going on and achieved excessive progress, certain limitations, especially in accessing the data source for pandemic modeling, is inevitable. Even when the data is accessible, there is no certainty that the data is complete, or in perfect condition, with full information available. As a result, despite currently having very few applications to mathematical modeling or pandemic prediction, the Grey Systems theory has tremendous potential for later development. Not only can it make accurate and reliable predictions for policy-making and controlling purposes, but Grey data analysis can also shed light on important insights that can help us understand much more about the pandemic in the near future, assisting researchers in containing this disease, at worldwide level.

References

1. Akay, D., Atak, M.: Grey prediction with rolling mechanism for electricity demand forecasting of Turkey. Energy **32**(9), 1670–75 (2007). https://doi.org/10.1016/j.energy.2006.11.014
2. Caydas, U., Hascalık, A.: Use of the grey relational analysis to determine optimum laser cutting parameters with multi-performance characteristics. Optics Laser Technol. **40**(7), 987–994 (2008). doi: https://doi.org/10.1016/j.optlastec.2008.01.004
3. Chang K.-C., Yeh M.-F.: Grey relational analysis based approach for data clustering (2015), IEE Proceedings online no. 20041209. doi: https://doi.org/10.1049/ip-vis:20041209
4. Chang, S.-C., Lai, H.-C., Yu, H.-C.: A Variable P value rolling grey forecasting model for Taiwan semiconductor industry production. Technol. Forecast. Social Change **72**(5), 623–40 (2005). https://doi.org/10.1016/j.techfore.2003.09.002
5. Chen, C.: Application of the novel nonlinear grey Bernoulli model for forecasting unemployment rate. Chaos, Solit. Fractals **37**(1), 278–287. doi: https://doi.org/10.1016/j.chaos.2006.08.024
6. Chen, L., Liu, Z., Ma, N.: Time-delayed polynomial with the fractional order accumulation. Math. Probl. Eng. (2018). https://doi.org/10.1155/2018/3640625
7. Chen, Y.-K., Tan, X.-R.: Grey relational analysis on serum markers of liver fibrosis. J. Grey Syst. **1**, 63 (1995)
8. China's State Council Information Office, Fighting COVID-19: China in Action, June 2020
9. Dang Y.-G., Liu, S.-F., Chen K-.J.: The GM model that x(n) be taken as initial value. Kybernetes **33**(2), 247–254 (2004). doi: https://doi.org/10.1108/03684920410514175
10. Delcea, C., Scarlat, E.: Grey relational analysis between social media engagement and users' decisions. In: 2015 IEEE International Conference on Grey Systems and Intelligent Services (GSIS), 2015. doi: https://doi.org/10.1109/gsis.2015.7301843
11. Deng, J.-L.: Introduction to Grey System Theory **1**, 1–24 (1989)
12. Deng, J.-L.: Control problems of grey systems. Syst. Control Lett. **1**(5), 288–94 (1982). https://doi.org/10.1016/s0167-6911(82)80025-x
13. Equbal, Md. I., Kumar, R., Shamim, M., Ohdar, R.K.: A grey-based Taguchi method to optimize hot forging process. Procedia Mater. Sci. **6**, 1495–1504 (2014). doi: https://doi.org/10.1016/j.mspro.2014.07.129
14. Guo, R.: A repairable system modelling: combining grey system theory with interval-valued fuzzy set theory. Int. J. Reliab. Qual. Safety Eng. **12**(03), 241–66 (2005). https://doi.org/10.1142/s0218539305001811
15. Hsin, P.-H. Forecasting Taiwan's GDP by the novel Nash nonlinear Grey Bernoulli model with trembling-hand perfect equilibrium, 2013. doi: https://doi.org/10.1063/1.4823908

16. Hollander, J.E., Carr, B.G.: Virtually Perfect? Telemedicine for Covid-19. New Engl. J. Med. **382**(18), 1679–1681. doi: https://doi.org/10.1056/nejmp2003539
17. Huang J-.C.: Application of grey system theory in telecare. Comput. Biol. Med. **41**(5), 302–306 (2011). doi: https://doi.org/10.1016/j.compbiomed.2011.03.007
18. Huang, W., Shi, H.-R., Tan, X.-R.: A grey relational study on determination of stroke volume with D and M echocardiography. J. Grey Syst. **3**, 203 (1994)
19. Jin, X.-Z.: Grey correlation cluster method and it's application study. J. Henan Med. Coll. Staff Workers **11**(4), 1–4 (1999)
20. Juan, L., Liu, W.-J.: Population forecasting in China based on the Grey-Markov model. In: 2011 International Conference on Information Management, Innovation Management and Industrial Engineering, 2011. doi: https://doi.org/10.1109/iciii.2011.315
21. Kalsi, N.S., Sehgal, R., Sharma, V.S.: Multi-objective optimization using Grey relational Taguchi analysis in machining. Int. J. Organ. Collect. Intell. **6**(4), 45–64 (2016). https://doi.org/10.4018/ijoci.2016100103
22. Keshvardoost, S., Bahaadinbeigy, K., Fatehi, F.: Role of telehealth in the management of COVID-19: lessons learned from previous SARS, MERS, and Ebola outbreaks. Telemedicine and E-Health. doi: https://doi.org/10.1089/tmj.2020.0105
23. Kose, E., Burmaoglu, S., Kabak, M.: Grey relational analysis between energy consumption and economic growth. Grey Syst.: Theory Appl. **3**(3), 291–304 (2013). https://doi.org/10.1108/gs-06-2013-0010
24. Kuo, Y., Yang, T., Huang, G.-W.: The Use of Grey Relational Analysis in Solving Multiple Attribute Decision-Making Problems. Computers & Industrial Engineering **55**(1), 80–93 (2008). https://doi.org/10.1016/j.cie.2007.12.002
25. Li, G.-D., Yamaguchi, D., Nagai, M.: A GM(1,1)-Markov chain combined model with an application to predict the number of Chinese International Airlines. Technol. Forecast. Soc. Change **74**(8), 1465–81 (2007). https://doi.org/10.1016/j.techfore.2006.07.010
26. Lin B.-Y., Gao, F., Wang, M., et al.: A parameter estimation of fractional order grey model based on adaptive dynamic Cat Swarm Algorithm (2018), arXiv:1805.08680
27. Liu, L., Wang, Q.-R., Wang, J.-Z., Liu, M.:A Rolling Grey Model optimized by particle swarm optimization in economic prediction. Comput. Intell. **32**(3), 391–419. doi: https://doi.org/10.1111/coin.12059
28. Liu, P.-J., Dong, G.-Y.: Applying grey relational grade in determining pharmacokinetic modeling. J. Chinese Hosp. Pharmacy **3**, 141 (1996)
29. Liu, S., Yi, L.: Grey Information: Theory and Practical Applications. England: Springer, London Ltd, 2010. doi: https://doi.org/10.1016/j.techfore.2006.07.010
30. Liu, S., Yi, L.: An introduction to grey systems: foundations, methodology and applications. Kybernetes **32**(4) (2003). doi: https://doi.org/10.1108/k.2003.06732dae.008
31. Lu, J.-S., Xie, W.-D., et al.: An optimized nonlinear grey Bernoulli model and its application. Neurocomputing **17**, 206–214 (2016). https://doi.org/10.1016/j.neucom.2015.11.032
32. Ma, X., Xie, M., Wu, W., Zeng, B., Wang, Y., Wu, X.: The novel fractional discrete multivariate Grey system model and its applications. Appl. Math. Modell. **70**, 402–24 (2019). https://doi.org/10.1016/j.apm.2019.01.039
33. Mao, S., Gao, M., Xiao, X., Zhu, M.: A novel fractional Grey system model and its application. Appl. Math. Modell. **40**(7–8), 5063–76 (2016). https://doi.org/10.1016/j.apm.2015.12.014
34. Ngo, H.-A., Hoang, T.-N.: A Rolling Optimized Nonlinear Grey Bernoulli model and application in predicting total COVID-18 infected cases (2020). Accepted paper at the 2020 International Congress for Grey Systems and Uncertainty Analysis, Nanjing
35. Nguyen, P.-H., Sheu, T.-W., Nguyen, P.-T., Pham, D.-H., Nagai, M.: Taylor approximation method in grey system theory and its application to predict the number of foreign students studying in Taiwan. Int. J. Innov. Sci. Res. **10**(2), 409–420 (2014)
36. Rausch N., Wright, T.: The role of data management techniques during COVID-19: 4 examples (2020), SAS Blogs
37. Reducing Ebola Virus Transmission: Improving Contact Tracing in Sierra Leone. (2020, March 19). Retrieved July 06, 2020, from https://www.poverty-action.org/study/reducing-ebola-virus-transmission-improving-contact-tracing-sierra-leone

38. Sahin, U., Sahin, T.: Forecasting the cumulative number of confirmed cases of COVID-19 in Italy, UK and USA using fractional nonlinear grey Bernoulli model. Chaos, Solit. Fractals **138**, 109948 (2020). https://doi.org/10.1016/j.chaos.2020.109948
39. Shen, X., Ou, L., Tan, X.: Applications of Grey prediction model for quantity prediction of medical supplies: a case study. In: Proceedings of 2013 IEEE International Conference on Grey systems and Intelligent Services (GSIS), 2013. doi: https://doi.org/10.1109/gsis.2013.6714772
40. Tan, G.-T.: The structure method and application of background value in grey system GM model (I), Syst. Eng.-Theory Pract. **4**, 98–103 (2000)
41. Tan, X.R., Deng, J.L., Pan, H.X., Liu, S.F.: Grey system and Grey data management in medicine. In: Proceedings of 2007 IEEE International Conference on Grey Systems and Intelligent Services. doi: https://doi.org/10.1109/GSIS.2007.4443258
42. Tan, X.-R., Deng, J.-L., Xu, Y.-C.: The statistical and grey relational analysis of the pressure-lowering effect of captopril. The academic seminar proceedings of the national clinical evaluation of the cardiovascular drugs. The expert committee of clinical drug evaluation of Chinese Medical Association, 1996: 127
43. Tan, X.-R., Li, Y.-G., Chen, M.-Z.: Applications of gray relational analysis in gastroenterology. World J. Gastroenterol. **11**(22): 3457–3460. doi: https://doi.org/10.3748/wjg.v11.i22.3457
44. Tien, T.-L.: A research on the grey prediction model GM(1, n). Appl. Math. Comput. **218**, 4903–4916 (2012). https://doi.org/10.1016/j.amc.2011.10.055
45. What is Telecare? A Definition of Services, Technologies & Equipment. (2020, January 28). Retrieved July 06, 2020, from https://evisit.com/resources/what-is-telecare/
46. Chia-Nan, W., Van-Thanh, P.: An improved nonlinear Grey Bernoulli model combined with fourier series. Math. Probl. Eng. **2015**, 1–7 (2015). https://doi.org/10.1155/2015/740272
47. Wang, Y., Tang, J., Cao, W.: Grey prediction model-based food security early warning prediction. Proceedings of 2011 IEEE International Conference on Grey Systems and Intelligent Services (2011). doi: https://doi.org/10.1109/gsis.2011.6043997
48. Wang, Z.-W., Dang, Y.-G., et al.: Solution of GM(1,1) power model and its properties. Syst. Eng. Electrion. **31**(10), 2380–2383 (2009)
49. Wang, Z.-X.: Nonlinear Grey prediction model with convolution integral NGMC (1, n) and its application to the forecasting of China's industrial SO_2 emissions. J. Appl. Math. 580161 (2014). doi: https://doi.org/10.1155/2014/580161
50. Wang, Z.-X., Hipel, K.W., Wang, Q., He, S.-W.: An optimized NGBM(1,1) model for forecasting the qualified discharge rate of industrial wastewater in China. Appl. Math. Modell. **35**(12), 5524–32 (2011). https://doi.org/10.1016/j.apm.2011.05.022
51. Wei, L., Dang, Y.-G.: The optimized grey model GM(l, N) based on the development trends of driving variables and its application. In: IEEE International Conference on Systems, Man, and Cybernetic (SMC), Budapest, Hungary (2016). doi: https://doi.org/10.1109/SMC.2016.7844247
52. Wu, L., Liu, S., Yao, L., Yan, S., Liu, D.: Grey system model with the fractional order accumulation. Commun. Nonlinear Sci. Numer. Simul. **18**(7), 1775–85 (2013). https://doi.org/10.1016/j.cnsns.2012.11.017
53. Wu, W.-H., Lin, C.-T., Peng, K.-H., Huang, C.-C.: Applying hierarchical grey relation clustering analysis to geographical information systems – A case study of the hospitals in Taipei City. Expert Syst. Appl. **39**, 7247–7254 (2012). https://doi.org/10.1016/j.eswa.2012.01.052
54. Wu, W.-Z., Zhang, T., Zheng, C.: A novel optimized nonlinear Grey Bernoulli model for forecasting China's GDP. Complexity **2019**, 1–10 (2019). https://doi.org/10.1155/2019/1731262
55. Yang, S.Q.: Public health statistics. the People's Health Press, Beijing (1978)
56. Yang, Y.J., Liu, S.F., Xie, N.M.: Uncertainty and grey data analytics. Marine Econ. Manag. (2019). https://doi.org/10.1108/MAEM-08-2019-0006
57. Yang, Y.-K.: Optimization of injection-molding process for mechanical and tribological properties of short glass fiber and polytetrafluoroethylene reinforced polycarbonate composites with Grey relational analysis: a case study. Polymer-Plastics Technol. Eng. **45**(7), 769–777 (2006). https://doi.org/10.1080/03602550600611826

58. Yang, Y.Y., Shie, J.R., Huang, C.H.: Optimization of dry machining parameters for high purity graphite in end-milling process. Mater. Manuf. Process. **21**, 832–7 (2006). https://doi.org/10.1080/03602550600728141
59. Zeng, B., Luo, C.: Forecasting the total energy consumption in China using a new-structure Grey system model. Grey Syst.: Theory Appl. **7**(2), 194–217 (2017). https://doi.org/10.1108/gs-05-2017-0011
60. Zeng, B., Duan, H., Zhou, Y.: A new multivariable grey prediction model with structure compatibility. Appl. Math. Modell. doi: https://doi.org/10.1016/j.apm.2019.05.044
61. Zhao, Y.-F., Shou, M.-H., Wang, Z.-X.: Prediction of the number of patients infected with COVID-19 based on rolling Grey Verhulst models. Int. J. Environ. Res. Public Health **17**, 4582 (2020). https://doi.org/10.3390/ijerph17124582
62. Mao, Z.-L., Sun, J.-H.: Application of Grey-Markov model in forecasting fire accidents. Procedia Eng. **11**, 314–18 (2011). https://doi.org/10.1016/j.proeng.2011.04.663
63. Zhou, W., He, J.-M.: Generalized GM (1, 1) model and its application in forecasting of fuel production. Appl. Math. Modell. **37**(9), 6234–43 (2013). https://doi.org/10.1016/j.apm.2013.01.002

Mathematical Analysis of Diagnosis Rate Effects in Covid-19 Transmission Dynamics with Optimal Control

Nasser Al-Salti, Ibrahim M. Elmojtaba, Jaqueline Mesquita, Dayse Pastore, and Maryam Al-Yahyai

Abstract Many countries around the world are trying to fight Covid-19, and their main methods are lockdown, quarantine, isolation, and awareness programs to encourage people to adopt social distancing and maintain personal hygiene. The lockdown is aimed to restrict the movement of humans from or to certain places. Quarantine is aimed toward separating the susceptible humans from infected or exposed humans as much as possible, whereas isolation is aimed toward keeping the confirmed cases of infected humans away from the rest of the population. The confirmed cases are mainly identified through the diagnosis of individuals who showed symptoms of Covid-19 and sometimes through random checking of individuals hoping to identify either asymptomatic or pre-symptomatic cases, which is generally an expensive method. In this chapter, we develop a mathematical model to investigate the role of diagnosis rate in the transmission dynamics of Covid-19 together with the combined effects of quarantine and isolation. Our model will be fully analyzed both qualitatively and quantitatively in order to gain insight about the role of different model parameters in the disease transmission dynamics, especially those related to diagnosis and quarantine. The analysis will include the estimation of both the basic and the control reproduction numbers, and sensitivity analysis of the reproduction numbers to the corresponding model parameters. The optimal control theory will be

N. Al-Salti · I. M. Elmojtaba · M. Al-Yahyai
Department of Mathematics, Sultan Qaboos University, Al-Khoudh 123, Oman
e-mail: nalsalti@squ.edu.om

I. M. Elmojtaba
e-mail: elmojtaba@squ.edu.om

M. Al-Yahyai
e-mail: alyahyai44@hotmail.com

J. Mesquita (✉)
Department of Mathematics, Universidade de Brasília, Brasília, Brazil

D. Pastore
Department of Mathematics, Centro Federal de Educaçåo Tecnológica Celso Suckow da Fonseca, Rio de Janeiro, Brazil
e-mail: dayse.pastore@cefet-rj.br

P. Agarwal et al. (eds.), *Analysis of Infectious Disease Problems (Covid-19) and Their Global Impact*, Infosys Science Foundation Series,
https://doi.org/10.1007/978-981-16-2450-6_11

also applied to the model to examine the role of some other optimal control strategies and to study the effect of diagnosis and quarantine rates in the effectiveness of these controls.

Keywords Covid-19 · Basic reproduction number · Sensitivity analysis · Optimal control

1 Introduction

Covid-19 is a severe acute respiratory syndrome (SARS) disease. First, it has been associated with severe pneumonia cases in Wuhan city, China, in December 2019 [18]. The early stage transmission was assumed to be from animal to human only; however, it has been proved that its major route of transmission is from human to human [33] as well as it has been reported that there is a possibility of transmission through contaminated environment [7, 12]. There is no approved treatment yet, which makes very difficult to control the disease especially due to its high transmission rate reaching over seven million cases by June 9, 2020 [35]. Nevertheless, some kind of treatment has been employed to reduce the symptoms and enhance the immune system, but until now none of them showed to be efficient and that is why many efforts around the world are being made in order to develop an effective vaccine to fight this disease, with some initial success so far.

The Covid-19 presents some particular aspects which turns its control a nontrivial challenge to deal. It is a known fact that Covid-19 may have a large incubation period, compared to other diseases, taking between 1 and 14 days for the first symptoms to appear into the individual body ([4, 33]), which represents a challenge to detect the infected individuals right at the beginning, especially because this period may vary a lot depending on the individual. Other aspect that should be pointed out concerns on the variety of ways that the novel coronavirus may manifest into the human body [15, 34], which seems to depend on several variables. This fact is still an object of extensive study by the scientists around the world. In addition to all these matters, even though the infected individuals do not present any symptoms, they can spread the virus to other individuals, hindering the disease containment [3, 5, 20, 24, 27, 30, 38].

All these aspects represent a barrier in the control and measurement of the pandemics, since they reveal the big deal behind of promoting cheap and general public policies to contain the spread of the disease. One of the most efficient policies addressed to this issue concerns on providing an extremely high accuracy testing policy for the population (see [28, 31]). Notice that if the number of testing is not enough, it is necessary to adopt high quarantine rate, even when the region has a low infection rate, since the real number of infected individuals is not known. Also, with the low testing rate, it is not possible for the local authorities to know the real dimension of the pandemics, hence it may have higher proportion than it is being measured.

In face of this context, the main methods which have been currently employed for fighting Covid-19 are lockdown, quarantine, isolation, and awareness programs to encourage people to adopt social distancing and maintain personal hygiene, while an effective treatment is still in development. The aim of lockdown is to restrict the mobility of individuals from or to certain places, and quarantine is aimed toward separating the susceptible humans from infected or exposed humans as much as possible to avoid the contagious. On the other hand, the aim of isolation is to keep the confirmed cases of infected humans away from the rest of the population. The confirmed cases are mainly identified through the diagnosis of individuals who showed the symptoms of Covid-19 and sometimes through contact tracing or random checking of individuals hoping to identify asymptomatic or pre-symptomatic cases.

The model that we present here shows the importance of adopting these methods, specially quarantine and social distancing, in order to control the pandemics, being one of the most efficient methods for its containment. In the simulations presented in this chapter, one can confirm this fact.

In [1], a comparison was made between the rigidity of the social distance measures adopted in Argentina, Spain, Italy, Brazil, and the USA. In this survey, carried out in April 2020, it was concluded that Argentina, Spain, and Italy adopted stricter social distance measures, while Brazil and USA adopted more flexible measures. When comparing the numbers of diagnosed cases, among these countries, in the months following the adoption of isolation measures, we see that the countries that have adopted a stricter isolation policy have a steady growth in the number of cases, while the other countries have had a marked growth, these data can be seen in [10]. This fact corroborates the results found in the model presented in this chapter.

Understanding the Covid-19 transmission dynamics using mathematical modeling plays an important role for disease control, management, and allowing the design of effective public policies to be employed by the several governments in different parts of the world. For this reason, in the last months, a huge number of mathematical models have been developed in order to comprehend the pandemic and control its transmission in a better way; see, for instance, [11, 16, 19, 21, 25, 26, 32, 36, 37]. The susceptible–exposed–infectious–recovered (SEIR) model is the most commonly investigated model, in which the infectious individuals are taken as one class or divided into a number of classes such as asymptomatic, pre-symptomatic, and symptomatic infectious classes.

In this chapter, we develop a mathematical model to investigate the role of diagnosis rate in the transmission dynamics of Covid-19 together with the combined effects of quarantine and isolation, and taking into account the routes of transmission from human to human as well as from environment to human, this last one is very important to consider in order to get a better description of the disease, since an individual can acquire the novel coronavirus when an individual has contact with contaminated surfaces, as some investigations and important studies have suggested (see [7, 12]). Our model is formulated in the next section and is fully analyzed both qualitatively and quantitatively in order to gain insight about the role of different model parameters in the disease transmission dynamics, especially those related to diagnosis and quarantine. The full mathematical analysis is given in Sect. 3, and it includes the calculation of the disease-free equilibrium and the estimation of both the basic and control reproduction numbers, and sensitivity analysis of the reproduction numbers to the corresponding model parameters. The stability of equilibrium points has been also addressed in this section, which is concluded with numerical simulation to demonstrate the obtained theoretical results. In Sect. 4, an optimal control model is developed and analyzed numerically to examine the role of some other optimal control strategies and study the effect of diagnosis and quarantine rates in the effectiveness of these controls. Finally, a brief conclusion is presented in Sect. 5.

2 Model Formulation

In this section, the goal is to present the model formulation and discuss its description and interpretation.

We start by considering both direct (from human to human) and indirect (from environment to human) routes of transmission. The human population $N(t)$ is divided into eight sub-population, namely susceptible $S(t)$, exposed $E(t)$, quarantined $Q(t)$, asymptomatic $A(t)$, pre-symptomatic $P(t)$, symptomatic infected $I(t)$, diagnosed (tested positive for Covid-19) $D(t)$, and recovered $R(t)$, so that

$$N(t) = S(t) + E(t) + Q(t) + A(t) + P(t) + I(t) + D(t) + R(t).$$

It is assumed that susceptible humans are recruited into the population at a constant rate Λ. Susceptible humans acquire Covid-19 by either contacted with a pre-symptomatic, an asymptomatic, a symptomatic infected human or from the contaminated environment with rates β_P, β_A, β_I, and $\dfrac{\beta_e B}{k + B}$, respectively, or they are quarantined at a rate λ_Q. Quarantined humans leave quarantine and rejoin the susceptible class at a rate λ_S. All newly infected humans enter a latent period and then either become pre-symptomatic or asymptomatic at a rate λ_P or λ_A, respectively. Then, pre-symptomatic individuals develop symptoms at a rate λ_I and become symptomatic infected. Pre-symptomatic, asymptomatic, and symptomatic infected individuals get diagnosed at rates ϵ_P, ϵ_A, and ϵ_I, respectively, and enter the diagnosed class. Here, we assume that susceptible individuals avoid contact with diagnosed individuals who are isolated at home or at health institutions till they have been recovered or die and, hence, they do not contribute to the disease transmission. Asymptomatic, symptomatic infected, and diagnosed (isolated) individuals recover from the disease with rates γ_A, γ_I, and γ_D, respectively. It is assumed that pre-symptomatic individuals will recover after they develop symptoms. All human sub-populations are subject to natural death which occurs at a rate μ. Moreover, symptomatic infected and diagnosed humans are subject to disease related to death that occurs at rates δ_I and δ_D, respectively. It is assumed that the environment gets contaminated from pre-symptomatic, asymptomatic, and symptomatic infected individuals with rates

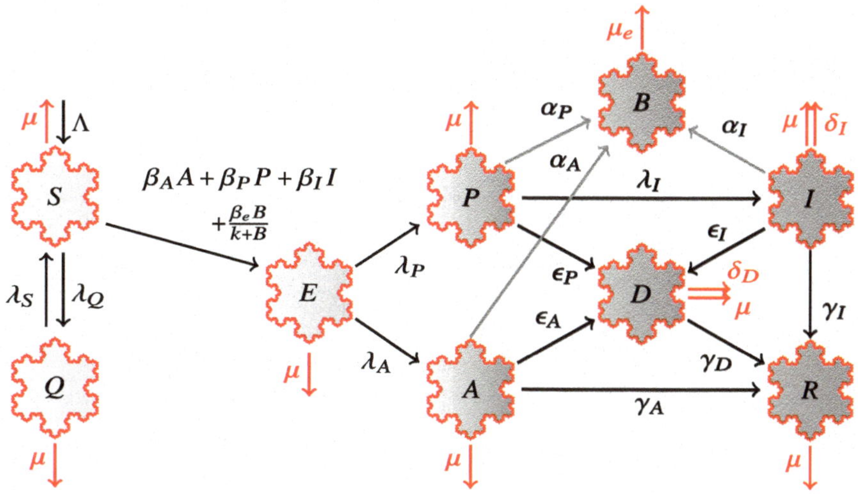

Fig. 1 Model flow diagram for Covid-19

α_P, α_A, and α_I, respectively. Covid-19 virus is cleared from the environment at a rate μ_e. The description of the model is illustrated in Fig. 1.

Using the above-mentioned description, and Fig. 1, the proposed mathematical model is given by the following set of differential equations:

$$
\begin{aligned}
\frac{dS}{dt} &= \Lambda - \beta_A A(t)S(t) - \beta_P P(t)S(t) - \beta_I I(t)S(t) - \frac{\beta_e B(t)S(t)}{k + B(t)} - \mu S(t) - \lambda_Q S(t) + \lambda_S Q(t) \\
\frac{dE}{dt} &= \beta_A A(t)S(t) + \beta_P P(t)S(t) + \beta_I I(t)S(t) + \frac{\beta_e B(t)S(t)}{k + B(t)} - \lambda_A E(t) - \lambda_P E(t) - \mu E(t) \\
\frac{dQ}{dt} &= \lambda_Q S(t) - \lambda_S Q(t) - \mu Q(t) \\
\frac{dA}{dt} &= \lambda_A E(t) - \gamma_A A(t) - \mu A(t) - \epsilon_A A(t) \\
\frac{dP}{dt} &= \lambda_P E(t) - \lambda_I P(t) - \mu P(t) - \epsilon_P P(t) \\
\frac{dI}{dt} &= \lambda_I P(t) - \gamma_I I(t) - \mu I(t) - \epsilon_I I(t) - \delta_I I(t) \\
\frac{dD}{dt} &= \epsilon_A A(t) + \epsilon_P P(t) + \epsilon_I I(t) - \gamma_D D(t) - \mu D(t) - \delta_D D(t) \\
\frac{dR}{dt} &= \gamma_A A(t) + \gamma_I I(t) + \gamma_D D(t) - \mu R(t) \\
\frac{dB}{dt} &= \alpha_A A(t) + \alpha_P P(t) + \alpha_I I(t) - \mu_e B(t)
\end{aligned}
\tag{1}
$$

where $N'(t) = \Lambda - \delta_I I(t) - \delta_D D(t) - \mu N(t)$, $B(t)$ represents the concentration of coronavirus at contaminated environment, and the constant k represents the minimum concentration of virus at environment capable of ensuring 50% chance of contracting the disease. All other parameters of model (1) are defined in Table 1.

Table 1 Parameters used in model (1)

Parameter	Description
Λ	Recruitment rate
μ	Natural death rate of humans
β_A	Transmission rate of the disease from asymptomatic
β_P	Transmission rate of the disease from pre-symptomatic
β_I	Transmission rate of the disease from symptomatic infected
λ_Q	quarantined rate
$1/\lambda_S$	Average number of day in quarantine
λ_A	Rate at which exposed becomes asymptomatic
λ_P	Rate at which exposed becomes pre-symptomatic
λ_I	Rate at which pre-symptomatic becomes symptomatic
ϵ_A	Diagnostic rate of asymptomatic
ϵ_P	Diagnostic rate of pre-symptomatic
ϵ_I	Diagnostic rate of symptomatic
γ_A	Recovery rate of asymptomatic
γ_I	Recovery rate of symptomatic
γ_D	Recovery rate of diagnosed
δ_I	Covid-19-related death rate of symptomatic
δ_D	Covid-19-related death rate of diagnosed
β_e	Contact rate with contaminated environment
α_A	Shedding rate from asymptomatic to environment
α_P	Shedding rate from pre-symptomatic to environment
α_I	Shedding rate from symptomatic to environment
$1/\mu_e$	Lifetime of the virus in the environment

3 Mathematical Analysis

3.1 *The Disease-Free Equilibrium and Control Reproduction Number*

The disease-free equilibrium (DFE) of the model is given by

$$E_0 = \left(\frac{(\mu + \lambda_S)\Lambda}{\mu(\mu + \lambda_Q + \lambda_S)}, 0, \frac{\lambda_Q \Lambda}{\mu(\mu + \lambda_Q + \lambda_S)}, 0, 0, 0, 0, 0, 0 \right).$$

Now, depending whether the term $\alpha_A A(t) + \alpha_P P(t) + \alpha_I I(t)$ is considered as new infection or not, one may get two different expressions for the control reproduction number $\mathcal{R}_c$ using the next-generation matrix method [13]. These expressions are, respectively, given by

$$\mathcal{R}_c = \frac{1}{2}\left(\mathcal{R}_{hh} + \sqrt{\mathcal{R}_{hh}^2 + 4\mathcal{R}_{he}}\right) \quad \text{or} \quad \mathcal{R}_c = \mathcal{R}_{hh} + \mathcal{R}_{he}$$

where

$$\begin{aligned}\mathcal{R}_{hh} = &\frac{(\mu+\lambda_S)\Lambda\beta_A\lambda_A}{\mu(\mu+\lambda_Q+\lambda_S)(\mu+\lambda_A+\lambda_P)(\mu+\gamma_A+\epsilon_A)} + \frac{(\mu+\lambda_S)\Lambda\beta_P\lambda_P}{\mu(\mu+\lambda_Q+\lambda_S)(\mu+\lambda_A+\lambda_P)(\mu+\lambda_I+\epsilon_P)}\\ &+\frac{(\mu+\lambda_S)\Lambda\beta_I\lambda_P\lambda_I}{\mu(\mu+\lambda_Q+\lambda_S)(\mu+\lambda_A+\lambda_P)(\mu+\lambda_I+\epsilon_P)(\mu+\gamma_I+\epsilon_I+\delta_I)}\\ \mathcal{R}_{he} = &\frac{(\mu+\lambda_S)\beta_e\alpha_A\lambda_A\Lambda}{\mu(\mu+\lambda_Q+\lambda_S)(\mu+\lambda_A+\lambda_P)(\mu+\gamma_A+\epsilon_A)} + \frac{(\mu+\lambda_S)\beta_e\lambda_P\alpha_P\Lambda}{\mu(\mu+\lambda_Q+\lambda_S)(\mu+\lambda_A+\lambda_P)(\mu+\lambda_I+\epsilon_P)}\\ &+\frac{(\mu+\lambda_S)\beta_e\alpha_I\lambda_P\lambda_I\Lambda}{\mu(\mu+\lambda_Q+\lambda_S)(\mu+\lambda_A+\lambda_P)(\mu+\lambda_I+\epsilon_P)(\mu+\gamma_I+\epsilon_I+\delta_I)}\end{aligned}$$

It is clear that $\mathcal{R}_{hh}$ gives the direct contribution from asymptomatic, pre-symptomatic, and symptomatic infected humans, whereas R_{he} gives the contribution from the contaminated environment. One should note here that both expressions of the control reproduction numbers have the same threshold, i.e., $\mathcal{R}_c = 1$ whenever $R_{hh} + R_{he} = 1$ and, hence, $\mathcal{R}_c \leqslant 1$ whenever $\mathcal{R}_{hh} + \mathcal{R}_{he} \leqslant 1$. In particular, if either $\mathcal{R}_{hh}$ or $\mathcal{R}_{he}$ is greater than 1, then $\mathcal{R}_c > 1$. We should also note here that the basic reproduction number $\mathcal{R}_0$ corresponds to the case when $\lambda_Q = \lambda_S = \epsilon_A = \epsilon_P = \epsilon_I = 0$.

Now, using [14, Theorem 2], we obtain the following result.

Theorem 1 *The disease-free equilibrium of model (1) is locally asymptotically stable if* $\mathcal{R}_c < 1$ *and unstable if* $\mathcal{R}_c > 1$.

3.2 Global Stability of DFE

In this subsection, we are interested to investigate the global behavior of system (1). To achieve our goal, we will need an auxiliary result, which was proved by Castillo–Chavez *et al.* in [8]. We state it here for the reader's convenience.

Theorem 2 ([8, Castillo–Chavez *et al.*]) *For the system:*

$$\begin{aligned}\frac{dX}{dt} &= F(X, Z)\\ \frac{dZ}{dt} &= G(X, Z) \qquad G(X, 0) = 0,\end{aligned} \tag{2}$$

where the components of the column vector $X \in \mathbb{R}^m$ *denote the number of uninfected individuals and the components of vector* $Z \in \mathbb{R}^n$ *denote the number of infected individuals.* $E_0 = (X^*, 0)$ *denotes the disease-free equilibrium of this system. The fixed point* $E_0 = (X^*, 0)$ *is a globally asymptotically stable equilibrium for this* *system provided that* $\mathcal{R}_0 < 1$ *(locally asymptotically stable) and the following two conditions are satisfied:*

(H1) *For* $\dfrac{dX}{dt} = F(X, 0)$, X^* *is globally asymptotically stable.*

(H2) $G(X, Z) = AZ - \hat{G}(X, Z)$, $\hat{G}(X, Z) \geq 0$ *for* $(X, Z) \in \Omega$, *where* $A = D_Z G(X^*, 0)$ *is an M-matrix (the off-diagonal elements of A are non-negative) and* Ω *is the region where the model has biological meaning.*

We can rewrite our system (1) using above notation, where

$$X = (S, Q, R) \quad \text{and} \quad Z = (E, A, P, I, D, B)$$

represent the uninfected and infected classes, respectively, and $F(X, Z)$ and $G(X, Z)$ are the corresponding right-hand side of model (1). Clearly, $G(X, 0) = 0$ and

$$F(X, 0) = \begin{pmatrix} \Lambda - (\mu + \lambda_Q)S + \lambda_S Q & \lambda_Q S - (\mu + \lambda_S)Q - \mu R \end{pmatrix}^T.$$

Moreover, the DFE E_0 can be written as $E_0 = (X^*, 0)$, where

$$X^* = \left(\frac{(\mu + \lambda_S)\Lambda}{\mu(\mu + \lambda_Q + \lambda_S)}, \frac{\lambda_Q \Lambda}{\mu(\mu + \lambda_Q + \lambda_S)}, 0 \right).$$

Now, solving the system of differential equations which appears in the first condition (H1), we obtain

$$\begin{aligned} S(t) &= c_1 \frac{\lambda_S}{\lambda_Q} e^{-\mu t} - c_2 e^{-(\mu+\lambda_Q+\lambda_S)t} + \frac{(\mu + \lambda_S)\Lambda}{\mu(\mu + \lambda_Q + \lambda_S)} \\ Q(t) &= c_1 e^{-\mu t} + c_2 e^{-(\mu+\lambda_Q+\lambda_S)t} + \frac{\lambda_Q \Lambda}{\mu(\mu + \lambda_Q + \lambda_S)} \\ R(t) &= c_3 e^{-\mu t} \end{aligned}$$

where c_1, c_2, and c_3 are arbitrary constants. Clearly, $X \to X^*$ as $t \to \infty$. Hence, X^* is globally asymptotically stable and condition (H1) is satisfied. For the second condition (H2), we have

$$A = \begin{pmatrix} -\kappa_1 & \beta_A S^* & \beta_P S^* & \beta_I S^* & 0 & \dfrac{\beta_e S^*}{k} \\ \lambda_A & -\kappa_2 & 0 & 0 & 0 & 0 \\ \lambda_P & 0 & -\kappa_3 & 0 & 0 & 0 \\ 0 & 0 & \lambda_I & -\kappa_4 & 0 & 0 \\ 0 & \epsilon_A & \epsilon_P & \epsilon_I & -\kappa_5 & 0 \\ 0 & \alpha_A & \alpha_P & \alpha_I & 0 & -\mu_e \end{pmatrix}$$

and

$$\hat{G}(X, Z) = \begin{pmatrix} \beta_A(S^* - S)A(t) + \beta_P(S^* - S)P(t) + \beta_I(S^* - S)I(t) + \dfrac{\beta_e S^* B^2 + \beta_e Bk(S^* - S)}{k(B+k)} \\ 0 \\ 0 \\ 0 \\ 0 \\ 0 \end{pmatrix}$$

where $\kappa_1 = \lambda_A + \lambda_P + \mu$, $\kappa_2 = \epsilon_A + \gamma_A + \mu$, $\kappa_3 = \epsilon_P + \lambda_I + \mu$, $\kappa_4 = \epsilon_I + \gamma_I + \delta_I + \mu$, $\kappa_5 = \gamma_D + \delta_D + \mu$ and $S^* = \dfrac{(\mu + \lambda_S)\Lambda}{\mu(\mu + \lambda_Q + \lambda_S)}$. It is clear that A is an M-matrix and $\hat{G}(X, Z) \geq 0$ for all $(X, Z) \in \Omega$, where

$$\Omega = \left\{(S, E, A, P, I, D, R, B) \in \mathbb{R}^8_+ : 0 < S + E + A + P + I + D + R \leq \frac{\Lambda}{\mu}, 0 < B \leq \frac{\alpha_P \Lambda}{\mu \mu_e}\right\}$$

is the region where the model makes biological sense. Hence, we obtain as a consequence the following result.

Theorem 3 *The disease-free equilibrium model (1) is globally asymptotically stable when* $\mathcal{R}_0 < 1$.

3.3 Existence and Local Stability of the Endemic Equilibrium

In this subsection, our goal is to prove the existence and the local stability of the endemic equilibrium. For it, we will use the center manifold theorem, namely [9, Theorem 4.1]. With this objective, we consider our system (1) in the following formulation

$$\begin{aligned}
\frac{dx_1}{dt} &= \Lambda - \beta_A x_4(t)x_1(t) - \beta_P x_5(t)x_1(t) - \beta_I x_6(t)x_1(t) - \frac{\beta_e x_9(t)x_1(t)}{k + x_9(t)} - \mu x_1(t) - \lambda_Q x_1(t) + \lambda_S x_3(t) \\
\frac{dx_2}{dt} &= \beta_A x_4(t)x_1(t) + \beta_P x_5(t)x_1(t) + \beta_I x_6(t)x_1(t) + \frac{\beta_e x_9(t)x_1(t)}{k + x_9(t)} - \lambda_A x_2(t) - \lambda_P x_2(t) - \mu x_2(t) \\
\frac{dx_3}{dt} &= \lambda_Q x_1(t) - \lambda_S x_3(t) - \mu x_3(t) \\
\frac{dx_4}{dt} &= \lambda_A x_2(t) - \gamma_A x_4(t) - \mu x_4(t) - \epsilon_A x_4(t) \\
\frac{dx_5}{dt} &= \lambda_P x_2(t) - \lambda_I x_5(t) - \mu x_5(t) - \epsilon_P x_5(t) \\
\frac{dx_6}{dt} &= \lambda_I x_5(t) - \gamma_I x_6(t) - \mu x_6(t) - \epsilon_I x_6(t) - \delta_I x_6(t) \\
\frac{dx_7}{dt} &= \epsilon_A x_4(t) + \epsilon_P x_5(t) + \epsilon_I x_6(t) - \gamma_D x_7(t) - \mu x_7(t) - \delta_D x_7(t) \\
\frac{dx_8}{dt} &= \gamma_A x_4(t) + \gamma_I x_6(t) + \gamma_D x_7(t) - \mu x_8(t) \\
\frac{dx_9}{dt} &= \alpha_A x_4(t) + \alpha_P x_5(t) + \alpha_I x_6(t) - \mu_e x_9(t)
\end{aligned} \tag{3}$$

Now, taking β_P to be the bifurcation parameter and $\beta_P = \phi$ to be the corresponding bifurcation value at $R_c = 1$, it follows that system (3) has the following Jacobian at the disease-free equilibrium E_0 and $\beta_P = \phi$:

$$J(\phi) = \begin{pmatrix} -(\lambda_Q+\mu) & 0 & \lambda_S & -\beta_A S^* & -\phi S^* & -\beta_I S^* & 0 & 0 & -\frac{\beta_e S^*}{k} \\ 0 & -\kappa_1 & 0 & \beta_A S^* & \phi S^* & \beta_I S^* & 0 & 0 & \frac{\beta_e S^*}{k} \\ \lambda_Q & 0 & -(\lambda_S+\mu) & 0 & 0 & 0 & 0 & 0 & 0 \\ 0 & \lambda_A & 0 & -\kappa_2 & 0 & 0 & 0 & 0 & 0 \\ 0 & \lambda_P & 0 & 0 & -\kappa_3 & 0 & 0 & 0 & 0 \\ 0 & 0 & 0 & 0 & \lambda_I & -\kappa_4 & 0 & 0 & 0 \\ 0 & 0 & 0 & \epsilon_A & \epsilon_P & \epsilon_I & -\kappa_5 & 0 & 0 \\ 0 & 0 & 0 & \gamma_A & 0 & \gamma_I & \gamma_D & -\mu & 0 \\ 0 & 0 & 0 & \alpha_A & \alpha_P & \alpha_I & 0 & 0 & -\mu_e \end{pmatrix}$$

where $\kappa_i, i = 1, 2, \cdots 5$ and S^* were defined earlier. One can easily verify that the above Jacobian has a simple zero eigenvalue. Then, computing the corresponding right and left eigenvectors, $w = [w_1 \quad w_2 \quad \cdots \quad w_9]^T$ and $v = [v_1 \quad v_2 \quad \cdots \quad v_9]$, respectively, we get

$$\begin{aligned} w_1 &= -\frac{k_1(\lambda_S+\mu)}{\mu(\lambda_Q+\lambda_S+\mu)} w_2 \\ w_3 &= -\frac{k_1\lambda_Q}{\mu(\lambda_Q+\lambda_S+\mu)} w_2 \\ w_4 &= \frac{\lambda_A}{\kappa_2} w_2 \\ w_5 &= \frac{\lambda_P}{\kappa_3} w_2 \\ w_6 &= \frac{\lambda_I\lambda_P}{\kappa_3\kappa_4} w_2 \\ w_7 &= \frac{1}{\kappa_5}(\epsilon_A w_4 + \epsilon_P w_5 + \epsilon_I w_6) \\ w_8 &= \frac{1}{\mu}(\gamma_A w_4 + \gamma_I w_6 + \gamma_D w_7) \\ w_9 &= \frac{1}{\mu_e}(\alpha_A w_4 + \alpha_P w_5 + \alpha_I w_6) \end{aligned}$$

and

$$
\begin{aligned}
v_1 &= v_3 = v_7 = v_8 = 0 \\
v_9 &= \frac{\beta_e S^*}{k\mu_e} v_2 \\
v_4 &= \frac{1}{\kappa_2}\left(\beta_A S^* v_2 + \alpha_A v_9\right) \\
v_6 &= \frac{1}{\kappa_4}\left(\beta_I S^* v_2 + \alpha_I v_9\right) \\
v_5 &= \frac{1}{\kappa_3}\left(\beta_P S^* v_2 + \lambda_I v_6 + \alpha_P v_9\right),
\end{aligned}
$$

where w_2 and v_2 are nonzero free parameters. Now, to calculate the values of a and b as defined in [9, Theorem 4.1], we need to compute the following second-order derivatives:

$$\frac{\partial^2 f_i}{\partial x_j \partial x_k} \quad \text{and} \quad \frac{\partial^2 f_i}{\partial x_j \partial \phi}, \quad i, j, k = 1, 2, \cdots 9,$$

where $f_i, i = 1, 2, \cdots 9$ denote the right-hand side of equation number i of system (3). We then have

$$
\begin{aligned}
\frac{\partial^2 f_1}{\partial x_1 \partial x_4} &= -\beta_A\,, & \frac{\partial^2 f_1}{\partial x_1 \partial x_5} &= -\phi \\
\frac{\partial^2 f_1}{\partial x_1 \partial x_6} &= -\beta_I\,, & \frac{\partial^2 f_1}{\partial x_1 \partial x_9} &= -\frac{\beta_e}{k} \\
\frac{\partial^2 f_2}{\partial x_1 \partial x_4} &= \beta_A\,, & \frac{\partial^2 f_2}{\partial x_1 \partial x_5} &= \phi \\
\frac{\partial^2 f_2}{\partial x_1 \partial x_6} &= \beta_I\,, & \frac{\partial^2 f_2}{\partial x_1 \partial x_9} &= \frac{\beta_e}{k} \\
\frac{\partial^2 f_1}{\partial \phi \partial x_5} &= -S^*\,, & \frac{\partial^2 f_2}{\partial \phi \partial x_5} &= S^*.
\end{aligned}
$$

Note that the rest of the second derivatives are all zero. Now, taking the free parameters w_2 and v_2 to be positive, the values and the signs of a and b are given, respectively, by

$$
\begin{aligned}
a &= -\frac{k_1(\lambda_S + \mu)}{\mu(\lambda_Q + \lambda_S + \mu)}\left[\beta_A w_4 + \phi w_5 + \beta_I w_6 + \frac{\beta_e}{k} w_9\right] w_2 v_2 \quad < \quad 0 \\
b &= \frac{S^* \lambda_P}{\kappa_3} w_2 v_2 \quad > \quad 0.
\end{aligned}
$$

Using [9, Theorem 4.1], the direction of the bifurcation is forward and, hence, it follows the result below.

Theorem 4 *If $\mathcal{R}_c > 1$, then there exists a unique endemic equilibrium point for system (1). Moreover, this point is locally asymptotically stable whenever it exists.*

3.4 Sensitivity Analysis

The impact of model (1) parameters on the model outcome is determined via sensitivity analysis [6, 22, 23]. Here, we adopt Latin hyper-cubic sampling (LHS) technique and partial rank correlation coefficient (PRCC). LHS is a stratified sampling without replacement method which allows for an efficient analysis of parameter variations across simultaneous uncertainty ranges in each parameter. PRCC measures the strength of the relationship between the model outcome and the parameters, stating the degree of the effect that each parameter has on the outcome [6, 22]. A total of 1000 simulations of model (1) per LHS run were carried out, using the ranges and baseline values given in Table 2 (with the control reproduction number, $\mathcal{R}_c$, and the basic reproduction number, $\mathcal{R}_0$, as the response functions).

In order to find the values of the parameters to be used for parameter's estimation, we fitted the Covid-19 published data from the Ministry of Health, The Sultanate of Oman, from February 24 to July 12, 2020, available at https://www.worldometers.info/coronavirus/country/oman/. The MATLAB function "fminsearch" was employ ed, and the sum of squares was used to measure the cost. The values of the parameters are then given in Table 2.

For the purpose of sensitivity analysis, each parameter value, an interval within 25% range of the parameter value is formed to test the sensitivity. Figures (2) and (3) depict the PRCC values for each parameter of the models using the reproduction numbers, $\mathcal{R}_c$ and $\mathcal{R}_0$, as the response functions, respectively. Parameters with the highest PRCC values have the largest impact on the response functions.

The parameters λ_Q, μ, and ϵ_P have the highest negative impact on $\mathcal{R}_c$, while the parameters β_P and λ_S have the highest positive impact on $\mathcal{R}_c$, which indicate that quarantine of susceptible humans and diagnosis of pre-symptomatic humans are very effective in decreasing $\mathcal{R}_c$, whereas the rate at which the susceptible humans leave the quarantine and the transmission of the virus from the symptomatic and pre-symptomatic individuals plays the most important role in increasing $\mathcal{R}_c$. This result shows that in order to control the disease, susceptible humans need to stay in quarantine or at least adopt social distancing. Moreover, pre-symptomatic humans need to be diagnosed through contact tracing, for example, and hence isolated.

The parameter with the highest positive impact on $\mathcal{R}_0$ is β_I, whereas the parameters with the highest negative impact on $\mathcal{R}_0$ are γ_I and μ. This result shows that when there is no control strategy applied to the system, then the transmission rate from symptomatic individuals is the key to increase $\mathcal{R}_0$, and the recovery rate of infected individuals is the key to reduce $\mathcal{R}_0$ (Fig. 3).

Table 2 Values of the estimated parameters

Parameters	Estimated value
Λ	202
μ	3.8×10^{-5}
β_I	7.479×10^{-7}
β_A	6.474×10^{-7}
β_P	8.418×10^{-7}
β_e	0.403
λ_Q	0.683
λ_S	0.391
λ_P	0.568
λ_A	0.289
λ_I	0.612
ϵ_A	0.009
ϵ_I	0.132
ϵ_P	0.0144
γ_A	0.606
γ_I	0.411
γ_D	0.51
δ_D	0.114
δ_I	0.57
α_I	0.487
α_P	0.169
α_A	0.216
μ_e	0.73

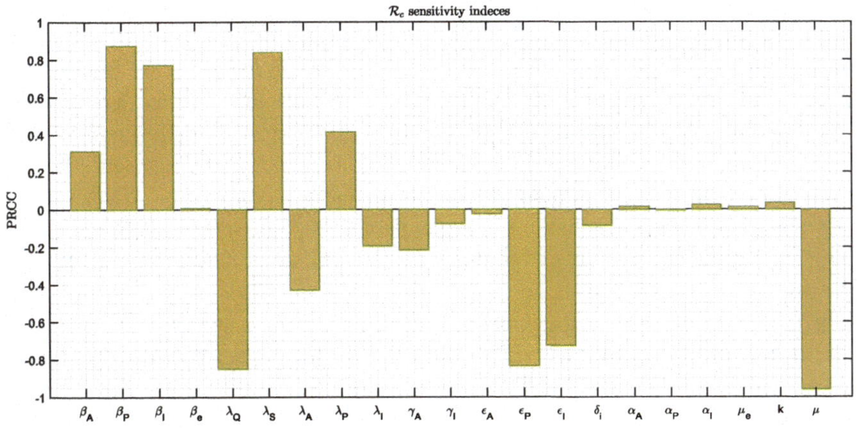

Fig. 2 PRCC values for model (1), using the control reproduction number ($\mathcal{R}_c$) as the response function

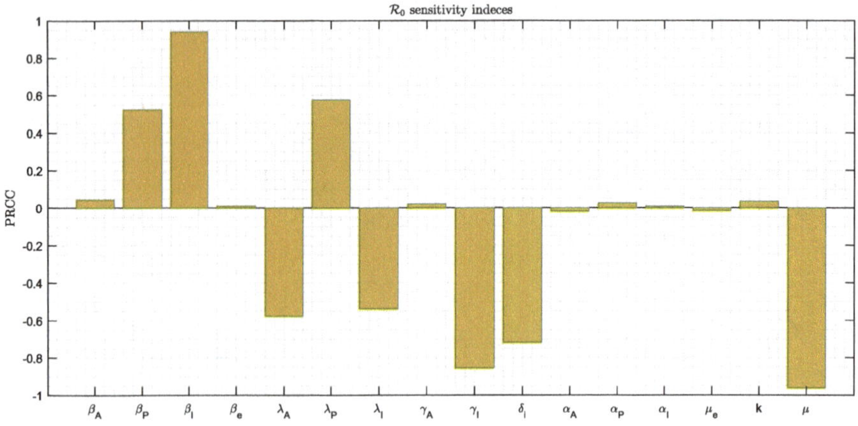

Fig. 3 PRCC values for model (1), using the basic reproduction number ($\mathcal{R}_0$) as the response function

3.5 Numerical Simulation

In this subsection, we will illustrate some numerical simulations in order to verify our theoretical results which were stated in the previous sections. The baseline values of the parameters were taken from Table 2, and some of the parameters were varied to investigate their role in the dynamics.

Figure 4 illustrates the effect of the diagnosis rates of symptomatic and pre-symptomatic individuals. For small values of ϵ_A, the maximum number of diagnosed individuals reaches above 2000, and as the value of ϵ_A increases, this number starts to decreases until it reaches less than around 1600 as ϵ_A reaches 0.132. Note that the baseline value of ϵ_A is really small (i.e., 0.009), and hence its effect starts to be clear as this value starts to increase, as one could see from Fig. 4 (left). Figure 4 (right) shows the effect of ϵ_P on the dynamics of diagnosed humans, and its effect is similar to the effect of ϵ_A; however, the effect of ϵ_P is much more clear and stronger than the effect of ϵ_A, as it is clear when comparing the two figures which are described in Figs. 4. By increasing ϵ_P to 0.132, the maximum number of diagnosed individuals reduces from over 2000 to around 600. This supports our theoretical results from the sensitivity analysis which indicate that ϵ_P is one of the parameters which have the most negative impact on $\mathcal{R}_c$; therefore, as ϵ_P increases $\mathcal{R}_c$ decreases and hence the prevalence of the disease decreases. This decrease is taking place, because once pre-symptomatic individuals are diagnosed, they are isolated and hence they do not contribute to the disease transmission and as a result the number of infected individuals (i.e., exposed, asymptomatic, pre-symptomatic, and symptomatic) decreases. This effect is illustrated in Fig. 5 for exposed individuals. This decrease in the exposed individuals will result in a decrease in all other infected individuals, which in turn leads to decrease the number of diagnosed individuals.

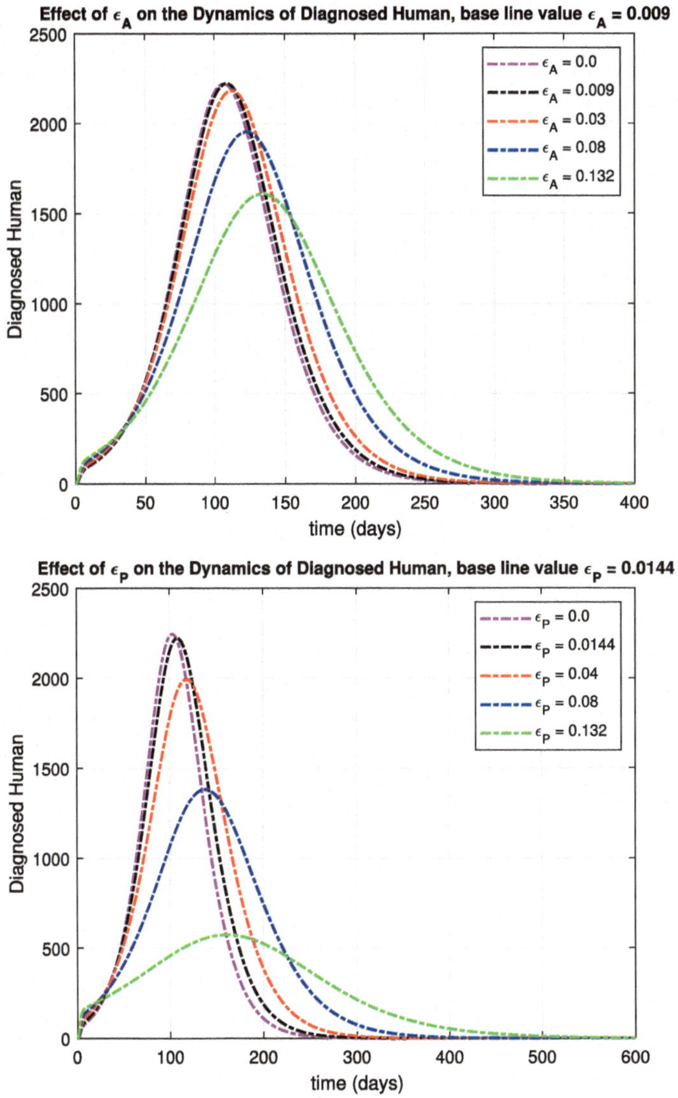

Fig. 4 Effect of varying ϵ_A (left) and ϵ_P (right) on the dynamics of the diagnosed humans

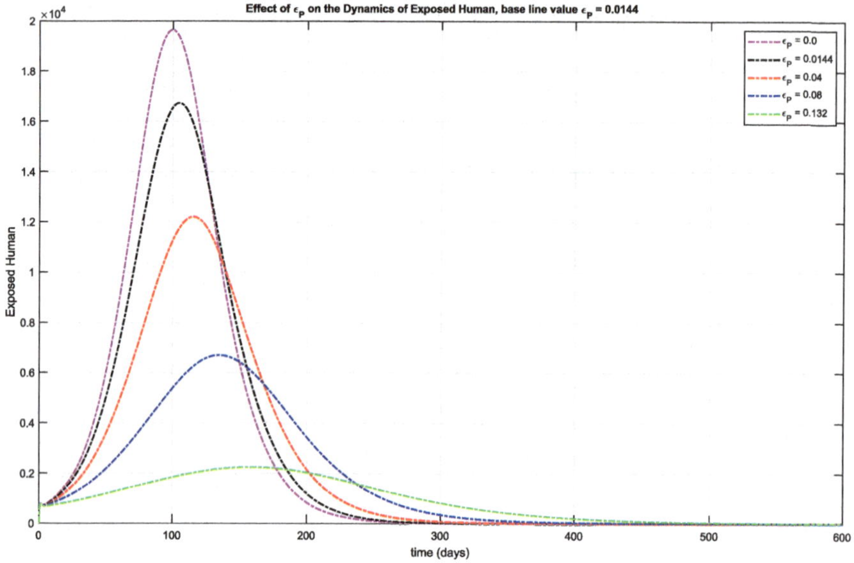

Fig. 5 Effect of varying ϵ_P on the dynamics of the exposed humans

The effect of the quarantine rate λ_Q and the rate by which individuals leave the quarantine is illustrated in Fig. 6. Clearly, the effects of λ_Q and λ_S are opposite to each other. When λ_Q increases, i.e., when the number of susceptible individuals who enter the quarantine increases, then the number of diagnosed humans decreases. When λ_S increases, i.e., when the number of quarantined individuals who return to the pool of susceptible individuals increases, the number of diagnosed humans increases. This again confirms that quarantine is one of the most important control strategies in fighting the disease.

4 Optimal Control

In this section, we introduce two time dependent controls into system (1) and examine their role in controlling the disease transmission. In particular, we introduce time-dependent treatment and sanitation of the environment, and our goal is to investigate the effect of diagnosis and quarantine rates in the effectiveness of these controls. We emphasize that treatment here should be understood as medical attendance in hospitals, but not as a specific treatment, since there is no successful treatment for Covid-19 so far.

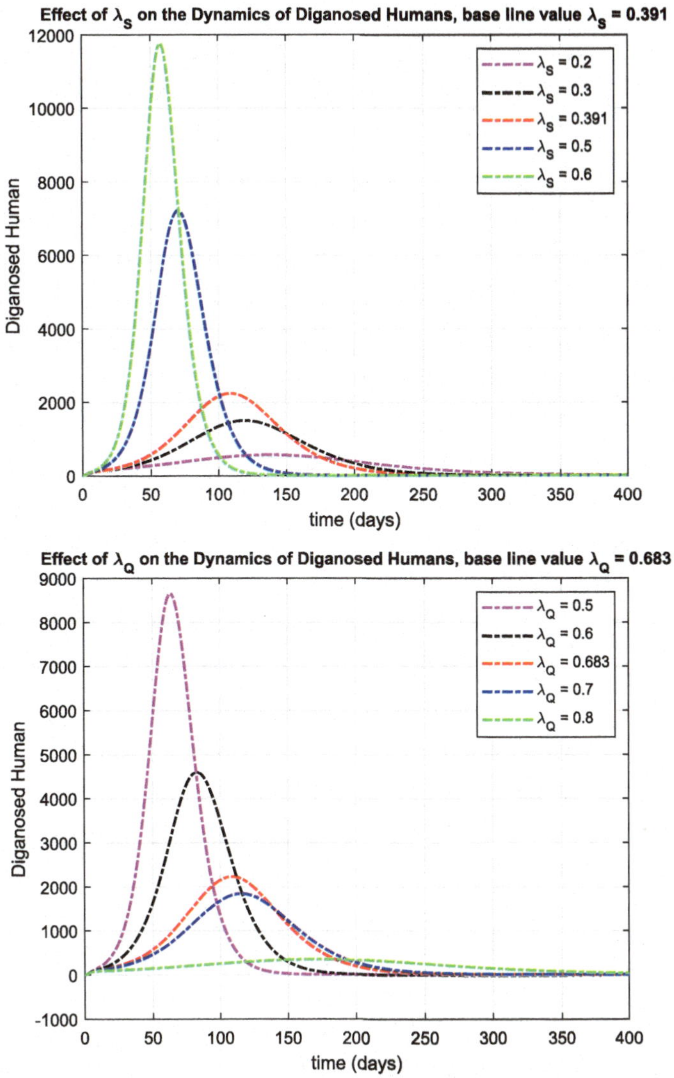

Fig. 6 Effect of varying λ_S (left) λ_Q (right) and on the dynamics of the diagnosed humans

4.1 Building the Optimal Control Problem

Let $u_1(t)$ be the time-dependent rate of treatment. It is assumed that this time-dependent treatment rate is applied to the symptomatic infected and diagnosed humans. Let $u_2(t)$ be the time-dependent sanitation of the environment. Then, the above system of ODEs (1) becomes

$$
\begin{aligned}
\frac{dS}{dt} &= \Lambda - \beta_A A(t)S(t) - \beta_P P(t)S(t) - \beta_I I(t)S(t) - \frac{\beta_e B(t)S(t)}{k + B(t)} - \mu S(t) - \lambda_Q S(t) + \lambda_S Q(t) \\
\frac{dE}{dt} &= \beta_A A(t)S(t) + \beta_P P(t)S(t) + \beta_I I(t)S(t) + \frac{\beta_e B(t)S(t)}{k + B(t)} - \lambda_A E(t) - \lambda_P E(t) - \mu E(t) \\
\frac{dQ}{dt} &= \lambda_Q S(t) - \lambda_S Q(t) - \mu Q(t) \\
\frac{dA}{dt} &= \lambda_A E(t) - \gamma_A A(t) - \mu A(t) - \epsilon_A A(t) \\
\frac{dP}{dt} &= \lambda_P E(t) - \lambda_I P(t) - \mu P(t) - \epsilon_P P(t) \\
\frac{dI}{dt} &= \lambda_I P(t) - u_1(t)I(t) - \gamma_I I(t) - \mu I(t) - \epsilon_I I(t) - \delta_I I(t) \\
\frac{dD}{dt} &= \epsilon_A A(t) + \epsilon_P P(t) + \epsilon_I I(t) - u_1(t)D(t) - \gamma_D D(t) - \mu D(t) - \delta_D D(t) \\
\frac{dR}{dt} &= \gamma_A A(t) + (u_1(t) + \gamma_I)I(t) + (u_1(t) + \gamma_D)D(t) - \mu R(t) \\
\frac{dB}{dt} &= \alpha_A A(t) + \alpha_P P(t) + \alpha_I I(t) - \mu_e B(t) - u_2(t)B(t)
\end{aligned}
\tag{4}
$$

We want to find the controls that minimize the total number of exposed, asymptomatic, pre-symptomatic, and symptomatic infected humans, the concentration of the virus in the environment, and the cost of controls; i.e., we want to find the optimal values (u_1^*, u_2^*) of the control variables that minimize the cost objective functional

$$
J(u_1, u_2) = \int_0^T \left[c_1 E + c_2 A + c_3 P + c_4 I + c_5 B + c_6 u_1^2 + c_7 u_2^2\right] dt. \tag{5}
$$

subject to the differential equations (4), where T is the final time. This performance specification involves the numbers of exposed, asymptomatic, pre-symptomatic, and symptomatic infected humans and the concentration of the virus in the environment, along with the cost of applying the controls ($u_1(t)$ and $u_2(t)$). The coefficients, $c_i, i = 1 \cdots 7$, are balancing cost factors. The control doubles, ($u_1(t)$ and $u_2(t)$), are bounded and Lebesgue integrable functions [2, 17].

4.2 Characterization of the Optimal Control

The necessary conditions that an optimal control double, (u_1^*, u_2^*), must satisfy come from the Pontryagin's maximum principle [29]. This principle converts equations (4) and (5) into a problem of minimizing pointwise Hamiltonian H, with respect to the controls (u_1, u_2). First, we formulate the Hamiltonian from the cost functional and the governing dynamics to obtain the optimality conditions

$$
H = c_1 E + c_2 A + c_3 P + c_4 I + c_5 B + c_6 u_1^2 + c_7 u_2^2 + \sum_{i=1}^{9} \phi_i g_i \tag{6}
$$

where g_i is the right-hand side of the ith equation of system (4).

The system of adjoint equations is found by taking the appropriate partial derivatives of the Hamiltonian equation (6) with respect to the associated state and control variables, i.e.,

$$\frac{d\phi_i}{dt} = -\frac{\partial H}{\partial V_i}$$

where $V_i, i = 1 \cdots 9$, is the ith variable in the system (4). Then, the adjoint system is given by:

$$\begin{aligned}
\frac{d\phi_1}{dt} &= \left(\beta_A A + \beta_P P + \beta_I I + \frac{\beta_e B}{k+B}\right)(\phi_1 - \phi_2) + (\lambda_Q + \mu)\phi_1 - \lambda_Q \phi_3 \\
\frac{d\phi_2}{dt} &= -c_1 + (\lambda_A + \lambda_P + \mu)\phi_2 - \lambda_A \phi_4 - \lambda_P \phi_5 \\
\frac{d\phi_3}{dt} &= (\lambda_S + \mu)\phi_3 - \lambda_S \phi_1 \\
\frac{d\phi_4}{dt} &= -c_2 + \beta_A S(\phi_1 - \phi_2) + (\gamma_A + \epsilon_A + \mu)\phi_4 - \epsilon_A \phi_7 - \gamma_A \phi_8 - \alpha_A \phi_9 \\
\frac{d\phi_5}{dt} &= -c_3 + (\lambda_I + \epsilon_P + \mu)\phi_5 + \beta_P S(\phi_1 - \phi_2) - \lambda_I \phi_6 - \epsilon_P \phi_7 - \alpha_P \phi_9 \\
\frac{d\phi_6}{dt} &= -c_4 + (\epsilon_I + u_1 + \delta_I + \mu + \gamma_I)\phi_6 + \beta_I S(\phi_1 - \phi_2) - \epsilon_I \phi_7 - (\gamma_D + u_1)\phi_8 - \alpha_I \phi_9 \\
\frac{d\phi_7}{dt} &= (u_1 + \delta_D + \mu)\phi_7 - u_1 \phi_8 + \gamma_D(\phi_7 - \phi_8) \\
\frac{d\phi_8}{dt} &= \mu \phi_8 \\
\frac{d\phi_9}{dt} &= -c_5 + \frac{\beta_e k S}{(k+B)^2}(\phi_1 - \phi_2) + (\mu_e + u_2)\phi_9
\end{aligned} \tag{7}$$

and with transversality conditions

$$\phi_i(T) = 0 \tag{8}$$

Furthermore, the control quadruple (u_1^*, u_2^*) is given as

$$\begin{aligned}
u_1^* &= min\left\{1, max\left[0, \frac{(\phi_6 - \phi_8)I + (\phi_7 - \phi_8)D}{2c_6}\right]\right\} \\
u_2^* &= min\left\{1, max\left[0, \frac{\phi_9 B}{2c_7}\right]\right\}.
\end{aligned} \tag{9}$$

4.3 Numerical Simulation of the Optimal Control Problem

Numerical solutions to the optimality system comprising the state equations (4), adjoint equations (7), control characterization equations (9), and corresponding initial/final conditions are carried out using the forward–backward sweep method (implemented in MATLAB) and using parameters set in Table 2.

In this subsection, we employ numerical simulations to the optimality system to provide examples about the dynamics of the disease under the controls and to assess the impact of the control variables on the disease dynamics. We use the following initial conditions $S_0 = 4.89 \times 10^6$, $E_0 = 0$, $Q_0 = 0$, $A_0 = 0$, $P_0 = 0$, $I_0 = 2$, $D_0 = 2$, $R_0 = 0$ and $B_0 = 10^3$.

In general, numerical simulations of the optimality system show that quarantine and diagnosis are the key stone for controlling the disease, and even when other control strategies are implemented, namely treatment of symptomatic infected and diagnosed humans, as well as sanitation of the environment. They play a major role in the effectiveness of these two controls as illustrated in the next two subsections.

4.3.1 Effect of Diagnosis

To study the effect of diagnosis on the optimal control model, we apply both controls with diagnosis to all infected classes and with diagnosis to symptomatic individuals only. Then, we remove the controls and simulate the system with diagnosis to all infected classes and with diagnosis of symptomatic individuals only. The results of this simulation show that including the diagnosis of asymptomatic and pre-symptomatic enhances the effectiveness of the used controls by reducing the maximum number of infected individuals and delaying the time it takes to reach this maximum as illustrated in Figs. 7, 8 and 9, which illustrate the dynamics of asymptomatic, pre-symptomatic, and symptomatic individuals, respectively, with the effects of optimal controls and diagnosis. Hence, it is very important to implement some methods that help in diagnosing asymptomatic and pre-symptomatic individuals, such as contact tracing.

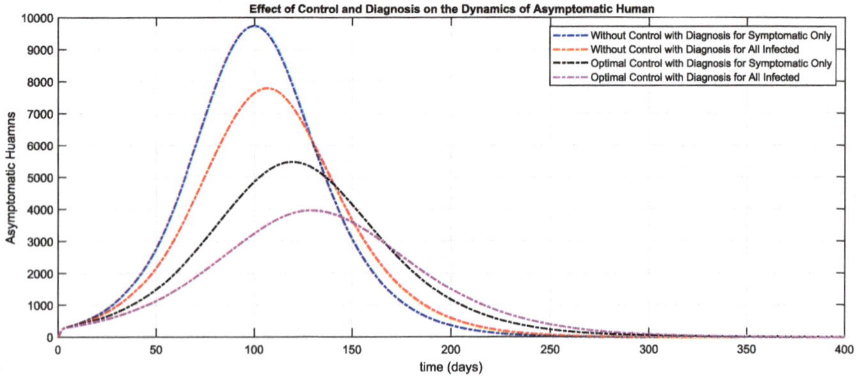

Fig. 7 Number of asymptomatic humans with and without control

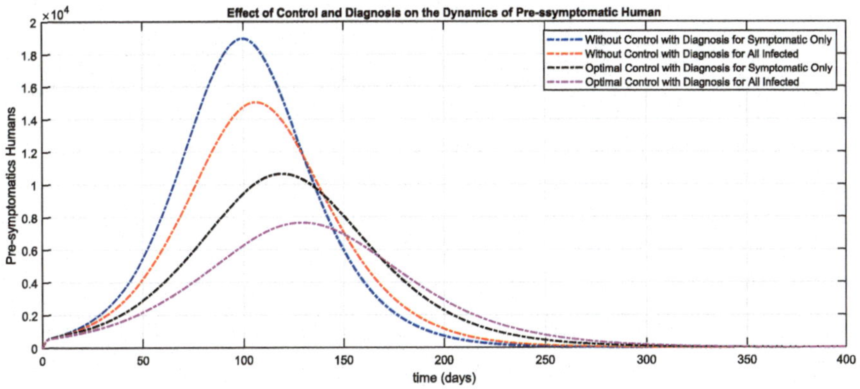

Fig. 8 Number of pre-symptomatic humans with and without control

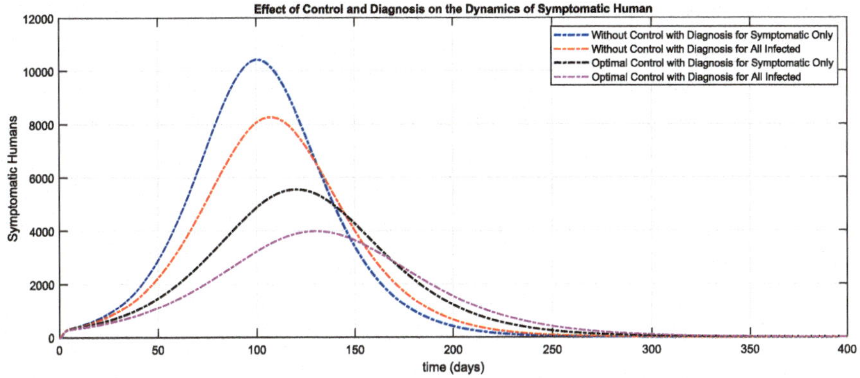

Fig. 9 Number of symptomatic infected humans with and without control

4.3.2 Effect of Quarantine

In order to investigate the effect of quarantine on the optimal control system, we apply both controls with quarantine and without quarantine, and then we remove both controls and simulate the system with quarantine and without quarantine. The results are illustrated in Figs. 10, 11 and 12, which show the effect of control and quarantine in the dynamics of asymptomatic, pre-symptomatic, and symptomatic individuals, respectively. Comparing parts (A) and (B) in these figures, it is clear that quarantine is much more important in controlling the disease transmission than the two introduced controls, as its effect in reducing the maximum number of infected individuals is much higher than the effect of controls. This result is very matching with the suggestion of WHO regarding quarantine of susceptible individuals as the

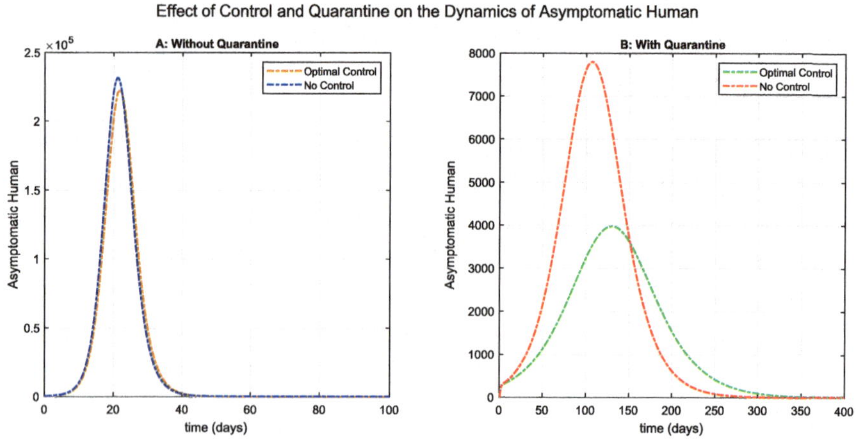

Fig. 10 Number of asymptomatic humans with and without control

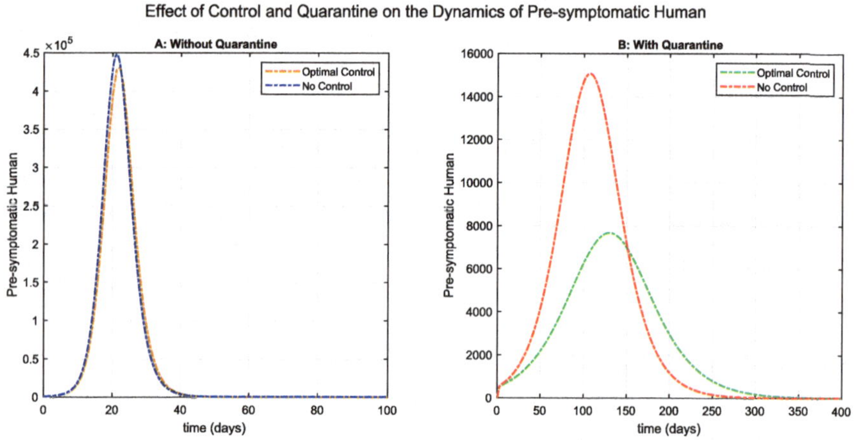

Fig. 11 Number of pre-symptomatic humans with and without control

best controlling strategy. Note that wearing face mask and keeping the social distancing could be also considered (to some extent) as quarantine, because they work toward reducing the contact between susceptible and infected individuals, avoiding the transmission.

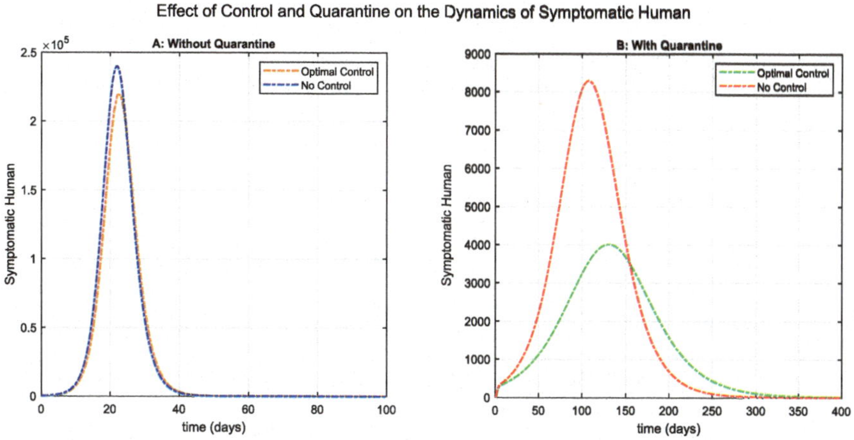

Fig. 12 Number of symptomatic infected humans with and without control

5 Conclusion

In this chapter, we have developed and analyzed a mathematical model for Covid-19 taking into account role of diagnosis and quarantine. The model includes both direct and indirect asymptomatic, pre-symptomatic, and symptomatic transmissions, and it has been analyzed both qualitatively and quantitatively. The analysis includes calculation of the control and basic reproduction numbers, stability of equilibrium points, sensitivity analysis, and numerical simulation to demonstrate the obtained theoretical results; the goal of them is to show that the disease-free equilibrium is globally asymptotically stable whenever $\mathcal{R}_c$ is less than unity and when $\mathcal{R}_c$ passes unity, the disease-free equilibrium loses its stability and a unique endemic equilibrium exists and becomes locally asymptotically stable. Sensitivity analysis shows that the parameters with the highest positive influence on $\mathcal{R}_c$ are the transmission rate from pre-symptomatic individuals, the rate at which humans leave the quarantine and the transmission rate from symptomatic infected individuals. On the other hand, the parameters with the highest negative influence on $\mathcal{R}_c$ are the rate at which humans enter the quarantine, the natural death rate of humans, and the diagnosis rate of pre-symptomatic individuals. This result shows that quarantine and diagnosis, especially for the pre-symptomatic humans, play the most crucial role in controlling the disease transmission. This effect has been demonstrated numerically as well. Numerical simulations show that both diagnosis and quarantine rates have the effect of reducing the maximum number of diagnosed individuals and delaying the time it takes to reach this maximum. Moreover, an optimal control problem has been developed and analyzed numerically. The optimal control result agrees with the sensitivity analysis result on the importance of diagnosis and quarantine rates in controlling the disease transmission. Moreover, it shows that without diagnosis and without quarantine, other control strategies (namely treatment of symptomatic infected and diagnosed individuals and sanitation of the environment) will not be enough to control the disease and reduce its catastrophic effect on the population.

References

1. 4, S.R.N.B.: Covid-19: Public policies and societyś responses (2020). http://www.iea.usp.br/pesquisa/nucleos-de-apoio-a-pesquisa/observatorio-inovacao-competitividade/boletim-oic-4-en
2. Agusto, F., ELmojtaba, I.: Optimal control and cost-effective analysis of malaria/visceral leishmaniasis co-infection. PLOS One **12**(2) (2017)
3. Arons, M.M., Hatfield, K.M., Reddy, S.C., Kimball, A., James, A., Jacobs, J.R., Taylor, J., Spicer, K., Bardossy, A.C., Oakley, L.P., Tanwar, S., Dyal, J.W., Harney, J., Chisty, Z., Bell, J.M., Methner, M., Paul, P., Carlson, C.M., McLaughlin, H.P., Thornburg, N., Tong, S., Tamin, A., Tao, Y., Uehara, A., Harcourt, J., Clark, S., Brostrom-Smith, C., Page, L.C., Kay, M., Lewis, J., Montgomery, P., Stone, N.D., Clark, T.A., Honein, M.A., Duchin, J.S., Jernigan, J.A.: Presymptomatic sars-cov-2 infections and transmission in a skilled nursing facility. New Engl. J. Med. **382**(22), 2081–2090 (2020)
4. Backer, J.A., Klinkenberg, D., Walling, J.: Incubation period of 2019 novel coronavirus (2019–ncov) infections among travellers from Wuhan, China, 20–28 January 2020. Eurosurveillance p. 25(5) (2020)
5. Bai, Y., Yao, L., Wei, T., Tian, F., Jin, D., Chen, L., Wang, M.: Presumed asymptomatic carrier transmission of covid-19. JAMA **323**(14), 1406–1407 (2020)
6. Blower, S., Dowlatabadi, H.: Sensitivity and uncertainty analysis of complex 448 models of disease transmission: an hiv model, as an example. Int. Stat. Rev., 229–243 (1994)
7. Carraturo, F., Del Giudice, C., Morelli, M., Cerullo, V., Libralato, G., Galdiero, E., Guida, M.: Persistence of sars-cov-2 in the environment and covid-19 transmission risk from environmental matrices and surfaces. Environmental pollution (Barking, Essex : 1987) (Pt B), 115010
8. Castillo-Chavez, C., Feng, Z., Huang, W.: On the computation of r_0 and its role on global stability. In:Mathematical approaches for emerging and re emerging infectious 458 diseases. An Introduction. Castillo-Chavez, C., Blower, S., van den Driessche, P., Kirschner, 459 D. and Yakubu, A.-A. (Eds.) pp. 229–250 (2002)
9. Castillo-Chavez, C., Song, B.: Dynamical models of tuberculosis and their applications. Math. Biosci. Eng. **1**(2), 361–404 (2004)
10. Center, J.H.U..M.C.R.: Cumulative cases (2020). https://coronavirus.jhu.edu/data/cumulative-cases
11. Chang, D., Mo, G., Yuan, X., Tao, Y., Peng, X., Wang, F.S., Xie, L., Charles, S., Dela Cruz, L.S., Qin, E.: Mathematical modeling and epidemic prediction of covid-19 of the state of sao paulo, brazil. Int. J. Adv. Eng. Res. Sci. (IJAERS) **7**, 338–347 (2020)
12. da Cruz, P.A., Cruz, L.C.C.: Time kinetics of viral clearance and resolution of symptoms in novel coronavirus infection. Am. J. Respir. Critical Care Med. **201**, 1150–1152 (2020). https://ijaers.com/uploads/issue_files/41IJAERS-05202019-Mathematical.pdf
13. Diekmann, O., Heesterbeek, J., Metz, J.: On the definition and the computation of the basic reproduction ratio r0 in models for infectious diseases in heterogeneous populations. J. Math. Biol. **28**(4), 365–382 (1990)
14. van den Driessche, P., Watmough, J.: Reproduction numbers and the sub-threshold endemic equilibria for compartmental models of disease transmission. Math. Biosci. **180**, 29–48 (2002)

15. Guan, W.j., Ni, Z.y., Hu, Y., Liang, W.h., Ou, C.q., He, J.x., Liu, L., Shan, H., Lei, C.l., Hui, D.S., Du, B., Li, L.j., Zeng, G., Yuen, K.Y., Chen, R.c., Tang, C.l., Wang, T., Chen, P.y., Xiang, J., Li, S.y., Wang, J.l., Liang, Z.j., Peng, Y.x., Wei, L., Liu, Y., Hu, Y.h., Peng, P., Wang, J.m., Liu, J.y., Chen, Z., Li, G., Zheng, Z.j., Qiu, S.q., Luo, J., Ye, C.j., Zhu, S.y., Zhong, N.s.: Clinical characteristics of coronavirus disease 2019 in china. New Engl. J. Med. **382**(18), 1708–1720 (2020). https://doi.org/10.1056/NEJMoa2002032. https://doi.org/10.1056/NEJMoa2002032
16. Jia, J., Ding, J., Liu, S., Liao, G., Li, J., Duan, B., Wang, G., Zhang, R.: Modeling the control of covid-19: impact of policy interventions and meteorological factors. Electron. J. Differ. Equ. **23**, 1–24 (2020)
17. Jung, E., Lenhart, S., Feng, Z.: Optimal control of treatments in a two-strain 490 tuberculosis model. Discrete Continuous Dyn. Syst.-Ser B **4**(2), 473–482 (2002)
18. Kong, W., Li, Y., Peng, M., Kong, D., Yang, X., Wang, L., Liu, M.: Sars-cov-2 detection in patients with influenza-like illness. Nat. Microbiol. **5**, 675–678 (2020)
19. Kucharski, A., Russell, T., Diamond, C., Liu, Y., Edmunds, J., Funk, S., Eggo, R., Sun, F., Jit, M., Munday, J., Davies, N., Gimma, A., van Zandvoort, K., Gibbs, H., Hellewell, J., Jarvis, C., Clifford, S., Quilty, B., Bosse, N., Abbott, S., Klepac, K., Flasche, F.: Early dynamics of transmission and control of covid-19: a mathematical modelling study. Lancet Infect. Dis. **3099**(20), 1–7 (2020)
20. Lavezzo, E., Franchin, E., Ciavarella, C., Cuomo-Dannenburg, G., Barzon, L., Del Vecchio, C., Rossi, L., Manganelli, R., Loregian, A., Navarin, N., Abate, D., Sciro, M., Merigliano, S., De Canale, E., Vanuzzo, M.C., Besutti, V., Saluzzo, F., Onelia, F., Pacenti, M., Parisi, S.G., Carretta, G., Donato, D., Flor, L., Cocchio, S., Masi, G., Sperduti, A., Cattarino, L., Salvador, R., Nicoletti, M., Caldart, F., Castelli, G., Nieddu, E., Labella, B., Fava, L., Drigo, M., Gaythorpe, K.A.M., Ainslie, K.E.C., Baguelin, M., Bhatt, S., Boonyasiri, A., Boyd, O., Coupland, H.L., Cucunubá, Z., Djafaara, B.A., Donnelly, C.A., Dorigatti, I., van Elsland, S.L., FitzJohn, R., Flaxman, S., Gaythorpe, K.A.M., Green, W.D., Hallett, T., Hamlet, A., Haw, D., Imai, N., Jeffrey, B., Knock, E., Laydon, D.J., Mellan, T., Mishra, S., Nedjati-Gilani, G., Nouvellet, P., Okell, L.C., Parag, K.V., Riley, S., Thompson, H.A., Unwin, H.J.T., Verity, R., Vollmer, M.A.C., Walker, P.G.T., Walters, C.E., Wang, H., Wang, Y., Watson, O.J., Whittaker, C., Whittles, L.K., Xi, X., Ferguson, N.M., Brazzale, A.R., Toppo, S., Trevisan, M., Baldo, V., Donnelly, C.A., Ferguson, N.M., Crisanti, A., Team, I.C.C.R.: Suppression of a sars-cov-2 outbreak in the italian municipality of vo'. Nature (2020)
21. Lin, Q., Zhao, S., Gao, Z., Lou, Y., Yang, S., Musa, S., Wang, M., Cai, Y., Weiming Wang, W., Yang, L., He, D.: A conceptual model for the coronavirus disease 2019 (covid-19) outbreak in wuhan, china with individual reaction and governmental action. Int. J. Infect. Dis. **93**, 211–216 (2020)
22. Marino, S., Hogue, I., Ray, C., Kirschner, D.: A methodology for performing global uncertainty and sensitivity analysis in systems biology. J. Theorit. Biol. **254**, 178–196 (2008)
23. McLeod, R., Brewster, J., Gumel, A., Slonowsky, D.: Sensitivity and uncertainty analyses for a sars model with time-varying inputs and outputs. Math. Biosci. Eng. **3**, 527–544 (2006)
24. Moghadas, S.M., Fitzpatrick, M.C., Sah, P., Pandey, A., Shoukat, A., Singer, B.H., Galvani, A.P.: The implications of silent transmission for the control of covid-19 outbreaks. Proc. Natl. Acad. Sci. **117**(30), 17513–17515 (2020)
25. Mwalili, S., Kimathi, M., Ojiambo, V., Gathungu, D., Mbogo, R.: Seir model for covid-19 dynamics incorporating the environment and social distancing. BMC Res. Notes **13**(352)
26. Ndaïrou, F., Area, I., Nieto, J., Torres, D.: Mathematical modeling of covid-19 transmission dynamics with a case study of wuhan. Chaos, Solit. Fractals **135**, 109846 (2020)
27. Oran, D.P., Topol., E.J.: Prevalence of asymptomatic sars-cov-2 infection: A narrative review. Ann. Intern. Med. (2020)
28. Peeling, R.W., Wedderburn, C.J., Garcia, P.J., Boeras, D., Fongwen, N., Nkengasong, J., Sall, A., Tanuri, A., Heymann, D.L.: Serology testing in the covid-19 pandemic response. The Lancet Infectious Diseases (2020)
29. Pontryagin, L.: Mathematical Theory of Optimal Processes. CRC Press (1987)

30. Qian G, Y.N., AHY, M., et al.: Covid-19 transmission within a family cluster by presymptomatic carriers in china. Clin. Infect Dis. **71**(15) (2020). https://doi.org/10.1093/cid/ciaa316
31. Studdert, D.M., Hall, M.A.: Disease control, civil liberties, and mass testing - calibrating restrictions during the covid-19 pandemic. New Engl. J. Med. **383**(2), 102–104 (2020)
32. Tang, B., Wang, X., Li, Q., Bragazzi, N.L., Tang, S., Xiao, Y., Wu, J.: Estimation of the transmission risk of the 2019-ncov and its implication for public health interventions. J. Clin. Med. **9**(2), 462 (2020)
33. Wang, W., Tang, J., Wei, F.: Updated understanding of the outbreak of 2019 novel coronavirus (2019-ncov) in wuhan, china. J. Med. Virol. **92**(4), 441–447 (2020)
34. WHO: What are the symptoms of covid-19? (2020). https://www.who.int/emergencies/diseases/novel-coronavirus-2019/question-and-answers-hub/q-a-detail/q-a-coronaviruses
35. WHO: Who coronavirus disease (covid-19) dashboard (2020). https://covid19.who.int
36. Wu, J., Leung, K., Leung, G.: Nowcasting and forecasting the potential domestic and international spread of the 2019-ncov outbreak originating in wuhan, china: a modelling study. Lancet **6736**(20), 675–678 (2020)
37. Yang, C., Wang, J.: A mathematical model for the novel coronavirus epidemic in wuhan, china. Math. Biosci. Eng. **17**(3), 2708–2724 (2020)
38. Zou, L., Ruan, F., Huang, M., Liang, L., Huang, H., Hong, Z., Yu, J., Kang, M., Song, Y., Xia, J., Guo, Q., Song, T., He, J., Yen, H., Peiris, M., Wu, J.: Sars-cov-2 viral load in upper respiratory specimens of infected patients. N. Engl. J. Med **382**, 1177–1179 (2020)

Development of Epidemiological Modeling RD-Covid-19 of Coronavirus Infectious Disease and Its Numerical Simulation

Rashmi Bhardwaj and Debabrata Datta

Abstract Coronavirus disease (Covid-19) occurred first in Wuhan city of Hubei province of China in December 2019. The World Health Organization (WHO) declared the spread or the transmission of this virus as a global pandemic. The virus was named as severe acute respiratory syndrome coronavirus 2 (SARS-CoV-2) by the International Committee on Taxonomy of Viruses on February 11, 2020. Disease due to this novel-coronavirus is infectious. Therefore, modeling such an infectious disease is essential to understand the method of its transmission, spread, and epidemic. Several researchers have found that the transfer of the virus occurs through human contact via their pathogens, such as coughing, sneezing, and breathing. With all sorts of preventive measures (social distancing, wearing mask and lockdown), there is a need to develop a dynamic model of epidemiology for infectious disease. In this article, we have developed a new epidemiological dynamical model named RD_Covid-19 (version 1.0) model. The traditional epidemiological model of an infectious disease known as susceptible-exposed-infected-recovered-dead (SEIRD) is modified to develop this new model. RD_Covid-19 is a networked epidemiological model in which a data-driven logistic model, traditional epidemiological models such as SIR (Susceptible, Infected, Recovered), SEIR and SEIQRDP are interlinked. The model forecasts the spread of the Covid-19. Nonlinear least-squares optimization technique is applied for fitting the model to estimate its parameters. The realistic data is taken from John Hopkins University and WHO dashboard. The outcome of the numerical simulation of the model generates the temporal profile of infected, recovered, and death cases. The severity of the model is measured by computing the basic reproduction number (R_0). The model executed to explore the corona outbreak in China, India, Brazil, and Russia. The estimated value of basic reproduction number,

R. Bhardwaj (✉)
Nonlinear Dynamics Research Lab, University School of Basic & Applied Sciences, Guru Gobind Singh Indraprastha University, Delhi, India
e-mail: rashmib@ipu.ac.in

D. Datta
Radiological Physics & Advisory Division, Bhabha Atomic Research Centre, Former Senior Scientist-H & Head, Mumbai, India

SRM Institute of Technology, Kattankulathur, Chennai, India

P. Agarwal et al. (eds.), *Analysis of Infectious Disease Problems (Covid-19) and Their Global Impact*, Infosys Science Foundation Series,
https://doi.org/10.1007/978-981-16-2450-6_12

R_0 is well in agreement with that obtained from the outcome of traditional models SIR and SEIR. The verification and validation (V & V) process of our model is carried out by comparing its results with an analogical logistic model.

Keywords Covid-19 · Epidemiological model · Optimization · Numerical Optimization · Nonlinear least square · Basic reproduction number

1 Introduction

Coronavirus disease (Covid-19) occurred first in Wuhan city of Hubei province of China in December 2019. The World Health Organization (WHO) has declared the spread or transmission of this virus as a global pandemic [1–4]. Initially, it has proposed that the transmission of the coronavirus is related to a seafood market (Wuhan Seafood Wholesale Market), and exposure took place whoever visited that market. Coronavirus genomic infection-2019 has been announced as a severe health emergency arising international awareness due to its spread to 201 countries at present. In April of the year 2020, it has undoubtedly been called the pandemic outbreak having approximately 11,16,643 infections confirmed, leading to around 59,170 deaths recorded all over the world. In general, human-affecting coronavirus contagions has some similarities with two Beta coronaviruses: severe-acute-respiratory-syndrome-coronavirus (SARS-CoV) and Middle-East-respiratory-syndrome-coronavirus (MERS-CoV) [5, 6].

In December 2019, the succession of pneumonia cases from an unknown cause appeared across the city of Wuhan, China, and clinical tests detected them as viral pneumonia. Deep-sequencing-analyzers depicted that the lower respiratory-tract samples indicated a novel-coronavirus coined as a 2019 novel coronavirus (2019-nCov). As of now, around 800 confirmed cases found among health-care workers from this genomic viral which exists in Wuhan along with the exported population in other provinces of China, Thailand, Japan, South Korea & the USA. The clinical findings, such as lower and upper respiratory symptoms of the infection, have been reported based on research findings from several countries. The pandemic situation has worsened at the national as well as at the international level. The outbreak of coronavirus (Covid-19) is categorized as incidence representing number of confirmed new cases, number of cases recovered and number of deaths occurred. Looking towards the daily outbreak of this virus and suspecting its transmission through contact of humans, various countermeasures such as social distancing and lockdown implemented to prevent its potential spread. Therefore, tasks about effective control of outbreak motivated us to develop a reasonable and feasible epidemic model for this infectious disease. Infectious disease epidemiology is characterized by the presence of at least one active player in addition to human population, namely, the infectious agent or parasite [7, 8]. The presence of this additional propagating population sets the stage for aspects specific to infectious disease epidemiology. First and foremost is transmission. Transmission from one host to another is fundamental to the survival strategy of the infectious agent, since any host will eventually either clear the infection or die, even if from an unrelated cause. A consequence of transmission is that, unlike non-infectious diseases, the occurrence of infectious diseases in individuals depends on the occurrence of those diseases in other members of the population. Sir Ronald Ross [9] called this dependence of disease events in infectious diseases as "dependent happenings".

Although most methods used in general epidemiology are applicable to the study of the infectious diseases, additional concepts are needed to describe the phenomena resulting from the dependence of disease events. These include infectiousness, the transmission probability, contact patterns and the basic reproduction number *(R_0)*. An intervention in infectious diseases can also have several different kinds of effects, including direct effects on a person receiving the intervention as well as indirect effects on other individuals. These different effects require additional parameters and study designs for their evaluation. Exposure to infection plays a special role because exposure to infection is necessary for infection and disease to occur. The components of exposure to infection, such as the contact and mixing patterns of the infective and susceptible hosts, as well as the degree and duration of the infectiousness, need to be taken into account in infectious disease epidemiology.

Even when conventional epidemiologic concepts are applicable, these should be used in infectious disease studies only after close examination of the underlying assumptions. Because the temporal evolution of the host population and the disease process under study can be quite rapid compared with the time frame of the study, conventional epidemiologic methods that assume stationarity can produce very biased estimates of effects in infectious disease epidemiology. Epidemiology of infectious disease is an extension of ecology and evolution. Since each infectious agent has its own life cycle, immunology, ecology, evolution and molecular biology, thus studies of infectious disease require the understanding of all these aspects [10]. Since present circumstances focus on the possibility of the spread of coronavirus, we have developed an epidemiological model named RD-Covid-19. With the help of the numerical simulation of RD-Covid-19 Model, the outburst for Covid-19 cases in several countries like China, India, Brazil and Russia has been simulated. RD Model provides the knowledge of basic reproduction number, $R_{0,}$ and with the help of $R_{0,}$ the rate of severity of the coronavirus disease in above mentioned countries has explored. Herd immunity computed from R_0. Case fatality rate (CFR) is an additional component of the epidemiology of infectious disease [10, 11], which was calculated using the RD-Covid-19 model. Modelling of the novel Coronavirus outbreak using data based transformations for epidemiology has been forecasted [12]. A Multi-risk SIR model with optimally targeted lockdown analyzed for the estimation of the transmission risk of 2019-nCov and its implication on public health interventions [13–15]. The corona theorem for differrnt functions analyzed and applied to study the spectral problems for predictive modelling [16, 17]. Predictive models for small molecules that target the severe acute respiratory syndrome human coronavirus nowcasted and forecasted for international spread of 2019-nCov [18, 19]. The clinical implications of Glycopeptide antibiotics that would inhibit Cathepsin L in the Late Endosome/Lysosome, and blocks entry of Ebola virus, MERS-CoV and SARS-CoV-2 discussed [20, 21].

The outburst of Covid-19 studied in detail through data-based modeling & forecast analysis with a detailed explanation of the mathematical perspective to understand the spread of infectious diseases [22, 23]. Estimation and spread of atmospheric pollutants through dynamic indicators, statistical simulations were modeled and analyzed in detail for prediction and forecasting [24–30]. Coronavirus data analyzed for forecasting and risk assessment [31]. Transmission dynamics using data analysis of the Covid-19 outbreak discussed for government interventaions and tracking the rate of transmission of the epidemic, dynamics of transmission and its control [32–37]. For 2019-nCoV pandemic, the efficiency of control strategies towards the reduction of social mixing and complexity with futuristic estimations for China modelled using supervised learning [38]. Time series forecasting of the spread of genomic virus using genetic programming for study of pandemic outbreak based on training testing of multimodal data predicted [39–41]. The molecules that enter into host cell and cause acute respiratory syndrome targeting towards coronavirus forecasted impending Covid-19 spread cases for China and some other regions using mathematical & traditional time-series prediction models [42–44].

In this chapter, we introduce a few important concepts of infectious disease epidemiology, focusing on the consequences of the dependent structure of disease events for measures of the effect. The detailed structure of RD-Covid-19 model with its numerical simulation also presented. Section 2 presents the various components of epidemiology of infectious disease such as time lines of infection, transmission probability, and secondary attack rate. Section 3 describes the basic reproduction number and its estimation methodologies. Incidence rate as a function of prevalence and contact rate is presented in Sect. 4. Section 5 describes the dynamic epidemic process in a closed population. Section 6 describes our RD-Covid-19 model and its various components (network). Numerical simulation of our model for countries, as mentioned, is presented in Sect. 7. Section 8 concludes the chapter with possible future research in this direction.

2 Infectious Disease Epidemiology Components

Its various components always understand the epidemiology of an infectious disease. These are (1) timelines of infection, (2) transmission probability, and (3) secondary attack rate. This section presents insight into these components.

2.1 Timelines of Infection

The time lines of infection within the host can be best described with reference to the dynamics of infectiousness and of disease (Fig. 1). Both start with the active disease

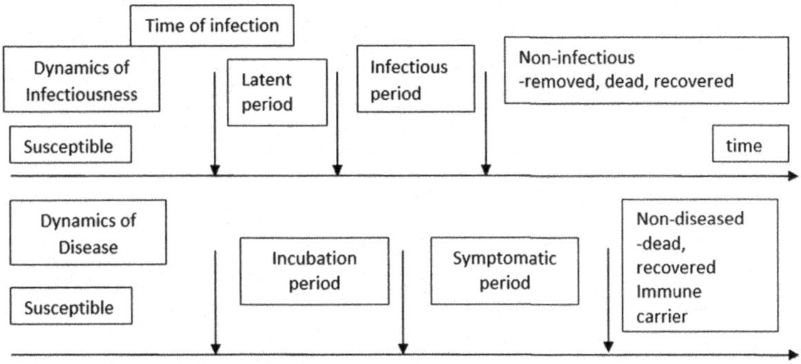

Fig. 1 Timeline for infection and disease

of the vulnerable host by the parasite. The time line of infectiousness includes the latent period, the time interval from infection to development of infectiousness and the period of infectiousness of the host, during which time the host could infect another host. Eventually, the host becomes noninfectious either by recovery from the infection, possibly developing immunity, or by death. The host can also become noninfectious while still alive and still harboring the parasite.

The time line of disease within the host includes the incubation period, the time from infection to development of symptomatic disease and the symptomatic period. The probability of developing symptoms or disease after becoming infected is the pathogenicity of the interaction of the parasite with the host. Eventually, the host leaves the symptomatic state either by recovering from the symptoms or by death. The host becomes an infectious carrier if he recovers from symptoms but remains infectious. The terminology used in infectious disease epidemiology always differs from that of non-infectious disease epidemiology. The term latent period refers the time corresponding to the period from development of asymptomatic disease to development of symptoms. The incubation period in infectious disease is a combination of what are called the induction and the latent periods in noninfectious diseases. The configuration of the two time lines in Fig. 1 and their relation to one another are specific to each parasite and can have important public health consequences and implications for study design.

2.2 Estimation of Transmission Probability

Transmission probability is an important parameter of infectious disease epidemiology which is defined as the probability that, given contact between two infective source and a susceptible host, successful transfer of the parasite will occur so that the susceptible host becomes infected (Fig. 2). Hence, estimation of transmission probability is very important from the point of knowing the outbreak of infectious disease Covid-19. The transmission probability depends on characteristics of the infective

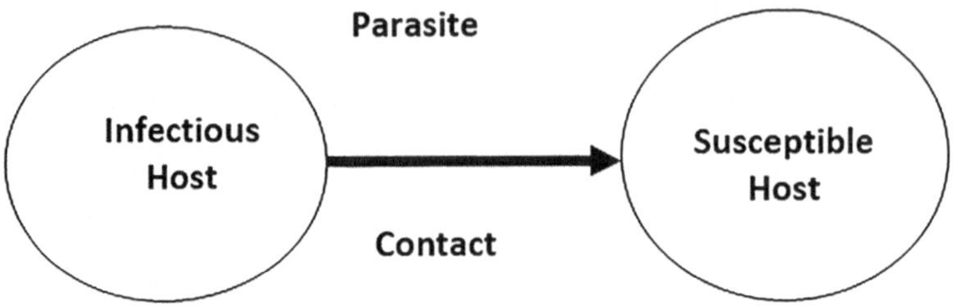

Fig. 2 Transmission from an infective to a susceptible host during contact

source, the parasite, the susceptible host and the type of definition of contact. The infectious source could be another person, as in Covid-19. The mode of transmission of a parasite determines what type of contact is potentially infectious.

It is worth to know the method of estimating transmission probability. In one method, infectious individuals are identified and the proportion of contacts that they make with susceptible hosts that result in transmission is determined. This approach can be explained further by introducing secondary attack rate.

Secondary Attack rate:

The conventional secondary attack rate (SAR) defined as the probability of the occurrence of disease among known susceptible persons following contact with a primary case:

$$SAR = \frac{n\ (number\ of\ \ persons\ exposed\ who\ develop\ disease)}{m\ (total\ number\ of\ susceptible\ exposed\ persons)}$$

2.3 The SAR is a Proportion, Not a Rate

In another technique, susceptible hosts are identified and data gathered on the number of contacts they make with infectives and outcomes of their infection. In this method binomial model is used to estimate the transmission probability. The probability of transmission during a contact between a susceptible and an infectious person is denoted by 'p' and the probability of a susceptible person's escaping infection during the contact is 'q = 1 – p'. The probability of escaping infection from all n potentially infective contacts is $q^n = (1-p)^{n}$. The probability of being infected after n contacts, that is, of not escaping infection from all n contacts is $1 - q^n = 1 - (1-p)^n$. The maximum likelihood estimate of the transmission probability under the binomial model can be written as

$$p = \frac{number\ of\ susceptibles\ who\ become\ infected}{total\ number\ of\ contacts\ with\ infectives}$$

It is required to note that, in the binomial model, the total number of potentially infectious contacts that susceptible individuals make, while in SAR, each vulnerable person had just one potentially infectious contact with the infective.

3 Estimation of Basic Reproduction Number/ Proliferation Number

Basic reproduction number, R_0 is defined as the expected number of new infectious hosts that one infectious host will produce during his or her period of infectiousness in a large population that is completely susceptible. R_0 does not include the new cases produced by the secondary cases which do not become infectious. For example, if $R_0 = 9$ for some infectious disease in a population, then one person with that infectious disease introduced to that population would be expected to produce nine new secondary infectious cases before recovering, if the population were completely susceptible. If the person produced two additional cases which did not become infectious, R_0 would still be 9. In general, for an epidemic to occur in a susceptible population, R_0 must be greater than one. If $R_0 < 1$, an average case will not produce itself, so an epidemic will not spread. Since R_0 is an average, it is possible that a particular infectious person will produce more than one infective case, even when $R_0 < 1$, so there may be a small cluster of cases. We would not, however, expect a self-sustaining outbreak.

The basic reproduction number, R_0 for infectious disease depends on three parameters, which are: (a) the rate of contacts c, (b) the duration of infectiousness d, and (c) the transmission probability per potentially infective contact p. Mathematical expression of R_0 hence can be written as

$$R_0 = \frac{numberofcontacts}{time} \times \frac{transmissionprobability}{numberofcontacts} \times duration(time) = cpd$$

By definition, R_0 assumes that all contacts are with susceptibles. Under these conditions, the expected number of new cases produced by an infectious person is less than R_0 and is called the effective reproductive number, R. If x is the proportion of a randomly mixing, homogeneous population that is susceptible, R is the product of R_0 times the proportion x of the contacts that are with susceptibles. So, $R = R_0$ x. For example, if $R_0 = 9$ and $x = 0.5$, then $R = 4.5$. So an infectious disease would produce on average only 4.5 new secondary cases in this population. We can also write $R = R_0 (1 - f)$, where fraction f is immunized before the age of first infection and $(1 - f)$ would be the maximum fraction of the population that is susceptible, disregarding immunity from previous disease. Therefore, to eliminate transmission, we should have, $R = R_0 (1 - f) < 1$. Therefore the fraction that needs to be immunized to eliminate transmission is $f > 1 - 1/R_0$. A higher R_0 requires immunization of a higher fraction to eliminate transmission.

Herd immunity [11] describes the collective immunologic status of a population of hosts, as opposed to an individual organism, with respect to a given parasite [9]. Herd immunity of a population may be high if many people have been immunized or have recovered from infection with immunity or may be low if most people are susceptible. As herd immunity increases, R will decrease.

3.1 *Estimation of R_0*

If the average life expectancy, L in a population is known, then R_0 can be estimated from the relation, $R_0 = L/A$, where $A = 1/I$ (incidence rate). R_0 can be calculated by computing the ratio of the rate of infection (β) to the rate of recovery (γ) for a standard SIR epidemic model. Maximum likelihood method can be the alternate method for estimating R_0. In case of a standard compartment epidemic model or networked model, R_0 is computed by next generation matrix method, where maximum eigenvalue of the next generation matrix is the value R_0.

3.2 *Virulence of R_0 and the Case Fatality Ratio (CFR)*

Virulence is a measure of the spread with which a virus (coronavirus) kills an infected host. Since R_0 is a function of the time spent in the infective state, R_0 could decrease as virulence increases. The case fatality ratio (CFR) is the probability of dying from a disease (Covid-19) before recovering or dying or something else [11]. Mathematically, CFR is defined as the ratio of number of deaths due to disease to the number of confirmed infectious cases. As virulence increases, the CFR increases.

4 Incidence Rate as a Function of Prevalence and Contact Rate

Apart from R_0, transmission probability, the incidence rate, also used in infectious disease epidemiology. Under the assumption of simple random mixing, constant contact rate, c, and the transmission probability p, the incidence rate I(t) expressed as a function of the prevalence P(t) at time t of infectious persons defined as

$$I(t) = cpP(t) = \frac{R_0}{d}P(t) \tag{1}$$

5 Dynamic Epidemic Process in a Closed Population

If the population is closed, then there are no births, immigration, deaths, or emigration. In a typical cohort study, we would not necessarily be concerned with how the individual people interact. In any study of infectious disease, the underlying contact and transmission process is essential, so we need to think about these processes in our model. If S is the susceptible population, I, the infected population, and R is the recovered population, we can have a SIR epidemic model [44–47] governed by following network diagram (Fig. 3) and equations as presented in Eq. (2).

$$\left.\begin{array}{c} \frac{dS}{dt} = -\beta\frac{SI}{N} \\ \frac{dI}{dt} = \beta\frac{SI}{N} - \gamma I \\ \frac{dR}{dt} = \gamma I \end{array}\right\} \quad (2)$$

where, β denotes the infection rate, γ indicates the rate of recovery and the total population is $N = S + I + R$.

The dynamics of the epidemic described by Eq. (2) The rate at which people leave the susceptible compartment S and become infected is simply the incidence rate. Prevalence of infectives at time t, P(t) is the number of infectious people I(t) divided by the size of population N, or I(t)/N. The incidence as a function of prevalence is given by

$$Incidence(t) = cpP(t) = cp\frac{I(t)}{N}$$

$$\frac{dS}{dt} = -Incidence(t)S(t) = -cp\frac{I(t)}{N}S(t) = -\beta\frac{SI}{N}$$

Therefore, the infection rate is given by $\beta = c\,p$. A cross-sectional study to estimate prevalence P(t) of current infection would yield an estimate of I(t)/N. We can write the differential equation representing the variation of the infected population for a variety of susceptible population of SIR model (Eq. 2) can be written as

$$\frac{dI}{dS} = \frac{\gamma}{\beta}\frac{N}{S} - 1 \quad (3)$$

Similarly, we can also write,

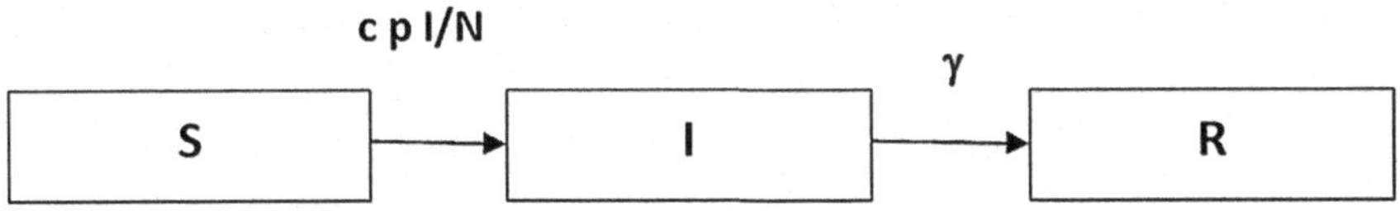

Fig. 3 Network diagram of SIR Model

$$\frac{dI}{dR} = \frac{\beta SI}{N} - 1 \quad (4)$$

Analytical solution of Eq. (3) with initial condition S(0) = N, I(0) = 0 and R(0) = 0 can be written as

$$I = f(S) = \frac{N\gamma}{\beta} ln\left(\frac{S}{N}\right) + (N - S) \quad (5)$$

Equation (5) utilized to reconstruct the phase of the infected-susceptible population. The epidemic process also depends on population biology. By using definition of R_0, for SIR model we can easily express $R_0 = c\ p/\gamma = \beta/\gamma$. The expected number of new cases per infective host decreases from R_0 to $R = R_0$ (S/N). The epidemic peaks begins to decrease when $R < 1$, so that $S(t)/N < 1/R_0$, that is, when the proportion of the population still susceptible becomes less than the reciprocal of the basic reproductive number. If an intervention (social distancing and lockdown) reduced some aspect of R_0, then the intervention would result in the epidemic peaking when a higher proportion of the population was still susceptible, and fewer people would become infected before the epidemic died out.

6 RD-Covid-19 Epidemiological Model

Looking towards the need of an epidemiological forecasting model for knowing the outbreak of coronavirus we have developed a hybrid model RD-Covid-19 which is a networked model of a data-driven logistic model, SIR model, SEIR model [43–48] and SEIQRDP (Susceptible, Exposed, Infected, Quarantine, Recovered, Dead, Protected) model. Epidemiological models are generally dynamic model and data dependency. Hence, forecasting the spread of the coronavirus disease (Covid-19) will change with the change or availability of new datasets addressing confirmed, recovered, and death cases. Moreover, every epidemiological model is the compartmental model, and the introduction of a fresh compartment always based on certain assumptions. The assumption based modeling motivates us to develop a data-independent epidemiological model to forecast the coronavirus outbreak optimally. Accordingly, this demands to develop an optimal model to predict the spread or transmission of Covid-19 optimally. Therefore, with a view to this demand, we developed a hybrid model by the networking of logistic Model with SIR, SEIR, and SEIQRDP Model [47, 48]. The fundamental concept behind this networked model is to cascade the output of one model into the input of another model. Every model in this work is calibrated with the help of the available data in a sense, that parameters of the specific model at every stage are estimated using nonlinear least square optimization method.

In the cascade, at first parameters (infection rate and rate of recovery) of a data-driven model (logistic model) are estimated. Estimated values of these parameters used as guess value of the parameters of the SIR model, which calibrated further using the same data set and generate an improved amount of rate of infection and rate of recovery parameters of the SIR model. In the next stage, again, those values are used as input to the SEIR model. It is considered that, at the input stage, values of the parameters of the model accepted as guess value. Finally, the estimated values of the parameters by fitting the SEIR model along with the other parameters of the SEIQRDP model used as a guess value (input) of the SEIQRDP epidemiological model. Finally, the Model SEIQRDP numerically solved with the fitted values of the model parameters. Since the estimated values of the rate of infection and rate of recovery are going through several stages for their improvement, our model provides optimal values of the rate of infection and rate of recovery. These two parameters of a dynamic epidemiological model are data-dependent. Other parameters, such as incubation rate, protection rate, and quarantine period, guessed based on model assumptions. Assumptions of SIR model are:

(1) The only way a person can leave the susceptible group is to become infected.
(2) The only way a person can leave the infected group is to recover from the disease.
(3) Once a person has recovered, the person received immunity.
(4) Age, sex, social status, and race do not affect the probability of being infected.

A schematic diagram of RD-Covid-19 model is as shown in Fig. 4.

The data-driven model estimates the growth curve of the epidemic by fitting the parameters of the model through the available data (confirmed cases of Covid-19) of the public for any country. As mentioned previously, hereafter, estimated values of the parameters (rate of infection and rate of recovery) from the logistic model fed as guess value of the parameters of the SIR model, and subsequently,

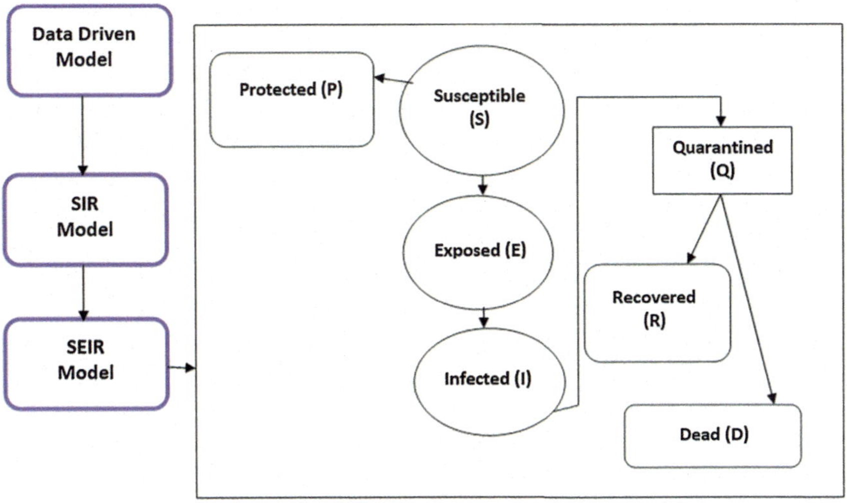

Fig. 4 Schematic Diagram of Networked RD-Covid-19 Model

similar trend follows for the other three networked model, viz., SEIR and SEIQRDP. Parameters of epidemiological models used in our work estimated by the nonlinear least-square fitting of the available data. Levenberg–Marquardt Algorithm [49] and an optimization technique of min-search (basically quadratic programming) used for fitting the model parameters. At the final stage, the SEIQRDP model is executed to compute the time-dependent profile of seven states of the model.

Let us discuss data-driven models that we have investigated, and finally, we have selected a specific model for the present work.

1. **Gompertz Model**

$$Q_t = cumulative\,confirmed\,cases = a * exp(-b * \exp(-c * (t - t_0))) \tag{6}$$

where, a = predicted maximum of confirmed, b and c are fitting coefficients, t represents the number of days since the first case, and t_0 signifies the time when the first case occurred.

2. **Logistic Model**
This model predicts the development and transmission trend of the epidemic. Governing equation of this data-driven model is given by

$$Q_t = \frac{a}{1 + exp(b - c(t - t_0))}, \tag{7}$$

where a = predicted maximum of confirmed cases, where b and c are the fitting coeffcients, t represents the number of days since the first case, t_0 signifies the time when the first case occurred.
The logistic model is used to explore the risk factors of particular disease and predict the probability of a specific disease according to the risk factors.

3. **Bertalanffy Model**
This model represents the growth curve model for a time series (cumulative or daily confirmed cases and death cases in case of Covid-19). It is a special case of generalized logistic function. Governing equation of this model is given by

$$Q_t = a(1 - exp(-b(t - t_0)))^c \tag{8}$$

where the symbols have usual significances, like previous other models as mentioned.

(4) **Monod Kinetic Growth Model**
This model is used to explore the growth of microorganisms. Form of this model is the same as Michaelis–Menten equation and is given by

$$Y_t = Y_{max} \frac{\theta}{K_\theta + \theta}, \tag{9}$$

Y_t specific growth rate of the microorganisms (in this case, coronavirus) Y_{max} = maximum value of the specific growth rate of microorganism, $\theta = concentration$ (cases) of the limiting substrate for growth, K_θ = half velocity constant. The present work follows the logistic model Monod Kinetic Growth model (Eq. 9) to explore the coronavirus outbreak of any country and the corresponding growth rate of the event in the same region.
The second stage of the networked model is SIR, which has already described in Eq. (2). The third stage of the networked model is SEIR model, where an extra compartment explaining the exposed population (E) introduced. The governing one-dimensional differential equation (ODE) of the SEIR epidemiological model is written (Eq. 10) as:

$$\begin{aligned} \frac{dS}{dt} &= -\frac{\beta SI}{N} \\ \frac{dE}{dt} &= \frac{\beta SI}{N} - \omega E \\ \frac{dI}{dt} &= \omega E - \gamma I \\ \frac{dR}{dt} &= \gamma I \end{aligned} \tag{10}$$

where, N = S + E + I + R = total population, β = rate of infection, which modeled as = β_0 K explaining β_0 as the probability of infection per encounter with an infected individual and K as the number of people encountered per day. The parameter ω is modeled as $1/T_e$, where T_e signifies the latent period (days). The average rate of recovery is denoted by the parameter $\gamma = 1/T_i$, where T_i is the average recovery time of infectives.

The last stage of networked RD-Covid-19 model is the SEIQRDP model, which is further networked by seven states. Those seven states are: (a) Susceptible (S), (b) Exposed (E), (c) Infected (I), (d) Quarantined (Q), (e) Recovered (R), (f) Dead (D) and (g) Protected (P) or in-susceptible population. This specific model contains six parameters which are defined as:

α—the protection rate,
β—the infection rate,
γ—the inverse of the average latent time,
δ—the rate at which infectious people enter in quarantine,
λ(t)—a time-dependent coefficient used to describe the recovery rate,
κ(t)—a time-dependent coefficient that describes the mortality rate.

The time-dependent coefficients, λ(t) and κ(t) further assumed in the following form:

$$\lambda(t) = \lambda_0(1 - e^{(-\lambda_1 t)})\, and\, \kappa(t) = \kappa_0 e^{(-\kappa_1 t)},\, where\, \lambda_0, \lambda_1, \kappa_0, \kappa_1\, are\, constants.$$

The values of λ(t) and κ(t) based on the empirical fitting of some provinces of China data indicate that the gradual increase of recovery rate and fast decrease of mortality rate. The assumptions are reasonably accepted by nature as pandemic always converges to zero while the recovery rate continues to increase towards a saturation level. The other parameters of the SEIQRDP model are constant because they do not fluctuate on time. The dynamic of each state is characterized mathematically by an ordinary differential equation given by (Eq. 11).

$$\begin{aligned}\frac{dS}{dt} &= -\alpha S - \frac{\beta SI}{N}\\ \frac{dE}{dt} &= \frac{\beta SI}{N} - \gamma E\\ \frac{dI}{dt} &= \gamma E - \delta I\\ \frac{dQ}{dt} &= \delta I - \lambda Q - \kappa Q\\ \frac{dR}{dt} &= \lambda Q\\ \frac{dD}{dt} &= \kappa Q\\ \frac{dP}{dt} &= \alpha S\end{aligned} \tag{11}$$

where N represents the total population and is written as N = S + E + I + Q + R + D + P.

The networked RD-Covid-19 model estimates the basic reproduction number R_0 at its networked stage. Therefore, in the first stage of the network, the output of data-driven (Monod Kinetic growth) and SIR models and the last stage of a network that is an output of SEIQRDP model-based estimated value of R_0 are mentioned, which is sufficient to know about the progress of coronavirus outbreak. The time evolution of reproduction number, R is modeled as $R_t = R_0 \exp(-\gamma t)$, γ signifies here the rate of recovery. There are many methods to estimate R_0. In our present work, we have used the next-generation matrix method for determining R_0. In the next-generation matrix method, the estimation of R_0 is based on the maximum eigenvalue of the product of two matrices F and V^{-1}, which are generated from the system of the differential equation of the specific model in matrix form.

7 Numerical Simulation of RD-Covid-19 Model

The general strategy of simulation of the infectious disease dynamics model for modeling and predicting the number of Covid-19 cases has carried out. The forecasting of RD-Covid-19 model validated with cases in Wuhan, China. Later on, our model implemented to forecast the coronavirus outbreak and epidemic profile of countries like India, Brazil, and Russia. Utilization of the numerical Model is of incredible managing hugeness to survey the effect of segregation of suggestive cases just as the perception of asymptomatic contact cases and to advance proof-based choices and strategy. We accepted no new transmissions from creatures, no distinctions in singular insusceptibility, the time-size of the pandemic is a lot quicker than trademark times for segment forms (normal birth and death), and no differences in common births and passings.

Numerical simulation of any dynamic model (a system of first-order coupled ODE) can be carried out either by the Runge–Kutta method or by explicit finite difference technique. Here we have adopted the fourth order Runge–Kutta method for simulating each networked node (epidemiological model). In the first stage of the RD-Covid-19 networked model we have fitted the Monod Kinetic Growth data-driven model. Subsequently, parameters of the SIR model fitted by Levenberg Marquardt nonlinear least square method based optimization technique. Data used for mounting the model and corresponding simulation captured from John Hopkins University and WHO dashboard [50]. Dataset preprocessed into three groups like (a) cumulative confirmed cases, (b) cumulative recovered cases, and (c) cumulative deaths. Dataset for daily new cases constructed by computing the forward difference of cumulative confirmed cases per day. Similarly, new deaths per day and new recovered cases per day also computed by following a similar strategy. Active cases per day generated by subtracting the cumulative recovered and cumulative deaths from cumulative confirmed cases.

We have divided numerical simulation of RD-Covid-19 into four parts. Part 1 presents the numerical outcome of India; Part 2 of China; Part 3 of Brazil and Part 4 of Russia.. Numerical simulation of each node of RD-Covid-19 model has been carried out with the fitted parameters at each stage, and finally, the simulated outcome of node 'SEIQRDP' of RD-Covid-19 shown in Fig. 11. We have developed computer code for numerical simulation of our RD-Covid-19 Model in R software (version 3.6.2) and MATLAB 2017a. The impact of various control measures (e.g., social distance, wearing a mask, and lockdown) implemented in code. In the process, S assumed to be the population of an individual country.

7.1 PART-1: Numerical Outcome of RD-Covid-19 Model Outcome for INDIA

Time histories profile of various events (confirmed cases, death cases, and recovered cases) and epidemic trend of coronavirus outbreak as the outcome of RD-Covid-19 Model for India during the period from January 22, 2020, to July-5, 2020 are shown in Figs. 5, 6, 7, 8, 9, 10 and 11. The results of the epidemic trend (plot) of coronavirus outbreak is as shown in Fig. 10 with a blue line (cases/day). Blue dots represent the actual infection rate (cases/day). A region with different colours separate the transmition phases of the epidemic like the red-colored zone signifies fast growth phase, yellow colored zone presents the transmition to steady state phase and green colored zone presents the ending phase.

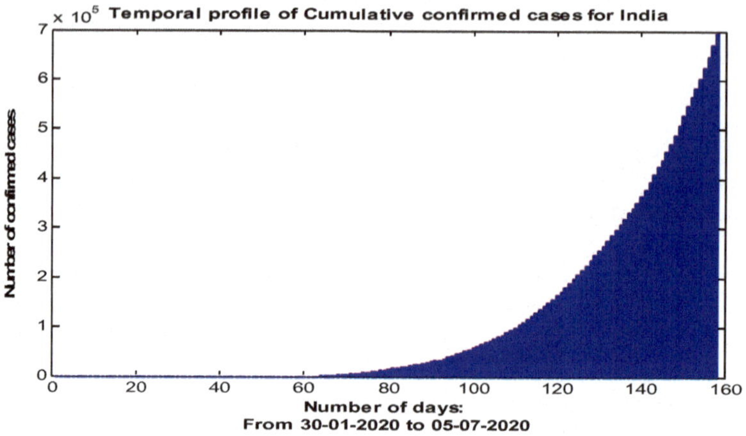

Fig. 5 Temporal profile of cumulative confirmed cases in India

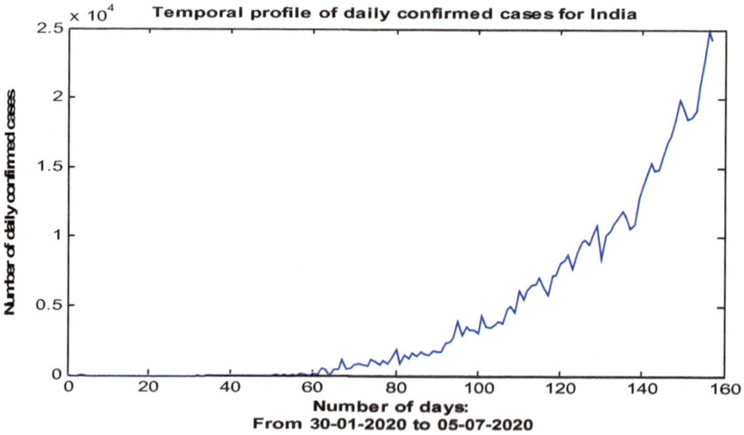

Fig. 6 Temporal profile of daily confirmed cases in India

7.2 PART-2: Numerical Outcome of RD-Covid-19 Model Outcome for CHINA

Time histories profile of various events (confirmed cases, death cases, and recovered cases) and epidemic trend of coronavirus outbreak as the outcome of RD-Covid-19 Model for China during the period during the period from January 22, 2020, to July-5, 2020 are shown in Figs. 12, 13, 14, 15, 16, 17 and 18. The result of the epidemic trend (plot) of coronavirus outbreak is as shown in Fig. 17 with a blue line (cases/day). Blue dots represent the actual infection rate (cases/day). A region with different colors

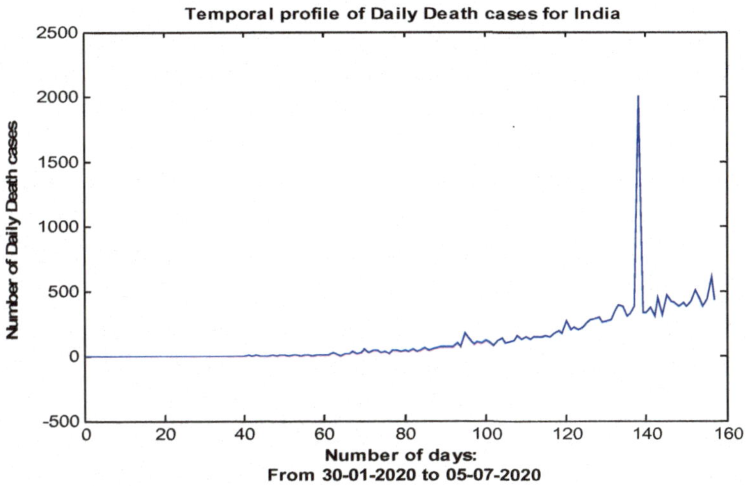

Fig. 7 Temporal profile of daily death cases in India

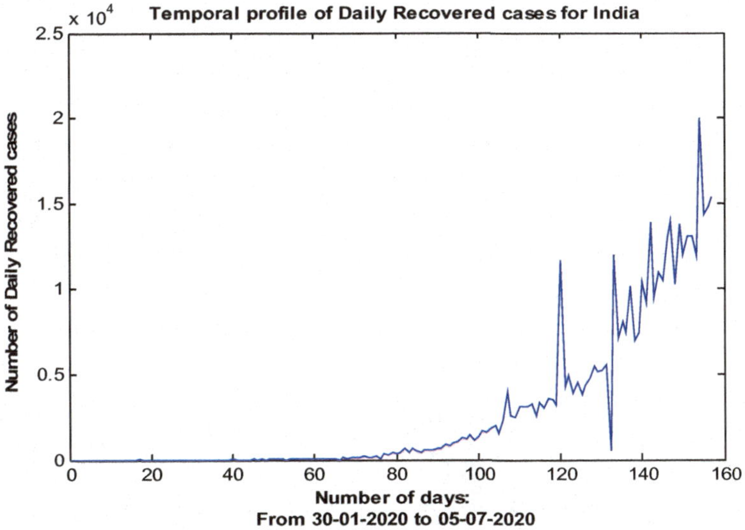

Fig. 8 Temporal profile of daily recovered cases in India

separate the transition phases of the epidemic like the red-colored zone signifies fast growth phase, yellow-colored zone presents the transition to steady-state phase, and green colored zone presents the ending phase.

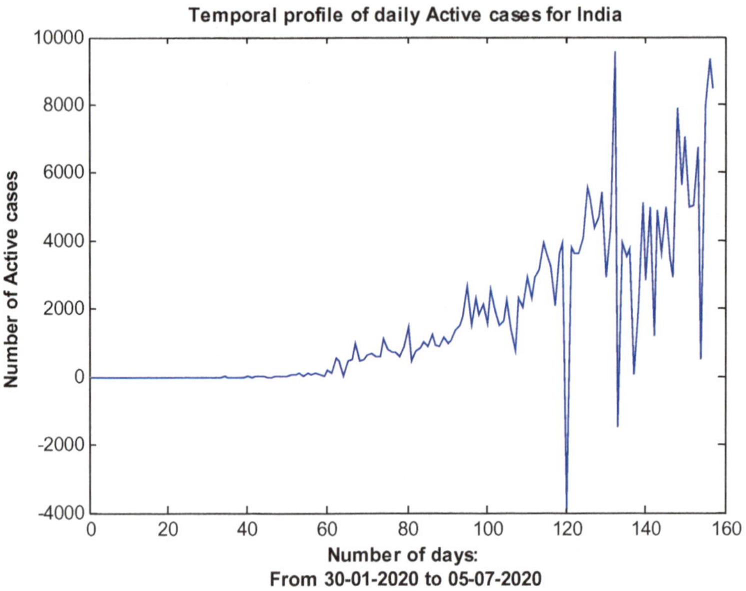

Fig. 9 Temporal profile of daily active cases in India

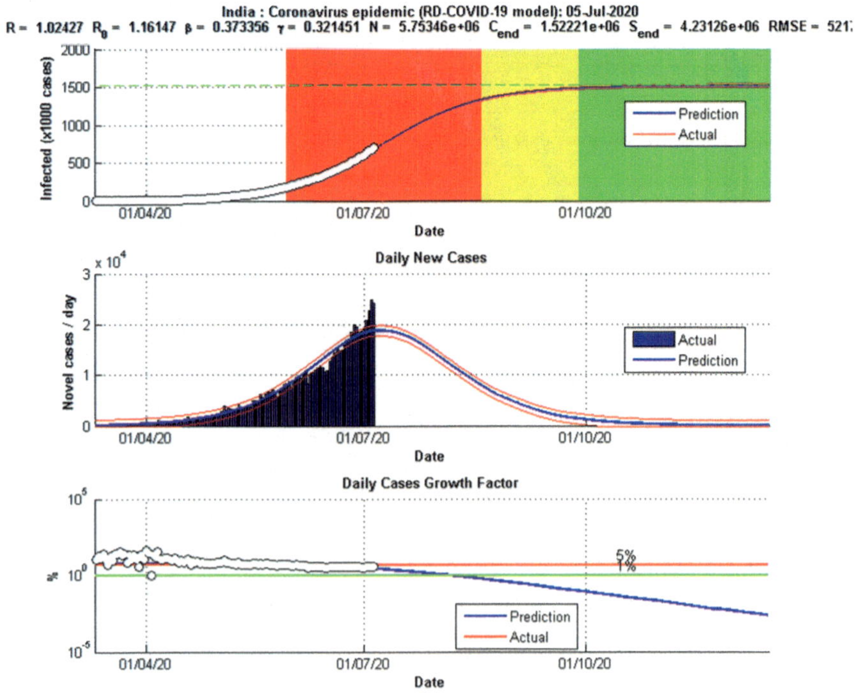

Fig. 10 Epidemic Trend of Coronavirus outbreak in India

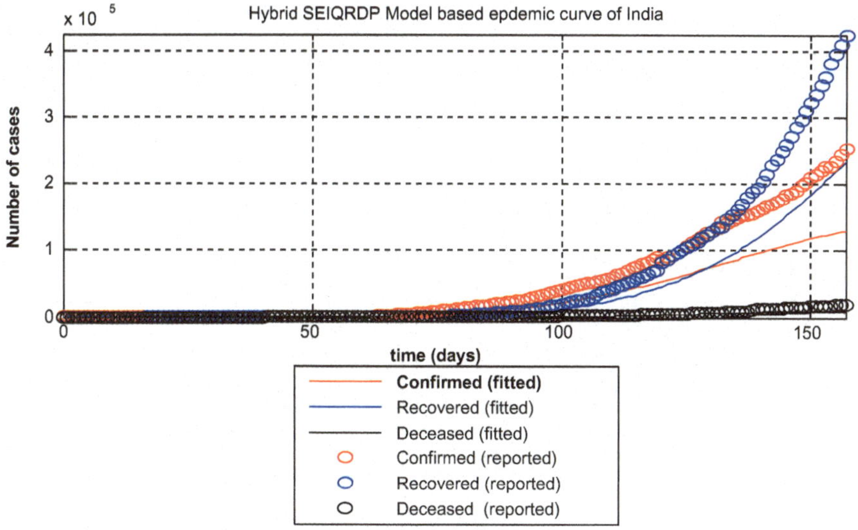

Fig. 11 Numerical simulation of Node SEIQRDP model of RD-Covid-19 (India)

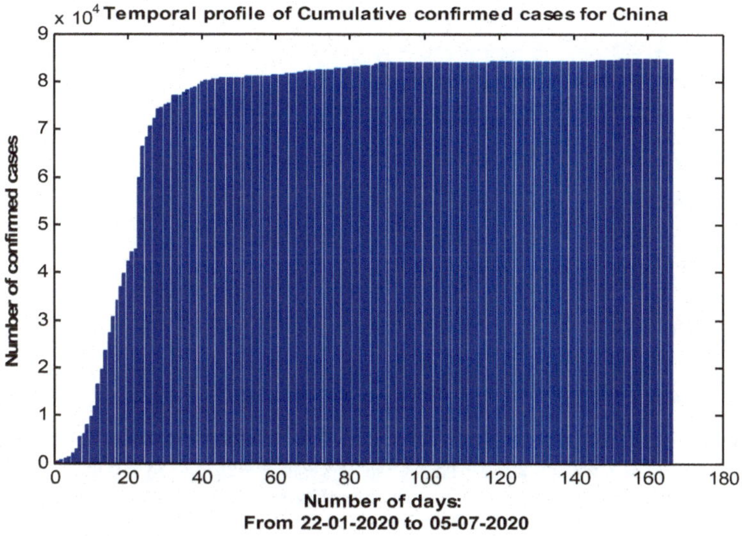

Fig. 12 Temporal profile of cumulative confirmed cases

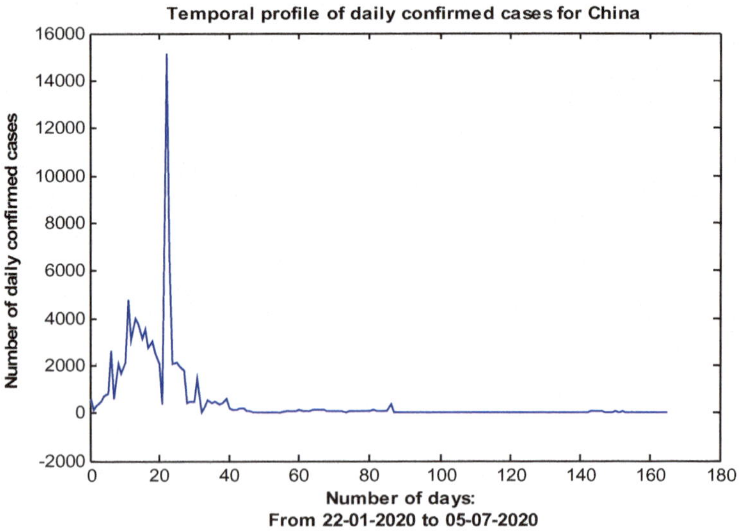

Fig. 13 Temporal profile of daily confirmed cases

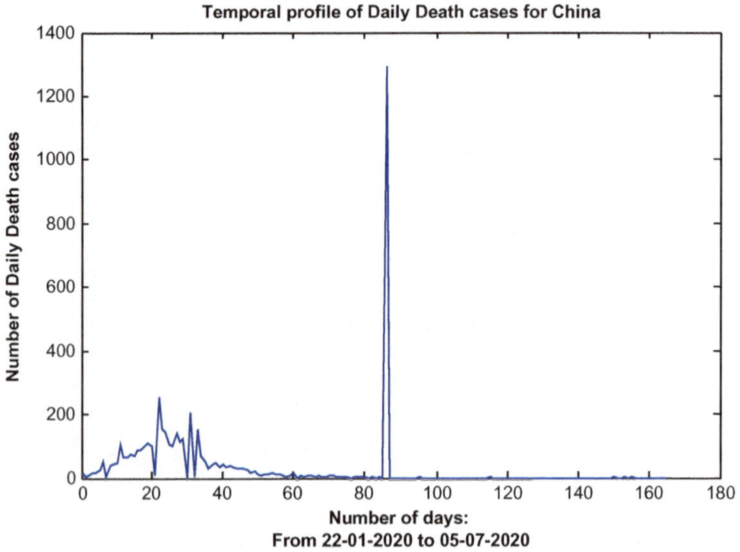

Fig. 14 Temporal profile of daily death cases

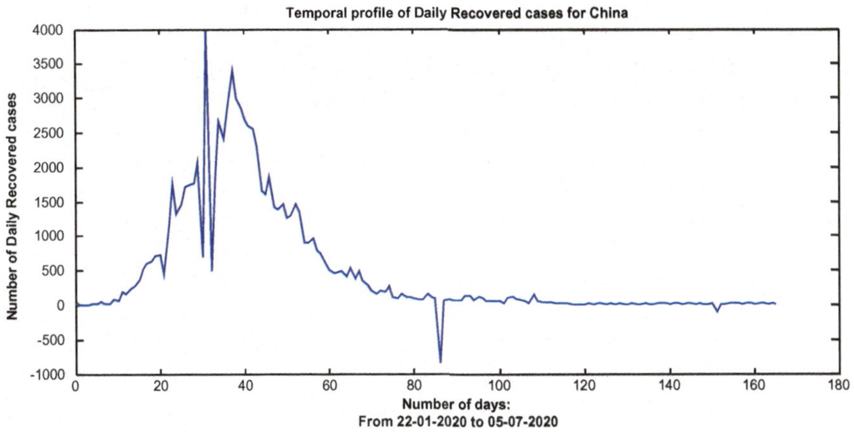

Fig. 15 Temporal profile of daily recovered cases

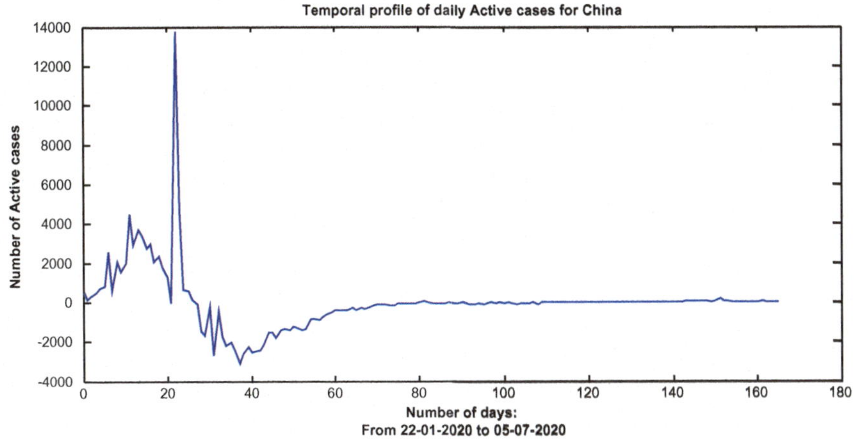

Fig. 16 Temporal profile of daily active cases

7.3 PART-3: Numerical Outcome of RD-Covid-19 Model Outcome for BRAZIL

Time histories profile of various events (confirmed cases, death cases, and recovered cases) and epidemic trend of coronavirus outbreak as the outcome of RD-Covid-19 Model for Brazil during the period during the period from January 22, 2020, to July-5, 2020 are shown in Figs. 19, 20, 21, 22, 23 and 24. The result of the epidemic trend (plot) of coronavirus outbreak is as shown in Fig. 23 with a blue line (cases/day). Blue dots represent the actual infection rate (cases/day). A region with different colors separate the transition phases of the epidemic like the red-colored zone signifies fast

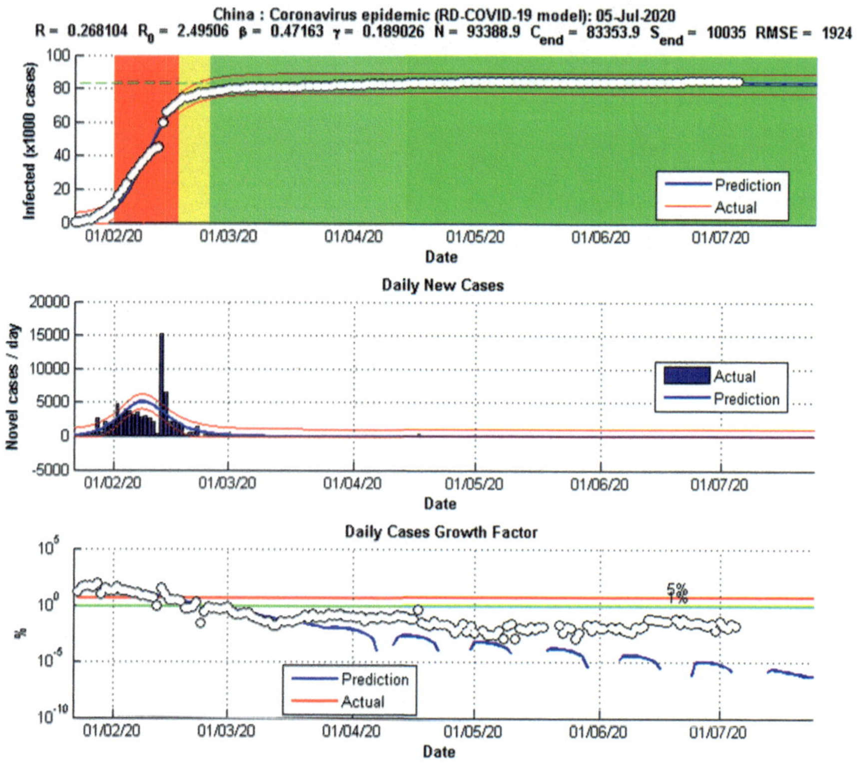

Fig. 17 Epidemic Trend of Coronavirus outbreak in China

growth phase, yellow-colored zone presents the transition to steady-state phase, and green colored zone presents the ending phase.

7.4 PART-4: Numerical Outcome of RD-Covid-19 Model Outcome for RUSSIA

Time histories profile of various events (confirmed cases, death cases, and recovered cases) and epidemic trend of coronavirus outbreak as the outcome of RD-Covid-19 Model for Russia during the period during the period from January 22, 2020, to July-5, 2020 are shown in Figs. 25, 26, 27, 28, 29 and 30. The result of the epidemic trend (plot) of coronavirus outbreak is as shown in Fig. 29 with a blue line (cases/day). Blue dots represent the actual infection rate (cases/day). A region with different colors separate the transition phases of the epidemic like the red-colored zone signifies fast growth phase, yellow-colored zone presents the transition to steady-state phase, and green colored zone presents the ending phase.

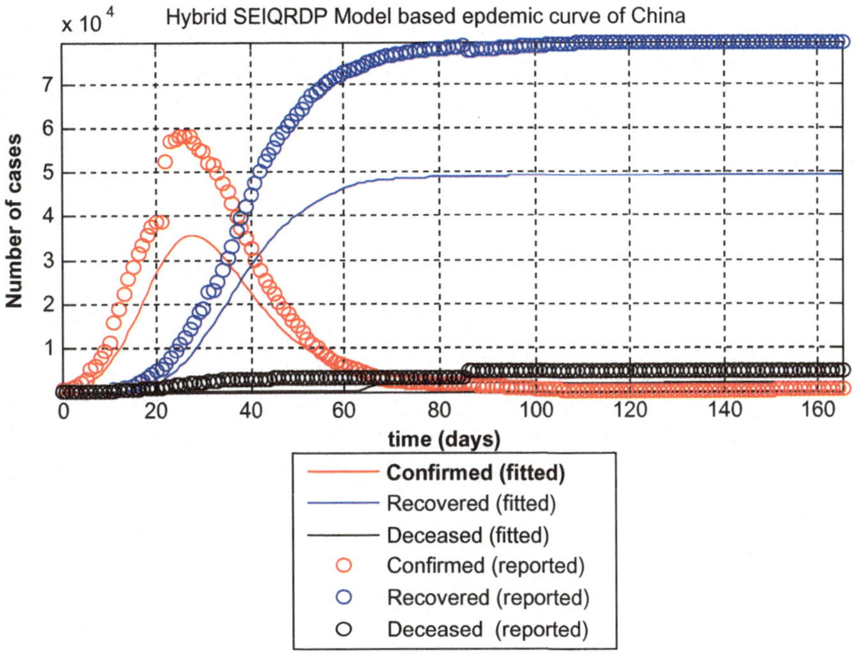

Fig. 18 Numerical simulation of Node SEIQRDP model of RD-Covid-19 (China)

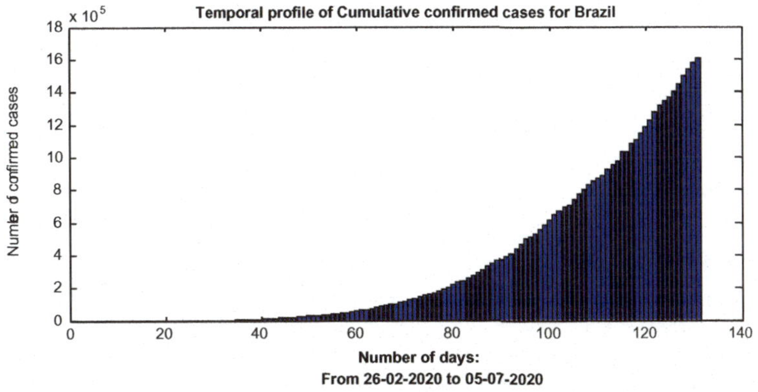

Fig. 19 Temporal profile of Cumulative confirmed cases in Brazil

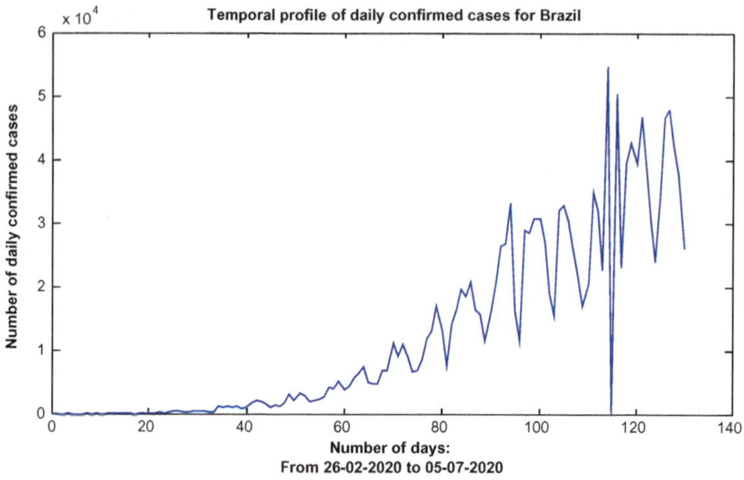

Fig. 20 Temporal profile of daily confirmed cases in Brazil

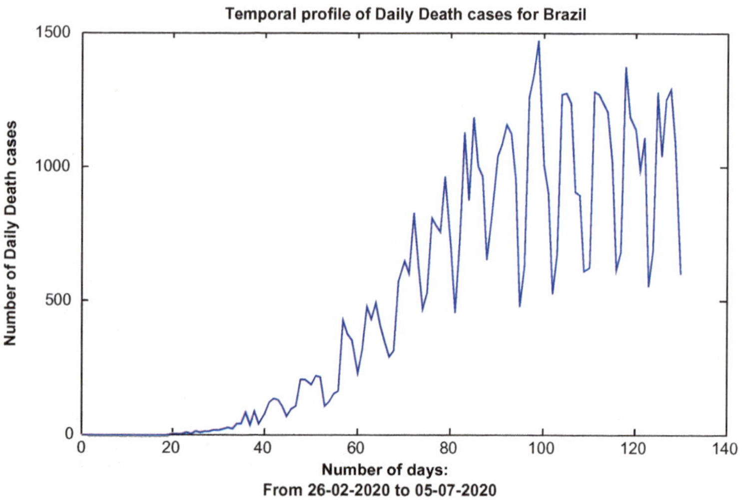

Fig. 21 Temporal profile of daily death cases in Brazil

Values of the fitted parameters of the last node SEIQRDP of RD-Covid-19 Model for various countries (China, India, Brazil, and Russia) tabulated in Table 1. Basic reproduction number (R_0), reproduction number (R), and herd immunity threshold concerning the epidemic curve of China, India, Brazil, and Russia tabulated in Table 2. The estimated duration of different stages of epidemic events presented in Table 3. Estimated datum (Dates) of the epidemic stage of China, India, Brazil, and Russia showed in Table 4. Table 5 presents the statistics of total and daily cases.

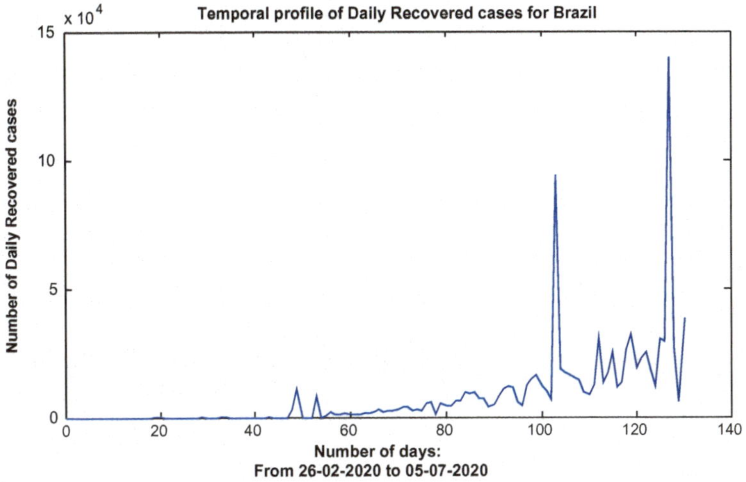

Fig. 22 Temporal profile of daily recovered cases in Brazil

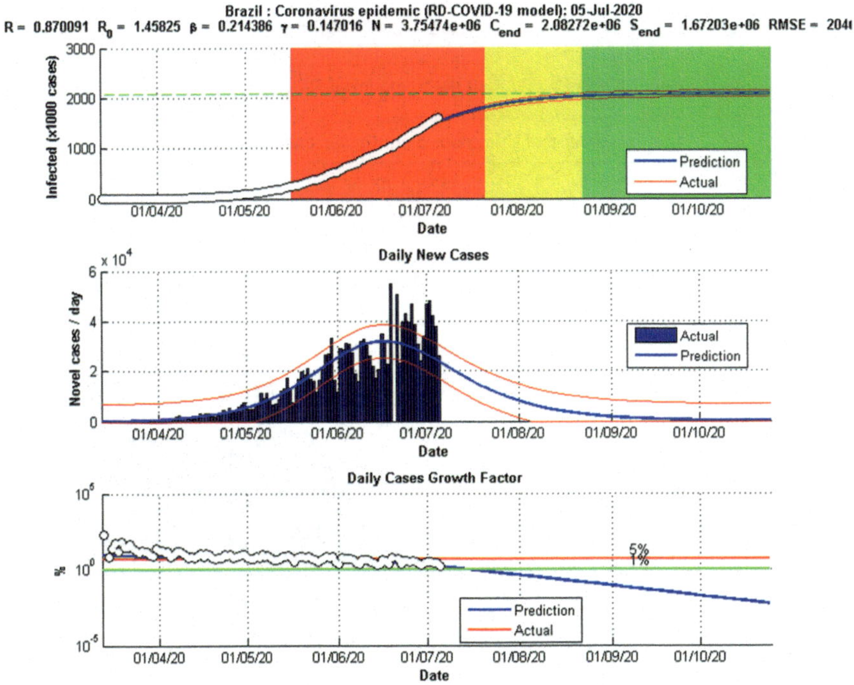

Fig. 23 Epidemic trend of Coronavirus outbreak in Brazil

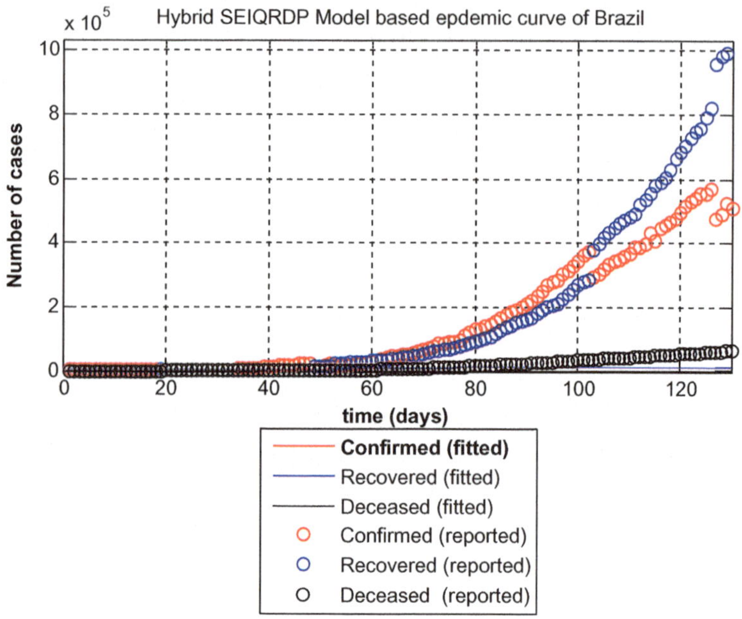

Fig. 24 Numerical simulation of Node SEIQRDP model of RD-Covid-19 (Brazil)

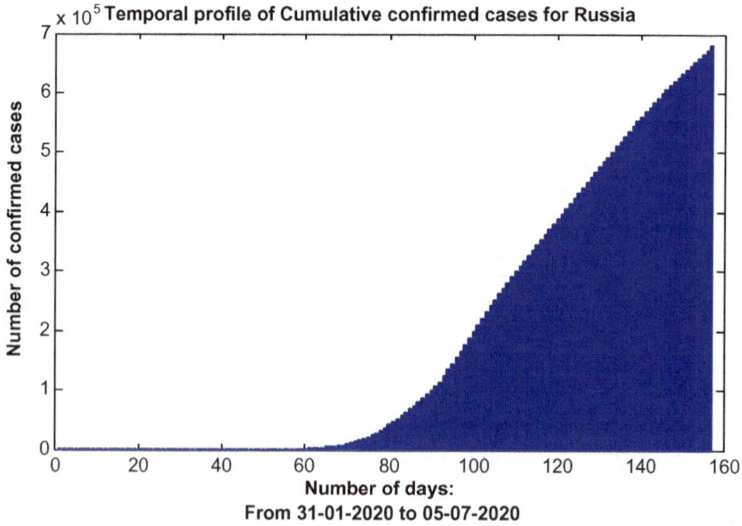

Fig. 25 Temporal profile of Cumulative confirmed cases in Russia

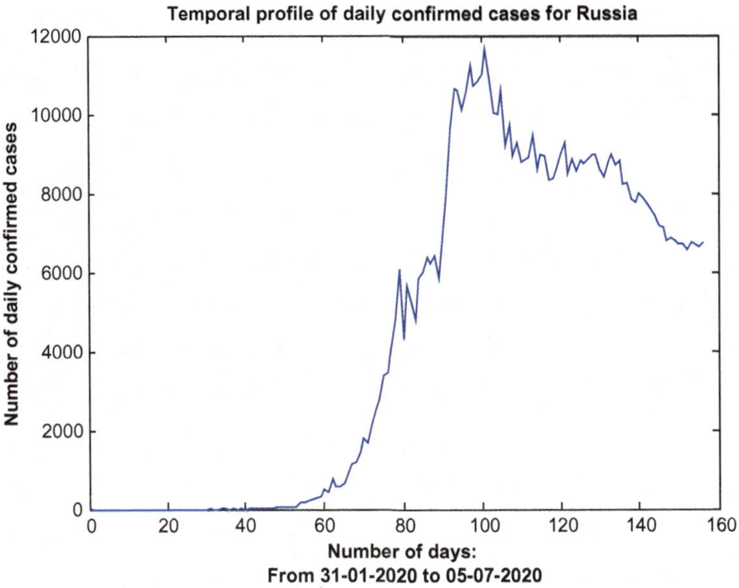

Fig. 26 Temporal profile of daily confirmed cases in Russia

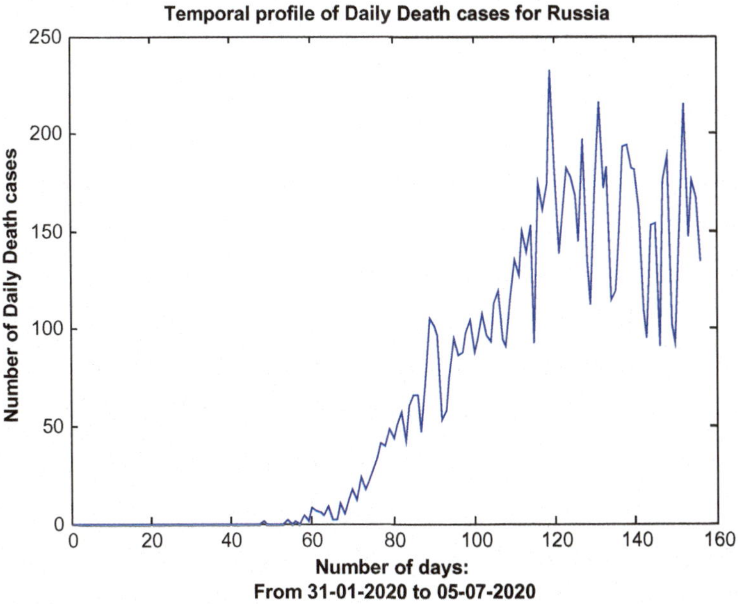

Fig. 27 Temporal profile of daily death cases in Russia

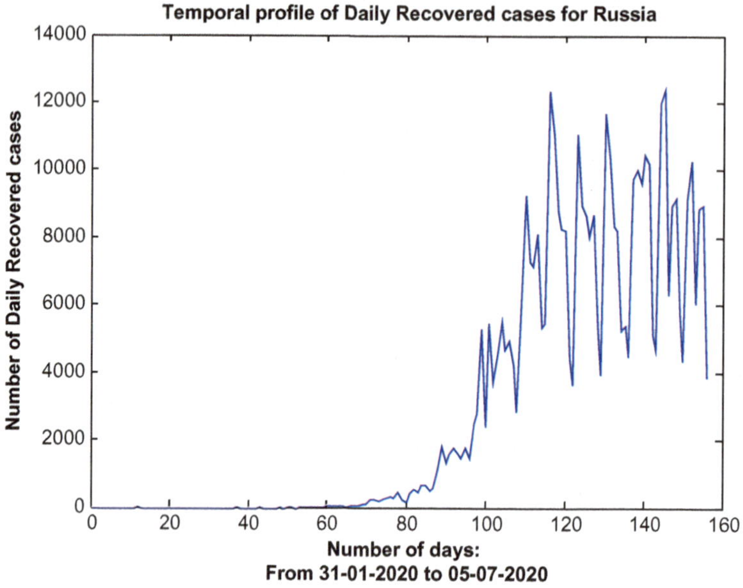

Fig. 28 Temporal profile of daily recovered cases in Russia

8 Conclusions

Epidemiological modeling of infectious diseases like Covid-19 has been discussed in detail in this chapter. The chapter discusses various issues associated with the fundamental aspects of the epidemiology of infectious diseases such as contact rate, attack rate, probability of transmission, basic reproduction number, and dynamic growth. Each traditional epidemiological models in this direction are compartmental model, and their evolution are discussed in the chapter. Here, in this chapter, we have presented the design, development and numerical simulation of an innovative networked RD-Covid-19 model. Various traditional models such as SIR, SEIR, and SEIQRDP are networked or cascaded to develop this RD-Covid-19. In our RD-Covid-19 Model, we have demonstrated the technique of fitting of model parameters using a nonlinear least square optimization method wherein we have used the Levenberg–Marquardt algorithm. Initially, guess the value of the model parameters required for fitting (mainly, infection rate and recovery rate) are guessed and subsequently iterated and improved by a data driven logistic growth model (Monod Kinetic Growth Model). Subsequently, guess values are used as input to the various stages of the network so that parameters have improved at every stage. Hence, the final stage of the system of RD-Covid-19 Model (SEIQRDP) generated the optimal values of the fitted parameter. The profile of various states (infected, quarantined, recovered, etc.) of the model have been created by using the optimal values of the parameters. The severity of the model is presented by estimating the basic reproduction number, R_0. The epidemic trend of four countries, viz. India, China, Brazil, and Russia is generated as an outcome of RD-Covid-19 model. Results are in agreement with the result

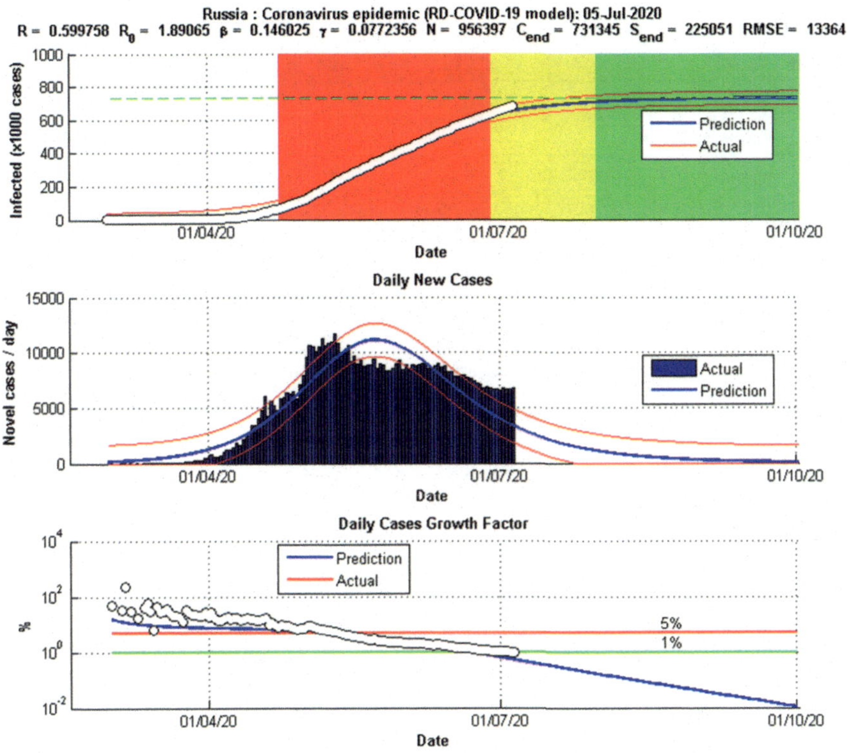

Fig. 29 Epidemic Trend of Coronavirus outbreak in Russia

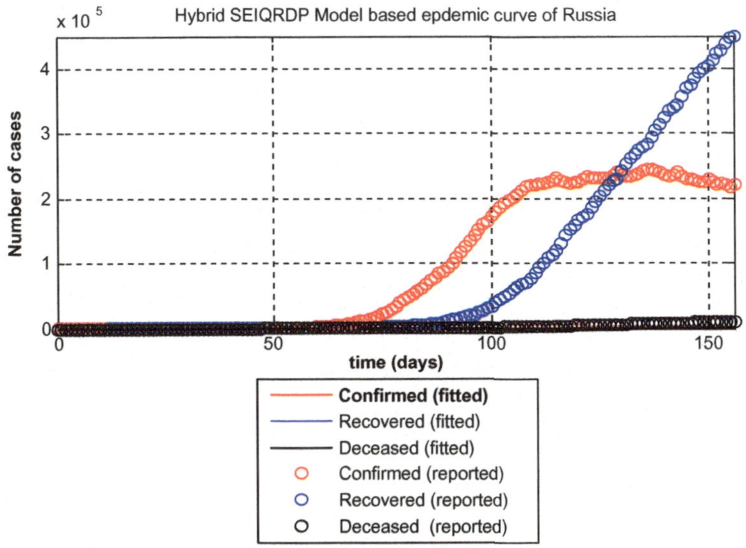

Fig. 30 Numerical simulation of Node SEIQRDP model of RD-Covid-19 (Russia)

Table 1 Fitted Value of Parameters of SEIQRDP node of RD-COVD-19 model

Event	China	India	Brazil	Russia
Fitted protection rate (alpha)	0.069	0.0116	0.0351	0.0208
Fitted infection rate (beta)	1.68	1.74	1.9279	1.4924
Fitted inverse of average latent time	0.68	0.0695	0.3327	0.2769
Fitted delta (rate of quarantine)	0.5937	0.27	0.3956	0.4333
Fitted recovery rate (lambda)	0.08	0.01	0.50	0.10
Fitted death rate (Kappa)	0.41	0.04	0.15	0.03

Table 2 Basic Reproduction number, Reproduction number and Herd Immunity

Event	China	India	Brazil	Russia
Basic reproduction number (R_0)	2.49	1.16	1.46	1.89
Reproduction number (R)	0.268	1.02	0.87	0.59
Herd immunity threshold	99.0	99.97	96.21	99.80

Table 3 Estimated duration of epidemic stage

Estimated duration (days)	China	India	Brazil	Russia
Turning day	17	158	109	84
Acceleration phase	7	39	31	30
Deceleration phase	9	41	35	36
Total growth phase duration	16	81	65	66
Total epidemic duration	92	461	388	388

Table 4 Estimated datum of epidemic stage

Estimated datum (Date)	China	India	Brazil	Russia
Outbreak	22-Jan-2020	30-Jan-2020	28-Feb-2020	31-Jan-2020
Start of acceleration	01-Feb-2020	30-May-2020	17-May-2020	24-Apr-2020
Turning point	08-Feb-2020	08-Jul-2020	16-Jun-2020	24-May-2020
Start of steady growth	17-Feb-2020	19-Aug-2020	21-Jul-2020	28-Jun-2020
Start of ending phase	25-Feb-2020	28-Sep-2020	23-Aug-2020	31-Jul-2020
End of epidemic (5 cases)	12-Apr-2020	03-Apr-2021	19-Feb-2021	15-Feb-2021
End of epidemic (1 case)	23-Apr-2020	07-May-2021	23-Mar-2021	24-Mar-2021

reported in the WHO dashboard. Future perspectives of this kind of study related to dynamic epidemiology will extend to compute risk management, including the cognitive behavior of humans facing this infectious disease under various control measures such as lockdown mainly and also social distance maintenance.

Table 5 Statistics of total and daily cases

	China	India	Brazil	Russia
Statistics (Total cases)				
Number of observations	166	156	129	127
Degrees of freedom	162	152	125	123
Root mean squared error	1924.35	5217.5	20,460.7	13,363.7
R^2	1	1	1	1
Adjusted R^2	1	1	1	1
F statistics vs. zero model	7997.59	58,808.5	21,400.2	12,597.6
p-value	9.01E-176	1.116E-112	3.058E-169	7.59E-153
Statistics (daily new cases)				
Number of observations	165	155	128	126
Degrees of freedom	161	151	124	122
Root mean squared error	1098.71	1025.52	6715.67	1502.51
R^2	1	1	1	1
Adjusted R^2	1	1	1	1
F statistics vs. zero model	65.79	1662.45	138.89	269.632
p-value	8.05E-28	2.15e-115	1.75E-39	1.21E-53

References

1. World Health Organization. WHO Statement January 19, 2020 Regarding Cluster of Pneumonia Cases in Wuhan, China, 2020. https://www.who.int/health-topics/coronavirus
2. World Health Organization. Novel Coronavirus—China. https://www.who.int/csr/don/12-january-2020-novel-coronavirus-china/en/
3. World Health Organization. Pneumonia of unknown cause—China 2020. https://www.who.int/csr/don/05-january-2020-pneumonia-of-unkowncause-china/en/
4. WHO. Novel Coronavirus(2019-nCoV) Situation Report—22
5. World Health Organization (WHO). Novel Coronavirus - Japan (ex-China). World Health Organization. cited January 20, 2020. https://www.who.int/csr/don/17-january-2020-novel-coronavirus-japan-ex-china/en/
6. World Health Organization (WHO). Middle East respiratory syndrome coronavirus (MERS-CoV) - update:2 December 2013. http://www.who.int/csr/don/2013_12_02/en/
7. Huang, C., et al.: Clinical features of patients infected with 2019 novel coronavirus in Wuhan, China. Lancet **395**(10223), 497–506 (2020). https://doi.org/10.1016/S0140-6736(20)30183-5
8. Huang, N.E., Qiao, F.: A data driven time-dependent transmission rate for tracking an epidemic: a case study of 2019-nCoV. Science Bulletin **65**, 425–427 (2020)
9. Ross, R.: "An application of the theory of probabilities in the study of a priori pathometry, part 1, proc. R Soc Series A **92**, 204–230 (1916)
10. Hethcote, H.W.: The Mathematics of Infectious Diseases. SIAM Rev. **42**(4), 599–653 (2000)
11. Brauer, F., Castillo-Chavez, C., Feng, Z.: Mathematical Models in Epidemiology. Springer, New York (2019)
12. Box, G.E.P., Cox, D.R.: An analysis of transformations. J. Roy. Stat. Soc. B **26**, 211–252 (1964)
13. Chen, T.-M., Rui, J., Wang, Q.-P., Zhao, Z.-Y., Cui, J.-A., Yin, L.: A mathematical model for simulating the phase-based transmissibility of a novel coronavirus. Infect. Dis. Poverty **9**(24), 1–8 (2020)

14. Chen, S.C., Chang, C.-F., Liao, C.-M.: Predictive models of control strategies involved in containing indoor airborne infections. Indoor Air **16**, 469–481 (2006)
15. Chen, N., et al.: Epidemiological and clinical characteristics of 99 cases of 2019 novel coronavirus pneumonia in Wuhan, China: a descriptive study. Lancet (2020). https://doi.org/10.1016/S0140-6736(20)30211-7
16. Rosenblum, M.A.: Corona theorem for countably many functions. Integral equations operator theory. **3**, 125–137 (1980)
17. Fuhrmann, P.A.: On the Corona Theorem and its Application to Spectral Problems in Hilbert Space. Trans. Am. Math. Soc. **132**(1), 55–66 (1968)
18. Wu, C.-Y., Jan, J.-T., Ma, S.-H., Kuo, C.-J., Juan, H.-F., Cheng, Y.-S.E., et al.: Small molecules targeting severe acute respiratory syndrome human coronavirus. Proceedings of National Academy of Sciences. **101**, 10012–10017 (2004)
19. Wu, J.T., Leung, K., Leung, G.M.: Nowcasting and forecasting the potential domestic and international spread of the 2019-nCoV outbreak originating in Wuhan, China: a modelling study. Lancet (London, England). **395**, 689–697 (2020)
20. Zhou, N., Pan, T., Zhang, J., Li, Q., Zhang, X., Bai, C., et al.: Glycopeptide Antibiotics Potently Inhibit Cathepsin L in the Late Endosome/Lysosome and Block the Entry of Ebola Virus, Middle East Respiratory Syndrome Coronavirus (MERS-CoV), and Severe Acute Respiratory Syndrome Coronavirus (SARS-CoV). J. Biol. Chem. **291**, 9218–9232 (2016)
21. Zhou, P., Yang, X.L., Wang, X.G., Hu, B., Zhang, L., Zhang, W., et al.: A pneumonia outbreak associated with a new coronavirus of probable bat origin. Nature **579**, 270–273 (2020)
22. Anastassopoulou, C., Russo, L., Tsakris, A., Siettos, C.: Data-based analysis, modelling and forecasting of the COVID-19 outbreak. PLoS ONE **15**(3), 1–21 (2020). https://doi.org/10.1101/2020.02.11.20022186
23. Bailey, N.T.J.: The Mathematical Theory of Infectious Diseases, 2nd edn. Hafner, New York (1975)
24. Bangia Aashima, Bhardwaj Rashmi and Jayakumar, K.V., (2020): River water quality estimation through Artificial Intelligence conjuncted with Wavelet Decomposition. 979. Numerical Optimization in Engineering and Sciences, pp 107–123. Springer. ISBN: 978–981–15–3214–6
25. Bhardwaj, R., Bangia, A.: Data Driven Estimation of Novel COVID-19 Transmission Risks through Hybrid Soft-Computing Techniques. Chaos, Soliton and Fractals. (2020). https://doi.org/10.1016/j.chaos.2020.110152
26. Bhardwaj, Rashmi and Datta, Debabrata (2020). Consensus Algorithm. 71, "Studies in Big Data" pp 91–107. ISBN: 978–3–030–38676–4. Springer
27. Bhardwaj, Rashmi. (2019). Nonlinear Time Series Analysis of Environment Pollutants. Mathematical Modeling on Real World Problems: Interdisciplinary Studies in Applied Mathematics. 71–102. Publisher: NOVA Publisher, New York, USA
28. Bhardwaj, Rashmi. (2016). Wavelets and Fractal Methods with environmental applications. Mathematical Models, Methods and Applications. pp. 173–195. ISBN: 978–981–287–971–4 Publisher: Springer Science + Business Media, Singapore
29. Bhardwaj, Rashmi; Bangia, Aashima and Mishra, Jyoti. (2020). Complexity Analysis of Pathogenesis of Coronavirus Epidemiology Spread in the China region. Mathematical Modelling and Soft Computing in Epidemiology, Taylor & Francis Publisher. Editors: Mishra Jyoti, Agarwal Ritu and Atangana Abdon
30. Bhardwaj, Shivam, Khanna Ashish and Gupta, Deepak (2020). "Water Quality Evaluation Using Soft Computing Method".. Advances in Intelligent Systems and Computing volume 1166. Editors. Deepak Gupta, Ashish Khanna, Siddhartha Bhattacharyya, Aboul Ella Hassanien, Sameer Anand, Ajay Jaiswal. Publisher: Springer
31. Chakraborty, T., Ghosh, I.: Real-time forecasts and risk assessment of novel coronavirus (COVID-19) cases: A data-driven analysis. Chaos, Solitons Fractals **135**(109850), 1–10 (2020)
32. Fang, Y., Nie, Y., Penny, M.: Transmission dynamics of the COVID-19 outbreak and effectiveness of government interventions: A data-driven analysis. J. Med. Virol. **92**, 645–659 (2020)

33. Kucharski, A.J., Russell, T.W., Diamond, C., Liu, Y., Edmunds, J., Funk, S., Eggo, R.M.: Early dynamics of Transmission and Control of COVID-19: A Mathematical Modelling Study. Lancet. Infect. Dis **20**(5), 553–558 (2020)
34. Melin, P., Monica, J.C., Sánchez, D., Castillo, O.: Analysis of Spatial Spread Relationships of Coronavirus (COVID-19) Pandemic in the World using Self Organizing Maps. Chaos, Solitons Fractals **138**, 109917–109917 (2020)
35. Pastor-, R., Vespignani, A.: Epidemic spreading in scale-free networks. Phys. Rev. Lett. **86**(14), 3200–3203 (2001)
36. Prem, K., Liu, Y., Russell, T.W., Kucharski, A.J., Eggo, R.M., Davies, N.: The effect of control strategies to reduce social mixing on outcomes of the COVID-19 epidemic in Wuhan, China: a modelling study. The Lancet Public Health. **5**(5), e261–e270 (2020)
37. Roda, W.C., Varughese, M.B., Han, D., Li, M.Y.: Why is it difficult to accurately predict the COVID-19 epidemic? Infectious Disease Modelling. **5**, 271–281 (2020)
38. Rustam, F., Reshi, A.A., Mehmood, A., Ullah, S., On, B.-W., Aslam, W., Choi, G.S.: COVID-19 Future Forecasting Using Supervised Machine Learning Models. IEEE Access **8**, 101489–101499 (2020)
39. Salgotra, R., Gandomi, M., Gandomi, A.H.: Time Series Analysis and Forecast of the COVID-19 Pandemic in India using Genetic Programming. Chaos, Solitons Fractals **138**(109945), 1–15 (2020)
40. Santosh, K.C.: AI-Driven Tools for Coronavirus Outbreak: Need of Active Learning and Cross-Population Train/Test Models on Multitudinal/Multimodal Data. J. Med. Syst. **44**, 1–5 (2020)
41. Sharma, S.K., Bhardwaj, S., Alowaidi, M., Bhardwaj, R.: Nonlinear Time series analysis of Pathogenesis of COVID-19 Epidemiology Spread in Saudi Arabia *Computers*. In press, Materials and Continua (2020)
42. Zhong, L., Mu, L., Li, J., Wang, J., Yin, Z., Liu, D.: Early Prediction of the 2019 Novel Coronavirus Outbreak in the Mainland China Based on Simple Mathematical Model. IEEE Access **8**, 51761–51769 (2020)
43. Acemoglu, Daron, Victor Chernozhukov, Iv´an Werning and Michael D. Whinston, (2020) "A Multi-Risk SIR Model with Optimally Targeted Lockdown," Technical Report, MIT 2020
44. Berger, David W, Kyle F Herkenhoff, and Simon Mongey, (2020) "An SEIR Infectious Disease Model with Testing and Conditional Quarantine," Working Paper 26901, National Bureau of Economic Research March 2020
45. Hui, D.S., et al.: The continuing 2019-nCoV epidemic threat of novel coronaviruses to global health—the latest 2019 novel coronavirus outbreak in Wuhan. China. Int. J. Infect. Dis. **91**, 264–266 (2020)
46. Kermack, William Ogilvy and A. G. McKendrick, (1927) "A contribution to the mathematical theory of epidemics, part I," Proceedings of the Royal Society of London. Series A, 115 (772), 700–721
47. Vynnycky, E., White, R.G. (eds.): An Introduction to Infectious Disease Modelling. Oxford University Press, Oxford (2010)
48. Li, Q., et al.: Early transmission dynamics in Wuhan, China, of novel coronavirus–infected pneumonia. N. Engl. J. Med. (2020). https://doi.org/10.1056/NEJMoa2001316
49. Gill, Philip E.; Murray, Walter (1978). "Algorithms for the solution of the nonlinear least-squares problem". SIAM Journal on Numerical Analysis. 15 (5): 977–992. Bibcode:1978SJNA...15..977G. https://doi.org/10.1137/0715063
50. Johns Hopkins University CSSE, "2019 Novel Coronavirus COVID-19 (2019-nCoV) Data Repository," 2020. Center for Systems Science and Engineering

Mediterranean Diet—A Healthy Dietary Pattern and Lifestyle for Strong Immunity

Anka Trajkovska Petkoska and Anita Trajkovska-Broach

Abstract The human health and the overall well-being are greatly affected by the individual's diet, lifestyle, age, and genetics, as well as the individual's response to stress, pathogens, and environmental pollution, which is mainly dictated by the immune system. A healthy gut microbiota plays a crucial role in the development and maintaining a healthy immune system. Numerous studies have shown that nutrients including vitamins, such as A, B6, B12, C, D, E, folate, and trace elements, such as zinc, iron, selenium, magnesium, and copper, and omega-3 fatty acids are complementary in maintaining a strong immune system. Besides nutrition, a healthy lifestyle including successful management of stress and anxiety, adequate sleep and rest, and physical activity are also crucial for boosting the immune system. A strong immune system would effectively respond to the attacks of pathogens (viruses, bacteria), such as the current *coronavirus* disease (Covid-19). The Mediterranean way of living seems an optimal dietary pattern and a lifestyle that could help in maintaining a healthy and diverse gut microbiota and thus strong immunity. Mediterranean diet is mainly a plant-based dietary pattern, which emphasizes consumption of fruits, vegetables, whole grains, nuts, legumes, and seeds followed by moderate consumption of fish, poultry, fermented dairy products, and extra virgin olive oil as a main source of healthy fats, while the use of processed red meat products and refined sugars is low. Plenty of water, fruit juices, and herb teas are also consumed with frequent, but moderate consumption of red wine usually with the meals. Taking rests, daily physical exercises, leisure, and social activities and be a part of the community are also common features of the Mediterranean lifestyle. Therefore, the Mediterranean diet rich in valuable phytonutrients, such as vitamins, minerals, dietary fibers, and antioxidant polyphenols, along with social aspects of the diet could help building a healthy gut and a strong immune system to effectively respond to the Covid-19 pandemic.

A. Trajkovska Petkoska
Faculty of Technology and Technical Sciences-Veles, University St. Kliment Ohridski-Bitola, Bitola, North Macedonia

A. Trajkovska-Broach (✉)
CSI: Create. Solve. Innovate. LLC, 2020 Kraft Dr., Suite 3007, Blacksburg, VA 24060, USA
e-mail: anita@createsolveinnovate.com

P. Agarwal et al. (eds.), *Analysis of Infectious Disease Problems (Covid-19) and Their Global Impact*, Infosys Science Foundation Series,
https://doi.org/10.1007/978-981-16-2450-6_13

Keywords Healthy dietary pattern · Lifestyle · Immunity

1 Introduction

It is of a vital importance to maintain a strong human immune system, which can defend the body from viruses, bacteria, and other pathogens. With more than 70% of the immune system located in the gut, the gut microbiota is responsible for developing and supporting a healthy immune system. Suppressed immunity and inflammation, which occurs as the immune system's response to the external invaders (viruses, bacteria) and subsequent cells' injuries, have been implicated as causes of many serious diseases. In fact, several chronic metabolic disorders and health outcomes, such as obesity, metabolic syndrome (MS), type 2 diabetes, cardiovascular diseases (CVDs), depression, Alzheimer's disease (AD), and certain types of cancers start in the gut and further progress as a result of a long-term inflammation.

As the viral Covid-19 pandemic is an "on-going" treat around the globe and there is uncertainty when this pandemic would "end," strategies to strengthen the immunity have been mainly directed toward a healthy and balanced nutrition that could help boosting the immune system necessary for prevention and management of viral and bacterial infections. These dietary recommendations usually involve consumption of mainly plant-based foods, such as foods rich in dietary fibers (vegetables, fruits, grains), proteins (fish, seafood), probiotics-rich food (fermented products), healthy fats (fish, seafood), and others. All of them provide diverse nutrients, viz. vitamins A, B6, B12, C, D, E, and folate, trace elements, including zinc, iron, selenium, magnesium, and copper, and omega-3 fatty acids playing important and complementary roles in supporting the immune system. Avoiding ultra-processed food containing refined sugars, salt, and unhealthy fats, known to promote inflammatory processes, is also recommended [1–10]. Beside the dietary recommendations, confinement and social distancing have been suggested for reduced spreading of the pandemic. This kind of restrictions significantly modifies the lifestyles of individuals and whole communities. Lack of relationships and social interactions, limited opportunities than those experienced before the pandemic, changes in circadian rhythms, more sedentary lifestyles, and other lifestyle restrictions are increasing the risks of overweight and obesity, CVDs, metabolic diseases, and many other issues, are just few of the consequences of the confinement measures. Anxiety, fear, stress, uncertainty for the future, and many other issues, whose real health consequences are yet to be determined, are surfacing. Taking all these factors into account, experts are suggesting lifestyle recommendations, which could keep the immune system strong. Among them, staying physically active and hydrated, maintaining healthy weight, having adequate rest and night sleep, keeping the stress under control, maintaining the social interactions (even remotely), and having optimistic attitude and positive mindset have been linked to have positive effects on gut microbiota, and thus, on immunity [11–14].

All of these dietary and lifestyle guidelines for strengthening the human immunity are actually in line with most of the principles of the traditional Mediterranean lifestyle.

2 Mediterranean Lifestyle

Mediterranean lifestyle, in general, refers to the traditional Mediterranean diet (MD) and the traditions of people living in the Mediterranean basin. It became a part of the UNESCO's intangible cultural heritage in 2010, where MD is defined as "*a set of skills, knowledge, rituals, symbols and traditions concerning crops, harvesting, fishing, animal husbandry, conservation, processing, cooking, and particularly the sharing and consumption of food*." Mediterranean lifestyle is often schematically presented as a MD pyramid, such as the one proposed by Oldways (Fig. 1) [15–18].

The MD pyramid (Fig. 1) is organized in a way that the foods consumed daily and in abundance are located in the base of the pyramid, followed by those that are moderately consumed, while the food items eaten in limited amounts or occasionally are at the top. MD emphasizes the use of plant-derived foods; in particular, daily consumption involves plenty of fruits and vegetables, whole grains, legumes, nuts,

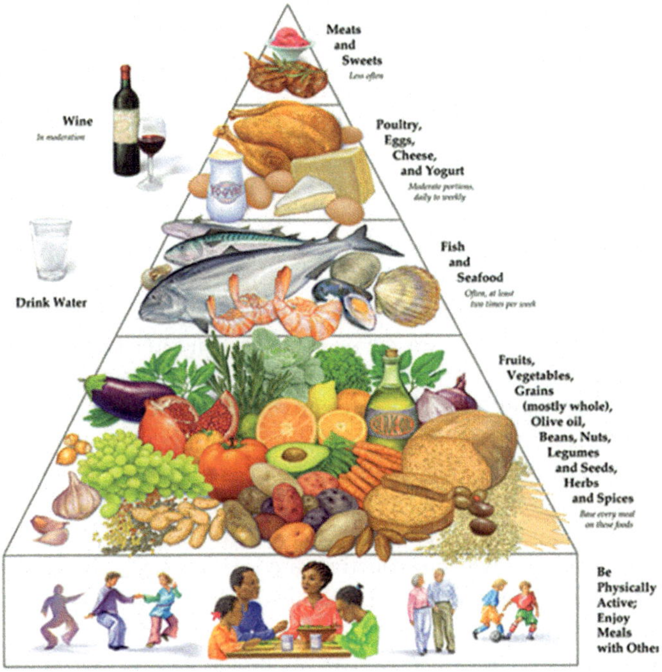

Fig. 1 Mediterranean Diet Pyramid (© *2009 Oldways Preservation and Exchange Trust*)

and seeds, extra virgin olive oil (EVOO), along with a moderate use (several times per week) of fermented milk products (sour milk, yogurt, cheese, curds), fish, poultry, lean red meat, and eggs while limited use, or use in special occasions (once–twice a week, or holidays) involves refined carbohydrates (sweets, cakes), and processed red meat products. Water, no sugar-added fruit juices, teas, soups, and broths are usually used to keep a good hydration during the day. Moderate red wine consumption with the meals is common in some of the Mediterranean countries depending on the religious beliefs.

The plant origin of the food in MD, rich in dietary fibers, antioxidants (polyphenols), vitamins, and minerals coupled with the probiotics, has been found to be responsible for the overall well-being of the people adhering to this diet and their reduced risks for many chronic diseases.

Seasonal plant-based foods, such as fruits and vegetables, whole grains, legumes, nuts, and seeds, are in the base of the pyramid, meaning their frequent consumption in abundance every day. The complex mixtures of phytochemicals found in the plants, i.e., in their roots, seeds, leaves, flowers, and fruits, give them their unique color, smell, and flavor, as well as dictate their bioactivities and bioavailability within the gut. Consuming variety of "bright colors and textures," i.e., a rainbow of colored fresh vegetables and fruits is usually recommended to ensure a broad spectrum of protective phytochemicals. For instance, vegetables are important sources of polyphenolic compounds (e.g., flavonols, flavones, stilbenes, etc.), dietary fibers, vitamins A, C, K, E, B6, folate, copper, potassium, magnesium, iron, and choline among many others. These phytochemicals have been proven to provide antimicrobial, anti-inflammatory, and antioxidant activities within the body. Moreover, the richness of the plants in dietary fibers promotes the feeling of satiety—the feeling of being and staying full for a longer time, which is good for the gut, digestion, and maintaining a healthy weight [19–24]

The phytochemicals, viz. polyphenols, carotenoids, tocopherols, tocotrienols, glutathione, vitamins, and enzymes, protect the cell damage from oxidative stress. The oxidative stress is a result of the generation of oxidative species (free radicals, reactive oxygen, and reactive nitrogen species) in the body, which is usually triggered by unhealthy diets and external factors, such as smoke, pollution, chemicals, drugs, and UV rays. The oxidative stress causes structural and functional damages of the main biomolecules in the body, including DNA, lipids, and proteins and has been implicated in the pathogenesis of many chronic degenerative diseases, inflammation, neurodegenerative disorders, and aging processes. In particular, the imbalance between the production of oxidative species in the body and the antioxidant defense could lead to many pathological situations (diseases). To counteract this oxidative stress caused by the reactive species, the body needs various types of antioxidants. The body fights with its own anti-oxidative defense mechanism, but de novo antioxidants' production in the human cells is limited. Therefore, it needs a continuous supply of external antioxidants, which to ensure better health is preferred to come from the diet (dietary antioxidants). The traditional MD is rich in antioxidants, such as vitamins (β-carotene, vitamin C, and vitamin E), natural folate, polyphenols (flavonoids), carotenoids, and selenium. Many of the MD food phytochemicals are also anti-inflammatory in nature and, thus, do not support the generation of pro-inflammatory molecules in the body [22, 24]. Representative food produces often used in the MD along with their phytonutrients are shown in Fig. 2.

The hallmark of MD, extra virgin olive oil (EVOO), is a main source of dietary lipids in the traditional MD. Its unique composition, the fatty acid composition, and the richness with bioavailable polyphenols give EVOO the health protective benefits and its resistance to elevated temperatures, which makes it a good candidate for both cooking and salad dressings. EVOO as one of the most studied oils to date has been associated with extended life expectancy and reduction of the risks of many age-related degenerative diseases. Reduction of the oxidative stress and suppression of chronic inflammation have been associated with EVOO in relation to the modulation of the aging processes and promotion of healthy aging. Moreover, EVOO has been reported to be inversely associated with the risks for several cancers and CVDs, as well as to positively affect blood lipids (i.e., cholesterol and triglyceride levels). All these benefits are due to the richness of the EVOO with valuable bioavailable phytochemicals, such as the optimal fatty acid profile, especially monounsaturated fatty acids (MUFA), viz. oleic, palmitic, linoleic, and a-linoleic acid, tocopherols (vitamin E), beta-carotene, and variety of polyphenols. Diversity of the polyphenols phenolic acids (caffeic, p-cumaric, ferulic acid), phenolic alcohols (hydroxytyrosol, tyrosol), secoiridoids (oleuropein), flavonoids (quercetin, luteolin, apigenin), lignans, and others, gives EVOO a strong anti-oxidative activity, capable of scavenging oxidative species, increasing cellular endogenous antioxidant defenses, and, thus, reducing the oxidative stress in the body [25–35].

Furthermore, the cooking practices are usually minimal, i.e., done in a way that does not destroy the nutritional profile of the used ingredients. Traditionally, in the Mediterranean cuisine, the vegetables along with herbs and spices are cooked in EVOO, namely onions (and garlic) cooked in EVOO are the base for many sauces and Mediterranean dishes, where the preparation process actually amplifies the nutritional value (the antioxidant capacity) of the sauce or the dish compared to that of the raw ingredients. The typical Mediterranean dish, tomato sofrito, for example, is rich with bioavailable lycopene, which is transformed from its natural form in the tomato by the cooking procedure in EVOO and the presence of onions, garlic, and herbs [36–40].

In addition, the food preparation and consuming the meals together with family and friends are common habits in the Mediterranean area. Adequate sleep, taking rests during the day, daily physical and leisure activities, and being a part of the community are features of the Mediterranean way of living, as well. The socializing aspect and the other characteristics of MD like moderate intake of red wine have been associated with the longevity and reduced risk of many diseases of the people living in the Mediterranean basin [41–48]. It is proven that red wine positively affects health and longevity due to its polyphenol (resveratrol) content [49–52].

Mediterranean way of living constitutes a set of lifestyle habits and behaviors, which have been associated with a better cognitive performance, well-being, and overall health of the people adhering to this lifestyle. In particular, the social interactions, the social support and the sense of community, the group participation in leisure and physical activities, and the adequate rest and sleep patterns have proven positive

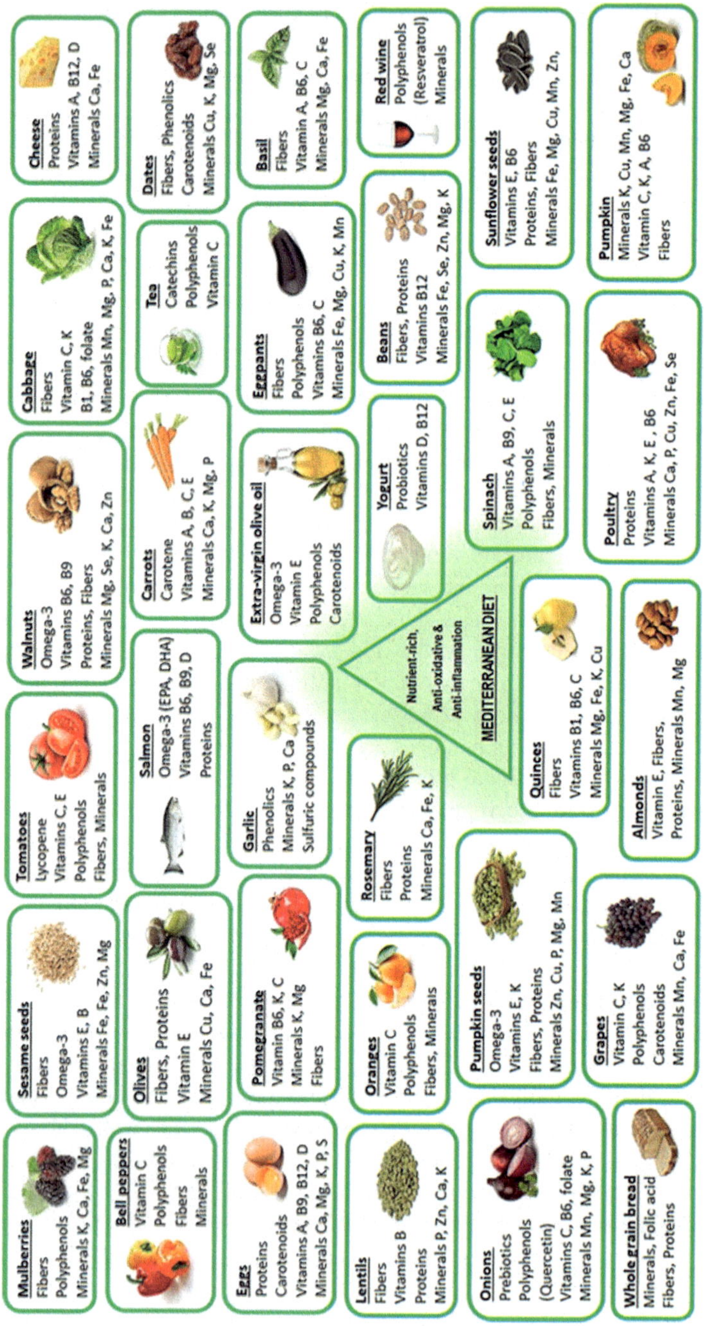

Fig. 2 Selected typical foods in the Mediterranean diet with their nutrients

effects on cognition [53–59]. The MD has been evolved over centuries by mostly "poor" people in the Mediterranean area working hard to produce food in mainly bad terrains for survival. Such hard work included a lot of physical activity with the crops in the "fields" and/or taking care of the farm animals [60–64]. The physical activity in combination with moderate portions of foods with different nutrients could yield healthy weight in people adhering to MD [65–67].

Although MD differs from country to country in terms of food choices and cooking practices, religious beliefs, and other traditions, it has a common set of features capturing the dietary and lifestyle habits of the people around the Mediterranean Sea. From a dietary aspect, MD is mostly a plant-based dietary pattern, which emphasizes consumption of fruits, vegetables, whole grains, nuts, legumes, and seeds, followed by moderate consumption of fish, poultry, fermented dairy products, and extra virgin olive oil as a main source of healthy fats, while the consumption of processed red meat products and products with refined sugars is limited. Daily intake of plenty of water, non-sugary drinks (juices, herbal teas), fermented drinks (yogurt), coffee, broths, and different soups is frequently consumed in the traditional MD during the day; hydration is important for an optimal health [68–70].

Overall, the nutritional value of the MD along with its associated social lifestyle aspects adds to a better management of stresses, reducing the sense of loneliness and isolation and increasing the sense of self-worth and the sense of contributing to the community, all together positively affecting the human health, mood, and cognitive functions.

3 Benefits of Mediterranean Diet

The health benefits of people adhering to the traditional Mediterranean diet were first reported in the seven countries study by Dr. Keys. Originally, MD was linked to significantly reduced rates of CVDs observed among the people residing in the Mediterranean region, but over the years MD has been also linked to reduced rates of many other chronic diseases, viz. several types of cancers [71–77], MS [77–80], obesity [74], diabetes [81–83], atherosclerosis] [84], cognitive impairment [85–90], depression] [43, 91–94], CVD [94–102], and other neurodegenerative disorders (AD, Parkinson's disease, PD) [103–105], as well as higher life expectancy in the Mediterranean populations compared to other population [93, 106–120].

Figure 3 summarizes the most important phytochemicals found in the traditional MD, which are responsible for the protective effects against multiple diseases, and the benefits that people enjoy by adhering to this diet.

The health benefits of MD have been mainly associated with the high intake of unprocessed nutrient-rich plant-based foods. In particular, the crucial dietary components of MD believed to be responsible for its health benefits are as follows: long-chain omega-3 fatty acids originating mainly from fresh fish, EVOO, nuts, and seeds; variety of powerful antioxidants, especially polyphenols (quercetin, resveratrol, hydroxytyrosol) originating from vegetables, fruits, EVOO, red wine, tea, etc.,

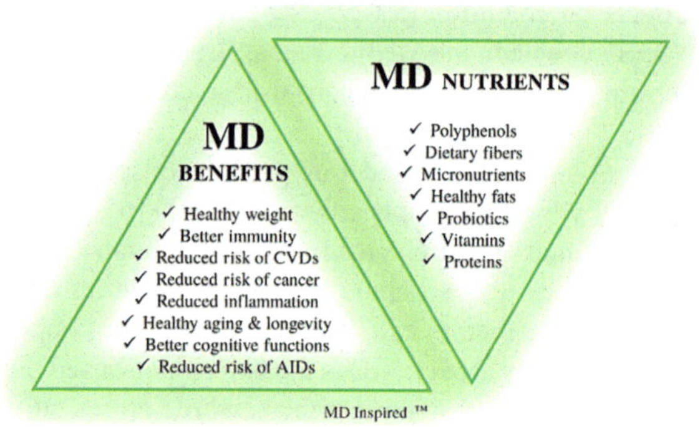

Fig. 3 Benefits of Mediterranean lifestyle: phytochemicals frequently found in Mediterranean diet could protect from a number of diseases

probiotics originating from fermented milk products (yogurt, sour curds, cheeses) and fermented vegetables; vitamins (A, D, E, C, B6, B9, B12), minerals (zinc, iron, selenium, magnesium, manganese), and other phytonutrients (carotenoids-lycopene) having strong antioxidant and anti-inflammatory activities originating from vegetables, fruits, herbs, and spices. Many institutions, like UNICEF, FAO, and WHO, also recommend the same nutrients in the current pandemic situation [121]. Recent studies have pointed out all of these MD nutrients as very beneficial in the fight against *coronavirus* [122–126]. In addition, two studies have linked the protective effects of the MD with its positive changes on the gut microbiota; in particular, participants adhering to the MD were found to have richer populations of beneficial bacteria and reduced pathogenic bacteria in their guts compared to the controls [127, 128].

4 Mediterranean Diet for a Healthy Gut

The human gut microbial communities are a mixture of different microorganisms collectively called the gut microbiota or "gut flora." The gut is comparable to an organ, because it contributes directly and/or indirectly in various vital physiological functions necessary for survival. Some of these functions include immunity, metabolism, fertility, development, aging, and antioxidant activities which promote health and fitness. A rich and diverse microbial community results in a balanced and healthy gut microbiota composition leading to an optimal host's health and well-being. This state of a healthy and balanced microbiota ecosystem, called *eubiosis,* is essential for proper metabolism of different dietary components, extraction of the nutrients, and their supply to the body. The microbiota ecosystem starts developing from early stages of life, with the baby's delivery and feeding practices, and is changing throughout the life depending on the lifestyle and habits, the environment, the antibiotics (and other drugs) use, and mostly by the nutrition choices [129–133].

Disruption and imbalance of the microbiota, known as *dysbiosis*, in most cases are characterized as a pathogenic state of the gut or gut with diminished microbiota. It usually happens via a loss of beneficial bacteria, overgrowth of harmful bacteria, and/or loss of the microbial diversity in the gut. In any case, it has been implicated as origin of many conditions and diseases, including MS [134], CVD [135, 136], obesity [137], autoimmune diseases (AID) [138], inflammatory bowel diseases (IBD) [139–141], and certain types of cancers [142]. The bidirectional communication between the gut microbiota and the brain, well-known as the *gut–brain axis*, has been shown to play a key role also in several neurological disorders, such as depression, AD, PD, autism spectrum disorders, and others [143–158].

The gut–brain axis is a complex communication system, which among others include the immune system. As it is known, the immune system protects the body by using both the innate and adaptive immune systems. More specifically, the innate immune system is comprising the physical barriers (skin, epithelial lining in gastrointestinal tract and respiratory tract) and the biochemical barriers (secretions and mucus), while the adaptive immune system consists of numerous different immune cells and antibodies. Depending on the nature of the insult (pathogen), certain levels of defense are triggered, and in general the innate immune system is activated first. If the pathogen manages to avoid the innate defenses, then the more complex, adaptive response is triggered, which produce antibodies to target and destroy the pathogen. The gut–brain communication is influenced by the composition and diversity of the gut microbiota, hormones, and immune- and neuropeptides produced in the gut, but also by the integrity of the intestinal wall serving as the physical barrier to the external environment. The integrity of this intestinal wall as a part of the gut mucosa is a functional barrier which controls the transfer of the nutrients through the intestinal wall into the bloodstream and defending the body from the penetration of unwanted dangerous molecules. The gut mucosa is a multilayered system consisting of an external "anatomical" barrier and an inner "functional" immunological barrier. This deeper, inner barrier consists of a complex network of immune cells, which could contain up to 70% of the body's total number of immunocytes; thus, it is involved in the body's response to the attack of pathogens (viruses and bacteria). Therefore, keeping the integrity of the barrier walls and the gut mucosa is crucial [130, 142, 155–158].

If the integrity of gut mucosa is impaired by a poor diet and/or other external insults, a condition known as a "leaky" gut will allow the passage of undigested food particles, toxic waste, and harmful bacteria into the blood circulation and, therefore, could affect the physiological, behavioral, cognitive, and memory functions of the brain, contributing to chronic diseases, mental health conditions, and neuropsychiatric disorders. For instance, intestinal dysbiosis and mucosal surfaces with impaired microbiota function and diversity have been related to the pathogenesis of several AIDs.

Furthermore, a close relationship between inflammation and suppressed immunity for various inflammation-caused diseases has been established. Maintaining a strong immune system could lead to reduced inflammation in the body and that can result in reduced risk of these diseases. Inflammation is a biological response of the immune system to events triggered by a variety of factors, including pathogens (viruses, bacteria), damaged cells, ionized pollution, toxic compounds, smoke, alcohol, etc. Like the oxidative stress, and sometimes caused by it, inflammation is a major factor in the pathology of many chronic diseases including CVD, cancer [142], type 2 diabetes, MS, AD[159] and obesity [160, 161], among others. Several immune-mediated inflammatory diseases, such as RA, IBD [139], multiple sclerosis, systemic lupus erythematosus, and psoriasis, have been determined to originate from suppressed immunity [159–162].

In this context, consumption of ultra-processed food, such as processed red meat products, products with refined sugars (cakes, cookies, refined sweetened cereals), prepacked and ready-to-eat meals, energy drinks, carbonated beverages with artificial sweeteners, high-fat milk products, can lead to severe dysbiosis. High intake of processed food containing animal-derived proteins, saturated and trans fats, refined sugars and salt, and poor in nutrients, such as natural antioxidants, omega-3 fatty acids, and fiber content, could stimulate the growth of pathogenic bacteria on the account of beneficial bacteria, leading to potential alterations of the gut and the intestinal barrier. For instance, Westernized diets [163–165] comprising mainly processed food have been shown to enhance *Escherichia coli* colonization and associated inflammation in mice by altering the host mucus layer, increasing intestinal permeability, and impairing immune function. Moreover, such dietary patterns may cause the activation of the innate immune system, most likely by excessive production of pro-inflammatory cytokines and reduced production of anti-inflammatory cytokines. The impaired gut epithelial barrier and disturbances in the intestinal microbiota will eventually result in a chronic mucosal inflammation and subsequent increases in chronic non-communicable diseases, such as obesity, CVDs, AIDs, type 2 diabetes, and colon cancer [165–171].

On the other hand, the protective effects of the Mediterranean diet against chronic diseases are attributed to the cumulative synergistic and interactive combination of its nutrients. In the context of gut health, MD promotes diverse and rich microbiota, and these positive changes have been attributed to MD as a consistent source of key nutrients, including dietary fibers, omega-3 fatty acids, and crucial vitamins, such as vitamins C, B6, B9, B12, and D, and minerals such as zinc, copper, selenium, potassium, iron, manganese, and magnesium**.** The consumption of dietary fibers and plant proteins has also been associated with an increase of beneficial bacteria quantity stimulating short-chain fatty acids (SCFA) production and other associated metabolites. Human enzymes are not able to digest most complex carbohydrates of the dietary fibers, but instead these polysaccharides are metabolized by gut microbes which generate short-chain fatty acids (SCFAs), such as acetate, propionate, and butyrate; they are actually produced by certain classes of beneficial bacteria among which are *Bacteroides, Bifidobacterium, Clostridium, and Eubacterium Lactobacillus* and are playing roles in different relationships of the gut with other organs in the body [172].

Comparison of consumption level of certain foods in the Mediterranean and Western diets is given in Table 1.

Two recent randomized controlled trials are linking MD to the positive changes in the gut—a more stable gut ecosystem characterized with richer populations of the bacteria that produce beneficial metabolites (e.g., SCFAs) and reduced levels of pathogenic bacteria. This statement is consistent with a study, which reported

Table 1 Comparison of consumption level of certain foods in Mediterranean and Western diets

Food	Mediterranean	Western
Fruits and vegetables (fresh, minimum-processed)	High	Low
Whole grains (unrefined cereals, oats, brown rice)	High	Low
Legumes (beans, lentils, chickpeas)	High	Low
Nuts (walnuts, hazelnuts, pistachio, peanuts)	High	Low / Moderate
Fish, seafood (salmon, tuna, shellfish)	Moderate	N/A
Poultry (chicken, turkey)	Moderate	Moderate / High
Processed red meats (sausages, hamburgers)	Low	High
Refined sugars (sweets, sweetened beverages)	Low	High
Extra virgin olive oil	High	Low
Red wine	Moderate	N/A

that high adherence to MD is related to decreased counts of *E. coli,* a representative of the pathogenic bacterium, as well as increased ratio of a typical beneficial *Bifidobacteria:E. coli,* which is considered an important indicator for gut microbiota equilibrium and overall health [127, 128]. Another recent study showed that a high-fiber-rich MD tested against an animal fat-rich low-fiber diet can alter the human gut microbiome composition in just four days. The dietary pattern low in fiber and high in sugar and saturated fat shifts the microbiome toward a profile that has been associated with chronic metabolic diseases, whereas the MD rich in fiber, unsaturated healthy fats (MUFA), polyphenols, and other phytonutrients shift the microbiome and plasma microbial metabolites toward a gut microbial profile that has been associated with beneficial health effects [173].

Due to the high consumption of plant-based foods, significantly higher levels of total SCFAs as metabolic products of the dietary fibers have been detected in people with high-level adherence to MD than in people on Western diets. Furthermore, bioactive substances such as polyphenols—plant compounds abundant in the Mediterranean dietary pattern, have been associated with enhanced microbial diversity that correlates with improved mood, cognition, and cardiovascular health, as well as enhanced blood flow to the brain. Omega-3 fatty acids and micronutrients in MD appear to have the potential to reduce the systemic inflammation and reduce intestinal permeability and further promote the gut microbiota diversity and stability. Toribio-Mateas [174] even coined the phrase "*Mediterranean gut*" for a healthy and resilient gut with diverse microbiota like those found in people adhering to the MD [173, 175–184].

Several studies have proved MD as an anti-inflammatory diet showing evidence that it reduces systemic inflammation by promoting a healthy microbiota. When compared to diets comprising mostly animal-based products, MD has shown to significantly reduce inflammatory biomarkers. MD as an anti-inflammatory diet is being also recommended to patients to enhance the effects of pharmacological therapies in treatment of several inflammatory diseases. For instance, MD has been shown to improve the quality of life and well-being of patients already having health issues, such as RA and irritable bowel disorder. MD can be neuroprotective, as well. Several dietary components consumed in the MD (omega-3 fatty acids, antioxidants) can inhibit neuro-inflammation processes associated with health-related outcomes, like AD [95, 185–194].

Chronic, systemic inflammation is believed to be one of the leading drivers of some of the most serious conditions, such as obesity, type 2 diabetes, MS, CVDs, AD, depression, and others. Obesity is a low-grade chronic inflammatory state that has been linked to an increased risk for viral and bacterial infections. In fact, the obesity can modify innate and adaptive immune responses, making the immune system more vulnerable to infections and less responsive to vaccinations, as well as can contribute to the onset of metabolic diseases. Therefore, maintaining a healthy weight can significantly benefit the immune system. A plant-based diet, like MD, is an effective diet for maintaining a healthy weight due to its abundance of dietary fibers, which helps the feeling of satiety, without adding extra calories [195].

Adequate sleep and undisturbed circadian rhythms are very important for maintaining strong immune system. Several studies have shown positive effects of MD on sleep patterns in different population groups [196–198]. Consuming foods containing tryptophan (roots, bananas, cherries, whole grain oats) during dinner time could improve the sleep quality. Tryptophan is an essential amino acid, which is actually involved in the metabolic production of serotonin and melatonin, important for the sleep quality. In fact, 95% of serotonin is produced and stored within the cells of gut [196].

Obviously, the interplay among the microbiota, genetics, age, diet, stress, physical activity, and environment is a complex process influencing both the mental and the physical health. By adopting a healthy diet and lifestyle, such as the Mediterranean way of living, healthy and diverse microbiota, strong immune system, and suppressed inflammatory processes are possible. It seems that the "*Mediterranean gut*" might be a solution to many metabolic diseases and mental disorders as well as a powerful weapon in the fight against Covid-19.

5 Conclusion

The discovery of high percentage of longer-living people with good cognitive functions and low incidence of cardiovascular, cancer, and metabolic diseases in the Mediterranean countries in 1960s, which was attributed to their diet and lifestyle, led to numerous studies on this diet making it one of the most studied diets in the world. The MD emphasizes consumption of fruits, vegetables, whole grains, legumes, nuts, seeds, and EVOO, while the consumption of animal-derived foods, such as processed red meat and products with refined sugars, is limited. Moderate consumption of fish, seafood, poultry, and fermented dairy and non-dairy products, sometimes accompanied with a glass of red wine, is also a characteristic of MD.

The efficacy of this diet has been attributed to its variety of nutrients and their anti-oxidative and anti-inflammation effects, which result in maintenance of a healthy gut and strong immune responses, and the overall good health in the Mediterranean populations.

To date, MD has been recognized as one of the healthiest dietary patterns in the world, not only due to its nutrient-packed dietary choices, but also due to the distinct lifestyle emphasizing conviviality, social interactions, adequate sleep, rest and leisure activities, and most importantly enjoying the life. Having positive mindset is what we need the most in this time of a worldwide pandemic. While social interactions are restricted at the moment, there are many ways that we could still stay socially connected, communicate with each other, take care, encourage and support each other, and, thus, experience the feeling of community—an important aspect of the Mediterranean way of living.

Mediterranean lifestyle is an affordable, easy-to-follow diet and habits for maintaining a healthy and resilient *"Mediterranean gut,"* which could protect us from infections and metabolic diseases. It has been also called an "*evergreen solution"* for optimal microbiota diversity and stability and even has been mentioned as a "*food pharmacy*" for immunological modulation through a diet [175, 176].

Moreover, MD is a remarkable representative of a sustainable food system (Fig. 4). It is a healthy diet that comprises the basic pillars of sustainability (environment, society, and economy) and is in line with the 17 Sustainable Development Goals (UN, 2015). The MD seems to be the best compromise between the need to reduce the environmental impact of food consumption and still maintains a healthy food consumption behavior. *A well fed nation is a healthy nation; it is a sustainable and productive nation* [199–205].

Hippocrates once said: *"Let food be thy medicine and medicine be thy food"*—this quote remains highly relevant after millennia. Surprisingly, the diet of his origin country—the Mediterranean diet—could be the perfect "medicine" that we all need

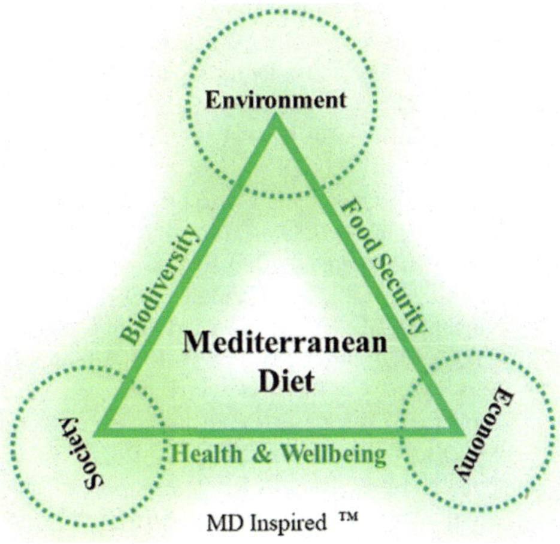

Fig. 4 MD positively affects the human health and well-being, society, economy, and environment, while maintaining the food security and biodiversity

today. With the Mediterranean healthy lifestyle and adequate nutrition, we could all emerge strong from the current pandemic situation and will be able to quickly adapt to "the new normal" life situations.

Acknowledgements The authors sincerely acknowledge the support of CSI: Create. Solve. Innovate. LLC and its MD Inspired™ concept for promoting the Mediterranean way of living outside the Mediterranean region.

References

1. Muscogiuri, G., Barrea, L., Savastano, S., Colao, A.: Nutritional recommendations for CoVID-19 quarantine. Eur. J. Clin. Nutr. **74**, 850–851 (2020). https://doi.org/10.1038/s41430-020-0635-2
2. Jayawardena, R., Sooriyaarachchi, P., Jeewandara, C., Ranasinghe, P.: Enhancing immunity in viral infections, with special emphasis on COVID-19: a review. Diabetes Metab. Syndr. **14**(4), 367–382 (2020). https://doi.org/10.1016/j.dsx.2020.04.015
3. Calder, P.C., Carr, A.C., Gombart, A.F., Eggersdorfer, M.: Optimal nutritional status for a well-functioning immune system is an important factor to protect against viral infections. Nutrients **12**(4), 1181 (2020). https://doi.org/10.3390/nu12041181
4. Gombart, A.F., Pierre, A., Maggini, S.: A review of micronutrients and the immune system - working in harmony to reduce the risk of infection. Nutrients **12**(1), 236 (2020). https://doi.org/10.3390/nu12010236
5. Islam, R., Parves, Md R., Paul, A. S., Uddin, N., Rahman, Md S., Al Malmun, A., Hosain Md Nayeem., Ali, Md A., Halim, M.A.: A molecular modeling approach to identify effective antiviral phytochemicals against the main protease of SARS-CoV-2. J. Biomol. Struct. Dyn., 1–12 (2020). DOI: https://doi.org/10.1080/07391102.2020.1761883.
6. Molloy, E.J., Murphy, N.: Vitamin D, Covid-19 and Children. Ir Med J. **113**(4), 59 (2020)
7. McCartney, D.M., Byrne, D.G.: Optimisation of Vitamin D status for enhanced immuno-protection against Covid-19. Ir Med J. **113**(4), 58 (2020)
8. Grant, W.B., Lahore, H., McDonell, S.L., Baggerly, C.A., French, C.B., Aliano, J.L., Bhattoa, H.P.: Evidence that Vitamin D supplementation could reduce risk of influenza and COVID-19 infections and deaths. Nutrients **12**(4), 988 (2020). https://doi.org/10.3390/nu12040988
9. Carr, A.C.: A new clinical trial to test high-dose vitamin C in patients with COVID-19. Crit. Care **24**, 133 (2020). DOI: https://doi.org/10.1186/s13054-020-02851-4.
10. Cheng, Z.R.: Can early and high intravenous dose of vitamin C prevent and treat coronavirus disease 2019 (COVID-19)? Medicine in Drug Discovery **5**,(2020). https://doi.org/10.1016/j.medidd.2020.100028
11. Galli, F., Reglero, G., Bartolini, D., Visioli, F.: Better prepare for the next one. Lifestyle lessons from the COVID-19 pandemic. Pharma Nutr. **12**, 100193 (2020). DOI: https://doi.org/10.1016/j.phanu.2020.100193.
12. Minni, A., Ralli, M., Candelori, F., Cialente, F., Ercoli, L., Parlapiano, C., Greco, A., De Vincentiis, M.: Lessons learned From COVID-19 pandemic in Italy. Bosn J. Basic Med. Sci. (2020). DOI: https://doi.org/10.17305/bjbms.2020.4847.
13. Muscogiuri, G., Pugliese, G., Barrea, L., Savastano, S., Colao, A.: Obesity: The "Achilles heel" for COVID-19? Metab., Clin. Exp. **108**,(2020). https://doi.org/10.1016/j.metabol.2020.154251
14. Conlon, M.A., Bird, A.R.: The impact of diet and lifestyle on gut microbiota and human health. Nutrients **7**(1), 17–44 (2015). https://doi.org/10.3390/nu7010017
15. https://oldwayspt.org/traditional-diets/mediterranean-diet. Accessed 16 June 2020

16. Willett, W.C., Sacks, F., Trichopoulou, A., Drescher, G., Ferro-Luzzi, A., Helsing, E., Trichopoulou, D.: Mediterranean diet pyramid: a cultural model for healthy eating. AJCN. **61**(6), 1402S-14066S (1995). https://doi.org/10.1093/ajcn/61.6.1402S
17. Bach-Faig, A.: Mediterranean diet pyramid today. Science and cultural updates, Public Health Nutrition **14**(12A), 2274–2284 (2011). https://doi.org/10.1017/S1368980011002515
18. Vitiello, V., Germani, A., Dolcetta, E.C., Donini, L.M., Del Balzo, V.: The new modern Mediterranean Diet Italian Pyramid. Ann Ig. **28**(3), 179–186 (2016). https://doi.org/10.7416/ai.2016.2096
19. Roman, G.C., Jackson, R.E., Gadhia, R., Roman, A.N., Reis, J.: Mediterranean diet: The role of long-chain v–3 fatty acids in fish; polyphenols in fruits, vegetables, cereals, coffee, tea, cacao and wine; probiotics and vitamins in prevention of stroke, age-related cognitive decline, and Alzheimer disease. Revue Neurologique **175**(10), 724–741 (2019). https://doi.org/10.1016/j.neurol.2019.08.005
20. Dreher, M.L., M. L. : Whole fruits and fruit fiber emerging health effects. Nutrients **10**(12), 1833 (2018). https://doi.org/10.3390/nu10121833
21. Alonso, A.: Fruit and vegetable consumption is inversely associated with blood pressure in a Mediterranean population with a high vegetable-fat intake: the Seguimiento Universidad de Navarra (SUN) Study. Br. J. Nutr. **92**(3), 311–319 (2004). https://doi.org/10.1079/BJN20041196
22. Leri, M., Scuto, M., Ontario, M.L., Calabrese, V., Calabrese, E.J., Bucciantini, M., Stefani, M.: Healthy effects of plant polyphenols: molecular mechanisms. Int. J. Mol. Sci. **21**, 1250 (2020). https://doi.org/10.3390/ijms21041250
23. Muralidharan, J., Galie, S., Hernandez-Alonso, P., Bullo, M., Salas-Salvado, J.: Plant-based fat, dietary patterns rich in vegetable fat and gut microbiota modulation. Front. Nutr. **6**, 157 (2019). https://doi.org/10.3389/fnut.2019.00157
24. Visioli, F., Galli, C.: The role of antioxidants in the Mediterranean diet. Lipids **36**(Suppl), S49-52 (2001). https://doi.org/10.1007/s11745-001-0682-z
25. Mazzocchi, A., Leone, L., Agostoni, C., Pali-Scholl, I.: The secrets of the Mediterranean Diet. Does [Only] Olive Oil Matter? Nutrients **11**(12), 2941 (2019). DOI: https://doi.org/10.3390/nu11122941.
26. Rossi, M., Caruso, F., Kwok, L., Lee, G., Caruso, A., Gionfra, F., Candelotti, E., Belli, S.L., Molasky, N., Raley-Susman, K.M., Leone, S., Filipsky, T., Tofani, D., Pedersen, J., Incerpi, S.: Protection by extra virgin olive oil against oxidative stress *in vitro* and *in vivo*. Chemical and biological studies on the health benefits due to a major component of the Mediterranean diet. PLOS ONE (2017). DOI: https://doi.org/10.1371/journal.pone.0189341.
27. Francisco V., Ruiz-Fernández, C., Lahera, V., Lago, F., Pino, J., Skaltsounis, L., Gonzalez-Gay, M.A., Mobasheri, A., Gomez, R., Scotece, M.'Gualillo, O.: Natural molecules for healthy lifestyles: Oleocanthal from extra virgin olive oil. J. Agric. Food Chem. **67**(14), 3845–3853 (2019). DOI: https://doi.org/10.1021/acs.jafc.8b06723.
28. Luisi, M.L.E., Lucarni, L., Biffi, B., Rafanelli, E., Pietramellara, G., Durante, M., Vidali, S., Provensi, G., Madiari, S., Gheri, C.F., Masini, E., Ceccherini, M.T.: Effect of Mediterranean diet enriched in high quality extra virgin olive oil on oxidative stress, inflammation and gut microbiota in obese and normal weight adult subjects. Front. Pharmacol. **10**, 1366 (2019). https://doi.org/10.3389/fphar.2019.01366
29. Sánchez-Villegas, A., Cabrera-Suárez, B., Molero, M., González-Pinto, A., Actis, C. C., Lahortiga-Ramos, F., Florido-Rodríguez, M., Vega-Pérez, P., Pia, J., M. J. Calviño-Cabada, M. J., Ortuno, F., Navarno, S., Almeida, Y., Hernández-Fleta, J.L.: Preventing the recurrence of depression with a Mediterranean diet supplemented with extra-virgin olive oil. The PREDI-DEP trial: study protocol. BMC Psychiatry **19**, 63 (2019). DOI: https://doi.org/10.1186/s12888-019-2036-4.
30. T. Wongwarawipat, T., Papageorgiou, N., Bertsias, D., Siasos, G., Tousoulis, D.: Olive Oil-related anti-inflammatory effects on atherosclerosis: potential clinical implications. Endocr. Metab. Immune Disord. Drug Targets. **18**(1), 51–62 (2018). DOI: https://doi.org/10.2174/1871530317666171116103618.

31. Fernandes, J., Fialho, M., Santos, R., Peixoto-Placido, C., Adeira, T., Sousa-Santos, N., Virgolino, Ana., Santos, O., Vaz Carneiro, A.: Is olive oil good for you? A systematic review and meta-analysis on anti-inflammatory benefits from regular dietary intake. Nutrition **69**, 110559 (2020). DOI: https://doi.org/10.1016/j.nut.2019.110559.
32. Cicerale, S., Lucas, L.J., Keast, R.S.J.: Antimicrobial, antioxidant and anti-inflammatory phenolic activities in extra virgin olive oil. Curr. Opin. Biotechnol. **23**(2), 129–135 (2012). https://doi.org/10.1016/j.copbio.2011.09.006
33. Serreli, G., Deiana, M.: Extra virgin olive oil polyphenols: modulation of cellular pathways related to oxidant species and inflammation in aging. Cells **9**(2), 478 (2020). https://doi.org/10.3390/cells9020478
34. Alkhatib, A., Tsang, C., Tuomilehto, J.: Olive oil nutraceuticals in the prevention and management of diabetes: from molecules to lifestyle. Int. J. Mol. Sci. **19**(7), 2024 (2018). https://doi.org/10.3390/ijms19072024
35. Lanza, B., Ninfali, P.: Antioxidants in extra virgin olive oil and table olives: connections between agriculture and processing for health choices. Antioxidants **9**(1), 41 (2020). https://doi.org/10.3390/antiox9010041
36. Ramírez-Anaya, J.P., Castañeda-Saucedo, M.C., Olalla-Herrera, M., Villalón-Mir, M., López-García de la Serrana, H., Samaniego-Sánchez, C.: Changes in the antioxidant properties of extra virgin olive oil after cooking typical Mediterranean vegetables. Antioxidants **8**(8), 246 (2019). DOI: https://doi.org/10.3390/antiox8080246.
37. Ramírez-Anaya, J.D., Samaniego-Sánchez, C., Castañeda-Saucedo, M.C., Villalón-Mir, M., López-García de la Serrana, H.: Phenols and the antioxidant capacity of Mediterranean vegetables prepared with extra virgin olive oil using different domestic cooking Techniques. Food Chem.**188**, 430–438 (2015). DOI: https://doi.org/10.1016/j.foodchem.2015.04.124.
38. Rinaldi de Alvarenga, J.F., Quifer-Rada, P., Juliano, F.F., Hurtado-Barroso, S., Illan, M., Torrado-Prat, X., Lamuela-Raventós, R.M.: Using extra virgin olive oil to cook vegetables enhances polyphenol and carotenoid extractability: a study applying the *sofrito* technique. Molecules **19**, 24(8), 1555 (2019). DOI: https://doi.org/10.3390/molecules24081555.
39. Rinaldi de Alvarenga, J. F., Tran, C., Hurtado-Barroso, S., Martinez-Huélamo, M., Illan, M., Lamuela-Raventos, R. M. Home cooking and ingredient synergism improve lycopene isomer production in Sofrito. *Food Res Int.* **2017**, 99(Pt 2), 851–861. DOI: https://doi.org/10.1016/j.foodres.2017.01.009.
40. Rinaldi de Alvarenga, J.F., Quifer-Rada, P., Westrin, V., Hurtado-Barroso, S., Torrado-Prat, X., Lamuela-Raventós, R.M.: Mediterranean Sofrito home-cooking technique enhances polyphenol content in tomato sauce. J. Sci. Food Agric. **99**(14), 6535–6545 (2019). DOI: https://doi.org/10.1002/jsfa.9934.
41. Diolintzi, A., Panagiotakos, D.B., Sidossis, L.S.: From Mediterranean diet to Mediterranean lifestyle: a narrative review. Public Health Nutr. **22**(14), 2703–2713 (2019). https://doi.org/10.1017/S1368980019000612
42. Lacatus, C.M.: The Mediterranean diet: from an environment-driven food culture to an emerging medical prescription. Int. J. Environ. Res. Public Health **16**(6), 942 (2019). https://doi.org/10.3390/ijerph16060942
43. Yannakoulia, M., Kontogianni, M., Scarmeas, N.: Cognitive health and Mediterranean Diet: Just diet or lifestyle pattern? Ageing Res. Rev. **20**, 74–78 (2015). https://doi.org/10.1016/j.arr.2014.10.003
44. Castro-Quezada, I., Román-Viñas, B., Serra-Majem, L.: The Mediterranean diet and nutritional adequacy: a review. Nutrients **6**(1), 231–248 (2014). https://doi.org/10.3390/nu6010231
45. Radd-Vagenas, S., Kouris-Blazos, A., Singh, M.F., Flood, V.M.: Evolution of Mediterranean diets and cuisine: concepts and definitions. Asia Pac. J. Clin. Nutr. **26**(5), 749–763 (2017). https://doi.org/10.6133/apjcn.082016.06
46. Davis, C., Bryan, J., Hodgson, J., Murphy, K.: Definition of the Mediterranean diet: a literature review. Nutrients **7**(11), 9139–9153 (2015). https://doi.org/10.3390/nu7115459

47. Trichopoulou, A., Lagiou, P.: Healthy traditional Mediterranean diet: an expression of culture, history, and lifestyle. Nutr. Rev. **55**(11), 383–389 (1997). https://doi.org/10.1111/j.1753-4887.1997.tb01578.x
48. Ortega, R.M.: Importance of functional foods in the Mediterranean diet. Public Health Nutr. **9**(8A), 1136–1140 (2006). https://doi.org/10.1017/S1368980007668530
49. Guerrero R.F., Maria, C., García-Parrilla, M.C., Puertas, B., Cantos-Villar, E.: Wine, resveratrol and health: a review. Nat. Prod. Commun. **4**(5), 635–658 (2009). DOI: https://doi.org/10.1177/1934578X0900400503.
50. López-Miranda, V., Soto-Montenegro, M.L., Vera, G., Herradón, E., Desco, M., Abalo, R.: Resveratrol: a neuroprotective polyphenol in the Mediterranean diet. Rev. Neurol. **54**(6), 349–356 (2012). https://doi.org/10.33588/rn.5406.2011611
51. Artero, A., Artero, A., Tarin, J.J., Cano, A.: The impact of moderate wine consumption on health. Maturitas **80**(1), 3–13 (2015). https://doi.org/10.1016/j.maturitas.2014.09.007
52. Amor, S., Pauline Châlons, P., Aires, V., Delmas, D.: Polyphenol extracts from red wine and grapevine: potential effects on cancers. Diseases **6**(4), 106 (2018). https://doi.org/10.3390/diseases6040106
53. Chatzianagnostou, K., Del Turco, S., Pingitore, A., Sabatino, L., Vassalle, C.: The Mediterranean lifestyle as a non-pharmacological and natural antioxidant for healthy aging. Antioxidants (Basel). **4**(4), 719–736 (2015). https://doi.org/10.3390/antiox4040719
54. Alessia Cavaliere, Cavaliere, A., Elisa De Marchi, E., Banterle, A.: Exploring the adherence to the Mediterranean diet and its relationship with individual lifestyle: the role of healthy behaviors, Pro-Environmental Behaviors, Income, and Education. Nutrients **10**, 141 (2018). DOI: https://doi.org/10.3390/nu10020141.
55. Mamalaki, E., Anastasiou, C.A., Kosmidis, M.H., Dardiotis, E., Hadjigeorgiou, G.M., Sakka, P., Scarmeas, N., Yannakoulia, M.: Social life characteristics in relation to adherence to the Mediterranean diet in older adults: findings from the Hellenic Longitudinal Investigation of Aging and Diet (HELIAD) study. Public Health Nutr. **23**(3), 439–445 (2020). https://doi.org/10.1017/S1368980019002350
56. Mamalaki, E., Anastasiou, C.A., Ntanasi, E., Tsapanou, A., Kosmidis, M.H., Dardiotis, E., Hadjigeorgiou, G.M., Sakka, P., Scarmeas, N., Yannakoulia, M.: Associations between the Mediterranean diet and sleep in older adults: Results from the hellenic longitudinal investigation of aging and diet study. Geriatr Gerontol Int **18**(11), 1543–1548 (2018). https://doi.org/10.1111/ggi.13521
57. Jenny Theorell-Haglöw, J., Lemming, E.W., Michaëlsson, K., Elmståhl, S., Lind, L., Lindberg, E.: Sleep duration is associated with healthy diet scores and meal patterns: results from the population-based EpiHealth study. J. Clin. Sleep Med. **16**(1), 9–18 (2020). https://doi.org/10.5664/jcsm.8112
58. Godos, J., Ferri, R., Caraci, F., Cosentino, F.I.I., Castellano, S., Fabio Galvano, F., Grosso, G.: Adherence to the Mediterranean diet is associated with better sleep quality in italian adults. Nutrients **11**, 976 (2019). https://doi.org/10.3390/nu11050976
59. Foscolou, A., D'Cunha, N.M., Naumovski, N., Tyrovolas, S., Rallidis, L., Matalas, A.L., Polychronopoulos, E., Sidossis, L.S., Panagiotakos, D.: Midday napping and succesful aging in older people living in the mediterranean region: The epidemiological Mediterranean Islands Study (MEDIS). Brain Sci. **10**(1), 14 (2020). https://doi.org/10.3390/brainsci10010014
60. Alvarez-Alvarez, I., Zazpe, I., de Rojas, J.P., Bes-Rastrollo, M., Ruiz-Canela, M., Fernandez-Montero, A., Hidalgo-Santamaría, M., Martínez-González, M.A.: Mediterranean diet, physical activity and their combined effect on all-cause mortality: The Seguimiento Universidad de Navarra (SUN) cohort. Prev. Med. **106**, 45–52 (2018). https://doi.org/10.1016/j.ypmed.2017.09.021
61. Katsagoni, C.N., Psarra, G., Georgoulis, M., Tambalis, K., Panagiotakos, D.B., Sidossis, L.S.: High and moderate adherence to Mediterranean lifestyle is inversely associated with overweight, general and abdominal obesity in children and adolescents: The MediLIFE-index. Nutr. Res. **73**, 38–47 (2020). https://doi.org/10.1016/j.nutres.2019.09.009

62. Galan-Lopez, P., Ries, F., Gisladottir, T., Domínguez, R., Sánchez-Oliver, A.J.: Healthy lifestyle: relationship between Mediterranean diet, body composition and physical fitness in 13 to 16-years old icelandic students. Int. J. Environ. Res. Public Health **15**(12), 2632 (2018). https://doi.org/10.3390/ijerph15122632
63. Zapala, G., Buscemi, S., Mulè, S., La Verde, M., D'Urso, M., Corleo, D., Marranzano, M.: High adherence to Mediterranean diet, but not individual foods or nutrients, is associated with lower likelihood of being obese in a Mediterranean cohort. Eat Weight Disord. **23**(5), 605–614 (2018). https://doi.org/10.1007/s40519-017-0454-1
64. D'Innocenzo, S., Biagi, C., Lanari, M.: Obesity and the Mediterranean diet: a review of evidence of the role and sustainability of the Mediterranean diet. Nutrients **11**(6), 1306 (2019). https://doi.org/10.3390/nu11061306
65. Castro-Barquero, S., Lamuela-Raventós, R.M., Doménech, M., Estruch, R.: Relationship between Mediterranean Dietary Polyphenol Intake and Obesity. Nutrients **10**(10), 1523 (2018). https://doi.org/10.3390/nu10101523
66. Bacopoulou, F., Landis, G., Rentoumis, A., Tsitsika, A., Efthymiou, V.: Mediterranean diet decreases adolescent waist circumference. Eur. J. Clin. Invest. **47**(6), 447–455 (2017). https://doi.org/10.1111/eci.12760
67. Galan-Lopez, P., Sanchez-Oliver, A.J., Pihu, M., Gísladóttír, T., Domínguez, R., Ries, F.: Association between adherence to the Mediterranean diet and physical fitness with body composition parameters in 1717 European Adolescents: The AdolesHealth Study. Nutrients **12**(1), 77 (2020). https://doi.org/10.3390/nu12010077
68. Giacosa, A., Barale, R., Bavaresco, L., Faliva, M.A., Gerbi, V., La Vecchia, C., Negri, E., Opizzi, A., Perna, S., Pezzotti, M., Rondanelli, M.: Mediterranean way of drinking and longevity. Crit. Rev. Food Sci. Nutr. **56**(4), 635–640 (2016). https://doi.org/10.1080/10408398.2012.747484
69. Ditano-Vázquez, P., Torres-Peña, J.D., Galeano-Valle, F., Pérez-Caballero, A.I., Demelo-Rodríguez, P., Lopez-Miranda, J., N., Katsiki, N., Delgado-Lista, J., Alvarez-Sala-Walther, L.A.: The fluid aspect of the Mediterranean diet in the prevention and management of cardiovascular disease and diabetes: the role of polyphenol content in moderate consumption of wine and olive oil. Nutrients **11**(11), 2833 (2019). DOI: https://doi.org/10.3390/nu11112833.
70. Naumovski N., Foscolou, A., D'Cunha, N.M., Tyrovolas, S., Chrysohoou, C., Sidossis, L.S., Rallidis, L., Matalas, A.L., Polychronopoulos, E., Pitsavos, C., Panagiotakos, D.: The Association between Green and Black Tea consumption on successful aging: a combined analysis of the ATTICA and MEDiterranean ISlands (MEDIS) Epidemiological Studies. Molecules **24**(10) (2019). DOI: https://doi.org/10.3390/molecules24101862.
71. Hernáez, A., Estruch, R.: The Mediterranean diet and cancer: what do human and molecular studies have to say about It? Nutrients **11**, 2155 (2019). DOI:https://doi.org/10.3390/nu11092155.
72. Mentella, M. C., Scaldaferri, F., Ricci, C., Gasbarrini, A., Giacinto Abele Donato Miggiano, G.A.D.: Cancer and Mediterranean diet: a review. Nutrients **11**(9), 2059 (2019). DOI: https://doi.org/10.3390/nu11092059.
73. Martínez-Poveda, B., Torres-Vargas, J.A., del Carmen Ocaña, M., García-Caballero, M., Medina, M.A., Quesada, A.R.: The Mediterranean diet, a rich source of angiopreventive compounds in cancer. Nutrients **11**, 2036 (2019). https://doi.org/10.3390/nu11092036
74. Kwan, H.Y., Chao, X., Su, T., Fu, X., Tse, A.K.W., Fong, W.F., Yu, Z.L.: The anti-cancer and anti-obesity effects of Mediterranean diet. Crit. Rev. Food. Sci. Nutr. **57**(1), 82–94 (2017). https://doi.org/10.1080/10408398.2013.852510
75. Maruca, A., Catalano, R., Bagetta, D., Mesiti, F., Ambrosio, F.A., Romeo, I., Moraca, F., Rocca, R., Ortuso, F., Artese, A., Costa, G., Alcaro, S., Lupia, A.: The Mediterranean Diet as source of bioactive compounds with multi-targeting anti-cancer profile. Eur. J. Med. Chem. **181**,(2019). https://doi.org/10.1016/j.ejmech.2019.111579
76. Pauwels, E.K.J.: The protective effect of the Mediterranean Diet: focus on cancer and cardiovascular risk. Med. Princ. Pract. **20**(2), 103–111 (2011). https://doi.org/10.1159/000321197

77. Di Daniele, N., Noce, A., Vidiri, M.F., Moriconi, E., Marrone, G., Annicchiarico-Petruzzelli, M., D'Urso, G., Tesauro, M., Rovella, V., De Lorenzo, A.: Impact of Mediterranean diet on metabolic syndrome, cancer and longevity. Oncotarget **8**(5), 8947–8979 (2017). https://doi.org/10.18632/oncotarget.13553
78. Bagetta, D., Maruca, A., Lupia, A., Francesco Mesiti, F., Raffaella Catalano, R., Romeo, I., Moraca, F., Francesca Alessandra Ambrosio, F.A., Giosuè Costa, G., Anna Artese, A., Ortuso, F., Alcaro, S., Rocca, R.: Mediterranean products as promising source of multi-target agents in the treatment of metabolic syndrome. Eur. J. Med. Chem. **186**, 111903 (2019). DOI: https://doi.org/10.1016/j.ejmech.2019.111903.
79. Finicelli, M., Squillaro, T., Di Cristo, F., Di Salle, A., Melone, M.A.B., Galderisi, U., Peluso, G.: Metabolic syndrome, Mediterranean diet, and polyphenols: evidence and perspectives. J. Cell Physiol. **234**(5), 5807–5826 (2019). https://doi.org/10.1002/jcp.27506
80. Garcia, M., Bihuniak, J.D., Shook, J., Kenny, A., Kerstetter, J., Huedo-Medina, T.B.: The effect of the traditional Mediterranean-style diet on metabolic risk factors: a meta-analysis. Nutrients **8**(3), 168 (2016). https://doi.org/10.3390/nu8030168
81. Granado-Casas, M., Martin, M., Martínez-Alonso, M., Alcubierre, N., Hernández, M., Alonso, N., Castelblanco, E., Mauricio, D.: The Mediterranean diet is associated with an improved quality of life in adults with Type 1 diabetes. Nutrients **12**(1), 131 (2020). https://doi.org/10.3390/nu12010131
82. G.-Casas, M., Alcubierre, N., Martín, M., Real, J., Ramírez-Morros, A.M., Cuadrado, M., Alonso, N., Falguera, M., Hernández, M., Aguilera, E., Lecube, A., Castelblanco, E., Puig-Domingo, M., Mauricio, D.: Improved adherence to Mediterranean diet in adults with type 1 diabetes mellitus. Eur. J. Nutr. **58**(6), 2271–2279 (2019). DOI: https://doi.org/10.1007/s00394-018-1777-z.
83. Marta Guasch-Ferré, M., Merino, J., Sun, Q., Fitó, M., Salas-Salvadó, J.: Dietary polyphenols, Mediterranean diet, Prediabetes, and Type 2 diabetes: a narrative review of the evidence. Oxid. Med. Cell Longev., 6723931 (2017). DOI: https://doi.org/10.1155/2017/6723931.
84. Schwingshackl, L., Missbach, B., König, J., Hoffmann, G.: Adherence to a Mediterranean diet and risk of diabetes: a systematic review and meta-analysis. Public Health Nutr. **18**(7), 1292–1299 (2015). https://doi.org/10.1017/S1368980014001542
85. Medina-Remón, A., Casas, R., Tressserra-Rimbau, A., Ros, E., Martínez-González, M.A., Fitó, M., Corella, D., Salas-Salvadó, J., Lamuela-Raventos, R.M., Estruch, R.: Polyphenol intake from a Mediterranean diet decreases inflammatory biomarkers related to atherosclerosis: a substudy of the PREDIMED trial. Br. J. Clin. Pharmacol. **83**(1), 114–128 (2017). https://doi.org/10.1111/bcp.12986
86. Petersson, S.D., Philippou, E.: Mediterranean diet, cognitive function, and dementia: a systematic review of the evidence. Adv. Nutr. **7**(5), 889–904 (2016). https://doi.org/10.3945/an.116.012138
87. Solfrizzi, V., Panza, F.: Mediterranean diet and cognitive decline. A lesson from the whole-diet approach: what challenges lie ahead? J. Alzheimers Dis. **39**(2), 283–286 (2014). DOI: https://doi.org/10.3233/JAD-130831.
88. Frisardi, V., Panza, F., Seripa, D., Imbimbo, B.P., Vendemiale, G., Pilotto, A., Solfrizzi, V.: Nutraceutical properties of mediterranean diet and cognitive decline: possible underlying mechanisms. J. Alzheimer's Dis. **22**(3), 715–740 (2010). DOI: https://doi.org/10.3233/JAD-2010-100942.
89. Aridi, Y.S., Walker, J.L., L Wright, O.R.L.: The association between the Mediterranean dietary pattern and cognitive health: a systematic review. Nutrients **9**(7), 674 (2017). DOI: https://doi.org/10.3390/nu9070674.
90. Feart, C., Samieri, C., Barberger-Gateau, P.: Mediterranean diet and cognitive health: an update of available knowledge. Curr. Opin. Clin. Nutr. Metab. Care. **18**(1), 51–62 (2015). https://doi.org/10.1097/MCO.0000000000000131
91. Yannakoulia, M., Kontogianni, M., Scarmeas, N.: Cognitive health and Mediterranean Diet: Just diet or lifestyle pattern? Ageing Res. Rev.**20**, 74–78 (2015). DOI: https://doi.org/10.1016/j.arr.2014.10.003.

92. Sadeghi, O., Keshteli, A.H., Afshar, H., Esmaillzadeh, A., Adibi, P.: Adherence to Mediterranean dietary pattern is inversely associated with depression, anxiety and psychological distress. Nutr. Neurosci. **11**, 1–12 (2019). https://doi.org/10.1080/1028415X.2019.1620425
93. Karstens, A.J., Tussing-Humphreys, L., Zhan, L., Rajendran, N., Cohen, J., Dion, C., Zhou, X.J., Lamar, M.: Associations of the Mediterranean diet with cognitive and neuroimaging phenotypes of dementia in healthy older adults. Am. J. Clin. Nutr. **109**(2), 361–368 (2019). https://doi.org/10.1093/ajcn/nqy275
94. Shafiei, F., Salari-Moghaddam, A., Larijani, B., Esmaillzadeh, A.: Adherence to the Mediterranean diet and risk of depression: a systematic review and updated meta-analysis of observational studies. Nutr. Rev. **77**(4), 230–239 (2019). https://doi.org/10.1093/nutrit/nuy070
95. Martínez-González, M.A., Gea, A., Ruiz-Canela, M.: The Mediterranean diet and cardiovascular health. A Critical Review. Circul. Res. **124**(5), 779–798 (2019). https://doi.org/10.1161/CIRCRESAHA.118.313348
96. Razquin, C., Martinez-Gonzalez, M.A.: A traditional mediterranean diet effectively reduces inflammation and improves cardiovascular health. Nutrients **11**(8), 1842 (2019). https://doi.org/10.3390/nu11081842
97. Minelli, P., Montinari, M.R.: The mediterranean diet and cardioprotection: historical overview and current research. J. Multidiscip. Healthc. **12**, 805–815 (2019). https://doi.org/10.2147/JMDH.S219875
98. Franquesa, M., Pujol-Busquets, G., García-Fernández, E., Rico, L., Shamirian-Pulido, L., Aguilar-Martínez, A., Medina, F.X., Serra-Majem, L.'; Bach-Faig, A.: Mediterranean diet and Cardiodiabesity: a systematic review through evidence-based answers to key clinical questions. Nutrients **11**(3), 655 (2019). DOI: https://doi.org/10.3390/nu11030655.
99. Martinez-Gonzaleza, M.A., Bes-Rastrollo, M.: Dietary patterns, Mediterranean diet, and cardiovascular disease. Curr. Opin. Lipidol. **25**(1), 20–26 (2014). https://doi.org/10.1097/MOL.0000000000000044
100. D'Almeida, K.S.M., Spillere, S.R., Zuchinali, P., Souza, G.C.: Mediterranean diet and other dietary patterns in primary prevention of heart failure and changes in cardiac function markers: a systematic review. Nutrients **10**(1), 58 (2018). https://doi.org/10.3390/nu10010058
101. Li, J., Guasch-Ferré, M., Chung, W., Ruiz-Canela, M., Toledo, E., Corella, D., Bhupathiraju, S.N., Tobias, D. K., Tabung, F.K., Hu, J. Zhao, T., Turman, C., Anne Feng, Y.C., Clish, C.B., Mucci, L., Eliassen, A.H., Costenbader, K.H., Karlson, E. W., Wolpin, B.M., Ascherio, A., Rimm, E.B., Manson, J.E., Qi, L., Martínez-González, M.A., Salas-Salvadó, J., Hu, F.B., Liang, L.: The Mediterranean diet, plasma metabolome, and cardiovascular disease risk. Eur. Heart J. 0, 1–14 (2020). DOI: https://doi.org/10.1093/eurheartj/ehaa209.
102. Paterson, K.E., Myint, P. K., Jennings, A., Bain, L.K.M., Marleen A.H. Lentjes, M. A.H., Khaw, K. T., MBBChir; Welch, A.A.: Mediterranean Diet reduces risk of incident stroke in a population with varying cardiovascular disease risk profiles. Stroke **49**(10), 2415–2420 (2018). DOI: https://doi.org/10.1161/STROKEAHA.117.020258.
103. Gu, Y., Luchsinger, J.A., Stern, Y., Scarmeas, N.: Mediterranean diet, inflammatory and metabolic biomarkers, and risk of Alzheimer's disease. J. Alzheimers Dis. **22**(2), 483–492 (2010). https://doi.org/10.3233/JAD-2010-100897
104. Sofi, F., Macchi, C., Abbate, R., Gian Franco Gensini, G.F., Casini, A.: Effectiveness of the Mediterranean diet: can it help delay or prevent Alzheimer's Disease? J. Alzheimer's Dis. **20**(3), 795–801 (2010). DOI: https://doi.org/10.3233/JAD-2010-1418.
105. Cassani, E., Barichella, M., Ferri, V., Pinelli, G., Iorio, L., Bolliri, C., Caronni, S., Faierman, S.A., Mottolese, A., Pusani, C., Monajemi, F., Pasqua, M., Lubisco, A., Cereda, E., Frazzitta, G., Petroni, M.L., Pezzoli, G.: Dietary habits in Parkinson's disease: Adherence to Mediterranean Diet. Parkinsonism Relat. Disord. **42**, 40–46 (2017). https://doi.org/10.1016/j.parkreldis.2017.06.007
106. La Verde, M., Mulè, S., Zappalà, G., Privitera, G., Maugeri, G., Pecora, F., Marranzano, M.: Higher adherence to the Mediterranean diet is inversely associated with having hypertension: is low salt intake a mediating factor? Int. J. Food Sci. Nutr. **69**(2), 235–244 (2018). https://doi.org/10.1080/09637486.2017.1350941

107. De Pergola, G., D'Alessandro, A.: Influence of Mediterranean Diet on Blood Pressure. Nutrients **10**(11), 1700 (2018). https://doi.org/10.3390/nu10111700
108. Davis, C.R., Hodgson, J.M., Woodman, R., Bryan, J., Wilson, C., Murphy, K.J.: Mediterranean diet lowers blood pressure and improves endothelial function: results from the MedLey randomized intervention trial. Am J Clin Nutr. **105**(6), 1305–1313 (2017). https://doi.org/10.3945/ajcn.116.146803
109. Martini, D.: Health benefits of Mediterranean diet. Nutrients **11**(8), 1802 (2019). https://doi.org/10.3390/nu11081802
110. Cena, H., Calder, P.C.: Defining a healthy diet: evidence for the role of contemporary dietary patterns in health and disease. Nutrients **12**(2), 334 (2020). https://doi.org/10.3390/nu12020334
111. Serra-Majem, L., Román-Viñas, B., Sanchez-Villegas, A., Guasch-Ferré, M., Corella, D., La Vecchia, C.: Benefits of the Mediterranean diet: epidemiological and molecular aspects. Mol. Aspects Med. **67**, 1–55 (2019). https://doi.org/10.1016/j.mam.2019.06.001
112. Schwingshackl, L., Morze, J., Hoffmann, G.: Mediterranean diet and health status: active ingredients and pharmacological mechanisms. Br. J. Pharmacol. **177**(6), 1241–1257 (2019). https://doi.org/10.1111/bph.14778
113. Martınez-Gonzalez, M.A., Salas-Salvadó, J., Estruch, R., Corella, D., Fitó, M., Ros, E.: Benefits of the Mediterranean diet: insights from the PREDIMED Study. Prog. Cardiovasc. Dis. **58**(1), 50–60 (2015). https://doi.org/10.1016/j.pcad.2015.04.003
114. Foscolou, A., D'Cunha, N.M., Naumovski, N., Tyrovolas, S., Chrysohoou, C., Rallidis, L., Polychronopoulos, E., Matalas, A.L., Sidossis, L.S., Panagiotakos, D.: The association between the level of adherence to the Mediterranean diet and successful aging: an analysis of the ATTICA and MEDIS (MEDiterranean Islands Study) epidemiological studies. Arch. Gerontol. Geriatr. **89**,(2020). https://doi.org/10.1016/j.archger.2020.104044
115. Capurso, C.: The Mediterranean diet slows down the progression of aging and helps to prevent the onset of frailty: a narrative review. Nutrients **12**(1), 35 (2020). https://doi.org/10.3390/nu12010035
116. Chatzianagnostou, K., Del Turco, S., Pingitore, A., Sabatino, L., Vassalle, C.: The Mediterranean lifestyle as a non-pharmacological and natural antioxidant for healthy aging. Antioxidants (Basel) **4**(4), 719–736 (2015). https://doi.org/10.3390/antiox4040719
117. Martinez-Gonzalez, M.A., Martín-Calvo, N.: Mediterranean diet and life expectancy; beyond olive oil, fruits and vegetables. Curr. Opin. Clin. Nutr. Metab. Care. **19**(6), 401–407 (2016). https://doi.org/10.1097/MCO.0000000000000316
118. Ferrer-Cascales, R., Albaladejo-Blázquez, N., Ruiz-Robledillo, N., Clement-Carbonell, V., Sánchez-SanSegundo, M., Zaragoza-Martí, A.: Higher Adherence to the Mediterranean diet is related to more subjective happiness in adolescents: the role of health-related quality of life. Nutrients **11**(3), 698 (2019). https://doi.org/10.3390/nu11030698
119. Morales-Ivorra, I., Romera-Baures, M., Roman-Viñas, B., Serra-Majem, L.: Osteoarthritis and the Mediterranean diet: a systematic review. Nutrients **10**(8), 1030 (2018). https://doi.org/10.3390/nu10081030
120. Keenan, T.D., Agrón, E., Mares, J.A., Clemons, T.E., van Asten, F., Swaroop, A., Chew, E.Y.: Adherence to a Mediterranean diet and cognitive function in the Age-Related Eye Disease Studies 1 & 2. Alzheimer's Dement., 1–12 (2020). DOI: https://doi.org/10.1002/alz.12077.
121. Christianne de Faria Coelho-Ravagnani: Flavia Campos Corgosinho, Fabiane La Flor Ziegler Sanches, Carla Marques Maia Prado, Alessandro Laviano, and Jo~ao Felipe Mota, Dietary recommendations during the COVID-19 pandemic. Nutr. Rev. , 1–14 (2020). https://doi.org/10.1093/nutrit/nuaa067
122. Shakoor, H., Feehan, J., Dhaheri, A.S.A., Ali, H.I., Platat, C., Ismail, L.C., Apostolopoulos, V., Stojanovska, L.: Immune-boosting role of vitamins D, C, E, zinc, selenium and omega-3 fatty acids: could they help against COVID-19? Maturitas (2020). https://doi.org/10.1016/j.maturitas.2020.08.003
123. Barrea, L., Pugliese, G., Laudisio, D., Colao, A., Savastano, S., Muscogiuri, G.: Mediterranean diet as medical prescription in menopausal women with obesity: a practical guide for

nutritionists. Crit. Rev. Food Sci. Nutr. (2020). https://doi.org/10.1080/10408398.2020.1755220
124. Zabetakis, I., Lordan, R., Norton, C., Tsoupras, A.: COVID-19: The Inflammation link and the role of nutrition in potential mitigation. Nutrients **12**, 1466 (2020). https://doi.org/10.3390/nu12051466
125. Cena, H., Chieppa, M.: Coronavirus Disease (COVID-19–SARS-CoV-2) and nutrition: Is Infection in Italy suggesting a connection? Front. Immunol. **11**, 944 (2020). https://doi.org/10.3389/fimmu.2020.00944
126. Stipp M. M., SARS-CoV-2: Micronutrient optimization in supporting host immunocompetence. Int. J. Clin. Case Rep. Rev. **2**(2)–024 (2020). DOI:https://doi.org/10.31579/2690-4861/024.
127. Ghosh, T.S., Rampelli, S., Jeffery, I.B., Santoro, A., Neto, M., Capri, M., Giampieri, E., Jennings, A., Candela, M., Turroni, S., Zoetendal, E.G., Hermes, G.D.A., Elodie, C., Meunier, N., Brugere, C.M., Pujos-Guillot, E., Berendsen, A.M., De Groot, L.C.P.G.M., Feskins, E.J.M., Kaluza, J., Pietruszka, B., Bielak, M.J., Comte, B., Maijo-Ferre, M., Nicoletti, C., De Vos, W.M., Fairweather-Tait, S., Cassidy, A., Brigidi, P., Franceschi, C., O'Toole, P.W.: Mediterranean diet intervention alters the gut microbiome in older people reducing frailty and improving health status: the NU-AGE 1-year dietary intervention across five European countries. Gut **69**, 1218–1228 (2020). https://doi.org/10.1136/gutjnl-2019-319654
128. Meslier, V., Laiola, M., Roager, H.M., De Filippis, F., Roume, H., Quinquis, B., Giacco, R., Mennella, L., Ferracane, R., Pons, N., Pasolli, E., Rivellese, A., Dragsted, L.O., Vitaglione, P., Ehrlich, S.D., Ercolini, D.: Mediterranean diet intervention in overweight and obese subjects lowers plasma cholesterol and causes changes in the gut microbiome and metabolome independently of energy intake. Gut , 1–11 (2020). https://doi.org/10.1136/gutjnl-2019-320438
129. Jandhyala, S.M., Talukdar, R., Subramanyam, C., Vuyyuru, H., Sasikala, M., Reddy, N.D.: Role of the normal gut microbiota. World J. Gastroenterol. **21**(29), 8787–8803 (2015). https://doi.org/10.3748/wjg.v21.i29.8787
130. Sirisinha, S.: The potential impact of gut microbiota on your health: current status and future challenges. Asian Pac. J. Allergy Immunol. **34**(4), 249–264 (2016). https://doi.org/10.12932/AP0803
131. Khan, R., Petersen, F.C., Shekhar, S.: Commensal bacteria: an emerging player in defense against respiratory pathogens. Front. Immunol. **10**, 1203 (2019). https://doi.org/10.3389/fimmu.2019.01203
132. Maggini, S., Pierre, A., Calder, P.C.: Immune function and micronutrient requirements change over the life course. Nutrients **10**(10), 1531 (2018). https://doi.org/10.3390/nu10101531
133. Maffei, V.J., Kim, S., Blanchard, E.T., Luo, M., Jazwinski, S.M., Taylor, C.M., Welsh, D.A.: Biological aging and the human gut microbiota. J. Gerontol. A Biol. Sci. Med. Sci. **72**(11) 1474–1482 (2017). DOI: https://doi.org/10.1093/gerona/glx042.
134. Velasquez, M.T.: Altered gut microbiota: a link between diet and the metabolic syndrome. Metab. Syndr. Relat. Disord. **16**(7), 321–328 (2018). https://doi.org/10.1089/met.2017.0163
135. Kazemian, N., Mahmoudi, M., Halperin, F., Wu, J.C., Pakpour, S.: Gut microbiota and cardiovascular disease: opportunities and challenges. Microbiomem. **8**(1), 36 (2020). https://doi.org/10.1186/s40168-020-00821-0
136. Busnelli, M., Manzini, S., Chiesa, G.: The gut microbiota affects host pathophysiology as an endocrine organ: a focus on cardiovascular disease. Nutrients **12**(1), 79 (2020). https://doi.org/10.3390/nu12010079
137. Kallus, S.J., Brandt, L.J.: The intestinal microbiota and obesity. J. Clin. Gastroenterol. **46**(1), 16–24 (2012). https://doi.org/10.1097/MCG.0b013e31823711fd
138. De Luca, F., Shoenfeld, Y.: The microbiome in autoimmune diseases. Clin. Exp. Immunol. **195**(1), 74–85 (2019). https://doi.org/10.1111/cei.13158
139. Fava, F., Danese, S.: Intestinal microbiota in inflammatory bowel disease: friend of foe? World J. Gastroenterol. **17**(5), 557–566 (2011). https://doi.org/10.3748/wjg.v17.i5.557

140. Mayer, E.A., Savidge, T., Shulman, R.J.: Brain-gut microbiome interactions and functional bowel disorders. Gastroenterology **146**(6), 1500–1512 (2014). https://doi.org/10.1053/j.gastro.2014.02.037
141. Bonaz, B.L., Bernstein, C.N.: Brain-gut interactions in inflammatory bowel disease. Gastroenterology **144**(1), 36–49 (2013). https://doi.org/10.1053/j.gastro.2012.10.003
142. Padoan, A., Plebani, M., Basso, D.: Inflammation and pancreatic cancer: focus on metabolism, cytokines, and immunity. Int. J. Mol. Sci. **20**(3), 676 (2019). https://doi.org/10.3390/ijms20030676
143. Rogers, G.B., Keating, D.J., Young, R.L., Wong, M.L., Licinio, J., Wesselingh, S.: From gut dysbiosis to altered brain function and mental illness: mechanisms and pathways. Mol. Psychiatry **21**(6), 738–748 (2016). https://doi.org/10.1038/mp.2016.50
144. Sommer, F., Anderson, J.M., Bharti, R., Raes, J., Rosenstiel, P.: The resilience of the intestinal microbiota influences health and disease. Nat. Rev. Microbiol. **15**(10), 630–638 (2017). https://doi.org/10.1038/nrmicro.2017.58
145. Christian, L.M., Galley, J.D., Hade, E.M., Schoppe-Sullivan, S., Kamp Dush, C., Bailey, M.T.: Gut microbiome composition is associated with temperament during early childhood. Brain Behav. Immun. **45**, 118–127 (2015). https://doi.org/10.1016/j.bbi.2014.10.018
146. Yang, T., Santisteban M. M., Rodriguez, V., Li, E., Ahmari, N,; Carvajal, J. M., Gut dysbiosis is linked to hypertension. Hypertension **65**(6), 1331–1340 (2015). DOI: https://doi.org/10.1161/HYPERTENSIONAHA.115.05315.
147. Yamashiro, K., Tanaka, R., Urabe, T., Ueno, Y., Yamashiro, Y., Nomoto, K., Takahashi, T., Tsuji, H., Asahara, T., Hattori, N.: Gut dysbiosis is associated with metabolism and systemic inflammation in patients with ischemic stroke. PLoS ONE **12**(2),(2017). https://doi.org/10.1371/journal.pone.0171521
148. Pereira, P.A.B., Aho, V.T.E., Paulin, L., Pekkonen, E., Auvinen, P., Scheperjans, F.: Oral and nasal microbiota in parkinson's disease. Parkinsonism Relat. Disord. **38**, 61–67 (2017). https://doi.org/10.1016/j.parkreldis.2017.02.026
149. Hopfner, F., Kunstner, A., Muller, S.H., Kunzel, S., Zeuner, K.E., Margraf, N.G., Deuschl, G., Baines, J.F., Kuhlenbaumer, G.: Gut microbiota in parkinson disease in a northern german cohort. Brain Res. **1667**, 41–45 (2017). https://doi.org/10.1016/j.brainres.2017.04.019
150. Spychala, M.S., Venna, V.R., Jandzinski, M., Doran, S.J., Durgan, D.J., Ganesh, B.P., Ajami, N.J., Putluri, N., Graf, J., Bryan, R.M., McCullough, L.D.: Age-related changes in the gut microbiota influence systemic inflammation and stroke outcome. Ann. Neurol. **84**(1), 23–36 (2018). https://doi.org/10.1002/ana.25250
151. Kleiman, S.C., Watson, H.J., Bulik-Sullivan, E.C., Huh, E.Y., Tarantino, L.M., Bulik, C.M., Carroll, I.M.: The intestinal microbiota in acute anorexia nervosa and during renourishment: Relationship to depression, anxiety, and eating disorder psychopathology. Psychosom. Med. **77**(9), 969–981 (2015). https://doi.org/10.1097/PSY.0000000000000247
152. Borgo, F., Riva, A., Benetti, A., Casiraghi, M.C., Bertelli, S., Garbossa, S., Anselmetti, S., Scarone, S., Pontiroli, A.E., Morace, G., Borghi, E.: Microbiota in anorexia nervosa: the triangle between bacterial species, metabolites and psychological tests. PLoS ONE **12**(6),(2017). https://doi.org/10.1371/journal.pone.0179739
153. Dinan, T.G., Stilling, R.M., Stanton, C., Cryan, J.F.: Collective unconscious: how gut microbes shape human behavior. J. Psychiatr. Res. **63**, 1–9 (2015). https://doi.org/10.1016/j.jpsychires.2015.02.021
154. Bauer, K.C., Huus, K.E., Finlay, B.B.: Microbes and the mind: emerging Hallmarks of the gut microbiota-brain axis. Cell Microbiol. **18**(5), 632–644 (2016). https://doi.org/10.1111/cmi.12585
155. Dockray, G.J.: Gastrointestinal hormones and the dialogue between gut and brain. J. Physiol. **592**(14), 2927–2941 (2014). https://doi.org/10.1113/jphysiol.2014.270850
156. Mayer, E.A., Tillisch, K., Gupta, A.: Gut/brain axis and the microbiota. J. Clin. Invest. **125**(3), 926–938 (2015). https://doi.org/10.1172/JCI76304
157. Bonaz, B., Bazin, T., Pellissier, S.: The vagus nerve at the interface of the microbiota-gut-brain axis. Front. Neurosci. **12** (2018). DOI: https://doi.org/10.3389/fnins.2018.00049.

158. Fernandez-Real, J.M., Serino, M., Blasco, G., Puig, J., Daunis-i-Estadella, J., Ricart, W., Burcelin, R., Fernandez-Aranda, F., Portero-Otin, M.: Gut microbiota interacts with brain microstructure and function. J. Clin. Endocrinol. Metab. **100**(12), 4505–4513 (2015). https://doi.org/10.1210/jc.2015-3076
159. McGrattan, A.M., McGuinness, B., McKinley, M.C., Kee, F., Passmore, P., Woodside, J.V., McEvoy, C.T.: Diet and inflammation in cognitive ageing and Alzheimer's disease. Current Nutrition Reports **8**(2), 53–65 (2019). https://doi.org/10.1007/s13668-019-0271-4
160. Han, J.M., Levings, M.K.: Immune regulation in obesity-associated adipose inflammation. J. Immunol. **191**(2), 527–532 (2013). https://doi.org/10.4049/jimmunol.1301035
161. Leocádio, P.C.L., Oriá, R.B., Crespo-Lopez, M.E., Alvarez-Leite, J.I.: Obesity: more than an inflammatory, an infectious disease? Front. Immunol. **10**, 3092 (2020). https://doi.org/10.3389/fimmu.2019.03092
162. Bibbò, S., Ianiro, G., Giorgio, V., Scaldaferri, F., Masucci, L., Gasbarrini, A., Cammarota, G.: The role of diet on gut microbiota composition. Eur. Rev. Med. Pharmacol. Sci. **20**(22), 4742–4749 (2016)
163. Zinöcker, M.K., Lindseth, I.A.: The western diet-microbiome-host interaction and its role in metabolic disease. Nutrients **10**(3), 365 (2018). https://doi.org/10.3390/nu10030365
164. Newman, T.M., Vitolins, M.Z., Cook, K.C.: From the table to the tumor: the role of Mediterranean and western dietary patterns in shifting microbial-mediated signaling to impact breast cancer risk. Nutrients **11**(11), 2565 (2019). https://doi.org/10.3390/nu11112565
165. Segata, N.: Gut Microbiome: westernization and the disappearance of intestinal diversity. Curr Biol. **25**(14), R611–R613 (2015). https://doi.org/10.1016/j.cub.2015.05.040
166. Collins, K.H., Paul, H.A., Hart, D.A., Reimer, R.A., Smith, I.C., Rios, J.L., Seerattan, R.A., Herzog, W.: A high-fat high-sucrose diet rapidly alters muscle integrity, inflammation and gut microbiota in male rats. Sci. Rep. **6**, 37278 (2016). https://doi.org/10.1038/srep37278
167. Cani, P.D., Bibiloni, R., Knauf, C., Waget, A., Neyrinck, A.M., Delzenne, N.M., Burcelin, R.: Changes in gut microbiota control metabolic endotoxemia-induced inflammation in high-fat diet–induced obesity and diabetes in mice. Diabetes **57**(6), 1470–1481 (2008). https://doi.org/10.2337/db07-1403
168. Hussain, M., Hussain, M., Umair Ijaz, M., Ahmad, M.I., Khan, I.A., Brohi, S.A., Shah, A.U., Shinwari, K.I., Zhao, D., Xu, X., Zhou, G., Li, C.: Meat proteins in a high-fat diet have a substantial impact on intestinal barriers through mucus layer and tight junction protein suppression in C57BL/6J mice. Food Funct. **10**(10), 6903–6914 (2019). https://doi.org/10.1039/c9fo01760g
169. Tomasello, G., Mazzola, M., Leonei, A., Sinagrad, E., Zummo, G., Farina, F., Damianic, P., Cappelloa, F., Geageaa, A.G., Jurjus, A., Assi, T.B., Messina, M., Carini, F.: Nutrition, oxidative stress and intestinal dysbiosis: Influence of diet on gut microbiota in inflammatory bowel diseases. Biomed. Pap. Med. Fac. Univ. Palacky Olomouc. Czech Repub. **160**(4), 461–466 (2016). DOI: https://doi.org/10.5507/bp.2016.052.
170. Del Chierico, F., Vernocchi, P., Dallapiccola, B., Putignani, L.: Mediterranean diet and health: food effects on gut microbiota and disease control. Int. J. Mol. Sci. **15**(7), 11678–11699 (2014). https://doi.org/10.3390/ijms150711678
171. Brown, K., DeCoffe, D., Molcan, E., Gibson, D.L.: Diet-Induced dysbiosis of the intestinal microbiota and the effects on immunity and disease. Nutrients **4**(8), 1095–1119 (2012). https://doi.org/10.3390/nu4081095
172. Morrison, D.J., Preston, T.: Formation of short chain fatty acids by the gut microbiota and their impact on human metabolism. Gut Microbes. **7**(3), 189–200 (2016). https://doi.org/10.1080/19490976.2015.1134082
173. Zhu, C., Sawrey-Kubicek, L., Beals, E., Rhodes, C.H., Houts, H.E., Sacchi, R., Zivkovic, A.M.: Human gut microbiome composition and tryptophan metabolites were changed differently by fast food and Mediterranean diet in 4 days: a pilot study. Nutr. Res. **77**, 62–72 (2020). https://doi.org/10.1016/j.nutres.2020.03.005
174. Toribio-Mateas, M.: Harnessing the power of microbiome assessment tools as part of neuroprotective nutrition and lifestyle medicine interventions. Microorganisms **6**(2), 35 (2018). https://doi.org/10.3390/microorganisms6020035

175. Rinninella, E., Cintoni, M., Raoul, P., Lopetuso, L.R., Scaldaferri, F., Pulcini, G., Miggiano, G.A.D., Gasbarrini, A., Mele, M.C.: Food components and dietary habits: keys for a healthy gut microbiota composition. Nutrients **11**, 2393 (2019). https://doi.org/10.3390/nu11102393
176. Molendijk, I., van der Marel, S., Maljaars, P.W.J.: Towards a food pharmacy: immunologic modulation through diet. Nutrients **11**(6), 1239 (2019). https://doi.org/10.3390/nu11061239
177. Garcia-Mantrana, I., Selma-Royo, M., Alcantara, C., Collado, M.C.: Shifts on gut microbiota associated to mediterranean diet adherence and specific dietary intakes on general adult population. Front. Microbiol. **9**, 890 (2018). https://doi.org/10.3389/fmicb.2018.00890
178. Krznarić, Ž, Bender, D.V., Meštrović, T.: The Mediterranean diet and its association with selected gut bacteria. Curr. Opin. Clin. Nutr. Metab. Care **22**(5), 401–406 (2019). https://doi.org/10.1097/MCO.0000000000000587
179. Lee, J., Pase, M., Pipingas, A., Raubenheimer, J., Thurgood, M., Villalon, L., Macpherson, H., Gibbs, A., Scholey, A.: Switching to a 10-day mediterranean-style diet improves mood and cardiovascular function in a controlled crossover study. Nutrition **31**(5), 647–652 (2015). https://doi.org/10.1016/j.nut.2014.10.008
180. De Filippis, F., Pellegrini, N., Vannini, L., Jeery, I.B., La Storia, A., Laghi, L., Serrazanetti, D.I., Di Cagno, R., Ferrocino, I., Lazzi, C., Turroni, S., Cocolin, L., Brigidi, P., Neviani, E., Gobbetti, M., O'Toole, P.W., Ercolini, D.: High-level adherence to a Mediterranean diet beneficially impacts the gut microbiota and associated metabolome. Gut **65**(11), 1812–1821 (2016). DOI: https://doi.org/10.1136/gutjnl-2015-309957.
181. Mitsou, E.K., Kakali, A., Antonopoulou, S., Mountzouris, K.C., Yannakoulia, M., Panagiotakos, D.B., Kyriacou, A.: Adherence to the Mediterranean diet is associated with the gut microbiota pattern and gastrointestinal characteristics in an adult population. Br. J. Nutr. **117**(12), 1645–1655 (2017). https://doi.org/10.1017/S0007114517001593
182. Bailey, M.A., Holscher, H.D.: Microbiome-Mediated Effects of the Mediterranean Diet on Inflammation. Adv. Nutr. **1**, 9(3), 193–206 (2018). DOI: https://doi.org/10.1093/advances/nmy013.
183. Lu, M.L.E., Lucarini, L., Biffi, B., Rafanelli, E., Pietramellara, G., Durante, M., Vidali, S., Provensi, G., Madiai, S., Gheri, C.F., Masini, E., Ceccherini, M.T.: Effect of Mediterranean diet enriched in high quality extra virgin olive oil on oxidative stress, inflammation and gut microbiota in obese and normal weight adult subjects. Front. Pharmacol. **10**, 1366 (2019). https://doi.org/10.3389/fphar.2019.01366
184. Shapira, N.: The Metabolic concept of meal sequence vs. satiety: glycemic and oxidative responses with reference to inflammation risk, protective principles and Mediterranean diet. Nutrients **11**(10), 2373 (2019). DOI: https://doi.org/10.3390/nu11102373.
185. Sureda, A., Del Mar Bibiloni, M., licia Julibert, A., Bouzas, C., Argelich, E., Llompart, I., Pons, A., Tur, J.A.: Adherence to the Mediterranean Diet and inflammatory markers. Nutrients **10**(1), 62 (2018). DOI: https://doi.org/10.3390/nu10010062.
186. Casas, R., Sacanella, E., Estruch, R.: The Immune Protective effect of the Mediterranean diet against chronic low-grade inflammatory diseases. Endocrine, Metabolic & Immune Disorders - Drug Targets **14**(4), 245–254 (2014). https://doi.org/10.2174/18715303146661409 22153350.
187. Milano, W., Pizza, V., Capasso, A.: Beneficial effects of mediterranean diet in neuroinflammation and related diseases. Integr Food Nutr Metab. **5**(1), 1–10 (2018). https://doi.org/10.15761/IFNM.1000207
188. Carvalho, K.M.B., Ronca, D.B., Michels, N., Huybrechts, I., Cuenca-Garcia, M., Marcos, A., Molnár, D., Dallongeville, J., Manios, Y., Schaan, B.D., Moreno, L., de Henauw, S., Carvalho, L.A.: Does the Mediterranean diet protect against stress-induced inflammatory activation in European Adolescents? The HELENA Study. Nutrients **10**(11), 1770 (2018). https://doi.org/10.3390/nu10111770
189. Dyer, J., Davison, G., Marcora, S.M., Mauger, A.R.: Effect of a Mediterranean type diet on inflammatory and cartilage degradation biomarkers in patients with osteoarthritis. J Nutr Health Aging. **21**(5), 562–566 (2017). https://doi.org/10.1007/s12603-016-0806-y

190. Oliviero, F., Spinella, P., Fiocco, U., Ramonda, R., Sfriso, P., Punzi, L.: How the Mediterranean diet and some of its components modulate inflammatory pathways in arthritis. Swiss Med Wkly. **145**,(2015). https://doi.org/10.4414/smw.2015.14190
191. Santangelo, C., Varì, R., Scazzocchio, B., De Sanctis, P., Giovannini, C., D'Archivio, M., Masella, R.: Anti-inflammatory activity of extra virgin olive oil polyphenols: which role in the prevention and treatment of immune-mediated inflammatory diseases? Endocrine, Metabolic & Immune Disorders - Drug Targets **18**, 36–50 (2018). https://doi.org/10.2174/187153031 7666171114114321
192. Gambino, C.M., Accardi, G., Aiello, A., Candore, G., Dara-Guccione, G., Mirisola, M.: Effect of extra virgin olive oil and table olives on the immune-inflammatory responses: potential clinical applications. Endocrine Metab. Immune Disord. - Drug Targets **18**(1), 14–22 (2017). DOI: https://doi.org/10.2174/1871530317666171114113822.
193. Hornedo-Ortega, R., Cerezo, A.B., de Pablos, R.M., Krisa, S., Richard, T., García-Parrilla, C.M., Troncoso, A.M.: Phenolic compounds characteristic of the Mediterranean diet in mitigating microglia-mediated neuroinflammation. Front. Cell. Neurosci. **12**, 373 (2018). https://doi.org/10.3389/fncel.2018.00373
194. Shah, R., Makarem, N., Emin, M., Liao, M., Jelic, S., Aggarwal, B.: Mediterranean diet components are linked to greater endothelial function and lower inflammation in a pilot study of ethnically diverse women. Nutr. Res. **75**, 77–84 (2020). https://doi.org/10.1016/j.nutres.2020.01.004
195. Luisi, M.L.E., Lucarini, L., Biffi, B., Rafanelli, E., Pietramellara, G., Durante, M., Vidali, S., Provensi, G., Madiai, S., Gheri, C.F. Masini, E., Ceccherini, M.T.: Effect of Mediterranean Diet enriched in high quality extra virgin olive oil on oxidative stress, inflammation and gut microbiota in obese and normal weight adult subjects. Front. Pharmacol. **10**(1366) (2019). DOI: https://doi.org/10.3389/fphar.2019.01366.
196. Martínez-Rodríguez, A., Rubio-Arias, J.Á., Ramos-Campo, D.J., Reche-García, C., Leyva-Vela, B., Nadal-Nicolás, Y.: Psychological and sleep effects of tryptophan and magnesium-enriched mediterranean diet in women with fibromyalgia. Int. J. Environ. Res. Public Health **17**(7), 2227 (2020). https://doi.org/10.3390/ijerph17072227
197. Godos, J., Ferri, R., Caraci, F., Cosentino, F.I., Castellano, S., Galvano, F., Grosso, G.: Adherence to the Mediterranean diet is associated with better sleep quality in italian adults. Nutrients **11**(5), 976 (2019). https://doi.org/10.3390/nu11050976
198. Gianfredi, V.: Sleep disorder, Mediterranean Diet and learning performance among nursing students: inSOMNIA, a cross-sectional study. Ann. Ig. **30**(6), 470–481 (2018). https://doi.org/10.7416/ai.2018.2247
199. Pairotti, M.B., Cerutti, A.K., Martini, F., Vesce, E., Padovan, D., Beltramo, R.: Energy consumption and GHG emission of the Mediterranean diet: a systemic assessment using a hybrid LCA-IO method. J. Clean. Prod. **103**, 507–516 (2015). https://doi.org/10.1016/j.jclepro.2013.12.082
200. Dernini, S., Berry, E.M.: Mediterranean diet: from a healthy diet to a sustainable dietary pattern. Front. Nutr. **2**, 15 (2015). https://doi.org/10.3389/fnut.2015.00015
201. Mantzioris, E., Villani, A.: Translation of a Mediterranean-style diet into the australian dietary guidelines: a nutritional. Ecological and Environmental Perspective, *Nutrients* **11**, 2507 (2019). https://doi.org/10.3390/nu11102507
202. Martínez-González, M.A., et al.: Transferability of the Mediterranean diet to non-Mediterranean countries. What Is and What Is Not the Mediterranean Diet, Nutrients **9**, 1226 (2017). https://doi.org/10.3390/nu9111226
203. Moore, S.E., et al.: Barriers to adopting a Mediterranean diet in Northern European adults at high risk of developing cardiovascular Disease. J. Hum. Nutr. Diet. **31**(4), 451–462 (2018)

204. Dernini S., Berry E.M., Serra-Majem L., La Vecchia C., Capone R., Medina F.X., Aranceta-Bartrina J., Belahsen R., Burlingame B., Calabrese G., Corella D., Donini L.M., Lairon D., Meybeck A., Pekcan A.G., Piscopo S., Yngve A., Trichopoulou A.: Med Diet 4.0: the Mediterranean diet with four sustainable benefits. Public Health Nutr. **20**(7), 1322–1330 (2016). doi:https://doi.org/10.1017/S1368980016003177.
205. Galanakis, C.M.: The food systems in the era of the Coronavirus (COVID-19) pandemic crisis. Foods **9**, 523 (2020). https://doi.org/10.3390/foods9040523

Rate-Induced Tipping Phenomena in Compartment Models of Epidemics

Jochen Merker and Benjamin Kunsch

Abstract The aim of this chapter is to explore non-autonomous compartment models of epidemics, like, e.g., SIR models with time-dependent transmission and recovery rates as parameters, and particularly the occurrence of rate-induced tipping phenomena. Specifically, we are interested in the question, whether there can exist parameter paths that do not cross any bifurcation points, but yet give rise to tipping if the parameters vary over time. From literature, it is known that such rate-induced tipping occurs, e.g., in two-dimensional models of ecosystems or predator–prey systems. We show in this chapter that rate-induced tipping can also occur in compartment models of epidemics. Thus, regarding the Covid-19 crisis, not only the measures established in a lockdown and the moment of the lockdown, but also the rate by which lockdown measures are implemented may have a drastic influence on the number of infectious.

Keywords Geometric methods in differential equations (34A26) · Nonlinear equations and systems (34A34) · Qualitative investigation and simulation of models (34C60) · Nonautonomous dynamical systems (37B55)

1 Introduction

Why do we see during the Covid-19 crisis in some states a very high relative number of infectious, while in other states the relative number of infectious is significantly lower, although the measures established by states in a lockdown are comparable? Maybe, this does not only depend on the moment in time at which a lockdown is decided, but also on the rate by which lockdown measures are implemented. In this chapter, we show that corresponding rate-induced tipping phenomena can occur in compartment models of epidemics with time-dependent parameters.

J. Merker (✉)
Leipzig University of Applied Sciences, PF 30 11 66, 04251 Leipzig, Germany
e-mail: jochen.merker@htwk-leipzig.de

B. Kunsch
Wilhelm-Ostwald-Gymnasium, Willi-Bredel-Straße 15, 04279 Leipzig, Germany

P. Agarwal et al. (eds.), *Analysis of Infectious Disease Problems (Covid-19) and Their Global Impact*, Infosys Science Foundation Series,
https://doi.org/10.1007/978-981-16-2450-6_14

The foundations of compartment models of epidemics, which divide the population into compartments and assume a certain form of the time rates for transfer from one compartment to another, were laid by ROSS (Nobel Prize in Medicine 1902) [13–15], MCKENDRICK and KERMACK [10–12] prior to 1935. Usually, spatial dependence is neglected in compartment models, and instead a homogeneous mixing of the population is assumed. Thus, mathematically a compartment model of an epidemic is usually given by a system of ordinary differential equations (ODEs) for continuous time, or by a system of finite difference equations for discrete time, or by a system of delay differential equations (DDEs) if, e.g., the period of temporary immunity is modeled, but not by a system of partial differential equations (PDEs) involving spatial derivatives. Therefore, autonomous compartment models for epidemics are not suitable for describing the beginning of a disease outbreak, because at the beginning the assumption of a homogeneous mixing of the population is invalid. Instead, models viewing the social network as a graph may be used. However, this graph is usually not known, and if it is considered as random, then compartment models and network models are related; see, e.g., [3, Sect. 9.4], [5, Sect. IV.B]. Particularly, this problem can be circumvented by using a time-dependent transmission rate, which at the beginning is significantly reduced in comparison with the transmission rate of the disease in a homogeneously mixed population.

The aim of using compartment models in epidemiology [2, 3] is to better understand the underlying mechanisms of the spread of a disease and to obtain during the mathematical analysis of the model threshold values [1]. A threshold for a parameter in a model is a value, where the system shows a different behavior below the threshold than above the threshold. Most mathematical epidemic models exhibit threshold behavior, e.g., for $R_0 < 1$ the disease will die out, while for $R_0 > 1$ there will be an epidemic. This behavior is consistent with observations and has been used, e.g., to estimate the effectiveness of vaccination policies and the likelihood that a disease may be eliminated or eradicated.

However, when calculating threshold values, one has to be very precise. One source of confusion is the interpretation of parameters. For example in a stochastic model, the basic reproduction number is defined as the expected number of infections caused by one infectious in a population where all individuals are susceptible to infection. However, if in a compartment model "the basic reproduction number is calculated by the Jacobian method," i.e., by linearizing the system about the state where all individuals are susceptible, and by writing the condition that this state is linearly unstable in the form $R_0 > 1$, then the so defined parameter R_0 may not be identical with the basic reproduction number, i.e., with the expected number of infections caused by one infectious, but just allows to test linear stability of the state where all individuals are susceptible. Thus, in general, it would be wrong to say that this parameter denoted by R_0 "is" the basic reproduction number. Yet, it resembles the basic reproduction number, as it allows to answer the question, whether the disease will become endemic or die out. Further, in reality, parts of the population may be immune to a disease. The basic reproduction number does not say anything about such a state of the population, but instead the effective reproduction number should be used, which is defined as expected number of new infections caused by one infectious in the actual state of the population.

Another source of confusion may be the interpretation what is meant by "different behavior" of a system below and above a threshold. The dynamics of an autonomous system below and above a threshold value are usually considered to be different, if they are not topologically equivalent, i.e., if crossing the threshold results in a (local or global) bifurcation of the system. Yet, for non-autonomous systems [4], particularly SIR models with time-dependent parameters studied, e.g., in [5], it is not so clear how to define different behavior, because if we start from the same initial value but at different times, then of course we usually obtain different solution curves. Remarkably, the dynamics in systems with time-dependent parameters may not only change drastically due to a bifurcation, but also due to other tipping phenomena. Particularly, transient resp. irreversible rate-induced tipping may occur, where the system fails to track a continuously changing quasi-static attractor uniformly resp. up to the end point due to a fast rate of change of parameters.

The focus of this chapter lies on such rate-dependent tipping phenomena in compartment models of epidemics with continuous time. From literature, it is known that rate-induced tipping occurs generically, e.g., in climate models [16], in two-dimensional models of ecosystems [7], in predator–prey systems [8] or in chaotic systems [6]. We show that irreducible rate-induced tipping can also occur in idealized compartment models of epidemics with $R_0 > 1$, where due to the slow dynamics near the stable endemic equilibrium (EE), the state may fail to track the EE for a fast parameter change and may leave its basin of attraction bounded by a homoclinic orbit resp. by the stable manifold connecting the boundary to the disease-free equilibrium (DFE), resulting in an eradication of the disease, while else the disease becomes endemic. Further, we show that artifacts of this tipping phenomenon can also be observed in non-idealized models.

1.1 Outline

In Sect. 2, we introduce basic facts about compartment models with continuous time and time-dependent parameters. Further, we derive basic properties of the classical SIR and SIRS models. In Sect. 3, we discuss linear compartment models of epidemics and particularly in the time-dependent case phenomena related to tipping. In Sect. 4, we turn to nonlinear compartment models of epidemics and discuss a typical bifurcation of compartment models at the DFE. By center manifold reduction, we obtain an idealized planar system, which governs the dynamics and shows irreducible rate-induced tipping. Finally, in Sect. 5, we study tipping phenomena in nonlinear compartment models of epidemics.

2 Preliminaries

Throughout this chapter, we consider compartment models with continuous time, and we normalize systems so that each state variable models the percentage of the whole population in the corresponding compartment.

2.1 Compartment Models with Time-Dependent Parameters

Definition 1 A compartment model with $n+1$ compartments is a semi-process on the n-dimensional probability simplex $\Sigma^n := \{x \in \mathbb{R}^{n+1} \mid x \geq 0\,,\ 1^T x = 1\} \subset \mathbb{R}^{n+1}$, i.e., a family of continuous maps $\Phi^{t,s} : \Sigma^n \to \Sigma^n$, $s \leq t$, such that $\Phi^{t,t} = \mathrm{Id}_{\Sigma^n}$ for all $t \in \mathbb{R}$ and the cocycle condition $\Phi^{t,r} = \Phi^{t,s} \circ \Phi^{s,r}$ holds for all $r \leq s \leq t$, and which is generated by an ODE $\dot{x}(t) = f(t, x(t))$ in the sense that $\Phi^{t,s}(x)$ is identical with the value $x(t)$ of the unique ODE solution to the initial value $x \in \Sigma^n$ at time s.

An ODE $\dot{x}(t) = f(t, x(t))$ with a time-dependent vector field $f : \mathbb{R} \times \mathbb{R}^{n+1} \to \mathbb{R}^{n+1}$ generates such a semi-process Φ on Σ^n, if the probability simplex Σ^n is positively invariant, and this is the case iff

(A1) $f_i(t, x) \geq 0$ holds for every $x \geq 0$ with $1^T x = 1$ and $x_i = 0$, and every $t \in \mathbb{R}$,
(A2) $1^T f(t, x) = 0$ holds for every $x \in \Sigma^n$ and every $t \in \mathbb{R}$.

Under these conditions, global existence of solutions forward in time to initial values in Σ^n holds for a continuous f due to compactness of Σ^n. Additionally, in compartment models of epidemics, we require that $(1, 0, \ldots, 0)$ is for all times an equilibrium, i.e.,

(A3) $f_i(t, (1, 0, \ldots, 0)) = 0$ holds for every $t \in \mathbb{R}$,

We call this equilibrium disease-free equilibrium (DFE) and correspondingly consider the first component of $x \in \Sigma^n$ as percentage of susceptibles in the population. Due to $1^T x = 1$, every compartment model can be reduced by one dimension to an n-dimensional ODE $\dot{\hat{x}} = \hat{f}(t, \hat{x})$ on the image $\hat{\Sigma}^n := \{\hat{x} \in \mathbb{R}^n \mid \hat{x} \geq 0\,,\ 1^T \hat{x} \leq 1\}$ of the diffeomorphism from Σ^n onto $\hat{\Sigma}^n$ given by $x = (x_1, \ldots, x_n, x_{n+1}) \mapsto (x_1, \ldots, x_n) = \hat{x}$ with inverse $\hat{x} \mapsto (\hat{x}, 1 - 1^T \hat{x}) = x$, i.e., by eliminating $x_{n+1} = 1 - \sum_{i=1}^{n} x_i$ from the ODE. The assumptions (A1)-(A3) then translate into

(A1)' $\hat{f}_i(t, \hat{x}) \geq 0$ holds for every $\hat{x} \geq 0$ with $1^T \hat{x} < 1$ and $\hat{x}_i = 0$ and every $t \in \mathbb{R}$,
(A2)' $\sum_{i=1}^{n} \hat{f}_i(t, \hat{x}) \leq 0$ holds for every $\hat{x} \geq 0$ with $1^T \hat{x} = 1$, and every $t \in \mathbb{R}$,
(A3)' $\hat{f}_i(t, (1, 0, \ldots, 0)) = 0$ holds for every $t \in \mathbb{R}$.

The longtime behavior of a semi-process Φ on Σ^n is governed by its global pullback attractor, i.e., by the time-dependent family of non-empty compact sets

$$A(t) := \bigcap_{s \leq t} \overline{\bigcup_{r \leq s} \Phi^{t,r}(D)}\,, \tag{1}$$

with $D := \Sigma^n$ chosen to be the whole state space. Note that $A(t)$ consists of all values of solutions at time t originating from D for times $s \to -\infty$, i.e., $A(t)$ is a kind of non-autonomous ω-limit set of orbits originating from D. The global pullback attractor is the minimal closed set which attracts all subsets $B \subset \Sigma^n$ at time $-\infty$, i.e., $\lim_{s\to-\infty} \operatorname{dist}(\Phi^{t,s}(B), A(t)) = 0$ holds for every subset $B \subset \Sigma^n$, and it is invariant, i.e., $\Phi^{t,s}A(s) = A(t)$ holds for all $s \leq t$. In the autonomous case, where $\Phi^{t,s} = \Phi^{t-s}$ is a continuous dynamical system on Σ^n and the vector field f in the generating ODE $\dot{x}(t) = f(x(t))$ does not depend on time, the global pullback attractor does not depend on time, i.e., $A(t) = A$ is a constant set, and A is identical with the global attractor of the autonomous dynamical system on Σ^n.

If D in (1) is not chosen as the whole space Σ^n but replaced by a locally pullback absorbing family of time-dependent sets $D(r)$, i.e., there exists a sufficiently small distance $\varepsilon > 0$ and a sufficiently large time $T > 0$ such that $\Phi^{t,r}(B_\varepsilon(D(r))) \subset D(t)$ holds for all (t, r) with $t \geq r + T$, where $B_\varepsilon(D) := \{x \in \Sigma^n \mid \operatorname{dist}(x, D) < \varepsilon\}$ denotes the ε-neighborhood of $D \subset \Sigma^n$, then $A(t)$ is called the local pullback attractor of the absorbing family $D(t)$. Given a local pullback attractor $A(t)$, the largest locally pullback absorbing family $D(t)$ of time-dependent sets is such that $A(t) \subset D(t)$ is called its time-dependent basin of attraction.

In this chapter, we are particularly interested in compartment models

$$\dot{x}(t) = f(x(t), \lambda(t)) \tag{2}$$

which are non-autonomous due to time dependence of parameters. Hereby, we assume that the system is driven, i.e., that we can write the system in skew-product form

$$\begin{aligned} \dot{x}(t) &= f(x(t), \lambda(t)) \\ \dot{\lambda}(t) &= rg(\lambda(t)) \end{aligned} \tag{3}$$

with parameter path induced by a vector field $g(\lambda)$ in parameter space for a fixed rate $r \geq 0$. Often, we assume that $\lambda(t)$ approaches constant values $\lambda_\pm$ for times $t \to \pm\infty$ with a flat derivative, i.e., $\lambda(t)$ is a heteroclinic orbit in parameter space connecting $\lambda_\pm$ and satisfies $\dot{\lambda}(t) \to 0$ as $t \to \pm\infty$ due to $g(\lambda_\pm) = 0$. We are mainly interested in the dependence of x on the rate r. Note that the derivative of $x(t)$ w.r.t. r is given by the solution y of

$$\begin{aligned} \dot{y}(t) &= \frac{\partial f}{\partial x}(x(t), \lambda(t))y(t) + \frac{\partial f}{\partial \lambda}(x(t), \lambda(t))\kappa(t) \\ \dot{\kappa}(t) &= rg'(\lambda(t))\kappa(t) + g(\lambda(t)) \end{aligned} \tag{4}$$

to the initial values $y(s) = 0$ and $\kappa(s) = 0$, where $\kappa = \frac{\partial \lambda}{\partial r}$. This equation can be used to obtain information about the dependence of x on the rate, e.g., if $y(t) = \frac{\partial x}{\partial r}(t) \to 0$ for $t \to \infty$, then a change of the rate does not lead to a different longtime behavior of the solution.

Example 1 For $g(\lambda) := -(\lambda - \lambda_-)(\lambda - \lambda_+)$ with $\lambda_\pm = \pm 1$, i.e., $g(\lambda) = 1 - \lambda^2$, the parameter path is given by

$$\lambda(t) = \tanh(rt) \tag{5}$$

due to $\tanh' = 1 - \tanh^2$. In this case, the second equation $\dot{\kappa}(t) = -2\lambda(t)r\kappa + 1 - \lambda(t)^2$ in (4) has for the rate $r = 1$ and the initial value $\kappa(-10) = 0$ the exact solution

$$\kappa(t) = (t + 10)\,\mathrm{sech}^2(t)\,. \tag{6}$$

Let us consider as one-dimensional example the parameter-dependent autonomous vector field $f(x, \lambda) := -x(x^2 + \lambda)$, i.e., a pitchfork. Depending on λ being positive resp. negative, $x = 0$ is the only equilibrium resp. there are additionally the two equilibria $x_\pm := \pm\sqrt{-\lambda}$. If $\lambda < 0$, then $x = 0$ is unstable and $x_\pm$ are asymptotically stable, while if $\lambda > 0$, then $x = 0$ is asymptotically stable. Now our parameter path $\lambda(t) = \tanh(rt)$ runs at $t = 0$ through the bifurcation point $\lambda = 0$, thus eventually the solution of

$$x'(t) = -x(t)(x(t)^2 + \tanh(rt)) \tag{7}$$

to the initial value $x(-10) = 0.1$ first tends to $x_+ \approx 1$, but at time $t = 0$ the bifurcation happens and merely the asymptotically stable equilibrium $x = 0$ survives. As (7) is a Bernoulli ODE, we can calculate the exact solution, which is given for the rate $r = 1$ by

$$x(t) = (\cosh(t)(2\sinh(t) + C\cosh(t)))^{-1/2} \tag{8}$$

with $C = \frac{100}{\cosh^2(-10)} - 2\tanh(-10) \approx 2 + 8.162 \cdot 10^{-7}$ put this solution $x(t)$, the parameter path $\lambda(t)$ from (5) and the function $\kappa(t)$ from (6) into the first equation of (4) and solve this linear inhomogeneous ODE to the initial value $y(-10) = 0$ to obtain as solution $y(t) = \frac{\partial x}{\partial r}(t)$ the derivative of the solution $x(t)$ w.r.t. r, without explicitly solving (7) for other rates than $r = 1$, see Fig. 1.

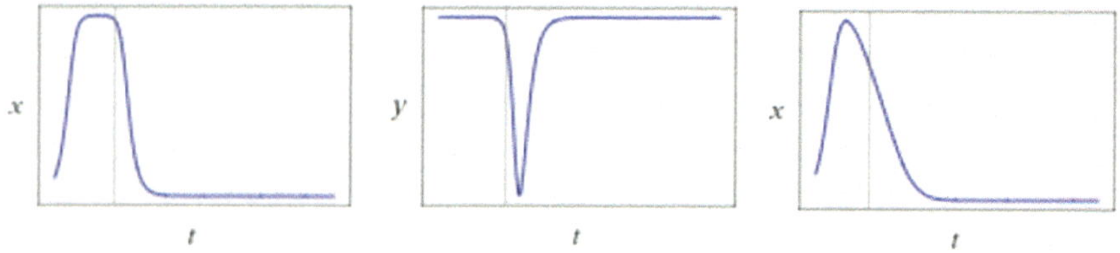

Fig. 1 On the left, the solution (8) of Eq. (7) with rate $r = 1$ to the initial value $x(-10) = 0.1$ is shown. In the middle, the derivative of this solution w.r.t. the rate is plotted, obtained by solving (4) for y. Observe that the rate mainly has an influence on the behavior of the solution shortly after the bifurcation at $t = 0$. Particularly, the rate does not have any influence on the long time behavior. This can also be seen by comparing the left picture to the right picture, which shows the solution of Eq. (7) with rate $r = 0.1$ to the same initial value $x(-10) = 0.1$

The sudden qualitative change of the state in Example 1 is mainly due to the bifurcation point $\lambda = 0$ of the autonomous system. To fix notation, if in (2) the parameter $\lambda(t) = \lambda$ is constant (or $r = 0$ in (3)), then we call

$$\dot{x}(t) = f(x(t), \lambda) \tag{9}$$

the autonomous frozen ODE. In such a parameter-dependent autonomous ODE, a sudden qualitative change of the behavior of the system at a threshold λ_0 can only occur due to a bifurcation. In fact, by definition, a bifurcation is said to occur at the parameter λ_0, if there are arbitrarily close parameters for which the generated dynamics are not topologically equivalent. The solution $x(t)$ of (9) to a fixed initial value $x(s) = x_0$ depends differentiably on the parameter λ, and moreover the derivative $\frac{\partial x}{\partial \lambda}$ of x w.r.t. λ solves

$$y' = \frac{\partial f}{\partial x}(x(t), \lambda_0)y + \frac{\partial f}{\partial \lambda}(x(t), \lambda_0) \tag{10}$$

to the initial value $y(s) = 0$. Compare Eq. (10) in the autonomous case with the corresponding first equation of (4) in the non-autonomous case to note that time dependence of parameters has a strong influence, if $\frac{\partial f}{\partial \lambda}$ is large. While for autonomous systems, a sudden qualitative change is related to a bifurcation, and for non-autonomous systems there are other sources of a sudden qualitative change. Particularly, rate-induced tipping may happen, where the system fails to track a continuously changing quasi-static attractor due to a fast rate of change of parameters.

Definition 2 For a non-autonomous ODE (2), a local attractor $A(\lambda)$ of the corresponding autonomous ODE (9) at parameter λ is called a local quasi-static attractor.

Let us assume that along $\lambda(t)$ there is no bifurcation, so that $A(\lambda_-)$ has a unique continuation $A(\lambda(t))$ for all times t. If the rate $r > 0$ is sufficiently small, then the local pullback attractor $A(t)$ originating form $A(\lambda_-)$ uniformly tracks $A(\lambda(t))$, i.e., $\sup_{t\in\mathbb{R}} \operatorname{dist}(A(t), A(\lambda(t)))$ is continuous w.r.t. to the rate r on which $\lambda(t)$ depends for small $r > 0$, and $\operatorname{dist}(A(t), A(\lambda(t)))$ tends to 0 as $t \to \pm\infty$. This property was obtained in [9] and allows to define rate-induced tipping. We use the following definition.

Definition 3 Under the assumption that along the path $\lambda(t)$ there is no bifurcation of the local quasi-static attractor $A(\lambda(t))$, we say that at points of discontinuity of $r \mapsto \sup_{t\in\mathbb{R}} \operatorname{dist}(A(t), A(\lambda(rt)))$ the system (2) has

1. transient rate-induced tipping, if $\lim\limits_{t\to\infty} \operatorname{dist}(A(t), A(\lambda(rt))) = 0$,
2. irreducible rate-induced tipping, if $\lim\limits_{t\to\infty} \operatorname{dist}(A(t), A(\lambda(rt))) > 0$.

In case of irreducible rate-induced tipping, the local pullback attractor $A(t)$ may tend for $t \to \infty$ to a local attractor at λ_+ different from $A(\lambda_+)$, while in case of transient rate-induced tipping $A(t)$ tends for $t \to \infty$ to $A(\lambda_+)$, but in between $A(t)$

approached another local attractor of the autonomous system. Rate-induced tipping is intimately related to basin instability; see [7, Definition 5.1]. Particularly, for equilibria the following definition makes sense.

Definition 4 Suppose $A(\lambda)$ is a stable equilibrium of the autonomous frozen ODE (9) for every λ on the chosen parameter path $\lambda(t)$, and let $B(A(\lambda))$ denote the basin of attraction of $A(\lambda)$. Then $A(\lambda)$ is said to be basin unstable on the parameter path, if there are two λ_1, λ_2 on the parameter path such that $A(\lambda_1)$ is outside the closure of the basin of attraction of $A(\lambda_2)$, i.e., $A(\lambda_1) \notin \overline{B(A(\lambda))}$.

The main result about basin instability is that it implies the existence of a parameter path along which rate-induced tipping happens.

Theorem 1 ([7]) *If a stable equilibrium $A(\lambda)$ of the autonomous frozen ODE* (9) *is basin unstable for all λ on the parameter path, then there is a time-varying external input $\lambda(t)$ of sufficiently fast rate that traces out the path and gives irreversible rate-induced tipping from $A(\lambda(t))$ in the non-autonomous system.*

Thus briefly, if the system is in a state where the dynamics is slow, but the actual parameter change is fast, then it may happen that the state may leave the basin of attraction of the continuation $A(\lambda(t))$ of the attractor $A(\lambda_-)$ and the local pullback attractor $A(t)$ tends to a different local attractor of the system.

Our main goal is to describe a mechanism how this kind of basin instability and the corresponding rate-induced tipping can happen in compartment models of epidemics. The difficulty hereby is that usually the endemic equilibrium (EE) is globally asymptotic stable, and then there is no way how basin instability can happen. Therefore, we consider idealized systems which has at least two different basins of attraction and argue that even in systems which do not have this idealized property, artifacts of rate-induced tipping can be seen. But first let us introduce basic compartment models of epidemics.

2.2 Autonomous SIR Model

The classical autonomous SIR model of McKendrick and Kermack [10–12] reads in full form as

$$\begin{aligned} S' &= -\beta S I \\ I' &= \beta S I - \alpha I \\ R' &= \alpha I \end{aligned} \tag{11}$$

with constant transmission rate $\beta > 0$ and recovery rate $\alpha > 0$, or in reduced form as

$$\begin{aligned} S' &= -\beta S I \\ I' &= (\beta S - \alpha) I \end{aligned} \tag{12}$$

with $R := 1 - S - I$. This system has a whole line segment $\{(S, 0) \mid 0 \leq S \leq 1\}$ of equilibrium points bounded to the right by the disease-free equilibrium (DFE) $(S, I) = (1, 0)$, and the parameter $R_0 := \frac{\beta}{\alpha}$ resembles the basic reproduction number: The Jacobian of the reduced model is

$$D\hat{f}(S, I) = \begin{pmatrix} -\beta I & -\beta S \\ \beta I & \beta S - \alpha \end{pmatrix}, \tag{13}$$

and therefore the linearization at the DFE

$$D\hat{f}(1, 0) = \begin{pmatrix} 0 & -\beta \\ 0 & \beta - \alpha \end{pmatrix} \tag{14}$$

has eigenvalues $\lambda = 0$ and $\lambda = \beta - \alpha$. Thus, linear instability holds if $R_0 := \frac{\beta}{\alpha} > 1$, but due to the degenerated eigenvalue $\lambda = 0$, which corresponds to the whole line segment of equilibria, even in the case $R_0 < 1$ we do not have local attractivity but just stability of the disease-free equilibrium $(S, I) = (1, 0)$. Nonetheless, in the case $R_0 < 1$, the system tends for every initial state (S_0, I_0) with $I_0 > 0$ to the disease-free equilibrium $(S, I) = (1, 0)$, i.e., the DFE attracts all states (S, I) with $I > 0$ and the disease dies out.

In the case $R_0 > 1$, solutions have a maximum number of infectious where $I' = 0$, i.e., at $S = \frac{\alpha}{\beta} = \frac{1}{R_0}$. Afterward the number of infectious decreases and tends for $t \to +\infty$ to an equilibrium with $S_\infty < 1$ and $I_\infty = 0$, i.e., the disease becomes epidemic. Let us calculate the value S_∞: By integration over $t \in [0, \infty)$ on the one hand $(S + I)' = -\alpha I$ implies $S_\infty - (S_0 + I_0) = -\alpha \int_0^\infty I(t)\, dt$, and on the other hand $S'/S = -\beta I$ implies $\ln(S_\infty/S_0) = -\beta \int_0^\infty I(t)\, dt$. Thus, $S_\infty - (S_0 + I_0) = \frac{\alpha}{\beta} \ln(S_\infty/S_0)$ holds and allows to calculate S_∞. Under the assumption that at the beginning, there are no recovered, we have to solve $S_\infty - 1 = \frac{\alpha}{\beta} \ln(S_\infty/S_0)$, and with the product log function $W(x)$, which solves $x = we^w$ for w, the solution can be written as $S_\infty = -\frac{\alpha}{\beta} W(-S_0 \frac{\beta}{\alpha} \mathrm{e}^{-\frac{\beta}{\alpha}})$.

2.3 Autonomous SIRS Model

Instead of a more appropriate DDE taking into account the period of temporary immunity, we consider in this subsection as model with temporary immunity the SIRS model given by

$$\begin{aligned} S' &= -\beta SI + \gamma R \\ I' &= \beta SI - \alpha I \\ R' &= \alpha I - \gamma R \end{aligned} \tag{15}$$

with an additional rate $\gamma > 0$ of loss of immunity. The reduced model

$$
\begin{aligned}
S' &= -\beta S I + \gamma(1 - S - I) \\
I' &= (\beta S - \alpha) I
\end{aligned}
\tag{16}
$$

has the disease-free equilibrium (DFE) $(S, I) = (1, 0)$, and for $\alpha < \beta$ additionally the endemic equilibrium (EE) $(S, I) = (\frac{\alpha}{\beta}, \frac{\gamma}{\alpha+\gamma}(1 - \frac{\alpha}{\beta}))$.

Particularly, for $\gamma \searrow 0$, we obtain $(S, I) = (\frac{\alpha}{\beta}, 0)$ as limit of the endemic equilibrium, i.e., a distinguished point on the line segment of equilibria of the autonomous SIR model. Thus, if the SIR model is considered as limit of the SIRS model with vanishing γ, then for $R_0 > 1$ the unique equilibrium with $S_\infty := \frac{\alpha}{\beta}$ on the whole line segment of equilibria should be considered as epidemic equilibrium in the SIR model. Again the parameter $R_0 := \frac{\beta}{\alpha}$ resembles the basic reproduction number: The Jacobian of the reduced model is

$$
D\hat{f}(S, I) = \begin{pmatrix} -(\beta I + \gamma) & -(\beta S + \gamma) \\ \beta I & \beta S - \alpha \end{pmatrix},
\tag{17}
$$

and we obtain that the linearization at the DFE

$$
D\hat{f}(1, 0) = \begin{pmatrix} -\gamma & -\beta - \gamma \\ 0 & \beta - \alpha \end{pmatrix}
\tag{18}
$$

has the eigenvalues $\lambda = -\gamma$ and $\lambda = \beta - \alpha$. Thus, the DFE is asymptotically stable if $R_0 := \frac{\beta}{\alpha} < 1$ and unstable if $R_0 > 1$. In the case $R_0 > 1$, the eigenvector $(-(\beta + \gamma), \beta + \gamma - \alpha)^T$ to $\lambda = \beta - \alpha > 0$ of sign structure $(-, +)^T$ has a second component which is smaller than the negative of the first component, thus the unstable manifold of the DFE points into the probability simplex $\hat{\Sigma}^n$. Further, the Jacobian at the EE

$$
D\hat{f}\left(\frac{\alpha}{\beta}, \frac{\gamma}{\alpha + \gamma}\left(1 - \frac{\alpha}{\beta}\right)\right) = \begin{pmatrix} -\gamma\frac{\beta+\gamma}{\alpha+\gamma} & -(\alpha + \gamma) \\ \gamma\frac{\beta-\alpha}{\alpha+\gamma} & 0 \end{pmatrix}
\tag{19}
$$

has for $R_0 > 1$ a negative trace as well as a positive determinant, i.e., the eigenvalues have negative real parts and thus the EE is asymptotically stable. The EE is a stable focus if $\gamma < 4(\beta - \alpha)(\frac{\alpha+\gamma}{\beta+\gamma})^2$, else it is a stable node. Observe that the linearization (18) at the DFE has for $\gamma = 0$ and $\beta = \alpha > 0$ a zero eigenvalue of algebraic multiplicity two and geometric multiplicity one. Therefore, when considered as a two-parameter system on whole $\mathbb{R}^2$, there is a bifurcation not very different from (but also not identical with) a Bogdanov–Takens bifurcation.

3 Linear Compartment Models

Linear compartment models of epidemics model the behavior near an endemic equilibrium. First, let us discuss the case of constant parameters and let us introduce some special names for matrices, which are unfortunately not used completely uniformly in the literature.

Definition 5 A matrix $A = (a_{ij}) \in \mathbb{R}^{n \times n}$ is called

1. Z-matrix, if $a_{ij} \leq 0$ holds for $i \neq j$,
2. Metzler matrix, if $a_{ij} \geq 0$ holds for $i \neq j$, or equivalently $-A$ is a Z-matrix,
3. M-matrix, if A is a Z-matrix and additionally $\Re(\lambda) \geq 0$ holds for every eigenvalue λ of A, or equivalently there is a non-negative matrix $B \geq 0$ and a scalar $\alpha \geq \rho(B)$ such that $A = \alpha E - B$.

These terms have to do a lot with non-negative linear flows. In fact, exactly the linear flows generated by Metzler matrices preserve the cone condition $x \geq 0$:

Theorem 2 *The non-negative cone* $\{x \in \mathbb{R}^n \mid x \geq 0\}$ *is positively invariant w.r.t. the linear flow generated by* $x' = Ax$, *iff* A *is a Metzler matrix.*

Proof On the one hand, if the non-negative cone $\{x \in \mathbb{R}^n \mid x \geq 0\}$ is positively invariant w.r.t. the linear flow $\exp(tA)$, then $0 \leq e_i^T \exp(tA) e_j = e_i^T e_j + t e_i^T A e_j + O(t^2)$ holds for i, j as $t \searrow 0$. Thus, $0 \leq e_i^T A e_j + O(t)$ is valid for $i \neq j$ as $t \searrow 0$, and this implies $a_{ij} = e_i^T A e_j \geq 0$ for $i \neq j$. On the other hand, if A is a Metzler matrix, then there is a scalar $\alpha \in \mathbb{R}$ and a matrix $B \geq 0$ such that $A + \alpha E = B$. Thus, $\exp(tA) = \mathrm{e}^{-\alpha t} \exp(tB)$, where $\exp(tB) \geq 0$, and hence $\exp(tA)x \geq 0$ for all $x \geq 0$. □

The invariance of the affine linear subspace consisting of all vectors whose entries sum up to 1 can be tested via the following criterion.

Theorem 3 *The affine linear subspace* $\{x \in \mathbb{R}^n \mid 1^T x = 1\}$ *is invariant w.r.t. the linear flow generated by* $x' = Ax$, *iff* $1^T A = 0$ *or equivalently* $A^T 1 = 0$, *i.e., the vector* 1 *containing just ones is an eigenvector of* A^T *to the eigenvalue* 0.

Proof If the flow generated by $x' = Ax$ preserves the condition $1^T x = 1$, then $0 = \frac{d}{dt} 1 = \frac{d}{dt} 1^T x = 1^T Ax$ for every solution $x(t)$ and thus $1^T A = 0$. On the other hand, if $1^T A = 0$ holds, then $\frac{d}{dt} 1^T x = 1^T Ax = 0$ so that $1^T x$ is constant. □

Of particular interest are matrices A, for which the linear flow generated by $x' = Ax$ is non-negative and leaves the subspace $\{x \in \mathbb{R}^n \mid 1^T x = 1\}$ invariant, as then the linear flow is a compartment model.

Corollary 1 *The probability simplex* $\Sigma^{n-1} := \{x \in \mathbb{R}^n \mid x \geq 0,\ 1^T x = 1\}$ *is positively invariant w.r.t. the linear flow generated by* $x' = Ax$, *iff* A *is a Metzler matrix with* $A^T 1 = 0$. *In this case,* $-A$ *is a M-matrix with semi-simple eigenvalue* 0. *If additionally* $A = B - \rho(B)E$ *for an irreducible matrix* $B \geq 0$, *then there is a unique equilibrium in the interior of the simplex, and this equilibrium is globally asymptotically stable.*

Proof The first claim follows from a combination of Theorems 2 and 3. A Metzler matrix A with $A^T 1 = 0$ is automatically an M-matrix, as $x \mapsto 1^T x$ is due to $1^T A = 0$ a Lyapunov function on the non-negative cone $\{x \in \mathbb{R}^n \mid x \geq 0\}$, i.e., 0 is a stable equilibrium of $x' = Ax$ on the non-negative cone as underlying space. Thus, all eigenvalues λ of A satisfy $\Re(\lambda) \leq 0$, and every eigenvalue with $\Re(\lambda) = 0$ is semi-simple. Additionally, the condition $A^T 1 = 0$ implies that A has the eigenvalue 0, too. Other eigenvalues $\lambda \neq 0$ of A with $\Re(\lambda) = 0$ cannot exist, because due to $A = B - \alpha E$ with $\alpha \geq \rho(B)$ for every eigenvalue λ of A with $\Re(\lambda) = 0$, there is an eigenvalue β of B with $\lambda = \beta - \alpha$, $\Re(\beta) = \alpha$, and $0 = \Re(\lambda) = \Re(\beta) - \alpha \leq \rho(B) - \alpha \leq 0$ implies $\alpha = \rho(B) = \beta$, i.e., $\lambda = 0$. Moreover, if $A = B - \rho(B)E$ holds with an irreducible non-negative matrix $B \geq 0$, then the last statement follows from Frobenius–Perron's famous theorem, which states that for an irreducible non-negative matrix B the spectral radius $\rho(B) > 0$ is an algebraically (as well as geometrically) simple eigenvalue of B and the only eigenvalue of B with positive eigenvector $x > 0$. Since for $A = B - \alpha E$ the equation $Ax = 0$ is equivalent to α being an eigenvalue of B with eigenvector x, there is exactly one point $x_0 > 0$ with $Ax_0 = 0$ and $1^T x_0 = 1$, namely the eigenvector normalized by $1^T x_0 = 1$ to the eigenvalue $\rho(B)$ of B. Since $-A$ is an M-matrix with a simple eigenvalue 0 and A otherwise has only eigenvalues with negative real part, the asymptotic stability of the equilibrium x_0 in the simplex follows. □

Example 2 The matrix $B := \begin{pmatrix} 0 & 0 & 0 \\ 1 & 0 & 1 \\ 0 & 1 & 0 \end{pmatrix}$ is non-negative, but not irreducible. It has eigenvalues $-1, 0, 1$, thus $A := B - E$ is a Metzler matrix with simple eigenvalue 0, and $A^T 1 = 0$ holds. Nonetheless, $x' = Ax$ has no equilibrium in the interior of the simplex $\{x \in \mathbb{R}^n \mid x \geq 0\,,\ 1^T x = 1\}$, because every eigenvector of A to the eigenvalue 0 is a multiple of the boundary point $x_0 = (0, 1/2, 1/2)^T$ of the simplex. This shows that in the final statement in Corollary 1, the irreducibility of B cannot be waived or replaced by the assumption that 0 is a simple eigenvalue of A.

Example 3 Two-dimensional linear compartment models have the full form

$$\begin{pmatrix} S' \\ I' \\ R' \end{pmatrix} = \begin{pmatrix} -\beta & \delta & \gamma - \zeta \\ \beta - \varepsilon & -\alpha & \zeta \\ \varepsilon & \alpha - \delta & -\gamma \end{pmatrix} \begin{pmatrix} S \\ I \\ R \end{pmatrix} \tag{20}$$

with constants $\alpha \geq \delta \geq 0$, $\beta \geq \varepsilon \geq 0$, $\gamma \geq \zeta \geq 0$. Here, we do not require (A3), because we consider the system (20) as linearization of a nonlinear system at the endemic equilibrium (EE). Let the transmission rate β of S be the maximum of the three constants α, β, γ, then the system matrix can be written as $A = B - \beta E$ with the non-negative matrix

$$B = \begin{pmatrix} 0 & \delta & (\gamma - \zeta) \\ (\beta - \varepsilon) & (\beta - \alpha) & \zeta \\ \varepsilon & (\alpha - \delta) & (\beta - \gamma) \end{pmatrix}$$

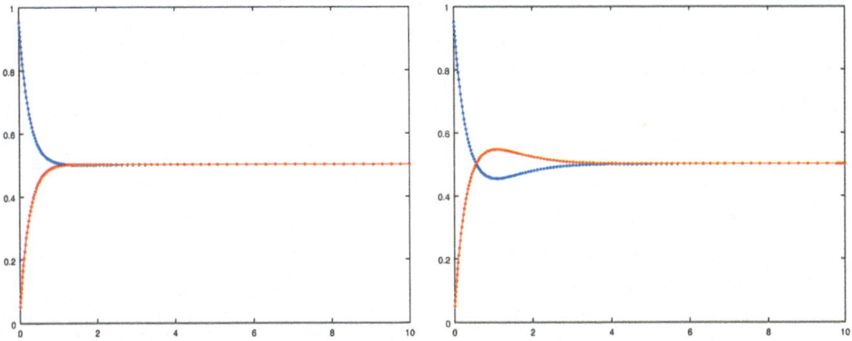

Fig. 2 Solution S in blue, I in red, of (21) to the initial value $(S_0, I_0) = (0.95, 0.05)^T$ for $\beta(rt) = (2 - \tanh(rt))$ decreasing from the value 2 at $t = 0$ to a value near $\alpha := 1$ approaches the equilibrium $(S, I) = (\frac{1}{2}, \frac{1}{2})$ for the fast rate $r = 2$ on the left directly, while for the slow rate $r = 1$ on the right there is a kind of overshooting. The critical rate lies between $r = 1.9$ and $r = 2$

This matrix is irreducible iff β is strictly larger than α, $\gamma > 0$ (even if $\delta = \varepsilon = \zeta = 0$).

3.1 Artifacts of Rate-Induced Tipping

Although linear compartment models cannot exhibit true rate-dependent tipping, because by Corollary 1 the unique equilibrium is globally asymptotically stable, some artifacts of rate-induced tipping in nearby nonlinear systems can be observed, as will be explained in more detail in Sect. 5. For example, consider the most simple one-dimensional non-autonomous SIS model

$$\begin{aligned} S' &= -\beta(rt)S + \delta I \\ I' &= \beta(rt)S - \delta I \end{aligned} \tag{21}$$

with a time-dependent transmission rate $\beta(rt) \geq 0$ of rate r and constant rate $\delta > 0$. The ODE (21) can be viewed as model of a disease, where susceptibles get ill without any contacts to infectious, and where there is no immunity. The reduced ODE reads as $\dot{S}(t) = -(\beta(rt) + \alpha)S(t) + \alpha$. If $\beta(t)$ connects β_- and β_+ with $\beta_- > \beta_+$ monotonely decreasing, then it depends on the rate r, whether the solution $S(t) = \left(S_0 + \int_0^t \exp(B(rs)/r + \alpha s)\alpha\, ds\right) \exp(-B(rt)/r - \alpha t)$, $B(t) := \int_0^t \beta(s)\, ds$, to the initial value $S(0) = S_0 \in [0, 1]$ has a local minimizer or not. For $r \to 0$, the solution tends to $\frac{\alpha}{\beta_-+\alpha} + (S_0 - \frac{\alpha}{\beta_-+\alpha}) \exp(-(\beta_- + \alpha)t))$ and thus is monotone decreasing for $S_0 > \frac{\alpha}{\beta_-+\alpha}$, while for $r \to \infty$ it tends to the same function with β_- replaced by β_+. Therefore, there is a threshold r_c, i.e., a critical rate, such that for rates $r < r_c$ there is a kind of overshooting when approaching the longtime equilibrium $\frac{\alpha}{\beta_-+\alpha}$, while for rates $r > r_c$ the solution does not show overshooting; see Fig. 2.

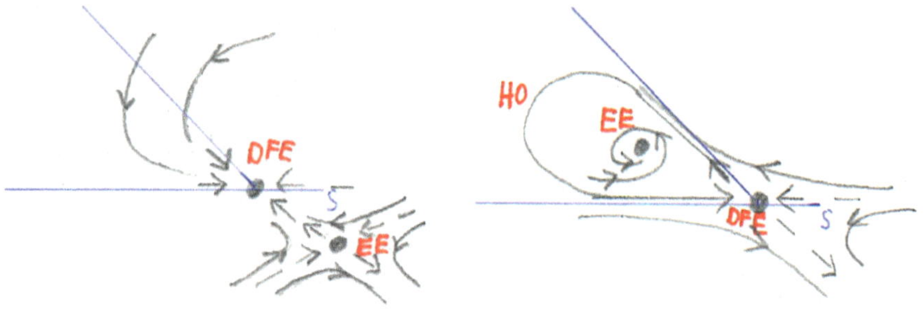

Fig. 3 On the left, the DFE is a stable node on a boundary vertex of the simplex, while the EE is an unstable saddle outside the simplex. On the right, the EE has entered the simplex through the boundary vertex and has become a stable focus, while the DFE lost its stability and has become an unstable saddle. Additionally, the unstable manifold of the DFE runs into the stable manifold and forms a homoclinic orbit HO surrounding the EE

4 Nonlinear Compartment Models

In this section, we consider autonomous nonlinear compartment models $\dot{x} = f(x)$ of epidemics on the probability simplex Σ^n and discuss the situation, where the asymptotically stable disease-free equilibrium (DFE) becomes unstable due to a local bifurcation. Note that the DFE does not lie in the interior but at a boundary vertex of the simplex Σ^n. As our knowledge about boundary equilibrium bifurcations is still a little patchy, the bifurcation theory of the DFE is not completely standard. Here we are mainly interested in a bifurcation of codimension two. In this case, by center manifold reduction we can consider the equation induced by $\dot{x} = f(x)$ on the two-dimensional center manifold, and this equation determines the dynamics of the full n-dimensional compartment model near the bifurcation point. However, center manifold reduction requires that f is sufficiently smooth, but as the DFE lies at a boundary vertex, the vector field f can be smooth in the interior but merely continuous up to the boundary. Then terms occur, which due to missing differentiability cannot be obtained by linearization, and we use such terms to obtain idealized models where after a transcritical bifurcation of the DFE the arising endemic equilibrium (EE) is surrounded by a homoclinic orbit (HO), see Fig. 3, or there is at least a trajectory from the boundary to the DFE such that the EE does not attract the whole interior of the simplex.

4.1 *Local Normal Form for a Bifurcation of Codimension Two*

Under the assumption that f is sufficiently smooth near the DFE, let us derive a normal form for the planar system on the two-dimensional center manifold of a compartment model $\dot{x} = f(x)$ of epidemics. If a two-parameter family of autonomous vector fields $\hat{f}(S, I)$ on $\hat{\Sigma}^2$ satisfying (A1)',(A2)',(A3)' has a local bifurcation at the DFE $(S, I) = (1, 0)$, then generically the linearization $A := D\hat{f}(1, 0)$ has a zero eigenvalue of algebraic multiplicity two, but geometric multiplicity one. Let q_0 be an eigenvector to the zero eigenvalue, i.e., $Aq_0 = 0$, and let q_1 be a corresponding generalized eigenvector, i.e., $Aq_1 = q_0$. Via a change of coordinates to

$$\begin{pmatrix} S-1 \\ I \end{pmatrix} = xq_0 + yq_1 ,$$

the Taylor expansion $T_2\hat{f}$ of second order of $\hat{f}$ around $(S, I) = (1, 0)$ reads as

$$\begin{aligned} T_2\hat{f}(S, I) &= \hat{f}(1, 0) + A\begin{pmatrix} S-1 \\ I \end{pmatrix} + \frac{1}{2}B\left(\begin{pmatrix} S-1 \\ I \end{pmatrix}, \begin{pmatrix} S-1 \\ I \end{pmatrix}\right) \\ &= yq_0 + \frac{1}{2}x^2B(q_0, q_0) + xyB(q_0, q_1) + \frac{1}{2}y^2B(q_1, q_1) \end{aligned}$$

with the second derivative $B := D^2\hat{f}(1, 0)$. Using an eigenvector p_1 of A^T to the zero eigenvalue and a corresponding generalized eigenvector p_0 with $A^T p_0 = p_1$ as dual basis vectors satisfying $\langle p_0, q_1\rangle = 0 = \langle p_1, q_0\rangle$ and $\langle p_0, q_0\rangle = 1 = \langle p_1, q_1\rangle$, we obtain due to (A3)', which excludes constant terms, under the genericity conditions

$$\langle p_1, B(q_0, q_1)\rangle \neq 0 , \qquad \frac{1}{2}\langle p_1, B(q_1, q_1)\rangle \neq 0 , \tag{22}$$

similar as in Bogdanov–Takens bifurcation the normal form

$$\begin{aligned} x' &= \langle p_0, x'q_0 + y'q_1\rangle = -\beta_1 x + y \\ y' &= \langle p_1, x'q_0 + y'q_1\rangle = \beta_2 y - xy - y^2 \end{aligned} \tag{23}$$

with parameters β_1, β_2 vanishing at the bifurcation. Beneath $(0, 0)$, there is a second equilibrium $(\frac{\beta_2}{1+\beta_1}, \frac{\beta_1\beta_2}{1+\beta_1})$ in $\hat{\Sigma}^2$ for $\beta_1 \geq 0$, $\beta_2 > 0$. This normal form differs from Bogdanov–Takens normal form

$$\begin{aligned} x' &= y \\ y' &= -\beta_1 + \beta_2 x - x^2 - xy \end{aligned} \tag{24}$$

mainly in that A is perturbed in the Bogdanov–Takens case to $\begin{pmatrix} 0 & 1 \\ \beta_2 & 0 \end{pmatrix}$, and the equilibrium $(0, 0)$ is split up into the two equilibria $(\frac{\beta_2}{2} \pm \frac{1}{2}\sqrt{\beta_2^2 - 4\beta_1}, 0)$ for $\beta_2^2 \geq 4\beta_1$, while our normal form (23) perturbs A to $\begin{pmatrix} -\beta_1 & 1 \\ 0 & \beta_2 \end{pmatrix}$ and leaves—as required by (A3)'—the DFE fixed. A coordinate transform of x, y, t and a substitution of the parameters in (23) leads to

$$\begin{aligned} x' &= -\gamma x + \alpha y \\ y' &= (\beta - \alpha - \delta - \beta x - \beta y)y\,, \end{aligned} \tag{25}$$

where the bifurcation happens at parameters $\gamma = 0$ resp. $\delta = \beta - \alpha$. Particularly, if $A = \begin{pmatrix} 0 & -1 \\ 0 & 0 \end{pmatrix}$ and correspondingly $q_0 = (-1, 0)^T, q_1 = (-1, 1)$, then $x = 1 - S - I = R$ and $y = I$ so that in the coordinates (S, I) the reduced normal form is given by

$$\begin{aligned} S' &= -\beta SI + \delta I + \gamma(1 - S - I) \\ I' &= (\beta S - \alpha - \delta)I\,, \end{aligned} \tag{26}$$

where additionally after an infection there may be partially no immunity due to $\delta > 0$. This normal form is a combination of SIRS and SIS models, wherein the SIS model $\alpha = 0, \gamma = 0$ so that all infectious become after the infect directly again susceptible. The Jacobian of the right-hand side of (26) is

$$D\hat{f}(S, I) = \begin{pmatrix} -\beta I - \gamma & \delta - \beta S - \gamma \\ \beta I & \beta S - \alpha - \delta \end{pmatrix}, \tag{27}$$

and for $\gamma > 0$ the DFE is asymptotically stable if $R_0 := \frac{\beta}{\alpha+\delta} < 1$ resp. unstable if $R_0 > 1$. In the case $R_0 > 1$, the EE has the coordinates $(\frac{\alpha+\delta}{\beta}, \frac{\gamma}{\alpha+\gamma}(1 - \frac{\alpha+\delta}{\beta}))$, and it is a stable focus for small $\gamma > 0$ resp. a stable node for large $\gamma > 0$.

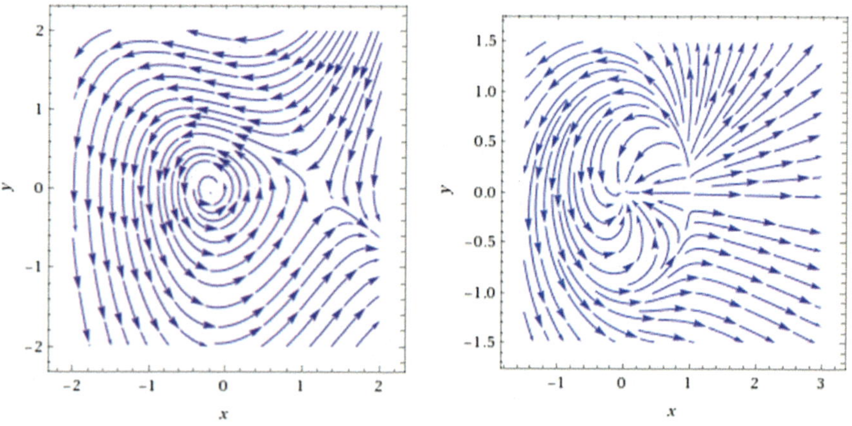

Fig. 4 On the left, the homoclinic orbit arising in (24) for $\beta_2 = 1, \beta_1 \approx -\frac{6}{25}\beta_2^2$, after a Bogdanov–Takens bifurcation. On the right, the homoclinic orbit occurring in (28). Note that trajectories outside but near to the homoclinic orbit miss the equilibrium and tend to infinity, while in our idealized model due to invariance of the axes they tend to the DFE

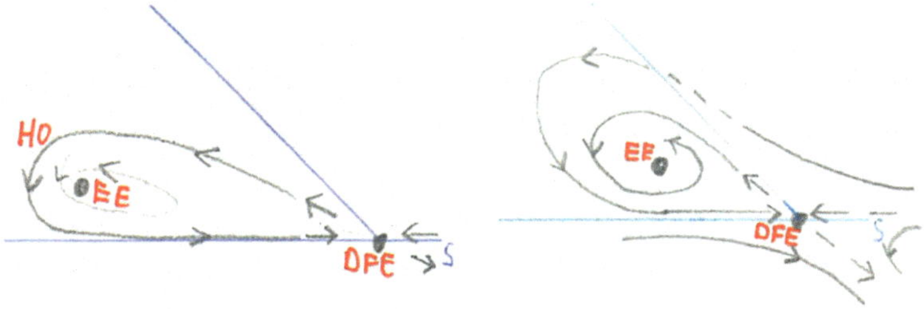

Fig. 5 On the left, compared to the right picture in Fig. 3 the EE has moved and the HO is a little deformed. On the right, it is shown that the HO vanishes for slight perturbations. Yet, due to the trajectory connecting the boundary with the DFE, the EE still is merely locally and not globally asymptotically stable

Yet, while in Bogdanov–Takens bifurcation a homoclinic orbit arises around the stable equilibrium for a rather specifically chosen combination of the two bifurcation parameters, see Fig. 4, this does not seem to be the case for (26) and parameters $\beta > \alpha + \delta$, $\alpha, \gamma, \delta \geq 0$. In the following subsection, we indicate how to construct compartment models of epidemics with this idealized behavior.

4.2 *Idealized Models*

In this subsection, we aim to construct an idealized system, where after a transcritical bifurcation of the DFE, the arising EE is surrounded by a homoclinic orbit HO; see Fig. 3. Although the HO may be deformed or may vanish for a slight perturbation of the two parameters, see Fig. 5, such idealized models will help us to explain tipping phenomena in compartment models of epidemics in Sect. 5. To obtain an idealized model with this behavior, we add non-smooth terms to the normal forms (25) resp. (26). Note that already the standard example of a system with a homoclinic orbit

$$\begin{aligned} x' &= -x + xy + (y - x)\sqrt{x^2 + y^2} \\ y' &= -y - x^2 + (x + y)\sqrt{x^2 + y^2} \end{aligned} \tag{28}$$

contains the non-smooth term $\sqrt{x^2 + y^2}$. In polar coordinates, this system (28) reads as

$$\begin{aligned} r' &= -r(1 - r) \\ \varphi' &= r(\cos(\varphi) - 1) \end{aligned} \tag{29}$$

and obviously has the circle $r = 1$ as invariant set, which consists of a homoclinic orbit and the equilibrium at $r = 1$, $\varphi = 0$, see Fig. 4.

Similarly, if we add the term $\varepsilon - \frac{x-y}{(x^2+y^2)^{1/2}} y$ to the right-hand side of the second equation in (25) for $\varepsilon := \frac{\alpha-\gamma}{(\alpha^2+\gamma^2)^{1/2}}$ chosen such that the term vanishes at the line where

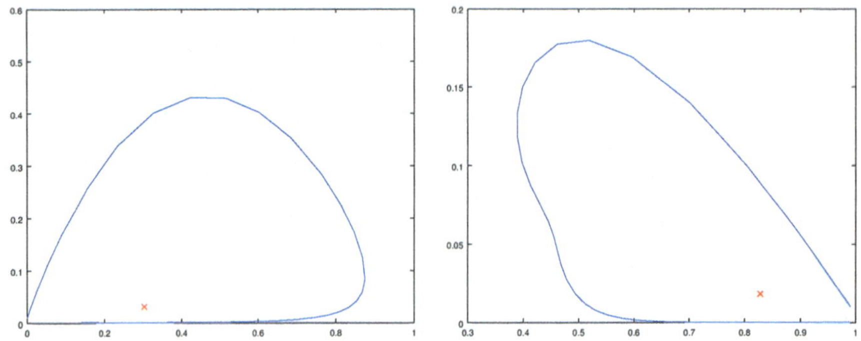

Fig. 6 On the left, for $\alpha := 1$, $\beta := 1.5$, $\gamma := 0.1$ and $\delta := 0$, the EE and the surrounding HO in (30) are shown. On the right, for $\alpha := 0.5$, $\beta := 1$ and $\gamma := 0.1$ and $\delta := 0$, the EE and the surrounding HO in (31) are shown

the first equation vanishes, i.e., for a rather specific combination of parameters, then the system

$$\begin{aligned} x' &= -\gamma x + \alpha y \\ y' &= \left(\beta - \alpha - \delta - \beta x - \beta y + \varepsilon - \frac{x-y}{(x^2+y^2)^{1/2}}\right) y\,, \end{aligned} \tag{30}$$

seems to have a HO at the DFE; see Fig. 6 on the left. Note that $\frac{x-y}{(x^2+y^2)^{1/2}}\,y$ is continuous due to $|\frac{x-y}{(x^2+y^2)^{1/2}}\,y| \leq |x-y|$. Yet, a disadvantage of this system is that trajectories starting far away from the HO may leave the simplex $\hat{\Sigma}^2$, but of course the vector field can be modified so that the simplex is positively invariant while the dynamics near the HO is not changed. Another example is the modification

$$\begin{aligned} S' &= -\beta S I + \gamma(1 - S - I) \\ I' &= \left(\beta S - \alpha\left(2 + \tanh\left(\frac{1-x}{2y} - 5\right)\right)\right) I\,, \end{aligned} \tag{31}$$

of (26) with $\delta := 0$, i.e., a modified SIRS system. Again, the term $\tanh(\frac{1-x}{2y} - 5)$ is smooth in the interior and continuous up to the boundary, as it tends to 1 for $(x, y) \to (x_0, 0)$ approaching the boundary. The HO and EE are given in Fig. 6 on the right. Yet, there seems to be an additional small instable periodic orbit around the EE, and again the system needs to be modified far away from the DFE.

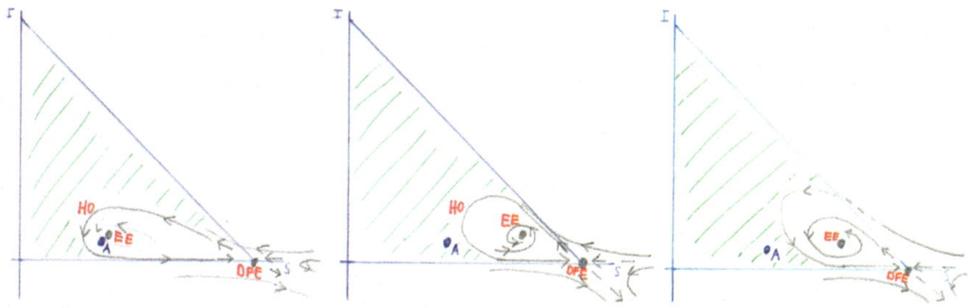

Fig. 7 On the left, the pullback attractor A lies near to the EE, but then the parameters are changed fast while the dynamics near A is slow. Therefore, the pullback attractor leaves the basin of attraction of the EE, which in the middle is the interior of the HO and on the right is separated by a trajectory from the boundary to the DFE. As A has entered the basin of attraction of the DFE marked in green, the disease will die out, while for a slow rate of parameter change the pullback attractor would have tracked the EE and the disease would have become endemic

5 Irreducible Rate-Induced Tipping in Non-autonomous Models

Regardless, whether there is a homoclinic orbit (HO) surrounding the endemic equilibrium (EE) after a transcritical bifurcation at the disease-free equilibrium (DFE) like in the idealized system on the left of Fig. 5, or whether there is an orbit connecting the boundary $R = 1 - S - I = 1$ with the DFE like in Fig. 5 on the right, if there are two different basins of attraction, one of the EE and one of the DFE, then irreducible rate-induced tipping may occur for time-dependent parameters. Hereby, starting with the pullback attractor $A(t_0)$ near the EE, if the parameters evolve so that the homoclinic orbit shrinks fast while the dynamics near $A(t)$ are slow, it may happen that $A(t)$ leaves the basin of attraction of the EE and enters the basin of attraction of the DFE; see Fig. 7. Then the disease will die out, while for a slower rate $A(t)$ would have tracked the EE and the disease would have stayed endemic. The critical rate for which $A(t)$ leaves the basin of attraction of the EE is a threshold for the occurrence of rate-induced tipping.

Of course, in application, it is necessary to estimate the time-dependent parameters from data. But this is not so difficult, e.g., in the SIR model (11) with time dependent $\beta = \beta(t)$ and $\alpha = \alpha(t)$, for S near 1 and small h as in [5] the parameters can be estimated by

$$\begin{aligned} \alpha(t) &\approx \frac{R(t+h) - R(t)}{hI(t)} \\ \beta(t) &\approx \frac{(I(t+h) - I(t)) + (R(t+h) - R(t))}{hI(t)} \end{aligned} \tag{32}$$

from time series for $I(t)$, $R(t)$, due to $\alpha = R'/I$ and $\beta = (I+R)'/SI$.

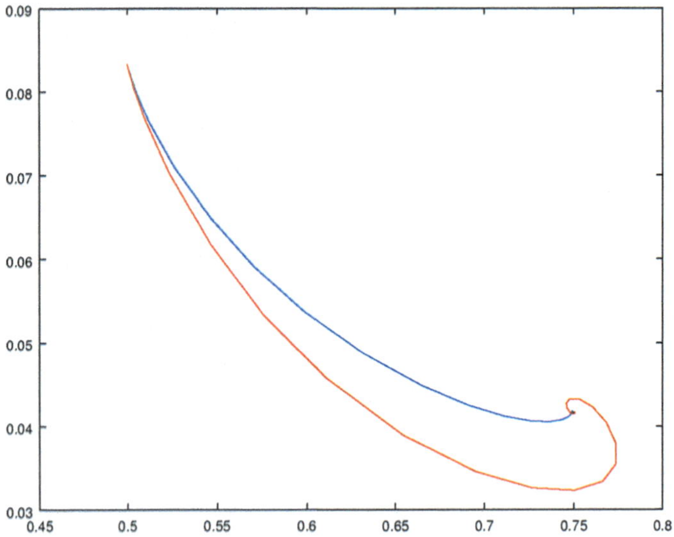

Fig. 8 For the slow rate $r = 0.05$, the blue solution curve (33) tracks the EE of the frozen system rather well, while for the higher rate $r = 0.1$ along the red curve, there is a reduced percentage of infectious in the middle part, and this can be considered as artifact of rate-induced tipping in a system where the red curve tends to the DFE. However, in (33), the EE attracts the whole interior of the simplex, and this enforces an additional turn at the end, i.e., a second wave with a little higher percentage of infectious than for the blue curve

5.1 Artifacts of Rate-Induced Tipping

Many compartment models in epidemics are not idealized, i.e., the DFE with its unstable manifold does not have a basin of attraction intersecting the interior of the simplex Σ. But even in the case, where the whole interior of the simplex belongs to the basin of attraction of the EE, artifacts of rate-induced tipping in nearby idealized systems can be seen. For example, instead of the SIRS model (15), consider

$$\begin{aligned} S' &= -\beta(t)SI + \gamma R \\ I' &= \beta(t)S - \alpha I \\ R' &= \alpha I \end{aligned} \tag{33}$$

with a time-dependent transmission rate $\beta = \beta(t) := 1 - \frac{1}{3}\tanh(rt)$ and constant $\alpha = 1/2, \gamma = 1/10$, i.e., $\beta(t)$ decreases from 1 at $t = 0$ to $2/3$ at time $t \to \infty$. Then Fig. 8 shows an artifact of rate-induced tipping in a nearby idealized systems where the red curve tends to the DFE.

6 Conclusion

We identified a mechanism which allows to have rate-induced tipping in idealized compartment models of epidemics with $R_0 > 1$, where not only the endemic equilibrium (EE) but also the disease-free equilibrium (DFE) has a basin of attraction intersecting the interior of the probability simplex. Moreover, even in the case that the compartment model is not idealized and the EE attracts every point in the interior of the simplex, we showed that artifacts of nearby idealized compartment models can be observed. Thus, in models it can happen that in two countries the same kind of lockdown measures is decided at the same time, corresponding to the same initial and final values of a parameter path at the same times, but that the measures are established by different rates so that the disease becomes endemic in a country where the measures are slowly established (or there is at least a high number of infectious), while in a country where the measures are established fast the disease is eradicated (or there is at least a lower number of infectious).

Yet, there are various open research questions: Is there an idealized compartment model of epidemics with polynomial right-hand side? How to determine the critical rate, i.e., the threshold for the rate below which a rate-induced tipping happens in idealized compartment models? Can (4) help to determine this threshold? Can we obtain quantitative and not only qualitative results for non-idealized systems? Maybe an answer to these questions can help us to better handle a pandemic disease like Covid-19 in future.

References

1. Hethcote, H.W.: The mathematics of infectious diseases. SIAM Rev **42**, 599–653 (2000)
2. Smith, R.: Modeling Disease Ecology with Mathematics. AIMS Series in Differential Equations & Dynamical Systems, vol. 2 (2008)
3. Brauer, F., Castillo-Chavez, C.: Mathematical Models in Population Biology and Epidemiology. Springer, New York (2012)
4. Kloeden, P., Rasmussen, M.: Nonautonomous Dynamical Systems. AMS Mathematical Surveys and Monographs, vol. 176 (2011)
5. Chen, Y.-C., Lu, P.-E., Chang, C.-S., Liu, T.-H.: A Time-dependent SIR model for COVID-19 with Undetectable Infected Persons. arXiv:2003.00122
6. Kaszás, B., Feudel, U., Tél, T.: Tipping phenomena in typical dynamical systems subjected to parameter drift. Sci. Rep. (2019). https://doi.org/10.1038/s41598-019-44863-3
7. O'Keeffe, P.E., Wieczorek, S.: Tipping phenomena and points of no return in ecosystems: beyond classical bifurcations. arXiv:1902.01796
8. Vanselow, A., Wieczorek, S., Feudel, U.: When very slow is too fast—collapse of a predator-prey system. J. Theor. Biol. **479**, 64–72 (2019)
9. Ashwin, P., Perryman, C., Wieczorek, S.: Parameter shifts for nonautonomous systems in low dimension: Bifurcation- and Rate-induced tipping
10. Kermack, W.O., McKendrick, A.G.: Contributions to the mathematical theory of epidemics I. Proc. R. Soc. A **115**, 700–721 (1927)
11. Kermack, W.O., McKendrick, A.G.: Contribution to the mathematical theory of epidemics II. Proc. R. Soc. A **138**, 55–83 (1932)

12. Kermack, W.O., McKendrick, A.G.: Contributions to the mathematical theory of epidemics III. Proc. R. Soc. A **141**, 94–122
13. Ross, R., Hudson, H.P.: An application of the theory of probabilities to the study of a priori pathometry II. Proc. R. Soc. A **92**, 204–230 (1916)
14. Ross, R., Hudson, H.P.: An application of the theory of probabilities to the study of a priori pathometry II. Proc. R. Soc. A **93**, 212–225 (1917)
15. Ross, R., Hudson, H.P.: An application of the theory of probabilities to the study of a priori pathometry III. Proc. R. Soc. A **93**, 225–240 (1917)
16. Ashwin, P., Wieczorek, S., Vitolo, R., Cox, P.: Tipping points in open systems: bifurcation, noise-induced and rate-dependent examples in the climate system. Phil. Trans. R. Soc. A **370**, 1166–1184 (2012)

Analysis of Impact of Covid-19 Pandemic on Financial Markets

Curt Burmeister, Alexander Kreinin, Rafael Mendoza-Arriaga, Hamed Rasouli, and Oleksandr Romanko

Abstract In this paper, we discuss impact of the Covid-19 pandemic on the North American financial markets and propose a framework for stress testing and financial scenario generation of market indicators. This framework includes the following main components:

- Epidemiological dynamic model describing evolution of the number of Susceptible, Infected, Recovered and Death cases with social distancing,
- Dynamical model describing dependence between financial indicators and growth of the pandemic in different geographical areas,
- Conditional stress scenario generation and financial portfolio analysis.

We apply an extended epidemiological model to analysis of Covid-19 pandemic spread and analyze its impact on some of the main financial indicators, including stock indices, credit spreads and FX rates, and characteristics of the pandemic process in different geographical areas. This analysis results in a model connecting the dynamics of the pandemic and that of the main financial indicators. The model allows one to generate pandemic scenarios under different assumptions on the parameters of the infectious disease and that of the social distancing policies. Once the pandemic scenarios are generated, one can transform them into a set of scenarios on macro-economic risk factors. Then, applying the conditional scenario technique we obtain a set of Monte Carlo scenarios on the risk factors driving the portfolio dynamics. The proposed dynamic models allow one to generate various financial stress scenarios on market indicators and compute the distribution of financial portfolio losses and their risk measures.

C. Burmeister
SS&C Technologies, Boston, MA, USA
e-mail: curt.burmeister@sscinc.com

A. Kreinin (✉) · H. Rasouli · O. Romanko
SS&C Technologies, Toronto, Ontario, Canada
e-mail: alex.kreinin@sscinc.com

R. Mendoza-Arriaga
SS&C Technologies, Austin, TX, USA
e-mail: rafael.mendoza@sscinc.com

P. Agarwal et al. (eds.), *Analysis of Infectious Disease Problems (Covid-19) and Their Global Impact*, Infosys Science Foundation Series,
https://doi.org/10.1007/978-981-16-2450-6_15

Keywords Geometric methods in differential equations (34A26) · Nonlinear equations and systems (34A34) · Qualitative investigation and simulation of models (34C60) · Nonautonomous dynamical systems (37B55)

1 Introduction

Over the first seven months in 2020, we have been facing dramatically increased social impacts of the Covid-19 (CV-19) pandemic: the number of cases already exceeds 13 million, the number of fatal outcomes exceeds 0.5 million and continues to grow.

The global spread of CV-19 has tremendous impact on all aspects of the international society including economy and financial markets. The first signs of market crash in North America (NA) were observed when the U.S. equity markets went down more than 30% from Feb. 14 through March 25. Similar market movements were observed in the European equity markets. At the same time, a sharp growth of the unemployment rate which accompanied the market drop, created an impression that the time of economic depression had come.

This pessimistic scenario has not occurred: in a relatively short time, financial markets managed to recover a substantial part of losses. We also observed that the start of the recovery process of the market appeared to be related to the time when social distancing policy was enforced in the US and Canada, and the CV-19 pandemic changed its growth rate.

Naturally, the latter observation raises the following question: is there a connection between pandemic dynamics and market behaviour and what kind of model can describe this relation?

In this paper, we answer this question using the NA data and describe our approach to this problem. We propose a framework linking together evolution of the pandemic and financial market movements. The main idea of our approach is to develop a robust statistical model for the processes describing the pandemic dynamics and that of the financial indicators of interest. Once this model is calibrated, one can generate non-financial scenarios simulating the pandemic growth and transform them into the scenarios on financial indices.

This approach is not the only one that can be used for developing financial stress scenarios during the pandemic growth. One can also produce historical scenarios by generating randomly permuted sequences of log-returns observed in the market.

The sentiment analysis also looks very attractive for developing CV-19 stress scenarios. The idea that sentiment and volume of market news and public opinion related to CV-19 development can forecast market movements underlies use of sentiment analysis for modeling financial market variables. Natural Language Processing (NLP) algorithms developed up to date can parse thousands of news articles and generate sentiments (positive or negative opinions) based on the frequency of positive and negative words in the text, on bag-of-words models, or on more complex word embeddings. If CV-19 sentiment can be extracted from the online news articles and related to movements of financial risk factors, we can build Machine Learning (ML) models to forecast financial risk drivers based on sentiment-based features extracted from online news.

Reliability of sentiment analysis models is subject to discussion as a sentiment score itself is subjective and depends on personal perceptions. As a result, NLP models for sentiment analysis may have errors, coming from sentiment subjectivity. Alternatively, measures such as volume of news that mention CV-19 in relation to financial markets may be more reliable. Building ML models that predict values of financial risk factors based on such features as sentiment scores and volumes of news, is in the plans for future research and development.

Another alternative methodology is the hypothetical scenario approach [20] providing the flexibility to evaluate the effect of a specific market view on the portfolio performance. This enables portfolio managers to impose specific constraints on the risk drivers and examine stress testing results. Unlike historical stress scenarios, hypothetical stress scenarios are constructed based on a specific view about stress events in the market. Value of the portfolio depends on its underlying risk factors. Elements, that affect portfolio value, are categorized into two groups: risk drivers and risk factors. In the first step, the risk driver shocks are computed. In the second step, the risk driver shocks are propagated to all risk factors. Implementation of this methodology requires calibration of a candidate probability distribution on the logarithmic return time series of risk drivers, and then using a linear regression model to propagate risk driver shocks to the risk factors.

In this paper we focus on the joint models of the pandemic processes and financial indices. The details of the historical and hypothetical scenario approaches as well as details of the sentiment analysis are not considered in the present paper.

The paper is organized as follows. In Sect. 2 the NA market behaviour during initial and intermediate pandemic phases is described. In Sect. 3 we describe the framework for modelling pandemic impact on financial markets. The first element of this framework is a set of models describing dynamics of the pandemic. We propose two models in this section. The first, deterministic model is an extension of the SIRD model describing the social distancing effect.

The second, stochastic model, is a combination of pure birth and pure death processes. This model also allows for simulation of social distancing. The model has simpler structure, but its explanatory power is not as high as that of the first model. In Sect. 3 we also describe the calibration algorithms developed for these models.

The second element of the framework is a mapping of the pandemic processes to the financial indices. We propose a regression model that links financial risk drivers such as DJI, TSX, $S\&P500$ and the VIX indices to a small subset of regularly observed epidemic variables. This mapping is expressed as a generalized regression model written for the log-price, auto-regressive process and the standardized pandemic variables.

In Sect. 4, we apply the constructed mapping to generation of stress scenarios on S&P500 and VIX indices. In conclusion, we provide some remarks on the extension of the framework and further research directions.

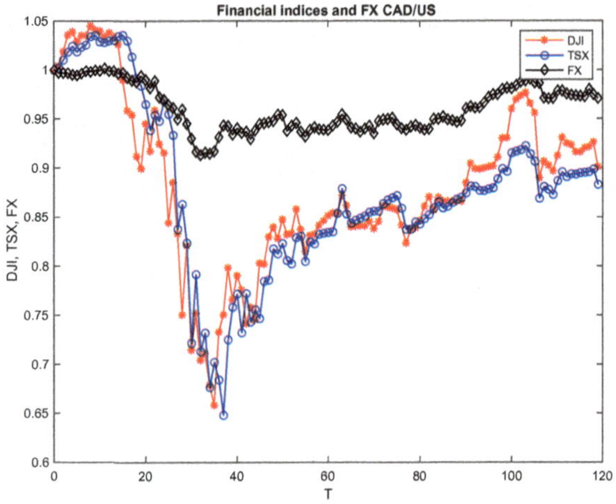

Fig. 1 Normalized financial indices

2 Market Behaviour During Initial and Intermediate Pandemic Phases

In this section we briefly inspect the time series of the following NA financial indices: Dow Jones Industrial index (DJI), TSX and FX CAD/USD. These observations are collected during the pandemic period starting 28 February and lasting next 4 months.

In Fig. 1 we display the normalized time series of the DJI and TSX indices and the normalized exchange rate CAD/USD. The normalization of the time series $\{X(t_n)\}_{n\geq 1}$ is obtained by the transformation $X(t_n)/X(t_1)$. The graphs of the financial indices have a V-shape in this Figure.[1] In the case of the volatility indices, their shape is a reflection of V-shape.

Several historical scenarios were studied and analyzed during the global CV-19 pandemic period. Here, we present two instances of these historical stress scenarios. Different countries were hit at different times, and similar pandemic scenarios can be constructed based on geographical areas.

2.1 *Covid-19 Market Crash (2020/02/19–2020/03/19)*

The coronavirus created such an uncertainty around the world that three of the largest single day drops in the Dow Jones and S&P500 are from March of 2020. On March 12, Dow Jones index lost almost 10% and S&P500 index dropped 9.5%. On March 16, the Dow Jones and S&P500 indices dropped 12% and 11.9%, respectively. Meanwhile the Chicago Board of Exchange Volatility Index rose steadily since the middle of February as the virus began to spread around the world [19]. VIX level reached 83

[1] Similar shape is observed in the case of the European indices MIB and FTSE100.

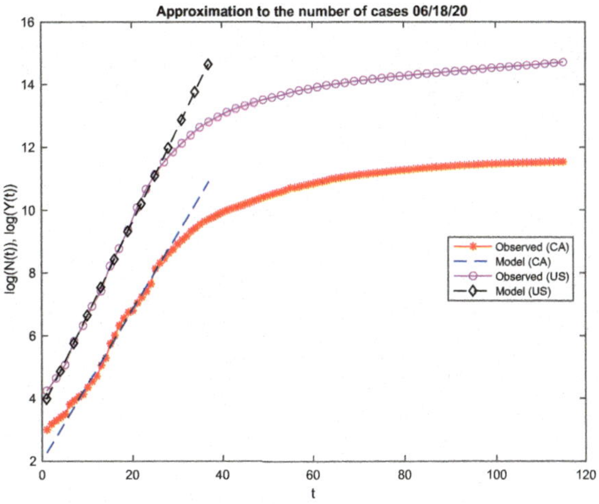

Fig. 2 Growth of the number of registered cases

points on March 16. Our analysis indicates that the correlation between different market indices got very close to one during this period which is a sign of severe financial stress.

Similar behaviour of the DJI and TSX indexes can be observed in Fig. 1.

2.2 *Market Recovery After Covid-19 Crash (2020/03/20 - 2020/03/26)*

Two major events contributed to the fast recovery of the market after the market crash due to CV19 pandemic. On March 23, 2019, federal reserve announced that it will remove its cap on the amount of government bonds buyback. This was previously set at \$700 billion. The US government two trillion-dollar aid package to assist Americans, who were affected by the virus pandemic, was another moving factor in the market. In the span of only three days, Dow Jones Index recovered as much as 21.3%, setting a record for the highest 3-day growth since the Great Depression.

2.3 *Pandemic Growth After 2020/03/18*

In Fig. 2 we depict the dynamics of the number of registered cases, in the US, and Canada, in the log-scale (that is the logarithm of the number of cases as a function of time).

It is known that the process $N(t)$ has initially exponential growth [1], [3]. For this reason, the choice of the function $\log N(t)$ is the most natural. Notice that after time $T_1 = 28^2$ the growth rate of the number of registered cases significantly deviates from exponential. During the same week the social distancing policies were enforced in the US and Canada.

3 Framework for Modelling Pandemic Impact

The modelling framework for analysis of pandemic impact on financial markets contains three main elements:

a. A set of models describing dynamics of the pandemic processes.
b. Calibration algorithms for tuning the model parameters.
c. A mapping of the pandemic process into the space of the standard financial risk factors.

We consider two pandemic models in this section. The first model is an extension of the classical SIRD model suitable for modelling social distancing effect on the pandemic spread. This model is a deterministic approximation to the Markov chain describing the dynamics of the pandemic. This approximation is close, in spirit, to the well-known Lunchester equations devised in 1916 to describe the relative strength of the military units in combat [17] as well as the famous Lottka-Volterra equations. The model allows us to introduce the social distancing policies by restricting the number of susceptible individuals.

The second model is a combination of the pure birth and pure death processes. The model has three phases each of which is calibrated to the corresponding historical scenario. One of the advantages of this model is its analytical tractability despite stochastic nature. The latter implies a relatively simple calibration. The effect of social distancing policies is also incorporated in the model dynamics.

These models allow us to generate pandemic scenarios. A generalized linear regression maps these scenarios into the space of financial risk factors and allows us to create stress scenarios on the financial indexes.

3.1 Susceptible, Infected, Recovered and Death (SIRD) Model with Time-Dependent Parameters and Social Distancing

The Susceptible, Infected, Recovered and Death (SIRD) Epidemiological Model is a compartmental model for describing spread of contagious diseases through a population. The SIRD model is based in the classic Susceptible, Infected and Recover (SIR) model introduced in the 1927, 1932, and 1933 series of papers by [14–16]. The only difference is that the SIRD model incorporates the *death (D)* compartment

[2] 28 days since the beginning of the pandemic.

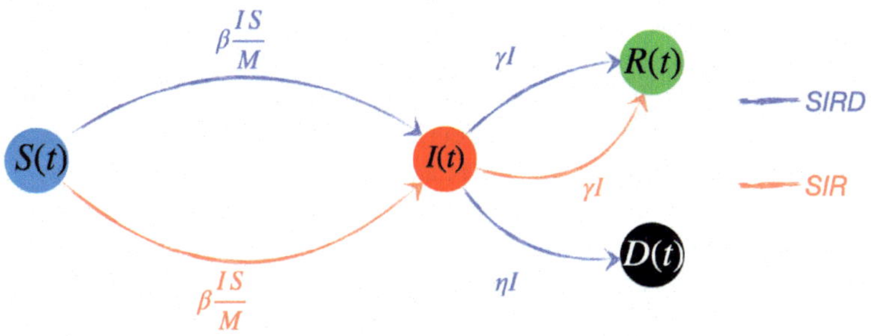

Fig. 3 SIRD and SIR transition dynamics

in order to keep track of the fatalities, which may occur at a different rate than the recoveries.

The SIRD model describes how in the presence of a contagious disease, individuals transition from one of the compartments to the next. Figure 3 illustrates the compartments of the SIR(D) model and the corresponding transition rates.

The compartments, or states, are defined as follows,

- *(S) Susceptible.* The part of the population who is likely to be infected with the disease. We denote the number of susceptible individuals at time t by $S(t)$.
- *(I) Infected.* The part of the population who is currently infected with the disease and is contagious. Specifically, this refers to the "actively" infected people.
- *(R) Recovered.* This is the population that survived the disease and becomes immune. The cumulative number of recovered individuals at time t is denoted by $R(t)$.
- *(D) Death.* This is the part of the population that succumbed to the disease, i.e., the number of fatalities. The cumulative number of fatal cases at time t is denoted by $D(t)$.

The number of actively infected people $I(t)$ can be obtained as

$$I(t) = N(t) - (R(t) + D(t)), \quad \text{with} \quad N(t) = \int_0^t c(u)du \tag{1}$$

where $N(t)$ refers to the cumulative number of infections at time $t \geq 0$, which is obtained as the time integral of the number of new registered cases $c(t)$.

There are two basic assumptions in this model. First, it is assumed that the birth rate and the (ex-disease) death rate are approximately the same and small compared to the rate of contagion. Hence, the total number M of individuals in the population is *constant* over time,

$$M = S(t) + I(t) + R(t) + D(t), \quad \forall t \geq 0. \tag{2}$$

Second, it is assumed that transition times are independent, exponentially distributed random variables. Typically, it is also assumed that the waiting times are identically distributed within each compartment; however, we do not make this assumption since we use time-dependent transition rates in order to obtain more accurate calibration results. One of the reasons for using time-dependent parameters is due to the fact that the number of cases is less certain at earlier stages of the epidemic event which may lead to different parameterization than on later stages. Another very important reason is that the rates of contagion change over time due to the implementation of different health policies. For example, when social distancing policies are implemented the rate of contagion is reduced but when these policies are lifted prematurely, the rate of contagion may increase again which in turn may cause a new wave of contagion.

The transitions of the SIRD model can be described using a continuous time Markov chain (CTMC). Since the total population M is constant, then one of the states is well defined by the remaining states. For instance, $D(t) = M - (S(t) + I(t) + R(t))$ for all $t \geq 0$. Hence, the SIRD epidemic processes is defined as a trivariate stochastic process on a continuous time scale, $t \in [0, \infty)$, with discrete states $(S, I, R)(t) = (S(t), I(t), R(t))$:

$$S(t), I(t), R(t) \in \{0, 1, \ldots, M\}. \tag{3}$$

The joint probability function of these states is denoted by,

$$P_{(s,i,r)}(t) = \mathbb{P}\left((S, I, R)(t) = (s, i, r)\right) \tag{4}$$

Since we do not assume time-homogeneity, the transition probabilities,

$$P_{(s,i,r),(s',i',r')}(u, t),$$

need to be defined using 2- parameter times $(u, t) \in [0, T] \times [u, T], T < \infty$. Hence, for a sufficiently small Δt the (forward) infinitesimal transition probabilities are given by

$$P_{(s,i,r),(s+h,i+j,r+m)}(t, t + \Delta t) \tag{5}$$

$$= \mathbb{P}\left((S, I, R)(t + \Delta t) = (s + h, i + j, r + m)\,|(S, I, R)(t) = (s, i, r)\right) \tag{6}$$

$$= \begin{cases} \beta(t)\frac{is}{M}\Delta t + o(\Delta t), & (h, j, m) = (-1, 1, 0) \\ \gamma(t)\, i\, \Delta t + o(\Delta t), & (h, j, m) = (0, -1, 1) \\ \eta(t)\, i\, \Delta t + o(\Delta t), & (h, j, m) = (0, -1, 0) \\ 1 - \left(\beta(t)\frac{S}{M} + \gamma(t) + \eta(t)\right) i\Delta t + o(\Delta t), & (h, j, m) = (0, 0, 0) \\ o(\Delta t) & \text{otherwise} \end{cases} \tag{7}$$

where, for all $t \geq 0$,[3]

- $\beta(t) > 0$ is the *transmission rate*. The factor $\beta\, I/M$ is called the *force of infection* which is the per-capita rate at which susceptible individuals leave the S compartment.
- $\gamma(t) > 0$ is the *per-capita recovery rate*. This is the rate at which an infected individual overcomes the disease and becomes immune.
- $\eta(t) > 0$ is the *per-capita death rate*. This is the rate at which an infected individual (i.e., a member of I) succumbs to the disease and becomes part of the death compartment D, which cannot be infected nor contagious.

From (7) we observe that: (a) an individual can only leave the susceptible compartment if she becomes infected (i.e., $(h, j, m) = (-1, 1, 0)$), (b) when the individual leaves the infected compartment it is either for recovered compartment (i.e., $(h, j, m) = (0, -1, 1)$) or the death compartment (i.e., $(h, j, m) = (0, -1, 0)$ and the fact that M is constant) and she no longer becomes susceptible to the disease again; and (c) no other transitions are possible. These are the dynamics of the SIRD process represented in Fig. 3.

In view of nonlinear nature of the SIRD model, we can only approximate the value of its moments. For example, the first moment can be approximated with the solution of the following deterministic non-linear ODE system:

$$\text{SIRD evolution} = \begin{cases} \frac{dS}{dt} = -\beta(t)\,\frac{I\,S}{M} \\ \frac{dI}{dt} = \beta(t)\,\frac{I\,S}{M} - (\gamma(t) + \eta(t))\,I \\ \frac{dR}{dt} = \gamma(t)\,I \\ \frac{dD}{dt} = \eta(t)\,I = -\left(\frac{dS}{dt} + \frac{dI}{dt} + \frac{dR}{dt}\right) \end{cases} \tag{8}$$

For more accurate approximations we refer to the moment closure procedures of [13, 18]. For the rest of this section, we use the solution of deterministic system as the expected value of the SIRD compartments since this is a commonly used approximation.

Strict Social Distancing. One possible way to study the effect of social distancing is obtained by introducing the parameter $\rho \in [0, 1]$ that defines the proportion of the susceptible population that *does not* or *cannot* follow the lockdown guidelines, and hence, remains vulnerable to the disease. On the other hand, $(1 - \rho) \in [0, 1]$ is the proportion of the susceptible population that follows a strict social distancing policy, and hence, it cannot be infected. The parameter ρ is called the *proportion of vulnerability*, such that $\rho = 0$ refers to the case of total lockdown (100% strict social distancing), meanwhile $\rho = 1$ refers to the base case in which no social distancing is applied whatsoever. Therefore, we can rewrite Eq (2) as,

---

[3] In order to have a well defined time-dependent process we restrict time-dependent parameters $(\beta(t), \gamma(t), \eta(t))$, $t \in [0, T]$, be continuous functions except for a finite number of discontinuities (e.g., stepwise function).

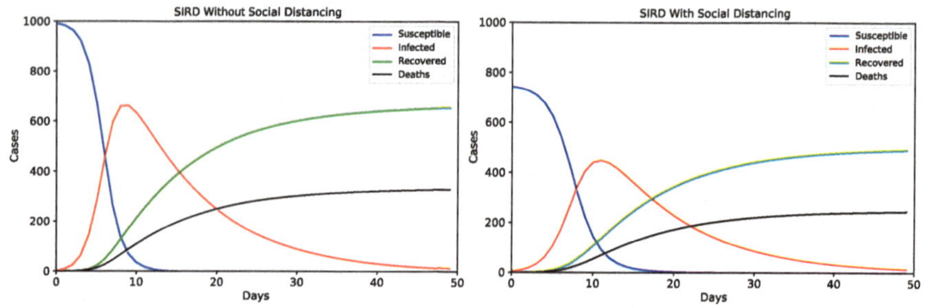

(a) $\rho = 1$ (b) $\rho = 0.75$

Fig. 4 SIRD Dynamics

$$\underbrace{\rho M}_{\text{vulnerable}} = S + I + R + D \tag{9}$$

As a result of the strict social distancing policy, the susceptible population is given by $S(t) = \rho M - I(t) - R(t) - D(t)$, and hence $S(0) = \rho M$, while for all $t > 0$, $S(t)$ is given by the dynamics described by Eqs. (7) and (8). For example, consider the case in which there are 5 actively infected people in a population of 1000 individuals. Moreover, assume that none has yet recovered or died. Hence, $M = 1000$. For convenience, assume that the model parameters $(\beta, \gamma, \eta) = (1, 1/15, 1/30)$ remain constant for all $t \geq 0$. Figure 4a, b show the expected values of the SIRD compartments with and without strict social distancing. Clearly, if the proportion of vulnerability was 75% of the total population then $(S, I, R, D)(0) = (745, 5, 0, 0)$ and the expected number of actively infected people would be significantly lower than without social distancing. This shows how social distancing may prevent the complete depletion of the available medical care.

3.2 *Calibration Algorithm*

Before we explain the calibration methodology, let us first mention some common difficulties that arise in the calibration of epidemiological models. The SIRD model, like many other epidemiological models, is useful for describing the epidemic dynamics in a well observed system. For example, in the case of a laboratory study, we can clearly observe each of the individuals transitioning across the SIRD compartments. However, in real life, these observations are much less accurate, specially when the virus is new and little information is known about its characteristics, and when it has spread across large populations since it is almost impossible to account for all the cases. For instance, in the current CV-19 pandemic event, we are not yet certain whether people who recover become completely immune or if the immunity is just temporary. Similarly, the actual number of cases is quite noisy, specially at early stages, this is due to the fact that different countries apply different testing policies, or because some countries tend to report fewer cases either for political or economical reasons or simply to avoid panic in the population. There is also the case of asymptomatic people or people who experienced only mild symptoms and never knew they were infected, and so they are not included in reported cases. Even if there is some level of certainty in the number of infected people and the number of fatalities, there is much less certainty in the number of recovered individuals, e.g., people may be released from the hospital prematurely in an effort to increase hospital availability. Nonetheless, the uncertainty in the number of cases decreases as time goes by, more data is gathered and there is more information about the features of the disease.

The set of complexities mentioned above is one of the reasons for using time-dependent parameters $(\beta(t), \gamma(t), \eta(t))$, for instance, the fact that the number of cases is less certain at earlier stages may lead to different parameterization than on later stages. Another very important reason for using time-dependent parameters is that, due to the implementation of different health policies, the rates of contagion change over time. For example, implementing social distancing reduces the rate of contagion, while reopening the city and its businesses may lead to a new rate increase, and subsequently, a new wave of contagion.

The data used in this calibration exercise are taken from the *Repository by Johns Hopkins CSSE*.[4] The advantage of this repository is that it contains the time series of the cumulative number of infected cases, recovered and deaths for almost all countries. Therefore, the actively infected number of cases can be directly obtained using Eq. (1).

Since it is our objective to calibrate multiple time series simultaneously, our problem is a multi-objective optimization. In this case, we simply use a *multi-objective weighted least squares* method in order to give more relevance to the most recent data. This problem can be formulated as follows:

$$\min_{[\beta,\theta,\eta]\in\mathbb{R}^3_+} \left(w_S^2 \sum_{i=0}^{K} \left(S_{t_i}^{obs} - S_{t_i}^{theo}\right)^2 + w_I^2 \sum_{i=0}^{K} \left(I_{t_i}^{obs} - I_{t_i}^{theo}\right)^2 \right. \tag{10}$$

$$\left. + w_R^2 \sum_{i=0}^{K} \left(R_{t_i}^{obs} - R_{t_i}^{theo}\right)^2 + w_D^2 \sum_{i=0}^{K} \left(D_{t_i}^{obs} - D_{t_i}^{theo}\right)^2 \right),$$

$$\text{where} \quad [w_S, w_I, w_R, w_D] \in \mathbb{R}^4_+, \tag{11}$$

and t_0 is the first time where an infected individual appears, K (in t_K) is the length of the time series, and $[w_S, w_I, w_R, w_D]$ are the weights for each objective function. Let $X_{[u,t]}^{obs} = [S_{[u,t]}^{obs}, I_{[u,t]}^{obs}, R_{[u,t]}^{obs}, D_{[u,t]}^{obs}]$ be the time series of the time interval $[u, t]$, $t > u \geq 0$, of the observed number of individuals in each compartment. Similarly, let $X_{[u,t]}^{theo} = [S_{[u,t]}^{theo}, I_{[u,t]}^{theo}, R_{[u,t]}^{theo}, D_{[u,t]}^{theo}]$ be the theoretical time series of the number

[4] We use the repository available in https://github.com/pomber/covid19, which in turn cleans and processes the data from Johns Hopkins CSSE (see also, https://github.com/CSSEGISandData/COVID-19).

of individuals in each compartment according to the dynamics prescribed in Eq. (8) during the same time interval $[u, t]$. Also, let $W = \text{diag}([w_S, w_I, w_R, w_D])$ be the diagonal matrix of weights for each time series. Lastly, we can solve a sequence of optimization problems

$$\left\{ \min_{[\beta_k, \gamma_k, \eta_k] \in \mathbb{R}^3_+} \quad \text{trace}\left((X^{diff}_{[t_k, t_{k+1}]} W)^T \, (X^{diff}_{[t_k, t_{k+1}]} W) \right) \right\} \Bigg|_{k=1}^{K-1} \tag{12}$$

over a time grid $0 = t_1 < t_2 < \cdots < t_K$. Such formulation implies that the time-dependent parameters $(\beta(t), \gamma(t), \eta(t))$ are specified by stepwise functions. Obviously, other kind of interpolation schemes can also be implemented.

Results. We calibrate the SIRD model to the US data available from February 1 to July 1, 2020. The calibration is done by solving the sequence of optimization problems of Eq. (12) over a semi-monthly grid.

Figure 5 illustrates the quality of our calibration procedure. We highlight the fact that we are able to capture the surge of the number of actively infected people that occurred in the second half of June. Figure 6 illustrates the step-wise profile of the time-dependent parameters $(\beta(t), \gamma(t), \eta(t))$ corresponding to our calibration procedure. We also highlight the fact that as time goes by, the parameters converge to a stable level. This is important, since it rules out possibility of over parameterizing estimation algorithm and confirms our assumption that the information on later stages is less noisy than on earlier stages of the epidemic event.

3.3 *Phenomenological Pandemic Model (PPM)*

This model describes development of the pandemic growth by the processes $N(t)$ and $I(t)$, in three phases: an initial pandemic growth, an intermediate growth and the final phase. In the initial phase, the pandemic growth is uncontrolled. In the intermediate phase, the social distancing rules restrict the growth. In the final phase, the number of registered cases does not change and the number of active cases decreases.

This model is a simplification of that considered in the previous section. At first, we introduce the stochastic process $N(t)$ describing the dynamics of the number of registered cases.

3.3.1 The Process $N(t)$

Consider the process $N(t)$ in the initial phase. Once the number of infected individuals becomes large enough, the social distancing measures get enforced and the population starts following the social distancing rules (SDR). The growth of the number of registered cases deviates from the exponential function marking the the end of the initial phase.

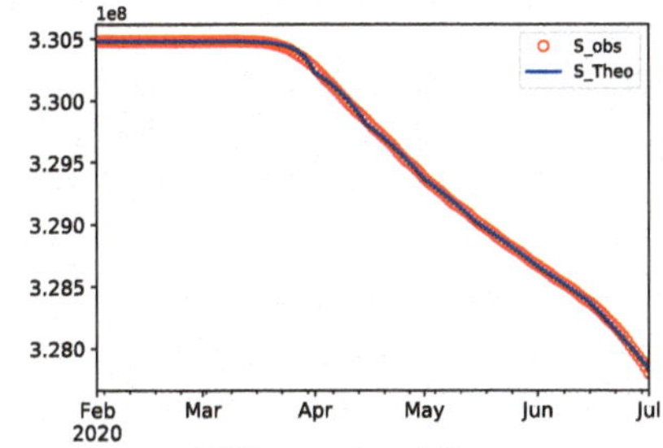

(a) Compartment S.

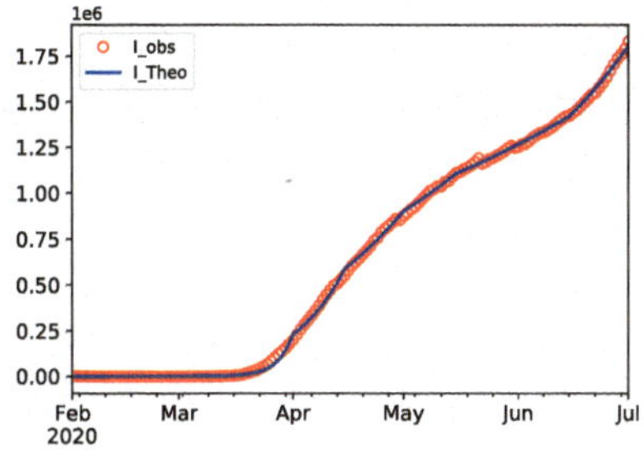

(b) Compartment I.

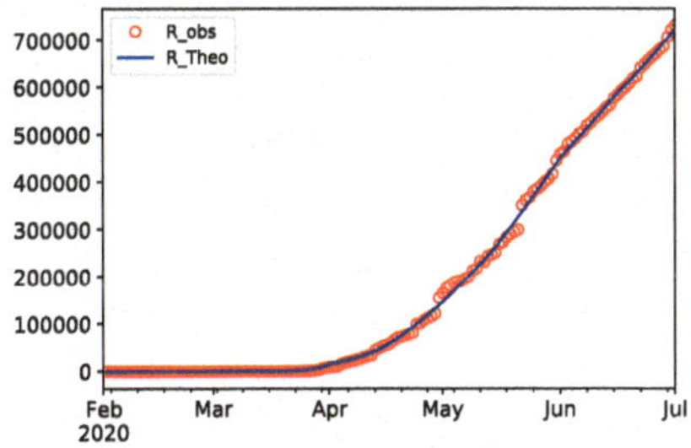

(c) Compartment R.

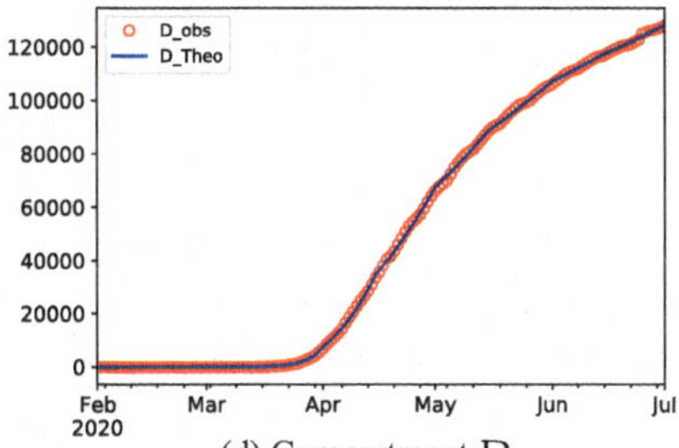

(d) Compartment D.

Fig. 5 Calibration of the SIRD model

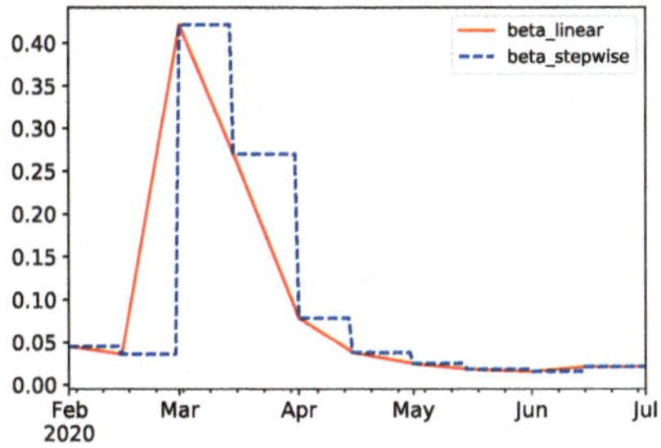

(a) Transmission rate, $\beta(t) > 0$.

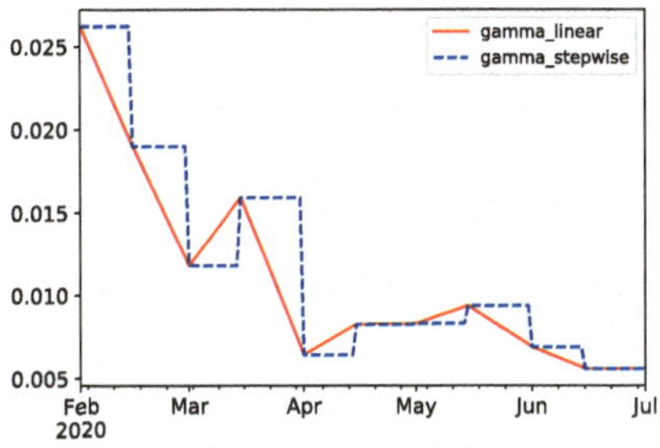

(b) Recovery Rate, $\gamma(t) > 0$.

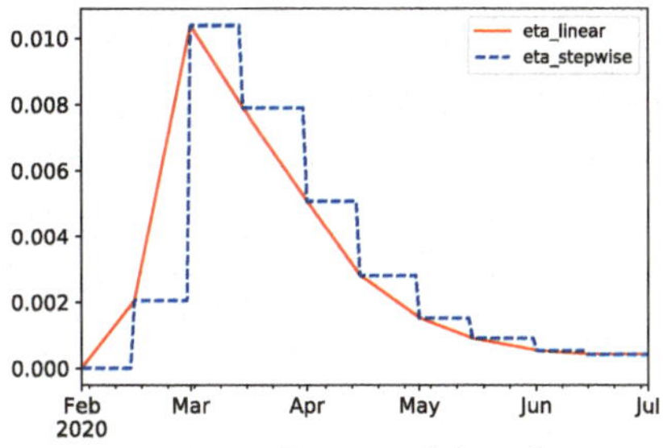

(c) Death Rate, $\eta(t) > 0$.

Fig. 6 Time-dependent coefficients

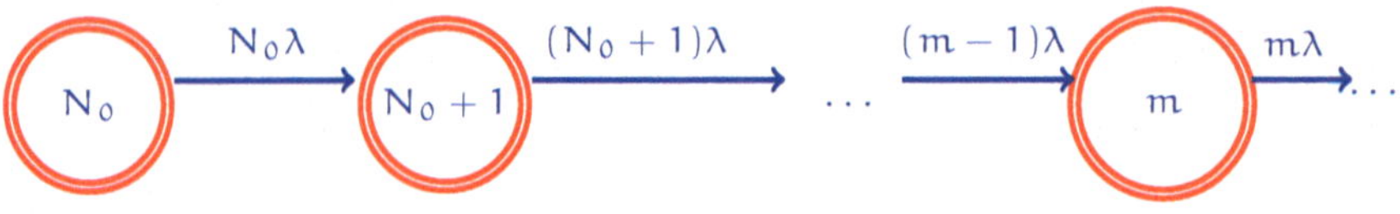

Fig. 7 Initial phase: the pure birth process, $N(t)$

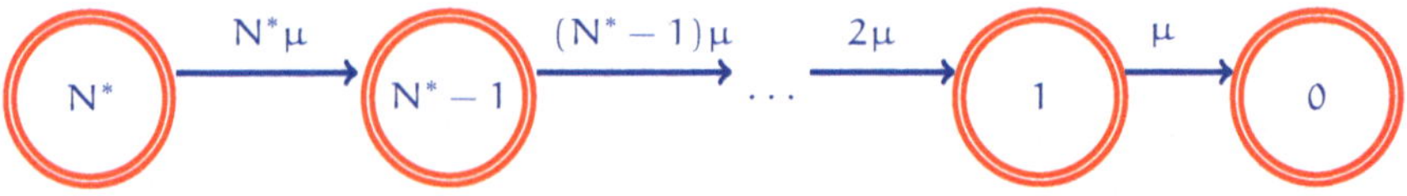

Fig. 8 Intermediate phase is described by the process $S(t)$, $t \geq T_1$

As before, we denote the cumulative number of infected individuals at time t by $N(t)$. We assume that $N(t)$ follows the pure birth process [7] in the interval $t \in [0, T_1]$. The process starts from the initial state N_0. The intensity of jump from the state m to the next state, $m + 1$, is $m\lambda$.

Fig. 7 describes the transition graph of the model in the initial phase. The probabilities $P_k(t) = \mathbb{P}(N(t) = k)$ satisfy for $t \in [0, T_1]$,

$$\frac{dP_k(t)}{dt} = -\lambda k P_k(t) + \lambda(k-1)P_{k-1}(t), \quad k = N_0 + 1, \ldots, \tag{13}$$
$$\frac{dP_{N_0}(t)}{dt} = -\lambda N_0 P_{N_0}(t),$$

and the initial condition

$$P_{N_0}(0) = 1.$$

The time of the SDR enforcement is denoted by T_1 in (13). The probability distribution, $P_k(t)$, is negative binomial on the set of non-negative integer numbers [7]:

$$P_{N_0+j}(t) = \binom{N_0 + j - 1}{j} e^{-N_0\lambda t} \left(1 - e^{-\lambda t}\right)^j, \quad j = 0, 1, \ldots. \tag{14}$$

The first moment and the variance of this process are also well-known:

$$\mathbb{E}[N(t)] = N_0 e^{\lambda t}, \qquad 0 \leq t \leq T_1, \tag{15}$$
$$\sigma^2(N_t) = N_0 \cdot \left(e^{2\lambda t} - e^{\lambda t}\right).$$

3.4 The Process $N(t)$ in an Intermediate Phase

We assume that during the initial phase of the pandemic a group of people following the SDR is formed. Individuals in this group will never be infected. The rest of the population is susceptible. The size of this group at time t is denoted by $S(t)$. We assume that $S(T_1) = N^*$. The number of infected individuals in this group increases from 0 to N^*. Therefore, the number of registered cases satisfies the relation

$$N(t) = N(T_1) + N^* - S(t), \quad t \geq T_1, \tag{16}$$

in the intermediate phase.

Remark 1 It is not difficult to see that the latter equation defines a monotonically increasing process $N(t)$ for $t \geq 0$.

The transition graph for S is presented in Fig. 8. The probabilities $Q_k(t) := \mathbb{P}(S(t) = k)$ satisfy for $t \geq T_1$ [7]

$$Q_k(t) = \binom{N^*}{k} e^{-k\mu(t-T_1)} \left(1 - e^{-\mu(t-T_1)}\right)^{N^*-k}, \quad k = 0, 1, \ldots, N^*, \tag{17}$$
$$Q_{N^*}(T_1) = 1.$$

The random time, T_{N^*}, of the transition from the state N^* to state 0 has the distribution [7]

$$\mathbb{P}(T_{N^*} > t) = 1 - (1 - e^{-\mu t})^{N^*}.$$

Then the expected value $\mathbb{E}[T_{N^*}] = \int_0^\infty \mathbb{P}(T_{N^*} > t)dt$ and we derive

$$\mathbb{E}[T_{N^*}] = \frac{1}{\mu} \sum_{m=1}^{N^*} \frac{1}{m} \tag{18}$$
$$\sim \frac{1}{\mu} \log N^*,$$

as $N^* \to \infty$. Therefore, for sufficiently large N^* the average length of the intermediate phase is proportional to the logarithm of N^*. The probability generating function

$$\hat{G}(t, z) := \mathbb{E}[z^{S(t)}], \quad |z| \leq 1,$$

satisfies for $t \geq T_1$

$$\hat{G}(t, z) = \left(ze^{-\mu(t-T_1)} + 1 - e^{-\mu(t-T_1)}\right)^{N^*}. \tag{19}$$

The expectation

$$\mathbb{E}[S(t)] = N^* e^{-\mu(t-T_1)}, \quad t \geq T_1$$

and

$$\sigma^2(S(t)) = N^* e^{-\mu(t-T_1)} \cdot (1 - e^{-\mu(t-T_1)}), \quad t \geq T_1.$$

If $N^* \to \infty$ such that $\lim_{N^* \to \infty} N^* e^{-\mu t} = \eta\tau$, we obtain

$$\lim_{N^* \to \infty} \hat{G}(t, z) = e^{\eta\tau(z-1)}. \tag{20}$$

Thus, the limiting stochastic process after a deterministic time change is just a Poisson process.[5]

We would like to stress that convergence result (20) seems to be related to the stage of the pandemic at which the number of individuals with a sufficient level of antibodies is sufficiently large.

3.4.1 The Process $I(t)$ and Distribution of Sickness Time

The second key element of the model is the process $I(t)$, the number of active cases at time t. The random variable $I(t)$ satisfies the equation

$$N(t) = I(t) + R(t) + D(t),$$

linking together the number of registered cases and the numbers of recovered and dead patients. Suppose that all individuals have the same deterministic sickness time τ. Then at time t all cases registered at time $t - \tau$ will be either recovered or dead. Therefore

$$I(t) = N(t) - N(t - \tau)$$

in this case. Naturally, this assumption on τ is unrealistic and we need a different line of reasoning. At the same time, the process $I(t)$ is observable and comparison of the processes N and I allows one to obtain an approximation to the sickness time distribution of all individuals recovered or dead at time t. The start time of sickness of the nth individual is

$$t_n = \min\{t : N(t) \geq n\}.$$

Denote $\hat{R}(t) = R(t) + D(t)$. Then

$$\tau_n = \min\{t : \hat{R}(t) \geq n\}$$

is the end of the sickness time of nth individual. Thus, for each n, $N_0 \leq n \leq R(t)$ we know the sickness time, $s_n = \tau_n - t_n$. We assume that $\{s_n\}_{n \geq N_0}$ is a sequence of independent identically distributed random variables. The distribution of the sickness

[5] Weak convergence of stochastic processes discussed in this section represents an independent interest. The rigorous presentation with the proof of (20) is deferred to a more specialized journal on stochastic processes.

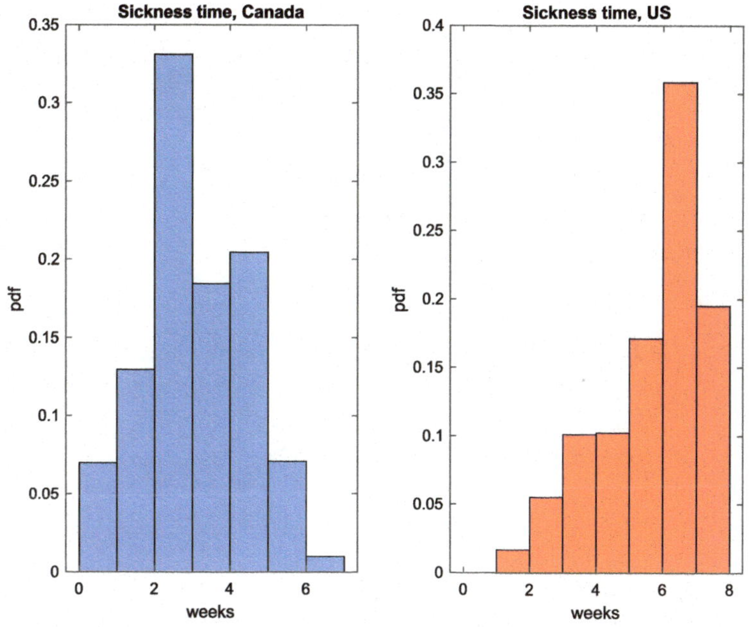

Fig. 9 Sickness time distributions

time, $F_s(x) = \mathbb{P}(s_n \leq x)$, depends on the geographical region, age, sex and many other individual parameters. For the purpose of our research, we aggregate the distribution of the sickness time at the country level. Figure 9 demonstrates distinction of the sickness times in Canada and the US. In particular, the maximal density in Canada has the group with 2 weeks sickness time. In the US, maximal density has the group of individuals with 6 weeks sickness time.[6]

3.5 Approximation to PPM

We consider a deterministic approximation to the process $N(t)$. It can be described by the equations representing the first two phases of the process $N(t)$. For $0 < t \leq T_1$, the number of registered cases, in accordance with (15), is $N(t) = N_0 \cdot e^{\lambda t}$.

After time T_1, the number of registered cases is approximated by the solution to the equation

$$\frac{\mathrm{d}N(t)}{\mathrm{d}t} = k(N(t)) \cdot N(t), \quad t > T_1,$$

[6] We hope that in the nearest future we will have more reliable data that would allow us to infer the statistical properties of the sickness time distribution.

Table 1 Parameters of the approximation, $Y(t)$

Country	k	b	σ	T_1 (days)
US	0.286	4.01	0.63	28
CA	0.223	2.394	0.44	28

with the initial condition

$$N(T_1) = N_0 \cdot \exp(\lambda T_1),$$

where $k(N) = k_0 \left(1 - \frac{N(t)}{N^*}\right)$. As $N(t) \to N^*$ the growth rate $k(N) \to 0$. Then we derive

$$N(t) = \frac{N^* \exp(k_0(t - T_1))}{\exp(k_0(t - T_1)) + N^*/N_1 - 1}, \quad t \geq T_1. \tag{21}$$

The process $\hat{R}(t)$ is computed using the sickness time distribution, F_s.

3.6 Calibration of PPM

The first step in the calibration procedure is estimation of the parameters of the process $N(t)$ in the initial pandemic phase. In Fig. 2 we depict the dynamics of the number of registered cases, in the US, and Canada, in the log-scale (that is the logarithm of the number of cases as a function of time).

It is known that initially the process $N(t)$ exhibits an exponential growth [1], [3], [8]. In Fig. 2 the least-square approximation to the observed values of $\log(N(t))$ is presented. In the initial phase, a deterministic approximation to the observed process $N(t)$ is described by the equation $Y(t) = e^{kt+b}$. The parameters k and b, are estimated using the Least Square Method. The values of these coefficients are shown in Table 1 [7]

The initial phase of the process $N(t)$ ends at T_1: after this time the growth rate deviates from the estimated value of k.

3.6.1 Calibration of Parameters of the Birth-Death Processes

Let us now show how to find the maximum likelihood estimator (MLE) of the parameter λ in the PPM to describe the pure birth process in the initial phase of the process $N(t)$. Assume that the process is observed at times $t = 0, \Delta t, \ldots, m\Delta t$ and denote the observations $N_0, N_1, \ldots, N_m$. It is also convenient to introduce the integer increments $n_k = N_k - N_{k-1}$, $(k = 1, 2, \ldots, m)$ of the observed process $N(k\Delta t)$. The

[7] The measurement date is 29/03/2020.

initial phase is the pure birth process having transition probabilities

$$\mathbb{P}_{\Delta t}\left(N_{k-1} \to N_k\right) = \binom{N_k - 1}{n_k} \cdot e^{-\lambda \Delta t N_{k-1}} \left(1 - e^{-\lambda \Delta t}\right)^{n_k}, \quad k = 1, 2, \ldots, m.$$

The process $N(t)$ is Markovian process. Its likelihood function

$$\mathcal{L}_m(\lambda) = \prod_{k=1}^{m} \binom{N_k - 1}{n_k} \cdot e^{-\lambda \Delta t N_{k-1}} \left(1 - e^{-\lambda \Delta t}\right)^{n_k}$$

can be written as

$$\mathcal{L}_m(\lambda) = C_m \cdot \exp\left(-\lambda \Delta t \sum_{k=1}^{m} N_{k-1}\right) \left(1 - e^{-\lambda \Delta t}\right)^{\sum_{k=1}^{m} n_k},$$

where

$$C_m = \prod_{k=1}^{m} \binom{N_k - 1}{n_k}.$$

For $\lambda > 0$, the function $\mathcal{L}_m(\lambda)$ has a unique point $\lambda_* = \text{argmax}_{\lambda > 0} \mathcal{L}_m(\lambda)$:

$$\lambda_* = -\frac{1}{\Delta t} \log\left(\frac{\sum_{k=1}^{m} N_{k-1}}{\sum_{k=1}^{m} N_k}\right). \tag{22}$$

Equation (22) defines the MLE for the process, $N(t)$ in the initial phase, starting from the state N_0, observed at $t_k = k \cdot \Delta t$.

The MLE for the process $N(t)$ in the intermediate phase is more challenging because the state of the Markovian, pure death process, $\mathcal{S}(t)$, is unknown at time T_1, $\mathcal{S}(T_1) = N^*$ (as well as at all times $t > T_1$). Again, we assume that the changes of the process are observed at times $t_k = T_1 + k\Delta t$, $k = 1, 2, \ldots, m$ and denote the observed decrements $\mathcal{D}_k := \mathcal{S}(t_{k-1}) - \mathcal{S}(t_k)$. Our goal is estimation of the parameters N^* and intensity μ.

Denote $p = e^{-\mu \Delta t}$. Then the likelihood function

$$\mathcal{L}_m^{\mathcal{S}}(N^*, p) = C_m \cdot p^{N^* m - K_m} \cdot (1 - p)^{K_m^*}, \tag{23}$$

where

$$C_m = \frac{N^*!}{\prod_{k=1}^{m} \mathcal{D}_k! \cdot (N^* - K_m^*)!},$$

$$K_m = \sum_{n=1}^{m} \mathcal{D}_n \cdot (m - n + 1), \quad \text{and } K_m^* = \sum_{n=1}^{m} \mathcal{D}_n.$$

The MLE of the parameters is a solution to the optimization problem

$$(\hat{N}, \hat{p}) = \operatorname{argmax} \mathcal{L}_m^S(N^*, p), \quad 0 < p < 1, \; N^* > K_m^*. \tag{24}$$

From the relation

$$\frac{\partial \mathcal{L}_m^S(N^*, \hat{p})}{\partial p} = 0, \tag{25}$$

we derive

$$\hat{p} = \frac{m\hat{N} - K_m}{K_m^* + m\hat{N} - K_m}. \tag{26}$$

The second equation needed to solve (24) can be conveniently obtained for the log-likelihood function if we consider N^* as a continuous variable and use Stirling's formula, $N! \approx \left(N \cdot e^{-1}\right)^N \sqrt{2\pi N}$, to approximate $\partial \log \mathcal{L}_m^S(N^*, p)/\partial N^*$ for large N^*.

We have

$$\begin{aligned} \log \mathcal{L}_m^S(N^*, p) \approx\; & N^*(\log N^* - 1) + \frac{1}{2}\log\left(\frac{N^*}{N^* - K_m^*}\right) + \tilde{\mathcal{D}}_m \\ & - (N^* - K_m^*)(\log(N^* - K_m^*) - 1) + (m \cdot N^* - K_m)\log p \\ & + K_m^* \cdot \log(1 - p), \end{aligned} \tag{27}$$

where

$$\tilde{\mathcal{D}}_m = \log\left(\prod_{k=1}^{m} \mathcal{D}_k!\right)$$

does not depend on p and N^*. Then (27) implies

$$\frac{\partial \log \mathcal{L}_m^S(N^*, p)}{\partial N^*} = \log\left(\frac{N^*}{N^* - K_m}\right) + \frac{1}{2}\left(\frac{1}{N^*} - \frac{1}{N^* - K_m^*}\right) + m\log p. \tag{28}$$

From (26) and (28) we derive that the root $\hat{N}$ of the equations (24) and (25) is a solution to the transcendental equation

$$\frac{\hat{N}}{\hat{N} - K_m} \cdot \left(\frac{m\hat{N} - K_m}{K_m^* + m\hat{N} - K_m}\right)^m = \exp\left(\frac{1}{2} \cdot \frac{K_m^*}{\hat{N}(\hat{N} - K_m^*)}\right). \tag{29}$$

Equation (29) has a unique solution that can be found numerically and after rounding delivers the MLE of the parameter N^*. Finally, from (26) we calculate the estimator of the probability $\hat{p}$ and find an estimate of intensity parameter

$$\hat{\mu} = -\frac{1}{\Delta t}\log \hat{p}.$$

3.6.2 Calibration of Parameters of Approximate Model

In the case of approximate PPM the dynamics of the process $N(t)$ are defined by Equation (21). The calibration algorithm for the approximate deterministic model solves numerically the optimization problem

$$(N^*, k_0) = \text{argmin} Y(\mathbf{t}; N^*, k_0), \quad \mathbf{t} = (t_1, \ldots, t_m), \ t_1 < t_2 < \cdots < t_m,$$

where

$$Y(\mathbf{t}; N^*, k_0) = \sum_{k=1}^{m} \left(N(t_k; N^*, k_0) - N^{ob}(t_k)\right)^2$$

is the distance between the theoretical values, $N(t_k; N^*, k_0)$, defined by (21), and the vector of observations, $N^{ob}(t_k)$, $(k = 1, 2, \ldots, m)$.

This problem requires global optimization techniques, since the objective function in (21) is not a convex function of the parameters N^* and k_0. Our implementation is based on the Quasi Monte Carlo sampling of the initial points of the Sequential Quadratic Programming solution algorithm.

3.7 *Mapping Epidemic Variables to Financial Risk Factors*

We propose a regression model that links financial risk drivers such as the $SP500$ and the VIX indices to epidemic variables such as the number individuals who are actively infected (I) and susceptible (S):

$$\widetilde{y}_t = \beta_0 \cdot \widetilde{y}_{t-1} + \beta_1 \cdot \widetilde{f(S_t, t)} + \beta_2 \cdot \widetilde{f(I_t, t)} + \epsilon_t, \quad \epsilon_t \sim N(0, \sigma_\epsilon). \tag{30}$$

where[8] y_t is the *natural logarithm* transformation of the risk driver price P, i.e., $y_t = \ln(P_t)$ where $P \in \{SPX500, VIX\}$. In addition, the quantity $\widetilde{x}$ indicates that variable x is standardized, i.e.,

$$\widetilde{x} = \frac{x - \mathbb{AVG}(x)}{\mathbb{STD}(x)}, \tag{31}$$

where $\mathbb{AVG}$ and $\mathbb{STD}$ refer to the arithmetic mean and standard deviation, respectively. The function $f(x_t, t)$ refers to the *running standartization* of the variable x_t, that is,

$$f(x_t, t) = \frac{x_t - \mathbb{AVG}_{(t)}(x_t)}{\mathbb{STD}_{(t)}(x_t)}, \tag{32}$$

[8] Recall that since we are not including the bias corrector β_0, then there may be a small, but insignificant, mean in the distribution of ϵ.

Table 2 SP500 calibration summary statistics

Dep. Variable:	$\widetilde{y_t} = \ln(\widetilde{P_t^{SP500}})$	**R-squared (uncentered):**	0.906
Model:	OLS	**Adj. R-squared (uncentered):**	0.903
Method:	Least Squares	**F-statistic:**	327.6
No. Observations:	105	**Prob (F-statistic):**	3.32e-52
Df Residuals:	102	**Log-Likelihood:**	-24.361
Df Model:	3	**AIC:**	54.72
		BIC:	62.68

	coef	**std err**	**t**	**P> |t|**	**[0.025**	**0.975]**
$\widetilde{f(I,t)}$	0.6658	0.278	2.392	0.019	0.114	1.218
$\widetilde{f(S,t)}$	0.8548	0.292	2.930	0.004	0.276	1.433
$\widetilde{y_{t-1}} = \ln(\widetilde{P_{t-1}^{SP500}})$	0.7764	0.053	14.533	0.000	0.670	0.882

where $\mathbb{AVG}_{(t)}$ and $\mathbb{STD}_{(t)}$ refer to the *running* arithmetic mean and standard deviation *up to time* $t > 0$, respectively. The difference between $\mathbb{AVG}$ and $\mathbb{AVG}_{(t)}$ is that the former calculates the mean over the whole sample while the latter calculates the mean only up to the running time t (the same applies to the standard deviation). The autoregressive term y_{t-1} captures the momentum of the most recent prices during the pandemic event ($\beta_0 \in (0, 1)$ implies that recent prices are more significant than older price levels).

Under this specification, the index price P_t has the solution,

$$P_t = \exp\Big(\mathbb{STD}(\ln(P))\big(\beta_0 \cdot \widetilde{y}_{t-1} + \beta_1 \cdot \widetilde{f(S_t,t)} + \beta_2 \cdot \widetilde{f(I_t,t)}\big) + \mathbb{AVG}(\ln(P)) + \mathbb{STD}(\ln(P)) \cdot \epsilon_t\Big), \qquad \epsilon_t \sim N(0, \sigma_\epsilon). \tag{33}$$

The solution implies that if we are able to (independently) forecast S and I we can simulate the index price P_t using Monte Carlo methods.

We illustrate our regression model of Eq. (30) by calibrating the S&P500 and VIX indices using the data available from February 1 to July 1, 2020. The regression summaries are shown in Tables 2 and 3. We can observe that for this estimation period all three parameters are significant. Figure 10 illustrates the index prices and the corresponding prediction values using (33). In conclusion, we can observe that the regression (30) provides us with a reasonable model to describe the dependency during the CV-19 pandemic crisis. We will use this model to shock our risk drivers.

Table 3 VIX calibration summary statistics

Dep. Variable:	$\widetilde{y_t} = \ln(\widetilde{P_t^{\text{VIX}}})$	**R-squared (uncentered):**	0.934
Model:	OLS	**Adj. R-squared (uncentered):**	0.932
Method:	Least Squares	**F-statistic:**	482.0
No. Observations:	105	**Prob (F-statistic):**	4.51e-60
Df Residuals:	102	**Log-Likelihood:**	-5.6967
Df Model:	3	**AIC:**	17.39
		BIC:	25.36

	coef	**std err**	**t**	**P> |t|**	**[0.025**	**0.975]**
$\widetilde{f(I,t)}$	-0.5972	0.233	-2.562	0.012	-1.060	-0.135
$\widetilde{f(S,t)}$	-0.6896	0.246	-2.798	0.006	-1.178	-0.201
$\widetilde{y_{t-1}} = \ln(\widetilde{P_{t-1}^{\text{VIX}}})$	0.8746	0.049	17.689	0.000	0.777	0.973

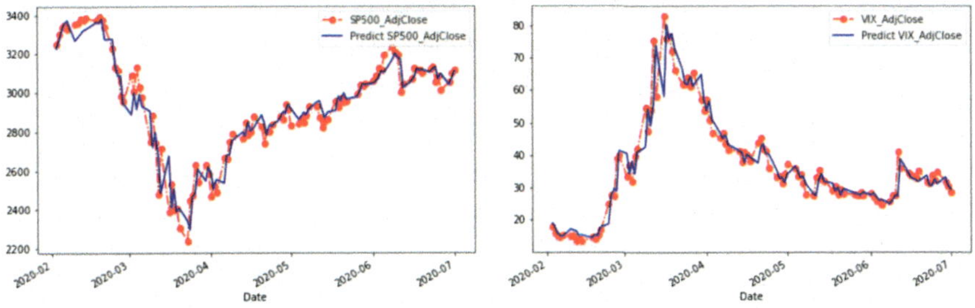

(a) SP500 Index. (b) VIX Index.

Fig. 10 Index price calibration

4 Simulation of Stress Scenarios

Let us now consider stress scenario generation in our framework.

4.1 *Simulation of Risk Drivers Under the SIRD Model*

The simulation of *risk drivers* according to (33) has two sources of uncertainty: the running standardized number of susceptible and actively infected people $(\widetilde{f(S_t,t)}, \widetilde{f(I_t,t)})$, and the error term ϵ_t, $(t > 0)$, where σ_ϵ is estimated as the residuals standard deviation of the regression model defined in (30).

Under the SIRD model of Sect. 3.1 the tuple $(\widetilde{f(S_t,t)}, \widetilde{f(I_t,t)})$ can be simulated using Monte Carlo techniques for CTMCs (e.g., we can approximate Eq. (7) to Poisson processes and simulate them using Euler schemes). Alternatively, one can simply assume that the dynamics of the SIRD compartments are deterministic using their expectation (i.e., use Eq. (8)), and hence, only simulate ϵ_t. Due to space limitations we focus our discussion on the second approach.

In order to generate sample paths of the risk driver $X_t \in \{SP\&500, VIX\}$ we use the following steps:

1. Consider the time grid $t_{grid} = (t_1, \ldots, t_N)$, where t_1 is the most recent date, and t_N is the end date for the simulation.
2. Forecast the SIRD compartments (e.g., in expectation), from time t_0 to time t_N by solving the ODE system (8) where the time-dependent parameters $(\beta_t, \gamma_t, \eta_t)$ are obtained from the calibration described in Sect. 3.2. One may use constant extrapolation for the parameters beyond the calibration horizon. The numerical solution to Eq. (8) can be easily implemented in Python using the *scipy.integrate.odeint* library.
3. Compute $(\widetilde{f(S_t,t)}, \widetilde{f(I_t,t)})$ for all $t \in t_{grid}$ using Eq. (32). Observe that these running standardized values are computed from an expanding window starting at time t_0, where t_0 is the initial pandemic date (i.e., $t_0 < t_1$).
4. For $i = 1$ to N:

   a. Draw $\epsilon_{t_i} \sim N(0, \sigma_\epsilon)$
   b. Compute P_{t_i} as in Eq. (33) using $P_{t_{i-1}}$ and $(\widetilde{f(S_{t_i}, t_i)}, \widetilde{f(I_{t_i}, t_i)})$. The parameters $(\beta_0, \beta_1, \beta_2)$ of Eq. (33) correspond to the regression parameters obtained from the regression model (30).

In this example, we simulate 1000 sample paths, from July 1st to August 3rd, 2020. In Figs. 11 and 12 we illustrate the sample paths of the S&P500 and VIX indices and the corresponding empirical confidence intervals, respectively. One can see that the sample paths imply high volatility levels. This can be explained by the fact that the dynamics of the model (33) are not from a geometric Brownian motion, but most importantly, by the fact that the residual's standard deviation σ_ϵ is estimated only during the pandemic event, which is quite high during this crisis period. Hence, we recommend the application of this methodology for short time horizons as one can argue that the assumptions are only valid during the pandemic crisis.

4.2 PPM Simulation

Similar approach is used when the simulation model is PPM. Once we constructed a regression model linking the pandemic variables to the market variables we generate a set of stress scenarios on the variables $N(t)$ and $I(t)$ using estimated values of the parameters. After that the regression model transforms the pandemic stress scenarios into the scenarios on financial indices.

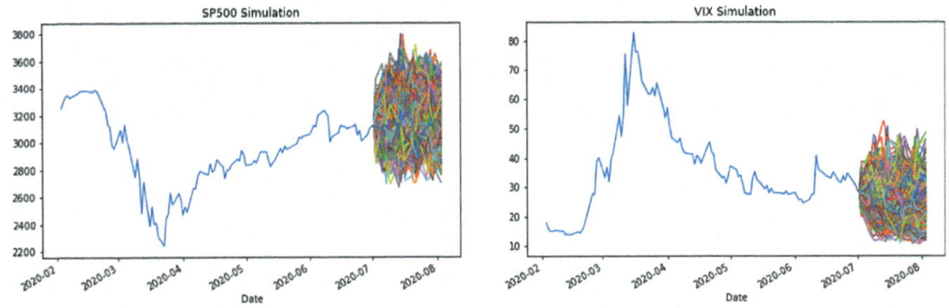

(a) S&P500 Index

(b) VIX Index

Fig. 11 Simulations

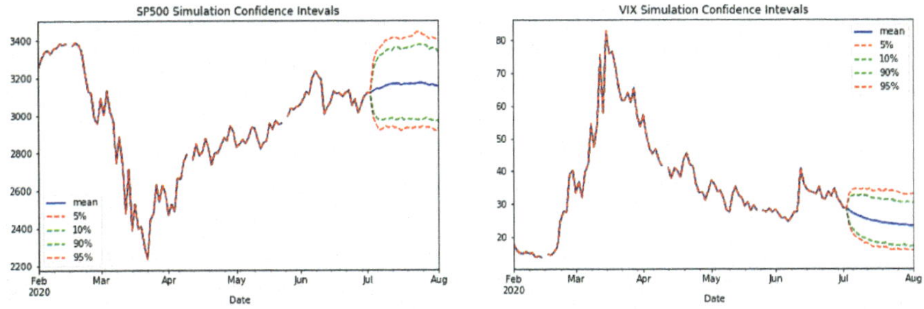

(a) SP500 Index

(b) VIX Index

Fig. 12 Confidence Intevals

This process is represented in Fig. 13 where a stress scenario on $N(t)$ and $I(t)$ is transformed into stress scenario on the financial indices DJI, TSX and CAD/USD FX rate. The explanatory power of the PPM is 10% lower than that of the SIRD model. For this reason, application of the regressed scenarios on the pandemic variables includes MC noise (the blue line representing the financial scenarios in the subfigures of Fig. 13. The red line in these subfigures describes the regression result.)

5 Conclusion

We proposed a framework for generation of stress scenarios on financial indices for analysis of the pandemic impact on financial markets. This framework includes pandemic models, their calibration algorithms and mapping of the non-financial pandemic processes to the financial indices driving the financial markets.

We think that the proposed models can be used not only for the purpose of this research but in a more general context. For instance, one can use the extended SIRD model or the PPM for the short-term prediction of the pandemic processes.

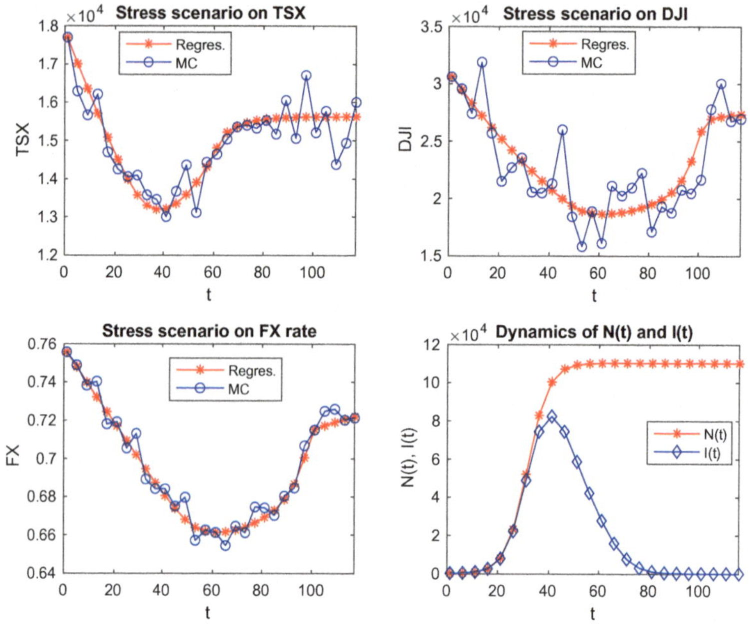

Fig. 13 Simulation of DJI, TSX and FX rate using PPM

Among the next steps we plan to analyze impact of Covid-19 on the European and Asian financial markets, extending both geography and the list of financial indices. The methods developed in this paper can be used for advanced historical and hypothetical scenario generation.

Acknowledgements We are very grateful to Rustom Barua, Yijun Jiang, Alan Yang, Ken Wang, Rob Seidman, Andrew Marchenko, Yuliy Koshevnik, Ken Jackson and Vladimir Vinogradov for the interesting discussions and suggestions.

References

1. Brauer, F., Driessche, P., Wu.: Mathematical Epidemiology. Springer, Berlin Heidelberg (2008)
2. Cushing, J.M.: Integro-differential Equations and Delay Models in Population Dynamic. Springer-Verlag, Berlin Heidelberg (1977)
3. Daley, D.J., Gani, J.: Epidemic Modeling: An Introduction. Cambridge University Press (2005)
4. Grassly, N.C., Fraser, C.: Mathematical models of infectious disease transmission. Nat. Rev. Microbiol. **6**(6), 477–487 (2008). https://doi.org/10.1038/nrmicro1845
5. Hoppensteadt, F.C.: Mathematical Methods of Population Biology. Cambridge University Press (1982)
6. Sameni, R.: Mathematical Modeling of Epidemic Diseases; A Case Study of the COVID-19 Coronavirus. Working paper, Grenoble, France 24 March (2020)

7. Feller, W.: An Introduction to Probability Theory ant its Applications. John Wiley & Sons, New York (1968)
8. IIDDA. The International Infectious Disease Data Archive, http://iidda.mcmaster.ca
9. The John Hopkins University coronavirus dash board. https://coronavirus.jhu.edu
10. Coronavirus Dashboard. https://ncov2019.live
11. Goldstein, J.A.: Abstract evolution equations. Trans. Am. Math. Soc. **141**, 159–185 (1969)
12. Isham, V.: Assessing the variability of stochastic epidemics. Math. Biosci. **107**(2), 209–224 (1991)
13. Keeling, M.J.: Meta-population moments: coupling, stochasticity and persistence. J. Animal Ecol. **69**(5), 725–736 (2000)
14. Kermack, W., McKendrick, A.: Contributions to the Mathematical Theory of Epidemics–I. 1927. Bull. Math. Biol. **53**(1-2), 33–55 (1991)
15. Kermack, W., McKendrick, A.: Contributions to the Mathematical Theory of epidemics–II. The Problem of endemicity.1932. Bull. Math. Biol. **53**(1-2), 57–87 (1991)
16. Kermack, W., McKendrick, A.: Contributions to the Mathematical Theory of epidemics–III. Further Studies of the Problem of Endemicity. 1933. Bull. Math. Biol. **53**(1-2), 89–118 (1991)
17. Lanchester, F.: Mathematics in Warfare. The World of Mathematics **4**, 2138–2157, (1956); anthologised from *Aircraft in Warfare* (1916)
18. Lloyd, A.L.: Estimating variability in models for recurrent epidemics: assessing the use of moment closure techniques. Theoret. Popul. Biol. **64**, 49–65 (2004)
19. https://www.theguardian.com/business/2020/mar/28/how-coronavirus-sent-global-markets-into-freefall
20. Aas, K., Haff, I.: The generalised hyperbolic skew student t-distribution. J. Finan. Econometr. **4**(2),(2006)
21. Breymann, W., Luthi, D.: Ghyp: a package on generalized hyperbolic distributions, November 2014

Symptom-Based Testing in a Compartmental Model of Covid-19

Ferenc A. Bartha, János Karsai, Tamás Tekeli, and Gergely Röst

Abstract Testing and isolation of cases is an important component of our strategies to fight SARS-CoV-2. In this work, we consider a compartmental model for Covid-19 including a nonlinear term representing symptom-based testing. We analyze how the considered clinical spectrum of symptoms and the testing rate affect the outcome and the severity of the outbreak.

Keywords Covid-19 · Compartmental model · Testing · Outbreak mitigation

Classifications 92D30 · 34H05 · 34C60

1 Introduction

Since a cluster of pneumonia cases of unknown origin was discovered in Wuhan, China in late 2019, Covid-19, the disease caused by the novel coronavirus SARS-CoV-2, has spread around the world giving rise to a pandemic. By early August 2020, around eighteen million cases and seven hundred thousand deaths have been reported worldwide [1].

One of the key difficulties in controlling Covid-19 is that many infections result in mild symptoms or none at all, making the detection of infectious Covid-19 cases particularly challenging [2]. Moreover, a considerable portion of secondary infec-

F. A. Bartha (✉) · J. Karsai · T. Tekeli · G. Röst
Bolyai Institute, University of Szeged, Szeged, Hungary
e-mail: barfer@math.u-szeged.hu

J. Karsai
e-mail: karsai@math.u-szeged.hu

T. Tekeli
e-mail: tekeli@math.u-szeged.hu

G. Röst
e-mail: rost@math.u-szeged.hu

P. Agarwal et al. (eds.), *Analysis of Infectious Disease Problems (Covid-19) and Their Global Impact*, Infosys Science Foundation Series,
https://doi.org/10.1007/978-981-16-2450-6_16

Table 1 Several key symptoms of Covid-19 and their prevalence among clinical Covid-19 cases

Name	Prevalence	Reference
Cough	67.8%	[9]
Fatigue	38.1%	[9]
Sputum production	33.7%	[9]
Diarrhea	3.8%	[9]
Fever	33.7%	[10]
Anosmia	70.2%	[8]
Ageusia	65%	[10]

tions, generated by those infectors who later develop symptoms, have been observed to take place before symptom onset, *i.e.* pre-symptomatic transmission occurs [3–5].

Covid-19 is classified as a respiratory disease, accordingly, it mainly affects the respiratory tract (similarly to other coronaviruses) but other classes of symptoms have been observed as well, *e.g.* affecting the gastrointestinal [6] and musculoskeletal systems [7]. In particular, the loss of smell (anosmia) and/or taste (ageusia) could be a key indicator symptom of Covid-19 [8]. We summarize findings of some recent studies regarding Covid-19 symptoms and their prevalence among clinical Covid-19 cases in Table 1.

The primary confirmation of Covid-19 infection, as of now, happens via real-time reverse transcription polymerase chain reaction (rRT-PCR) based testing of samples taken from *e.g.* nasopharyngeal or oropharyngeal swabs, sputum, lower respiratory tract aspirates, etc. [11].

A classical approach for modeling and understanding epidemics is constructing a system of ordinary differential equations (ODE) having a compartmental structure. Also, such models are widely utilized as an important tool of assessing the effectiveness of various control strategies [13, 14].

In particular, the transmission dynamics of the spread of Covid-19 has been analyzed via compartmental ODE models in a vast number of studies. Yang and Wang [15] investigated the outbreak of Covid-19 in Wuhan, China considering multiple transmission pathways in the infection dynamics. Non-constant transmission rates were employed, changing with the epidemiological status and environmental conditions reflecting the impact of the ongoing disease control measures. Boldog et al. [16] developed a tool comprised of three major components to assess the risk of global spread of Covid-19 with origin from Wuhan. A time-dependent *SEIR* model (Suceptible-Exposed-Infectious-Removed) was used to estimate the cumulative number of cases in China from which probability distributions were obtained for the number of potential disease spreaders outside China. Finally, for a given destination country, the initial spread of Covid-19 was approximated via a Galton-Watson process. Berger et al. [17] utilized an extended *SEIR* model to understand the role of testing and case-dependent quarantine with fixed rates and compared simple testing and quarantine policies. Weitz [18] developed an extended, age-stratified model analyzing both asymptomatic and severe courses of the disease in order to estimate the burden on the healthcare system by modeling hospital and intensive care unit (ICU) bed needs. Röst et al. [19] studied an age-stratified compartmental model and presented a comprehensive analysis exploring several post-lockdown scenarios with age-specific measures, seasonality, and spatial heterogeneity.

In this work, we consider an extended *SEIR*-type compartmental model for the transmission dynamics of Covid-19. We incorporate symptom-based testing of patients and isolation upon positive result *i.e.* removal from the infectious chain. The clinical symptoms that trigger the testing of individuals is referred to as *indicator symptom*. The *force of testing* is defined as the rate at which infected individuals are tested, see Sect. 2. It is described by a nonlinear function of the state of the epidemic and of all individuals displaying the indicator symptom at a given time, with or without Covid-19 infection, hence, it is considerably different from previous approaches. Our goal is to understand the impact, and especially the limitations of this testing strategy, hence we model neither contact-tracing of patients with positive tests nor the testing of a fraction of non-symptomatic contacts, both of which are common and efficient improvements and result in removal of additional patients from the infectious chain. Moreover, we assume perfect testing, that is we do not consider false positive or false negative results.

According to the current understanding of the disease, none of the symptoms are specific solely for Covid-19, thus, the chosen indicator symptom may and will be present amongst other individuals not infected with SARS-CoV-2. All patients, with or without Covid-19 infection, displaying the indicator symptom form the so-called *primary symptom pool*, whilst, those without Covid-19 infection (but with the same indicator symptom) are members of the *secondary symptom pool*, see Sect. 2. Naturally, choosing the indicator symptom for a testing campaign should be affected by its prevalence and by the historical statistics for the size of the associated secondary symptom pool. We emphasize that the latter might undergo seasonal variations as is typical with respiratory symptoms peaking in influenza season [20]. This is a common but not uniform feature of Covid-19 symptoms, *e.g.* gastrointestinal symptoms might show no seasonal variations, depending on age-groups [21].

The chapter is structured as follows. Section 2 presents the compartmental epidemic model and its parametrization. In addition, the next generation matrix computations are included that are used to derive formulae for the reproduction number. Then, Sect. 3 establishes several boundedness and monotonicity-type results on key characteristics of the epidemic model. The results of numerical simulations are discussed in Sect. 4. Finally, we present our conclusions in Sect. 5.

2 The Epidemic Model of Indicator Symptom-Based Testing

To assess the effectiveness of indicator symptom based testing in controlling the spread of Covid-19, we developed a compartmental population model based on the general *SEIR* formulation without vital dynamics.

We divide the population into five classes: susceptible (S), latent (L), pre-symptomatic (P), infected (I), and removed (R). Susceptibles are those who can get infected by SARS-CoV-2. The members of the latent compartment L have already been infected, but are not yet infectious nor do they display any symptoms. After that, latent individuals move to the pre-symptomatic class P meaning that, due to the increased viral load, they are able to infect susceptible individuals, even though, they still not display any symptoms. The existence of pre-symptomatic transmission is of particular importance in analyzing Covid-19 as it is one of the key features of the disease that makes controlling the outbreak difficult. Then, in our model, after the incubation period, at disease onset, members of P move to the infected class I. We note that another challenge with Covid-19 is that many patients will develop mild symptoms or none at all, yet being infectious. It is thus customary to collect these individuals in a separate compartment of asymptomatic individuals [18, 19]. Nevertheless, this distinction is not needed in our model as we will explain later in this section. Finally, patients transit to the removed compartment R by either recovery or by isolation after testing positive for Covid-19.

The above considerations are formulated in the following system of ordinary differential equations

$$\begin{aligned}
S'(t) &= -\beta \frac{S(t)}{N(t)} (P(t) + I(t)), \\
L'(t) &= \beta \frac{S(t)}{N(t)} (P(t) + I(t)) - \alpha L(t), \\
P'(t) &= \alpha L(t) - \rho P(t), \\
I'(t) &= \rho P(t) - \gamma I(t) - k \frac{pI(t)}{pI(t) + \sigma}, \\
R'(t) &= \gamma I(t) + k \frac{pI(t)}{pI(t) + \sigma}.
\end{aligned} \tag{1}$$

The disease transmission rate is denoted by the parameter β, the *incubation period* is $\alpha^{-1} + \rho^{-1}$, which is the sum of the duration of the latent period and the *pre-symptomatic* period, and, finally, γ^{-1} stands for the symptomatic infectious period. The transmission diagram of (1) is depicted on Fig. 1.

The *force of infection* is the rate associated with the outward flow from S to L, namely,

$$\lambda = \beta \frac{1}{N}(P + I).$$

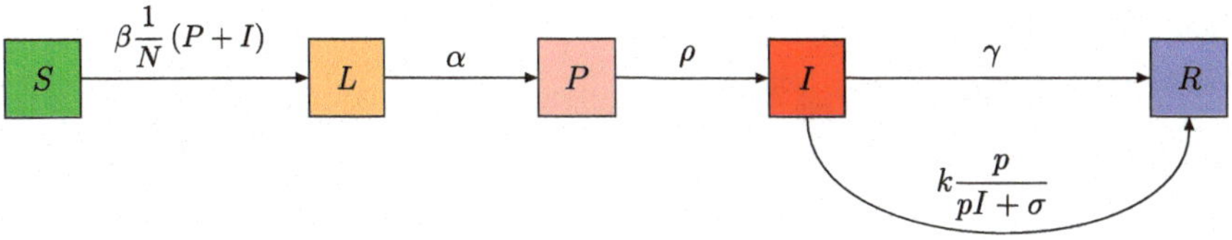

Fig. 1 The transmission diagram of the *SLPIR* model (1). Arrows represent the transition rates between the compartments

The indicator symptom-based testing is represented by the term

$$k\frac{pI}{pI+\sigma},$$

where k gives the number of tests done per unit time also referred to as the *testing rate*, the probability p describes how likely is that a member of compartment I displays the chosen indicator symptom. Note that this probability removes the need for an asymptomatic/mild compartment as it is straightforward to adjust p to account for all Covid-19 patients. The final term σ (possibly time-dependent) represents those individuals who are not infected by Covid-19, yet they show the very same symptom we base our testing upon. In this chapter, we refer to σ as the *secondary symptom pool*, whereas, the *primary symptom pool* Σ is composed of all members (with or without Covid-19 infection) of the population displaying the indicator symptom at a given time, that is

$$\Sigma = pI + \sigma.$$

The testing rate k has a natural upper bound, namely,

$$k \leq \Sigma$$

as we solely test patients displaying the indicator symptom. By reformulating the testing term as

$$k\frac{pI}{pI+\sigma} = \frac{k}{\Sigma}\cdot p\cdot I,$$

it is interpreted as the removal of the $\frac{k}{\Sigma}$ fraction of Covid-19 patients displaying the indicator symptom.

The rate of the testing-induced outward flow from I to R is referred to as the *force of testing* given by

$$\tau_{k,p,\sigma} = k\frac{p}{pI+\sigma}. \tag{2}$$

Finally, we introduce the *positivity rate* of testing as

Table 2 Parameters of the *SLPIR* model

Parameter	Notation	Value
Transmission rate	β	Sect. 2.1.
Latent period	α^{-1}	2.5 days
Pre-symptomatic (infectious) period	ρ^{-1}	3 days
Infectious period	γ^{-1}	4 days
Testing rate	k	varies
Secondary symptom pool	σ	varies
Probability of symptom amongst Covid-19 patients	p	varies

$$\theta = \frac{pI}{pI + \sigma}, \tag{3}$$

that may serve as a real-time indicator of the severity of an ongoing epidemic, and the adequateness of the testing rate.

Note that (1) is, in part, simpler than many other variants that have been used to assess the spread of Covid-19 as the infectious and latent compartments are not split into multiple stages [16, 18, 19, 22, 23]. However, these additional classes carry little significance for the testing strategies and to the analysis presented in this chapter. Hence, we chose to use this less complicated structure so that the emphasis is put on the testing itself.

We have parametrized (1) following [14]. From the infectivity profile of Covid-19 [3–5], we can see that most transmissions occur between 3 days prior to and 4 days after symptom onset, with the pre-symptomatic infection fraction being 43.7%. Thus, it is a reasonable approximation to set the pre-symptomatic period ρ^{-1} as 3 days, and the symptomatic infectious period γ^{-1} as 4 days, with the same infectiousness β during this period. The estimated mean incubation period of Covid-19 is 5.5 days [24], thus, the latent period α^{-1} is taken as 2.5 days, see Table 2. The choice of the transmission rate β is discussed in Sect. 2.1 and the testing parameters k, p, σ are varied throughout the analysis.

2.1 Choosing the Transmission Rate β

Now, we concentrate on establishing the relationship between the transmission rate β in (1) and the basic reproduction number $\mathcal{R}_0$ of the epidemic. We shall follow the terminology and techniques of [25] to compute the Next Generation Matrix (NGM) and the $\mathcal{R}_0$ as its spectral radius.

First, let us consider the infectious subsystem of (1), namely, equations describing $L(t)$, $P(t)$, and $I(t)$. Linearizing this subsystem w.r.t. the disease free equilibrium

Table 3 The basic reproduction number $\mathcal{R}_0$ and the corresponding transmission rate β

$\mathcal{R}_0$	2.2	1.8	1.3	1.1
β	0.338	0.277	0.2	0.169

yields the linearized infectious subsystem

$$X'(t) = (\mathbf{F} + \mathbf{V}) \cdot X(t),$$

where the matrices **F** and **V** are referred to as the *transmission part* and *transitional part*, respectively; the state is described by

$$X(t) = \begin{bmatrix} L(t) \\ P(t) \\ I(t) \end{bmatrix}.$$

The transmission matrix **F** has the form

$$\mathbf{F} = \begin{bmatrix} 0 & \beta & \beta \\ 0 & 0 & 0 \\ 0 & 0 & 0 \end{bmatrix},$$

and the transitional matrix **V** is, clearly, written as

$$\mathbf{V} = \begin{bmatrix} -\alpha & 0 & 0 \\ \alpha & -\rho & 0 \\ 0 & \rho & -\gamma \end{bmatrix}.$$

The basic reproduction number $\mathcal{R}_0$ is then obtained by computing the spectral radius of $-\mathbf{F}\mathbf{V}^{-1}$ that is

$$\mathcal{R}_0 = \rho(-\mathbf{F}\mathbf{V}^{-1}).$$

Therefore, as

$$-\mathbf{F}\mathbf{V}^{-1} = \begin{bmatrix} \frac{\beta}{\gamma} + \frac{\beta}{\rho} & \frac{\beta}{\gamma} + \frac{\beta}{\rho} & \frac{\beta}{\gamma} \\ 0 & 0 & 0 \\ 0 & 0 & 0 \end{bmatrix},$$

it follows that

$$\mathcal{R}_0 = \beta\left(\frac{1}{\rho} + \frac{1}{\gamma}\right),$$

providing a scheme for computing β. We list the corresponding transmission rates for the sample values of $\mathcal{R}_0$ used for illustrations in Table 3.

The basic reproduction number $\mathcal{R}_0$ is descriptive for the epidemic at the very beginning of an outbreak and in absence of control measures. For simplicity, we use the phrase basic reproduction number even if social distancing is in place, and by control measure in this chapter we mean the testing, the absence of which is modeled by $k = 0$. Similar key characteristics are the *control reproduction number* $\mathcal{R}_c$ and the *effective reproduction number* $\mathcal{R}_t$. The former describes the epidemic incorporating the effect of interventions, in our case indicator symptom-based testing, but still at the beginning of the outbreak. In contrast, the latter is suitable to measure the spread of the disease as the epidemic is progressing. The corresponding formulae may be obtained via analogous computations to those above as

$$\mathcal{R}_c = \beta\left(\frac{1}{\rho} + \frac{1}{\gamma + k\frac{p}{\sigma}}\right) = \beta\left(\frac{1}{\rho} + \frac{\sigma}{\sigma\gamma + kp}\right) \tag{4}$$

and

$$\mathcal{R}_t = \beta\,\frac{S(t)}{N}\left(\frac{1}{\rho} + \frac{1}{\gamma + \tau_{k,p,\sigma}}\right) = \beta\,\frac{S(t)}{N}\left(\frac{1}{\rho} + \frac{\Sigma}{\Sigma\gamma + kp}\right) = \beta\,\frac{S(t)}{N}\left(\frac{1}{\rho} + \frac{1}{\gamma + \frac{k}{\Sigma}p}\right).$$

As the testing rate k is bound by the size of the primary symptom pool Σ, it is apparent that both of the above reproduction numbers satisfy

$$\beta\frac{S}{N}\left(\frac{1}{\rho} + \frac{1}{\gamma + p}\right) \le \mathcal{R}_c, \mathcal{R}_t \le \mathcal{R}_0. \tag{5}$$

3 Dependence of Key Epidemic Quantities on the Testing Strategy

This section analyzes the symptom-based testing strategy with emphasis on how the force of testing and the effective reproduction number are affected by the particular choice of strategy. Repeatedly, we shall utilize the monotonicity of

$$f(x) = \frac{a + x}{b + x}, \qquad x_1 \le x_2 \Rightarrow f(x_1) \le f(x_2),$$

where $0 < a \le b$ and $0 \le x$.

First, we summarize trivial monotonicity properties of the force of testing $\tau_{k,p,\sigma}$.

Proposition 1 *Given a fixed state of* (1), *the force of testing* $\tau_{k,p,\sigma}$ *is*

(a) monotonically increasing in k,
(b) monotonically increasing in $\frac{k}{\Sigma}$.

In particular, as $\tau_{k,p,\sigma} = \frac{kp}{\Sigma}$, if $\frac{k}{\Sigma} = \text{const}$, then $\tau_{k,p,\sigma} = \text{const}$, *i.e.* the force of testing strongly correlates to what portion of the primary symptom pool is being tested.

As the epidemic is progressing, we may want to maintain the force of testing by increasing the testing rate k that is testing the same portion of individuals displaying the indicator symptom. Clearly, the required adjustment is linear w.r.t. the size of compartment I, thus, the given constant force of testing may be maintained as long as other logistical constraints make increasing the testing rate feasible.

The choice of the indicator symptom that serves as a basis for selecting patients for testing is clearly of importance. Different indicator symptoms typically have different associated probabilities and secondary symptom pools of non-equal sizes. Thus, it is natural to ask what (p, σ) pair is optimal.

Proposition 2 *The force of testing* $\tau_{k,p,\sigma}$ *is monotonically increasing in* $\frac{\sigma}{p}$.

Proof Clearly,

$$k\frac{p_1}{p_1 I + \sigma_1} = \tau_{k,p_1,\sigma_1} \leq \tau_{k,p_2,\sigma_2} = k\frac{p_2}{p_2 I + \sigma_2}$$

is equivalent to

$$\frac{1}{I + \frac{\sigma_1}{p_1}} \leq \frac{1}{I + \frac{\sigma_2}{p_2}}$$

that, in turn, simplifies to

$$\frac{\sigma_2}{p_2} \leq \frac{\sigma_1}{p_1}$$

yielding the required result. □

As we have seen, keeping the fraction $\frac{k}{\Sigma}$ constant results in constant force of testing $\tau_{k,p,\sigma}$. The authorities might obtain some data on the size of the primary symptom pool Σ during an outbreak and use this information for adjusting k on-the-go. When planning for a second wave, historical data on the size of the secondary symptom pool σ may give information on the required level of preparedness. Namely, if we know that σ has now a different size compared to the former outbreak, *e.g.* due to a seasonal variation, we may utilize the size difference of the secondary symptom pools as a guidance for the need for testing capacities as follows.

Proposition 3 *Given a fixed state of* (1), *consider two secondary symptom pools,* $0 \leq \sigma_1 \leq \sigma_2$ *for the same indicator symptom that appears amongst members of the compartment* I *with probability* p. *Let* k_1 *and* k_2 *be two testing rates corresponding to the testing strategies for* σ_1 *and* σ_2, *respectively. Then,*

$$\frac{k_2}{k_1} = \frac{\sigma_2}{\sigma_1}$$

implies

$$\tau_{k_1,p,\sigma_1} \leq \tau_{k_2,p,\sigma_2}.$$

Proof As the state is fixed, the two strategies having equal effect corresponds to the equality

$$k_1 \frac{p}{pI + \sigma_1} = \tau_{k_1,p,\sigma_1} = \tau_{k_2,p,\sigma_2} = k_2 \frac{p}{pI + \sigma_2}$$

that simplifies to

$$\frac{k_2}{k_1} = \frac{pI + \sigma_2}{pI + \sigma_1}.$$

Then, using the aforementioned monotonicity of $f(x)$, we obtain

$$k_2 \leq \frac{\sigma_2}{\sigma_1} k_1.$$

Finally, the monotonicity of $\tau_{k,p,\sigma}$ in k completes the proof. □

Recall, that the force of testing $\tau_{k,p,\sigma}$ explicitly appears in the formula for the effective reproduction number $\mathcal{R}_t$ as

$$\mathcal{R}_t = \beta \frac{S}{N} \left(\frac{1}{\rho} + \frac{1}{\gamma + \tau_{k,p,\sigma}} \right).$$

Accordingly, $\mathcal{R}_t$ may be kept decreasing by varying k as discussed in the first half of this section that is by keeping $\tau_{k,p,\sigma}$ constant or increasing. However, in practice, increasing k may eventually become infeasible. At that point, the force of testing will decrease, hence, $\mathcal{R}_t$ may increase temporarily, within the bounds given in (5), despite the constantly decreasing number of susceptible individuals $S(t)$.

A reasonable goal for the authorities is to keep $\mathcal{R}_t$ close to a designated value, ideally close to 1 to suppress the epidemic. Running estimates of the actual $\mathcal{R}_t$ might be obtained [19, 27, 28], hence, we investigate if, by an increase of the testing rate, we can alter $\mathcal{R}_t$ as desired.

Proposition 4 *Let* $0 \leq k_1 \leq k_2$ *be two testing rates. Consider an epidemic described by* (1) *with daily testing rate* k_1*, and the associated effective reproduction number* $\mathcal{R}_t(k)$ *as a function of* k*.*

Then, the ratio of the effective reproduction numbers corresponding to altering the testing rate from k_1 *to* k_2

$$r = \frac{\mathcal{R}_t(k_2)}{\mathcal{R}_t(k_1)}$$

satisfies the following inequality

$$\max \left\{ \frac{k_1}{k_2}, \frac{\gamma}{\rho + \gamma} \right\} \leq r \leq 1.$$

Proof The right bound is trivial as $\mathcal{R}_t$ is monotonic in k. Now, observe that

$$r = \frac{\frac{\Sigma}{k_2 p + \Sigma\gamma} + \frac{1}{\rho}}{\frac{\Sigma}{k_1 p + \Sigma\gamma} + \frac{1}{\rho}}.$$

Then,

$$r = \frac{\frac{\Sigma\rho + \Sigma\gamma + k_2 p}{k_2 p\rho + \Sigma\gamma\rho}}{\frac{\Sigma\rho + \Sigma\gamma + k_1 p}{k_1 p\rho + \Sigma\gamma\rho}} = \frac{\Sigma(\rho+\gamma)+k_2 p}{\Sigma(\rho+\gamma)+k_1 p} \cdot \frac{k_1 p\rho + \Sigma\gamma\rho}{k_2 p\rho + \Sigma\gamma\rho} = \frac{\Sigma(\rho+\gamma)+k_2 p}{\Sigma(\rho+\gamma)+k_1 p} \cdot \frac{k_1 p + \Sigma\gamma}{k_2 p + \Sigma\gamma}.$$

The first term is ≥ 1, thus,

$$r \geq \frac{k_1 p\rho + \Sigma\gamma\rho}{k_2 p\rho + \Sigma\gamma\rho} \geq \frac{k_1 p}{k_2 p} = \frac{k_1}{k_2}$$

using the monotonicity of $f(x)$ noted at the beginning of this section.

Now, consider reordering the product as

$$r = \frac{\Sigma(\rho+\gamma)+k_2 p}{k_2 p + \Sigma\gamma} \cdot \frac{k_1 p + \Sigma\gamma}{\Sigma(\rho+\gamma)+k_1 p}.$$

Again, the first term is ≥ 1, therefore,

$$r \geq \frac{k_1 p + \Sigma\gamma}{\Sigma(\rho+\gamma)+k_1 p} \geq \frac{\Sigma\gamma}{\Sigma(\rho+\gamma)} = \frac{\gamma}{\rho+\gamma}$$

holds using, again, the monotonicity of $f(x)$.

Combining the two inequalities above completes the proof. □

The implications of Proposition 4 on goals for the testing strategy are rather important as they point out some hard limitations. Clearly, as

$$0.43 \sim \frac{\gamma}{\rho+\gamma},$$

no matter our testing capacity or indicator symptom, we may not suppress the epidemic any further. As an example, if our current estimates for $\mathcal{R}_t$ are above 2.4, then we cannot expect the pure indicator symptom-based testing strategy (without contact-tracing) to be able to suppress the epidemic as $2.4 \cdot 0.43 \sim 1.03$. Additionally, as the indicator symptom limits our testing rate to $k \leq \Sigma = pI + \sigma$, we obtain another hard constraint, namely,

$$r \geq \frac{k_1}{\Sigma}$$

that is the ratio describing what proportion of the primary symptom pool is being tested directly limits the factor which the effective reproduction number may be decreased with via larger testing rates. Finally, we note that reordering the inequality yields $k_2 \geq \frac{k_1}{r}$ as a lower requirement for the required testing rate—given that the reduction by factor r is achievable.

We have discussed from various aspects that increasing the testing rate k decreases the effective reproduction number $\mathcal{R}_t$ that is it has a positive effect on the severity of the epidemic. Nevertheless, this positive effect is gradually decreasing as described by the following Proposition.

Proposition 5 *Consider the logarithmic derivative of $\mathcal{R}_t$ w.r.t. the testing rate k that is*

$$\mathcal{R}_t^* = \frac{\partial}{\partial k} \log(\mathcal{R}_t).$$

Then, $\mathcal{R}_t^*$ is negative and monotonically increasing in k.

Proof Clearly,

$$\mathcal{R}_t^* = \frac{\frac{\partial \mathcal{R}_t}{\partial k}}{\mathcal{R}_t} = \frac{-\Sigma \rho p}{(kp + \Sigma\gamma)(kp + \Sigma(\rho + \gamma)} \leq 0.$$

Then,

$$\frac{\partial \mathcal{R}_t^*}{\partial k} = \frac{(\Sigma \rho p)(2kp + \Sigma p(\rho + 2\gamma))}{(kp + \Sigma\gamma)^2(kp + \Sigma(\rho + \gamma)^2} \geq 0$$

completes the proof. □

This logarithmic derivative is a measure of the relative change in $\mathcal{R}_t$ w.r.t. the testing rate k. Proposition 5 states that the relative change is decreasing in absolute value as k increases.

4 Numerical Simulations

This section presents the results from several numerical simulations demonstrating the impact of the key parameters of the epidemic model (1). All simulations were executed with a sample population of size 10,000,000 with initial conditions placing 1000 individuals into the class L and the rest into S.

First, Sect. 4.1 presents the numerical analysis of the control reproduction number $\mathcal{R}_c$. Then, we investigate the connection between the progress of an outbreak and the positivity rate of testing in Sect. 4.2. We study the implications of maintaining a constant force of testing $\tau_{p,k,\sigma}$ in Sect. 4.3. The significance of the seasonality of the secondary symptom pool σ is analyzed in Sect. 4.4. Finally, in Sect. 4.5, we assess how an increased testing rate may delay the progress of Covid-19.

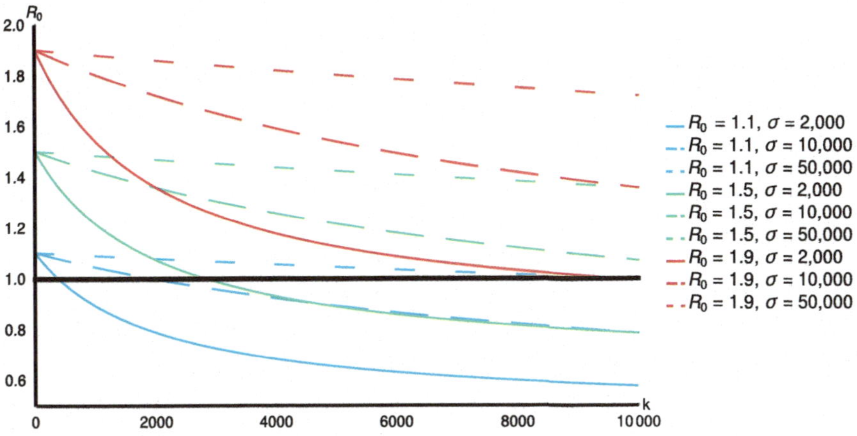

Fig. 2 The effect of indicator symptom-based testing on $\mathcal{R}_c$ for $p = 0.25$

4.1 *The Effect of Testing on the Control Reproduction Number $\mathcal{R}_c$*

The control reproduction number $\mathcal{R}_c$, given in (4), describes the initial progress of the epidemic at its very beginning. Figure 2 demonstrates what effect of indicator symptom-based testing has on $\mathcal{R}_c$ for various values of $\mathcal{R}_0$ and σ.

Clearly, larger maximal testing rate k results in lower $\mathcal{R}_c$. The size of the secondary symptom pool σ apparently greatly affects the decrease we may achieve by larger k.

4.2 *The Progress of an Outbreak and the Positivity Rate θ*

Recall that the positivity rate θ, see (3), is a key feature of the testing strategy that may be readily observed during an outbreak. If the efforts aimed at suppressing Covid-19 are not successful, the rate θ will increase as the term $pI(t)$ will eventually dominate the secondary symptom pool σ. Figure 3 demonstrates that the changes in θ are in close connection with the dynamics of $I(t)$. This relationship between θ and $I(t)$ carries a certain benefit for the authorities as the increase of the positivity rate precedes that of the epidemic curve, hence, it may serve as a primary indicator for the progress of an epidemic.

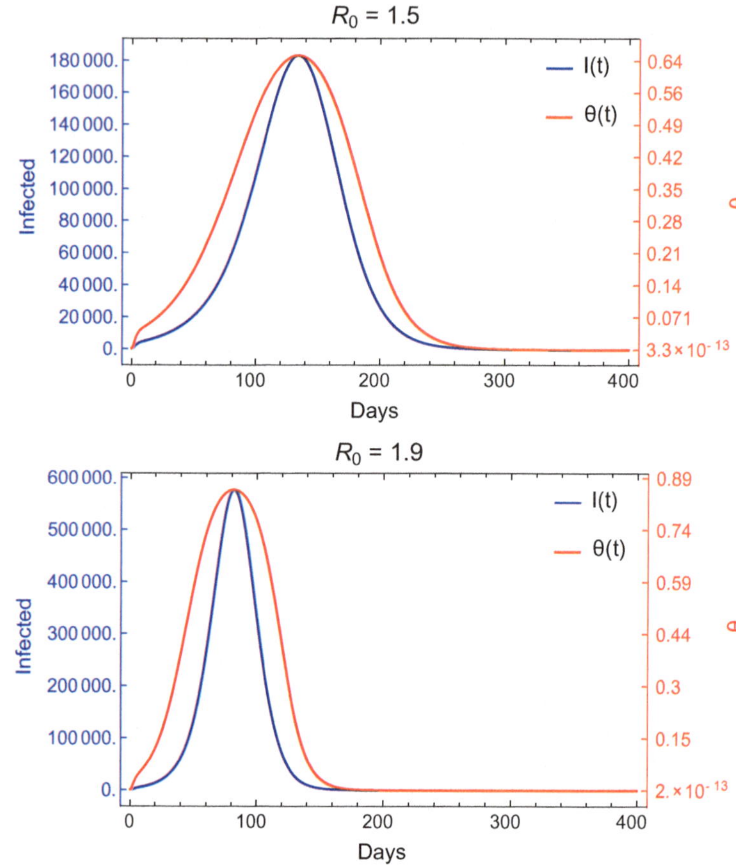

Fig. 3 Evolution of the positivity rate during outbreaks of different magnitudes. The prevalence of the indicator symptom is $p = 0.1$ with a maximal testing capacity $k = 10{,}000$ and secondary symptom pool $\sigma = 10{,}000$

4.3 Implications of Constant Force of Testing $\tau_{p,k,\sigma}$

As we have discussed in Sect. 3, a constant force of testing $\tau_{p,k,\sigma}$ is achieved by testing a fixed portion of the primary symptom pool Σ, *i.e.* $\frac{k}{\Sigma}$ is constant. For an ongoing epidemic this results in a constant increase in the required daily testing rate k. We have analyzed the maximal required testing capacity w.r.t. Covid-19 patients in Fig. 4.

Note that for constant $\tau_{p,k,\sigma}$, the system (1) is independent of the secondary symptom pool σ, thus, this requirement must be adjusted based on historical data on the size of σ to obtain the total maximal required capacity.

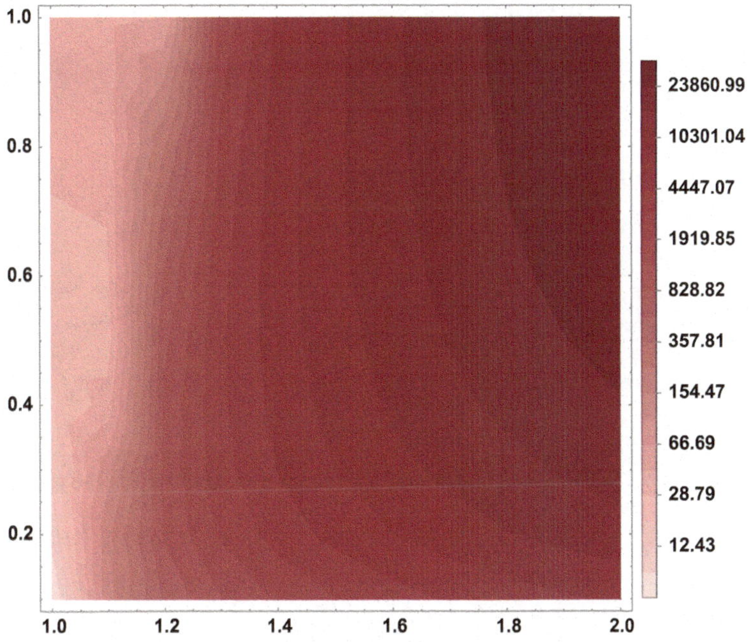

Fig. 4 Required testing capacity to maintain a constant force of testing $\tau_{p,k,\sigma}$. The vertical axis describes the desired portion for testing the primary symptom pool and the horizontal axis represents the underlying basic reproduction number $\mathcal{R}_0$. The prevalence of the indicator symptom is set to $p = 0.1$

4.4 Seasonality of the Secondary Symptom Pool σ

Now, let us investigate the epidemic curves in case of a periodically varying secondary symptom pool. To that end, we employ a commonly used seasonality function

$$\omega(t) = 365 \cdot \frac{10^{b\cos\left(\frac{2\pi(t-c)}{365}\right)}}{\int_0^{365} 10^{b\cos\left(\frac{2\pi(t-c)}{365}\right)} dt},$$

with $b = 0.5$ and consider $\sigma = \sigma_{\text{avg}} \cdot \omega(t)$. The parameter c is used to model shift in the seasonality, *i.e.* to analyze the differences between an outbreak starting at minimal or maximal secondary symptom pools. The function $\omega(t)$ is displayed on Fig. 5 for the case of minimal secondary symptom pool at time $t = 0$ that is for a shift $c = 183$.

Figure 6 demonstrates the effect of having seasonality in σ and the Covid-19 outbreak beginning around the minimal size of the secondary symptom pool. This comparison shows that we may expect a slight, but notable, delay in this scenario compared to the non-seasonal setting.

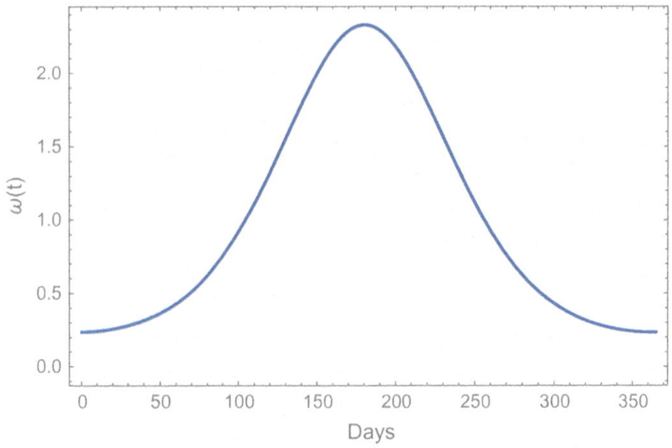

Fig. 5 The seasonality function $\omega(t)$ with $c = 183$. This corresponds to minimal secondary symptom pool at the beginning of an outbreak

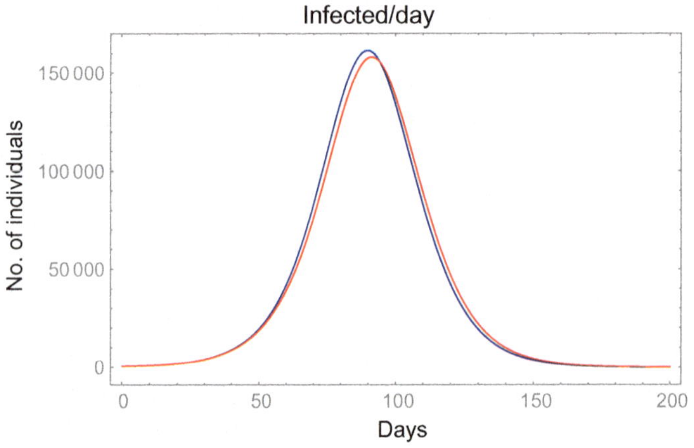

Fig. 6 The impact of seasonal σ with minimal size at the beginning of the outbreak. $\mathcal{R}_0 = 1.9$, $p = 0.1$, $k = 10{,}000$, $\sigma = 10{,}000$. The blue curve corresponds to assuming a constant (average) secondary symptom pool, whilst, the red curve depicts the effect of seasonality

A similar shift in the opposite direction takes place if we consider the beginning of the outbreak to coincide with the maximal state of σ, see Fig. 7.

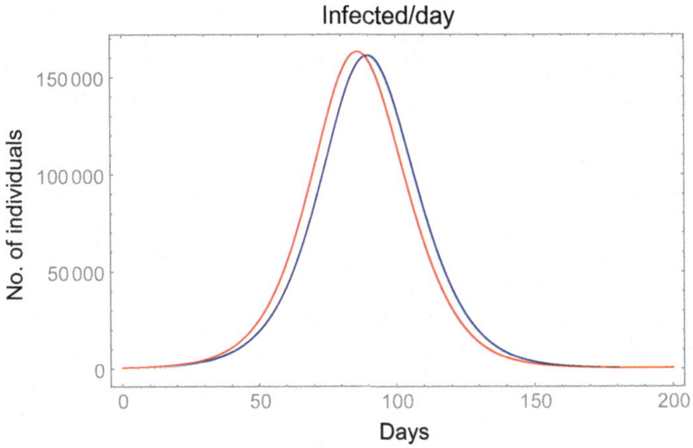

Fig. 7 The impact of seasonal σ with maximal size at the beginning of the outbreak. $\mathcal{R}_0 = 1.9$, $p = 0.1$, $k = 10{,}000$, $\sigma = 10{,}000$. The blue curve corresponds to assuming a constant (average) secondary symptom pool, whilst, the red curve depicts the effect of seasonality

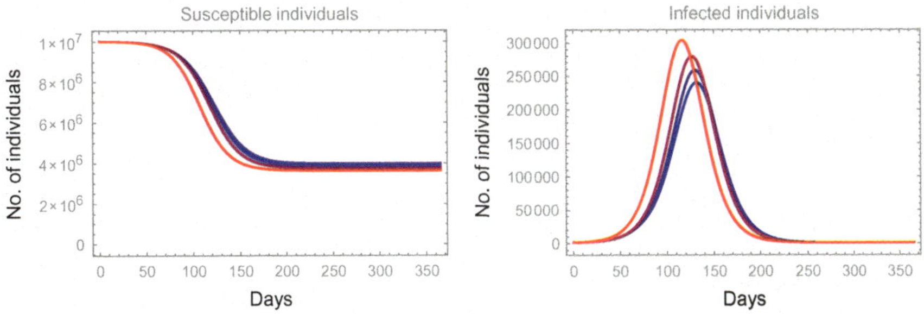

Fig. 8 The impact of increasing the testing rate from 1,000 (red) to 10,000 (blue) using parameters $\mathcal{R}_0 = 1.6,\ p = 0.1,\ 1,000 \leq k \leq 10{,}000,\ \sigma = 10{,}000$

4.5 The Effect of Varying the Testing Rate k

Increasing the testing rate k has a beneficial effect. We demonstrate this via transitional plots on Fig. 8. Note that a larger maximal k both delays in time and decreases in size the peak of the epidemic.

5 Conclusions

We have investigated the effects of indicator symptom-based testing on Covid-19. The benefits of increasing the testing rate k are demonstrated, suggesting that, as long as other logistical constraints allow, the authorities should aim to keep it as high as possible. The choice of the indicator symptom is of importance. We have shown that not just its prevalence p should be taken into account but the size and seasonality of the associated secondary symptom pool σ as well. Note that the analysis in this chapter did not directly consider contact/transmission-reducing nonpharmaceutical interventions (NPIs), *i.e.* curfew, closures of schools, wearing of masks, etc. Naturally, these interventions would affect not just the spread of Covid-19, but of other diseases, hence, potentially decreasing the secondary symptom pool σ as well. Such NPIs may be fitted into the presented framework by varying the basic reproduction number $\mathcal{R}_0$ and σ, as seen in Sect. 4.1.

The quality of tests was not considered. The false negativity rate could be easily modeled by a reduction factor in k. Handling the false positivity rate is more involved as susceptible individuals (susceptible to Covid-19, but still displaying the indicator symptom, *i.e.* members of σ) may be temporarily removed from the infectious chain just to reappear later, after a precautionary quarantine. However, rRT-PCR-tests have very high specificity, hence, false positives are rare.

We have modeled the transmission of Covid-19 using identical rates for the presymptomatic P and symptomatic I classes. This choice is influenced by the current understanding that according to the inferred infectivity profiles, the transmissibility prior to and after the onset of symptoms is of similar magnitude, and the ratio of presymptomatic transmissions is almost 50% [3–5]. Nevertheless, using different rates for the two compartments would not alter the computations heavily.

It is clear from the numerical simulations that indicator symptom-based testing, alone, cannot prevent an outbreak. It has a modest effect in delaying and slowing down the epidemic. Thus, symptom based testing alone may have clinical importance by providing guidance about how to treat a given patient, but its impact as epidemic mitigation is negligible. Therefore, in practice, authorities should opt to perform agile contact-tracing based on positive Covid-19 tests. The effect of this additional intervention is not included in our analysis. Nevertheless, it is safe to claim that the addition of contact-tracing would considerably increase the benefits of any testing strategy, in particular, some individuals would get removed from the presymptomatic compartment P and the latent compartment L as well via additional testing or general quarantine for contacts of Covid-19 patients with positive test result.

In summary, testing and isolation of cases is a key tool in combating the pandemic. However, symptom-based testing alone is not sufficient to control Covid-19. To significantly ease the disease burden on the society, it must be used in combination with other measures.

Acknowledgements This work was done in the framework of the Hungarian National Development, Research, and Innovation (NKFIH) Fund 2020-2.1.1-ED-2020-00003 and of the grants TUDFO/47138-1/2019-ITM and EFOP-3.6.2-16-2017-00015. Some authors were also supported by NKFIH KKP 129877 (J.K.), NKFIH FK 124016 (T.T.), János Bolyai Research Scholarship of the Hungarian Academy of Sciences (F.B.).

References

1. WHO. Novel Coronavirus (2019-nCoV): situation reports. *World Health Organization* **2020**. https://www.who.int/emergencies/diseases/novel-coronavirus-2019/situation-reports
2. Vetter, P., Vu Diem, L., L'Huillier, A.G., Schibler, M., Kaiser, L., Jacquerioz, F., et al.: Clinical features of COVID-19. BMJ **2020**, 369: 1470. https://doi.org/10.1136/bmj.m1470
3. He, X., et al.: Temporal dynamics in viral shedding and transmissibility of COVID-19. Nat. Med. **26**, 672–675 (2020). https://doi.org/10.1038/s41591-020-0869-5
4. Ashcroft, P., Huisman, J.S., Lehtinen, S., Bouman, J.A., Althaus, C.L., Regoes, R.R., Bonhoeffer, S.: COVID-19 infectivity profile correction. Swiss Med. Wkly, 150:w20336 (2020) https://doi.org/10.4414/smw.2020.20336
5. He, X., et al.: Author Correction: Temporal dynamics in viral shedding and transmissibility of COVID-19. Nat Med. **26**, 1491–1493 (2020). https://doi.org/10.1038/s41591-020-1016-z
6. R. Mao *et al.* Manifestations and prognosis of gastrointestinal and liver involvement in patients with COVID-19: a systematic review and meta-analysis. The Lancet **5**(7), 667–678 (2020). https://doi.org/10.1016/S2468-1253(20)30126-6
7. Docherty, A.B., et al.: Features of 16,749 hospitalised UK patients with COVID-19 using the ISARIC WHO Clinical Characterisation Protocol. medRχ iv 2020.04.28. https://doi.org/10.1101/2020.04.23.20076042
8. ECDC. Clinical characteristics of COVID-19. European Centre for Disease Prevention and Control (2020). https://www.ecdc.europa.eu/en/covid-19/latest-evidence/clinical
9. Guan, W., et al.: Clinical Characteristics of Coronavirus Disease 2019 in China. N. Engl. J. Med. **382**, 1708–1720 (2020). https://doi.org/10.1056/NEJMoa2002032
10. Menni, C., et al.: Real-time tracking of self-reported symptoms to predict potential COVID-19. Nat. Med. **26**, 1037–1040 (2020). https://doi.org/10.1038/s41591-020-0916-2
11. CDC. Real-Time RT-PCR Panel for Detection 2019-nCoV. Centers for Disease Control and Prevention 2020.01.29.
12. Lia, M.Y., Graef, J.R., Wang, L., Karsai, J.: Global dynamics of a SEIR model with varying total population size. Math. Biosci. **160(2)**, 191–213 (1990). https://doi.org/10.1016/S0025-5564(99)00030-9
13. Feng, Z.: Applications of epidemiological models to public health policymaking: the role of heterogeneity in model predictions. World Scientific (2014)
14. Péni, T., Csutak, B., Szederkényi, G., Röst, G.: Nonlinear model predictive control for COVID-19 management. Nonlinear Dyn. in press
15. Yang, C., Wang, Y.: A mathematical model for the novel coronavirus epidemic in Wuhan, China. Math. Biosci. Eng. **17(3)**, 2708–2724 (2020). https://doi.org/10.3934/mbe.2020148
16. Boldog, P., Tekeli, T., Vizi, Zs., Dénes, A., Bartha, F.A., Röst, G.: Risk Assessment of Novel Coronavirus COVID–19 Outbreaks Outside China. J. Clin. Med. **9(2)**, 571. https://doi.org/10.3390/jcm9020571
17. Berger, D.W., Herkenhoff, K.F., Mongey, S.: An SEIR infectious disease model with testing and conditional quarantine. NBER Working Paper No. 26901 (2020). https://doi.org/10.3386/w26901
18. Weitz, J.S.: COVID-19 Epidemic Risk Assessment for Georgia. Github 2020.03.24. https://github.com/jsweitz/covid-19-ga-summer-2020
19. Röst, G., et al.: Early phase of the COVID-19 outbreak in Hungary and post-lockdown scenarios. Viruses **12(7)**, 708 (2020). https://www.mdpi.com/1999-4915/12/7/708
20. Lofgren, E., Fefferman, N.H., Naumov, Y.N., Gorski, J., Naumova, E.N.: Influenza seasonality: underlying causes and modeling theories. J. Virol. **81(11)**, 5429–5436 (2007). https://doi.org/10.1128/JVI.01680-06
21. Olson, K.L., Mandl, K.D.: Seasonal patterns of gastrointestinal illness. Adv. Dis. Surveill. **4**, 262. http://faculty.washington.edu/lober/www.isdsjournal.org/htdocs/articles/2188.pdf
22. Giordano, G., et al.: Modelling the COVID-19 epidemic and implementation of population-wide interventions in Italy. Nat. Med. **26**, 855–860 (2020). https://doi.org/10.1038/s41591-020-0883-7

23. Barbarossa, M.V., et al.: Modeling the spread of COVID-19 in Germany: Early assessment and possible scenarios. PLOS ONE **15(9)**, e0238559 (2020). https://doi.org/10.1371/journal.pone.0238559
24. Lauer, S.A., et al.: The incubation period of coronavirus disease 2019 (COVID-19) from publicly reported confirmed cases: estimation and application. Ann. Intern. Med. **172(9)**, 577–582 (2020). https://doi.org/10.7326/M20-0504
25. Diekmann, O., Heesterbeek, J.A.P., Roberts, M.G.: The construction of next-generation matrices for compartmental epidemic models. J. R. Soc. Interface **7(47)**, 873–885 (2020). https://doi.org/10.1098/rsif.2009.0386
26. Chowell, G., Fenimore, P., Castillo-Garsow, M., Castillo-Chavez, C.: SARS outbreaks in Ontario, Hong Kong and Singapore: the role of diagnosis and isolation as a control mechanism. J. Theor. Biol. **224(1)**. https://doi.org/10.1098/rsif.2007.1036
27. Cori, A., Ferguson, N.M., Fraser, C., Cauchemez, S.: A new framework and software to estimate time-varying reproduction numbers during epidemics. Am. J. Epidemiol. **178(9)**, 1505–1512 (2020). https://doi.org/10.1093/aje/kwt133
28. Wallinga, J., Lipsitch. M.: How generation intervals shape the relationship between growth rates and reproductive numbers. Proc. R. Soc. B: Biol. Sci. **274(1609)**, 599–604 (2020). https://royalsocietypublishing.org/doi/full/10.1098/rspb.2006.3754

Challenges in Modeling of an Outbreak's Prediction, Forecasting and Decision Making for Policy Makers

Altaf H. Khan

Abstract In this work an attempt has been made to review the current state of arts in epidemiological modeling, assessment of predictive models as well as forecasting of new pathogen. The primary concern is the containment of the outbreak from wide spread of the disease among the whole population. This article also focuses for the development of management tools and techniques in decision making for policy makers that are based on scientific evidence. Moreover, the identification, detection and reporting for outbreak of an infectious disease particularly a new pathogen in timely manner is quite challenging and tedious. Apparently understanding and reporting of such events are commonly rely on statistical and mathematical tools and both these approaches commonly depend upon a priory estimates as well as some reliable data. For example: statistical models requires a sizable number of events to develop predictive models, which is impossible at the outset of an outbreak of the disease to collate enough number of samples. Whereas, the mathematical models are reliable as well as have better predictive behavior, but they also require better initial guess apart from some rigid constraints to fully satisfy the model's assumptions. Apart from these issues, the other important features to study in epidemiology of the disease is how fast and quickly the scientific community promptly can pinpoint and able to address any causal factor which may suffice to account for the magnitude and severity of the epidemics of new pathogen that may have been taken place to any geographic locations. Hence in this work, first of all the SIR model (susceptible: S, infected: I, and recovered: R) will be outlined, as it is the most commonly used model in epidemiology of infectious diseases. Moreover, the applicability and utilization of R_0 in public health domain especially adaptive policy with management tools will be developed for the healthcare workers as well as the higher management of healthcare facility.

Keywords Covid-19 · Compartmental model · Testing · Outbreak mitigation

---

A. H. Khan (✉)
Department of Biostatistics and Bioinformatics, King Abdullah International Medical Research Center, National Guard Health Affairs, Riyadh, Kingdom of Saudi Arabia

P. Agarwal et al. (eds.), *Analysis of Infectious Disease Problems (Covid-19) and Their Global Impact*, Infosys Science Foundation Series,
https://doi.org/10.1007/978-981-16-2450-6_17

1 Introduction

The infectious diseases related acute respiratory infections (ARIs) are the primary source of morbidity and mortality around the world, since each and every year approximately 5 to 6 million people die due to ARIs, and 98% of these deaths are due to lower respiratory tract infections see: Fig. 1 (the percentage of fatality rate on log-scale for some influenza types are shown, Source: New York Times). Mortality rates are higher among infants, children, and the elderly, and it's commonly prevalent in low-income and middle-income countries [6–8]. Influenza may also cause of an increase risk of strokes and heart attacks apart from disease complications [9–11]. The emergence of the current outbreak of the new pathogen started from Wuhan City, Hubei Province, China. This new outbreak cases were reported in the *1*st week of December, 2019, and the World Health Organization (WHO) on December 31, 2019 had declared this new pathogen as a 'Global-Pandemic'. It was soon identified as a novel coronavirus and termed as Covid-19, and belongs to the family of viruses that include the common cold and viruses such as SARS and MERS. On January 20, 2020, this has been also confirmed that the coronavirus can be transmitted between humans, and has wider risk of spread globally. Hence, the identification, detection and reporting for outbreak of an infectious disease particularly a new pathogen in timely manner is vital for the safety of general public health. Apparently reporting of such events are quite challenging and difficult, since it requires a complete understanding of the new pathogen. And to comprehend and stop from spreading any new such vicious viruses (like Covid-19) commonly rely on statistical and mathematical tools. Both these approaches commonly depend upon a priory estimates and some reliable data. For example: statistical models requires a sizable number of events to develop predictive models, which is impossible at the outset of an outbreak of the disease to collate enough number of samples. Whereas, the mathematical models are reliable as well as have better predictive behavior, but they also require better initial guess apart from some rigid constraints to fully satisfy the model's assumptions. Apart from these issues, the other important features to study in epidemiology of the disease is how fast and quickly the scientific community can pinpoint any causal factor which may suffice to account for the magnitude and severity of the epidemics of new pathogen that may have been taken place to any geographic locations. Moreover, some commonly utilized modeling tools in infectious diseases will be outlined here, whereas taking into account the primary aim of infectious disease modeling is: (i) to understand the mechanisms of spread, (ii) to estimate the time period of the latent and infectious periods, and (iii) the size of the epidemic, and the main focus is to determine strategies for disease control. Some of the commonly utilized approaches to model epidemic diseases are briefly outline here:

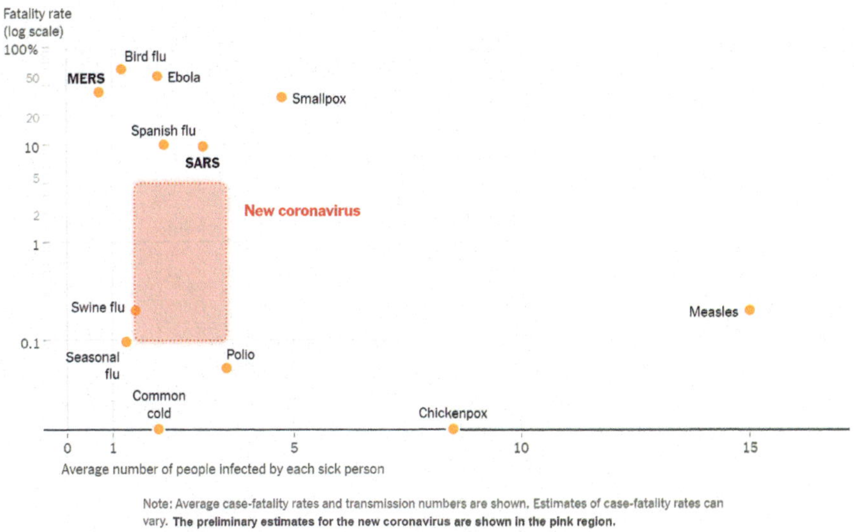

Fig. 1 The figure describes the percentage of different respiratory syndromes,the percentage of fatality rate is log scale: (*Source* New York Times)

1.1 Deterministic Compartmental Models (DCMs)

The DCMs based models are based on systems of differential equations which take into account the movement of the population through discrete states, including entry into and exit from the population, at specified rates. DCMs models are the most commonly used in the field of mathematical epidemiology, and can be solved analytically, or using numerical analysis. They can represent discrete forms of heterogeneity in the population. With DCMs, once the structure and parameters have been set explicitly, then there is no variation in model outcomes. In 1776, Daniel Bernoulli developed a model to analyze the life expectancy and death rates based on the inoculation or variolation in a public health enivironment, see: Dietz (2000) [37]. Some other scientists, for example namely: Philip-Charles Alexandre Louis, William Farr, Ronald Ross had made tremendous work in epidemiological sciences. Lately, epidemiologist now applying and utilizing new computational algorithms to analyze the infectious diseases based on modeling, and simulation of the dynamics of disease generation and propagation, see: Koopman (1996) [38].

1.2 Stochastic Individual Contact Models (ICMs)

The stochastic individual contact models (ICMs), also known as individual-based or agent based models, explicitly represent individual units in the population and the

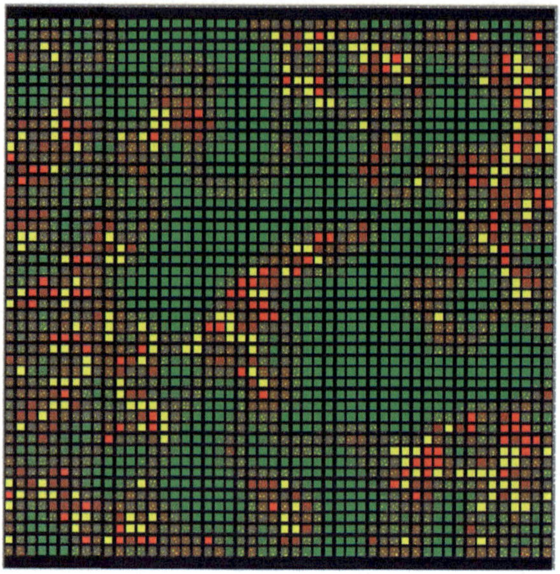

Fig. 2 Visual display of a two-dimensional agent-based model. Each square represents an individually programmable, mobile agent. Color-coding allows easy visual tracking of agents with different properties. *Source* https://www.ncbi.nlm.nih.gov/books/NBK221490/figure/mmm00027/?report=objectonly

contacts between them are unique with discrete events. In contrast to DCMs, they allow heterogeneity while specifying the contact process and other epidemiologically relevant events, and their stochasticity provides information on the range of plausible outcomes resulting from a given set of parameters. The setbacks with these models are they may require large amounts of input data that is needed for parameterization as well as the computational burden associated with running multiple stochastic simulations. Agent-based modeling are used extensively in biology such as: spread of epidemics, population dynamics, stochastic gene expression, plant-animal interactions, vegetation ecology, as well as modeling 3D breast tissue formation/morphogenesis etc. They are agent-based computational models using computer programs in which a population of individual entities is created, and each individual is endowed with simple rules for interactions with the environment and with other individuals, see: Holland (1995) [41]. They are used to model all manner of complex scientific phenomena. Some important studies had used the agent-based modeling to examine infectious diseases (e.g., influenza) and the immune response, see: Hofmeyr and Forrest (2000), [40]. For example, the Swarm Development Group (ref: http://www.swarm.org/wiki/Main_Page) had made the development of a wide variety of infectious disease modeling using the agent-based modeling, see: Figure 2 display of two-dimensional agent based model.

1.3 Network Models

Network models are also stochastic and represent individual units, but unlike ICMs, they providea flexible framework for representing repeated contacts with the same person or persons over time. These repeated contacts may give rise to persistent network configurations for example: pairs, triples, and larger connected components which in turn establishes the temporally ordered pathways for infectious disease transmission across a population. The R-package 'EpiModel' is a good tools for simulation of models for network analysis. It provides a generalized framework for both estimation and simulation of dynamically evolving networks. Network models provide the most accurate control over the contact process, but have greater computational burden than ICMs, both because they require statistical estimation of the network model parameters. Network models offer a versatile means of capturing heterogeneity in populations during an epidemic. In this approach, highly connected individuals tend to be infected at a higher rate early during an outbreak than those with fewer connections, see: Romanescu and Deardon [39]. Figure 3 shows the representation of evolving bit strings in a fitness landscape, and its clear that network models inspired by the Internet will productively inform the modeling of microbial pathogen networks, Albert et al. (2000) [42], Pastor-Satorras and Vesignani (2001) [43], and Lloyd and May (2001) [45]. As we know that the social networks had made a major role to determine the rate and pattern of epidemic spread of microbial diseases in human societies. Although it had been primarily focused in the role of population heterogeneity and sub-networks to study the spread of sexually transmitted diseases, especially HIV/AIDS. However, not too much attention had been paid in role of network topology to monitor the spread of other infectious diseases. Currently, computer scientists as well as physicists are more concerned about the spread of infectious agents, for example: computer viruses, worms, etc., through the Internet and the World Wide Web. This had made the development of new interest in network topology that have evolve as a revolution in network modeling, see Fig. 3, for references see the work of Barabasi (2002) [44], and Watts (1999).

1.4 Harmonic Decomposition Analysis

It should be noted that the biological scientists particularly in health-care's though were lagging behind to utilize sophisticated mathematical tools such as: Fourier transform as well as the wavelets theory, etc. but now these powerful analytical tools are also utilized by them for example: Fourier analysis has been used to decompose dengue and malaria data sets to reveal the weather-independence of interepidemic variability, Rogers et al. (2002) [47]; Hay et al. (2000) [48]. The power of wavelet analysis is evident as it was used to decompose measles epidemic harmonics to reveal recurrent spatial spreading patterns which were not evident in the undecomposed epidemic data, see Fig. 4 . With this successes the decompositional technique made

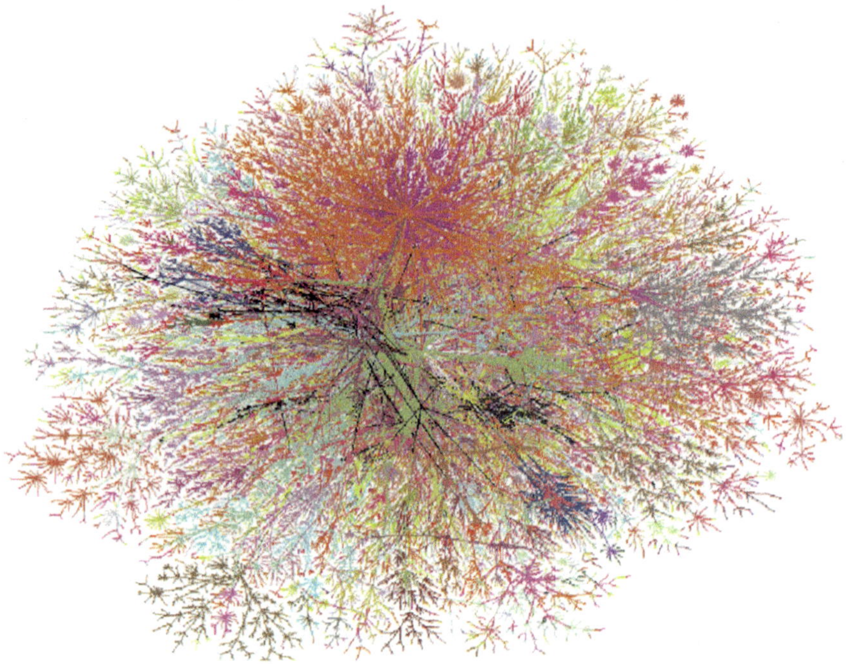

Fig. 3 Internet routing map (80,000 nodes). See http://www.cs.bell-labs.com/~ches/map/

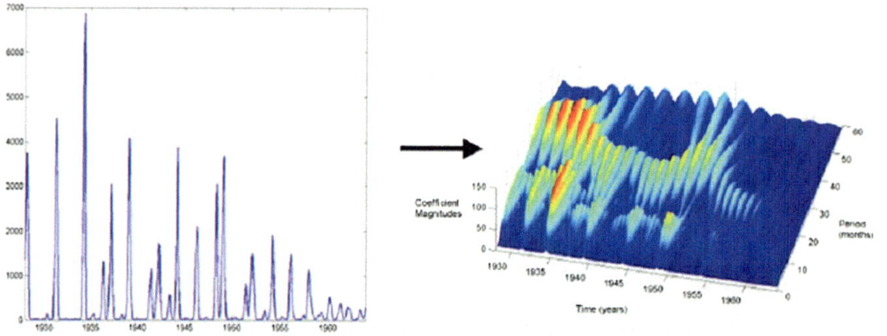

Fig. 4 Continuous wavelet transform decomposition of 1928–1964 Baltimore measles time series data showing that the incidence curve is decomposable into a shorter component with a periodicity of 12 months, and a longer component with a variable periodicity of 24–36 months. The longer component correlates closely with changes in birth rates. *Source* https://www.ncbi.nlm.nih.gov/books/NBK221490/figure/mmm00026/?report=objectonly

it possible to analyze and explain the dynamics of many infectious diseases, see: Grenfell et al. (2001) [49]; Strebel and Cochi (2001) [50].

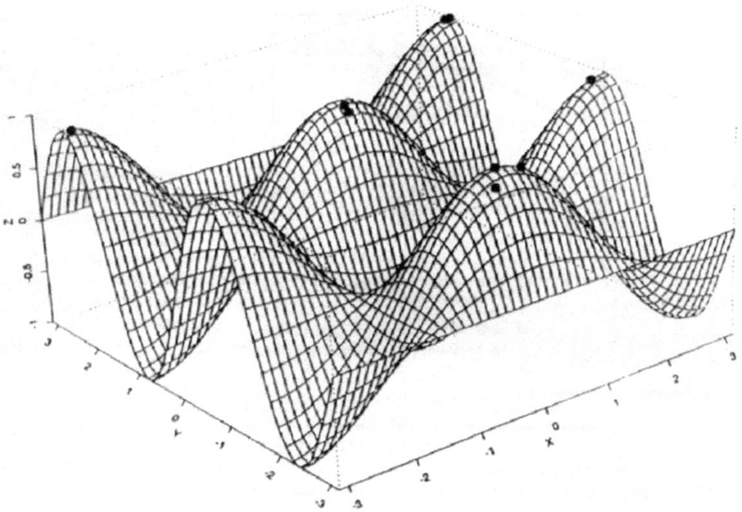

Fig. 5 Representation of evolving bit strings in a fitness landscape. In this example populations of strings are shown as dots colonizing local fitness optima in sequence space, *Source* https://www.ncbi.nlm.nih.gov/books/NBK221490/figure/mmm00029/?report=objectonly

1.5 Digital Microbes

The last decade had seen a see change after it's initial downfall in early nineties that evolutionary techniques would now be incorporated into machine learning, artificial intelligence, and computer programming. The genetic algorithms is the first and now a standard evolutionary computational technique—code strings are iteratively mutated, recombined, and selected for fitness, just as if they were nucleic acid strings evolving in nature, Burke et al. (1998) [51], see Fig. 5. This algorithms are widely employed to solve practical computationally intensive problems, such as protein folding, but only a few studies have appeared in which evolving code strings are used to simulate microbial evolution and adaptation. Preliminary studies suggest that the rules governing code string evolution may be independent of the stuff from which the evolving code strings are made, and that experiments on digital microbes with code string evolution and epidemiology "in silicon" may be a productive way to understand and solve problems that are difficult to study in nature, Ray (1995) [52]; Wilke et al., Adami et al. (2000) [53]; Radman et al. (1999) [54].[1]

In following sections: SIR model (susceptible: S, infected: I, and recovered: R) based on ordinary differential equations (ODEs) will be outlined, and it is the most

[1] Agent based, network based, harmonic decomposition analysis, and digital microbes notes were adopted from: Computational Modeling and Simulation of Epidemic Infectious Diseases Donald S. Burke (M.D.) Bloomberg School of Public Health, Johns Hopkins University (USA), and appendix from: Microbial Threats to Health: Emergence, Detection, and Response (2003), National Academic Press.

commonly used model in epidemiology of infectious diseases. The basic reproduction number known as: R_0 pronounced as R-naught will be estimated for the basic SIR and the extended SIR models and computed estimates of R_0 will be compared in different scenarios as well as computational algorithms will be outlined for solving SIR model. Next, the stochastic modeling will be briefly discussed.The applicability and utilization of R_0 in public health domain especially adaptive policy with management tools will be described for the healthcare workers as well as for higher management of healthcare facility.

2 Mathematical Modeling: The Basic SIR Model

The basic compartment models are: SIS, SIR, and SEIR, where the different compartments are symbolically denoted as letters S, E, I, and R. S: individual subjects in a population are susceptible to the disease, similarly E, I, and R mean that subjects are exposed (E), infected (I) from the disease and able to transmits to others, and R compartment signifies subjects have recovered from the disease, immune or have died. The disease parasite or virus dictates the choice or selection of the compartments and depends on the characteristics of the particular disease.It ought to be also noted that the inclusion of too many compartments into the model could be computationally intensive as well as tedious apart from risk of making unreliable prediction as well as may pose greater challenges in policy and decision making.

Historically, Daniel Bernoulli had formulated and solved a model for smallpox in 1760, and based on this he evaluated the efficacy by inoculating on healthy subjects the smallpox virus [12]. A discrete time model by Hamer in 1906 was formulated to understand the recurrence of the outbreak of measles [13]. Sir Ronald Ross was awarded the Nobel Prize, as he had developed a mathematical model for malaria as a host-vector disease in 1911 which was based on the differential equation differential [14]. Another interesting model was developed by Kermack and McKendrick [1] on epidemic models and introduced the threshold result that the density of susceptible must exceed a critical value in order for an epidemic outbreak to occur [8]. Moreover, recent development in mathematical modeling are numerous such as passive immunity, gradual loss of vaccine [3] and disease-acquired immunity, stages of infection, vertical transmission, disease vectors, vaccination, quarantine, social and sexual mixing groups and age structure [15–21]. The SIS, SIR, and SEIR models are graphically shown in Fig. 1. In SIR modeling the population is divided into three groups namely: (i) the group of individuals who are not infected and susceptible (S) of catching the disease, the group of individuals who are infected (I) by the concerned pathogen, and (iii) the group of recovered (R) individuals who have acquired a permanent immunity to the disease. Some of the basic ideas, assumptions, transmission, and recovery for an SIR model (adopted from [22]) are summarized in Table 1. Moreover, a system of differential equations for an SIR model for three compartments are modeled as follows:

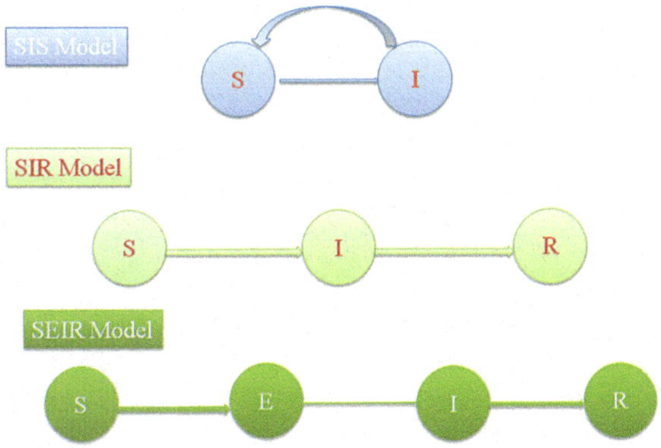

Fig. 6 The compartmental model: S represents the group of the subjects not infected and susceptible to the risk of the disease, I is the group of the subjects are infected by the new pathogen: virus or bacteria and R are those group of people who recovered and acquired immunity from the new pathogen

$$\frac{dS}{dt} = -\beta IS \tag{1}$$

$$\frac{dI}{dt} = -\beta IS - \gamma I \tag{2}$$

$$\frac{dR}{dt} = -\gamma I \tag{3}$$

where in the above equations: S denotes the number of susceptible, I the number of infected individuals and R the number of immune individual at time t, and the total population is given by: $N = S + I + R$ is constant by assumption as we have: $\frac{dN}{dt} = \frac{dS}{dt} + \frac{dI}{dt} + \frac{dR}{dt} = 0$. In equations (1) and (2): the first term βIS represents the disease transmission rate by contact between susceptible and infected individuals. This rate is assumed to be proportional to the sizes of both groups with a proportionality coefficient β and equations (2) and (3) the parameter γ is the specific rate at which infected individuals recover from the disease. For example: consider an epidemic outbreak in a population where, at the initial time, only a few individuals are infected, then the initial conditions for SIR model can be assumed as: $S(0) \approx N,\ I(0) = N - S(0) \approx 0,\ R(0) = 0$.

2.1 Phase Analysis

Sometimes, it's desired to have the dynamics in the phase-plane via deriving the isocline's and divide the plane into regions of increase and decrease of the various state variables. The phaseR package is a wrapper around ode that makes it easy to analyze 1D and 2D ode's. The R-state in the SIR model does not influence the dynamics, so we can rewrite the SIR model as a 2D system. So divide equation (1) by (2) gives the ODE:

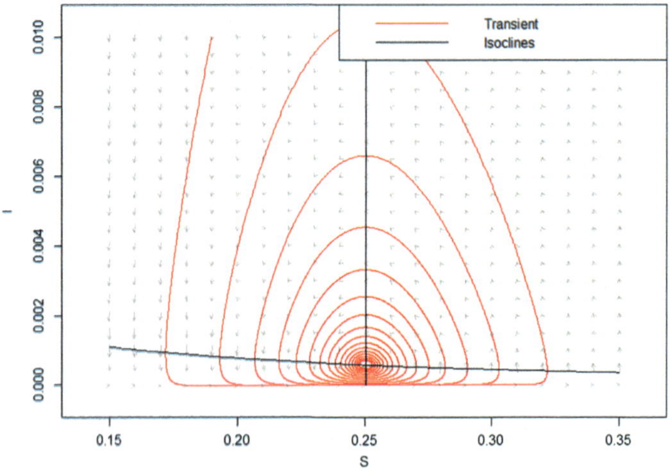

Fig. 7 The phase-plane diagram for the SI model

$$\frac{dS}{d}I = \frac{-\beta SI}{\beta SI - \gamma I} \tag{4}$$

The solution of the above ODE can be found analytically, using separation of variables the above equation can be rewritten as (for I > 0):

$$\int \frac{\beta S - \gamma}{\beta S} dS = - \int dI \tag{5}$$

After integrating the above equation and for every $t \geq 0$

$$I(t) + S(t) - \frac{\gamma}{\beta} log S(t) = I(0) + S(0) - \frac{\gamma}{\beta} log S(0) \tag{6}$$

The above expression gives the solutions (S(t), I(t)) in the S-I plane contains the level curves of the function (S(t); I(t)) viewed in the S–I plane (orbits) are contained in the level curves curves of this function $F(S; I) = I(t) + S(t) - \frac{\gamma}{\beta} log S(t)$, and it's shown in Fig. 7.

2.2 *Endemic of the Disease*

The above SIR model describes the long term state of the epidemic. The question may naturally arise: *"How long the pandemic may last?"*. It should be noted that always there will be a some portion of the population of susceptible individuals can never get infected. Mathematically, this can be answered by the SIR model by dividing Eq.

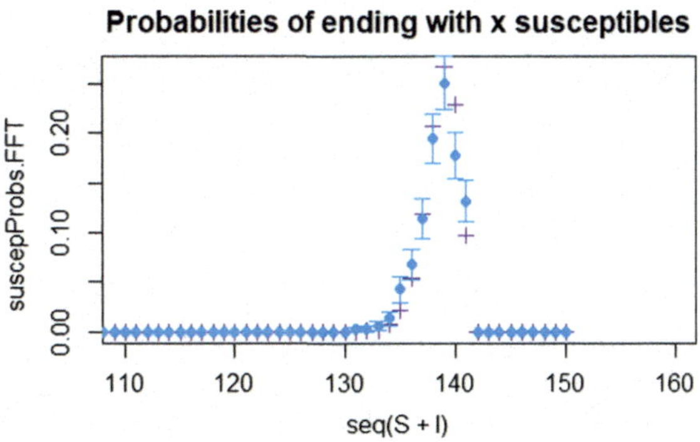

Fig. 8 The stochastic model for the endemic of the disease based on SIR branching approximation

(1) by Eq. (3), and integrating with respect to R, we have

$$S(t) = S(0)e^{-R(t)R_0} \tag{7}$$

From the above expression $S(0)$ will be always positive, whereas the exponential term $R(t)R_0$ has negative sign, ultimately there will no susceptible individual get infected over the time, and pandemic will be ceased to an end. Using stochastic SIR branching approximation and the MultiBD an R-package https://cran.r-project.org/web/packages/MultiBD/.

2.3 *Computational Methods for Solving SIR Model*

The SIR model's equations can be solved numerically using: Explicit time, Backward Euler, and Crank-Nicolson discretization schemes. The Explicit time discretization are explicit ODE (ordinary differential equation) methods, for example Forward Euler scheme, Runge-Kutta methods, Adams-Bashforth methods, and all these schemes evaluate the function at time levels. The Backward Euler method is an implicit method, also used to solve ODEs. The Crank-Nicolson method is based on the finite difference scheme and commonly used to solve ODEs/PDEs, and is a 2nd order method in time. This method is implicit in time and can be written as an implicit Runge–Kutta method, and this method has numerically stability. Rewriting the SIR model as follows:

$$S' = -\beta SI \tag{8}$$

$$I' = \beta SI - \gamma I \tag{9}$$

$$R' = \gamma I \tag{10}$$

where S(t) , I(t), and R(t) are susceptible, infected and recovered respectively, whereas the constants, $\beta > 0$ and $\gamma > 0$ should be given as the initial conditions: S(0), I(0),

Table 1 The assumptions for SIR model (*Source* lecture notes by V. A. Bokil, "Mathematical Modeling and Analysis of Infectious Disease Dynamics")

SIR model's basic assumptions transmission, and recovery		
Basic ideas and assumptions	**Transmission assumptions**	**Recovery assumptions**
1. Populations under study are divided into compartments.	1. β is the average number of adequate contacts (i.e., contacts sufficient for transmission) of a person per unit time.	1. A fraction α of infectives leave the infective class in unit time.
2. Rates of transfer between compartments are expressed mathematically as derivatives with respect to time of the sizes of the compartments: systems of ordinary differential equations	2. $\frac{\beta I}{N}$ is the average number of contacts with infectives per unit time of one susceptible.	2. There is no entry or departure from the population except possibly through death from the disease.
3. The community size is constant over the duration of the epidemic and is a large number, N	3. $(\frac{\beta I}{N})S$ is the number of new cases per unit time due to the S susceptibles. (Horizontal Incidence)L	
4. The infection is transmitted primarily by person-to person contacts (e.g., measles)		
5. Individuals are homogeneous and mix uniformly.		
Ignore demography, i.e., births and deaths		

and R(0). Now, applying the Implicit time discretization for the Crank-Nicolson scheme will make a 33 system of non-linear algebraic equations in the unknowns as: S^{n+1}, I^{n+1}, and R^{n+1}, and they are written below

$$\frac{S^{n+1}-S^n}{\Delta t} = \beta[SI]^{n+0.5} \approx 0.5\beta(S^n I^n + S^{n+1} I^{n+1}) \tag{11}$$

$$\frac{I^{n+1}-I^n}{\Delta t} = \beta[SI]^{n+0.5} - \gamma I^{n+0.5} \approx 0.5\beta(S^n I^n + S^{n+1} I^{n+1}) - 0.5\gamma(I^n + I^{n+1}) \tag{12}$$

$$\frac{R^{n+1}-R^n}{\Delta t} = \gamma I^{n+0.5} \approx 0.5\gamma(I^n + I^{n+1}) \tag{13}$$

Denoting S for S^{n+1}, $S^{(1)}$ for S^n, I for I^{n+1}, $I^{(1)}$ for I^n, and R for R^{n+1}, $R^{(1)}$ for R^n, now writing the system of equations as

$$F_S(S, I, R) = S - S^{(1)} + 0.5\Delta t\beta(S^{(1)}I^{(1)} + SI) = 0 \tag{14}$$

$$I_S(S, I, R) = I - I^{(1)} - 0.5\Delta t\beta(S^{(1)}I^{(1)} + SI) + 0.5\Delta t\gamma(I^{(1)} + I) = 0 \tag{15}$$

$$R_S(S, I, R) = R - R^{(1)} - 0.5\Delta t\gamma(I^{(1)} + I) = 0 \tag{16}$$

Applying Picard's iterative approximation method and assume that $\hat{S}$, $\hat{I}$ and $\hat{R}$, for S, I, and R as to linearize the non-linear terms., and solving the above equations with respect to the unknowns: S, I, and R.

$$S = \frac{S^{(1)} - 0.5\Delta t\beta S^{(1)}I^{(1)}}{1 + 0.5\Delta t\beta\hat{I}} \tag{17}$$

$$I = \frac{I^{(1)} + 0.5\Delta t\beta S^{(1)}I^{(1)} - 0.5\Delta t\gamma I^{(1)}}{1 - 0.5\Delta t\beta\hat{S} + 0.5\Delta t\gamma} \tag{18}$$

$$R = R^{(1)} - 0.5\Delta t\gamma(I^{(1)} + \hat{I}) \tag{19}$$

The non-linear system of equation (10), (11), and (12) can be written as G(u) = 0, where G =G_S, G_I, G_R), so the Jacobian can computed as

$$J = \begin{bmatrix} \frac{\partial G_S}{\partial S} & \frac{\partial G_S}{\partial I} & \frac{\partial G_S}{\partial R} \\ \frac{\partial G_I}{\partial S} & \frac{\partial G_I}{\partial I} & \frac{\partial G_I}{\partial R} \\ \frac{\partial G_R}{\partial S} & \frac{\partial G_R}{\partial I} & \frac{\partial G_R}{\partial R} \end{bmatrix} = \begin{bmatrix} 1 + 0.5\Delta t\beta I & 0.5\Delta t\beta S & 0 \\ 0.5\Delta t\beta I & 1 - 0.5\Delta t\beta S + 0.5\Delta t\gamma & 0 \\ 0 & 0.5\Delta t\gamma & 0 \end{bmatrix} \tag{20}$$

Updating after each iteration with new updates, using Newton method to solve the Jacobian as an algebraic equation, the solution could be obtained for unknowns S, R, and R. Moreover, for the above SIR model, an explicit time integration approaches work well, the 4th order Runge-Kutta method is a suitable choice since it is efficient, accurate and is based on the simple algorithms. Moreover, in order to fit the model with the observed or real data, broadly, two things need to be taken into account, first a solver for the system of differential equations and an optimizer. For solving DEs the function'ode' from the'deSolve' an R package, and to optimize'optim' function from base R; both these functions are also available in other software MATLAB, MAPLE, R and Mathematica (computational packages). So to minimize the sum of the squared differences between the number of infected I at time t and the corresponding number of predicted cases by our model $\hat{I(t)}$.

$$RSS(\beta, \gamma) = \sum_t (I(t) - \hat{I}(t))^2 \tag{21}$$

Using these tools from COVID19.analytic and R-package, the estimated cases for susceptible,infected, and recovered are shown below in Fig. 9, the plots on the right side are on semi-log- scale, the plots show that the model fit with the observed data quite well.

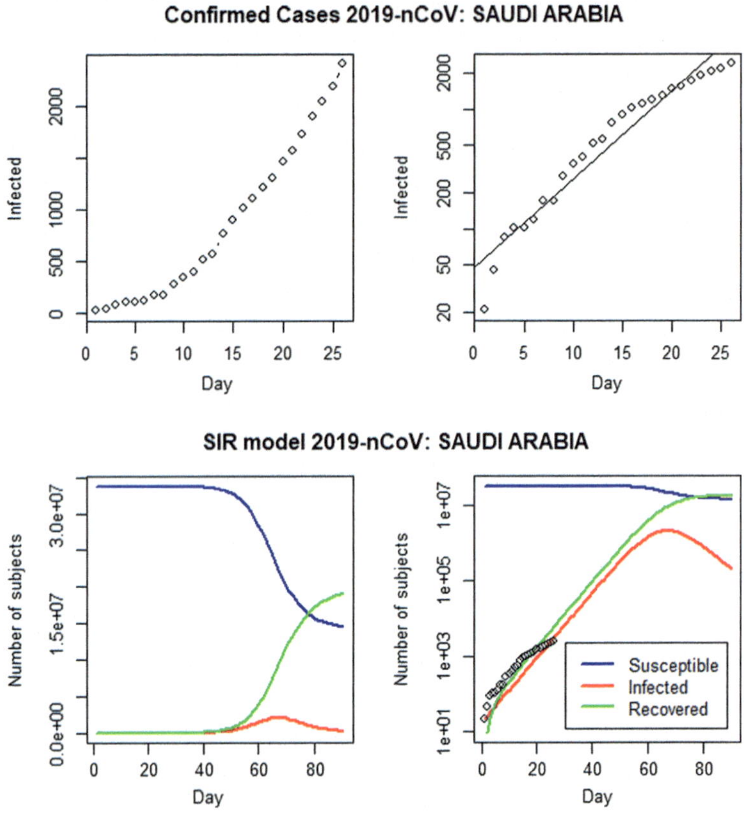

Fig. 9 Based on the SIR model the susceptible, infected, and recovered cases for Saudi Arabia is shown right hand side graphs on log-scale

Moreover, if the graphical plots do not fit well due to algorithm does not converge to the optimal solution. The reason could be the'optim' stops too early before it could not find an appropriate solution. Now, further explore the'optim' algorithm, the optim function uses the gradient algorithms such as:" "BFGS (by Broyden, Fletcher, Goldfarb and Shanno)", "CG (Fletcher and Reeves developed the conjugate gradients method" and "L-BFGS-B (method is by Byrd et al.)" methods. as well as a finite-difference approximation algorithms. These gradient based algorithms may try to find an optimum estimate via repeatedly improving the current estimate and finding a new solution with a lower residual sum of squares (RSS) each time. Gradient methods do this by computing for a small change of the parameters in which direction the RSS will change the fastest and is based on the linear search approach.

2.4 Estimating the Reproducing Number R_0

The basic reproduction number was introduced in 1886 by (the Director of the Statistical Office of Berlin) Richard Bockh, see: [23] and [24]. The basic reproduction number also commonly known as R_0 pronounced as 'R-nought' could be defined as the expected number of secondary cases produced by a single individual infected subject in a completely susceptible population [25]. It is a dimensionless number and not a rate. We can use the fact that R0 is a dimensionless number to help us in calculating it

$$R_0 \propto \left(\frac{infection}{contact}\right) \times \left(\frac{contact}{time}\right) \times \left(\frac{time}{infection}\right) \tag{22}$$

R_0 can be estimated from the above SIR model's equations (1) to (3), since it depends on the transmissibility, contact rates and expected duration of infection. Based on the model's assumption the population N is closed have N number of subjects, whereas number of susceptible S and infected I , and R subjects are removed, So rewriting the SIR model in terms of proportion, we have

$$\frac{ds}{dt} = -\beta is \tag{23}$$

$$\frac{di}{dt} = -\beta is - \gamma i \tag{24}$$

$$\frac{dr}{dt} = -\gamma i \tag{25}$$

where $s = \frac{S}{N}$, $i = \frac{I}{N}$, and $r = \frac{R}{N}$. The trajectory of the system solution in the $I - S$ plane is presented in Fig. 2; from this the existence of a 'threshold effect' can be observed. The maximum value of the curve occurs at $S = \frac{\gamma}{\beta}$. It implies that an epidemic will start and amplify only if $S(0) \approx N$ is larger than $\frac{\gamma}{\beta}$, or equivalently if

$$R_0 = \frac{N\beta}{\gamma} > 1$$

So under this condition, the number of infectious people will increase until the number of susceptible is reduced to $\frac{\gamma}{\beta}$ and will decrease thereafter. Thus the number R_0 represents a threshold for an epidemic to happen, and this number is also commonly known as 'basic reproduction ratio', since it represents the average number of susceptible which are contaminated by one infectious person. now divide Eq. 2 by 1, we get:

$$\frac{dI}{dS} = (\frac{\gamma}{\beta S} - 1)$$

Integrating this equation, we get:

$$I = \frac{\gamma}{\beta} log S - S + C \;\; with \;\; C \approx N - \frac{\gamma}{\beta} log N$$

From the above equation, the instantaneous maximum number of infectious subjects can computed as:

$$I_{max} = N(1 - \frac{1 + log R_0}{R_0})$$

The trajectory terminates on the S-axis at a positive value as shown in Fig. 7, which can be seen from Eq. 4 that I must vanish at some positive value of S. So the epidemic terminates before all susceptible have become infected and some individual subjects escape the new pathogen completely. Further, we can estimate how many susceptible subjects remain or equivalently the final value $R(\infty)$ of immune population size. Divide Eq. 2 by Eq. 3, so we have:

$$\frac{dS}{dR} = -\frac{\beta}{\gamma} S \implies S(R) = S(0)e^{-\frac{\beta}{\gamma}R} \approx Ne^{-\frac{\beta}{\gamma}R}$$

So

$$\frac{dS}{dt} = \gamma I = \gamma(N - S - R) = \gamma(N - Ne^{-\frac{\beta}{\gamma}R})$$

Therefore

$$t \to \infty \implies I \to 0 \implies \frac{dR}{dt} = 0 \implies N[1 - e^{-\frac{\beta}{\gamma}R(\infty)}] = R(\infty) \qquad (26)$$

Eq. 5 has unique solution $R(\infty)$ between 0 and N as long as $R_0 > 1$. Denote $x = \frac{R(\infty)}{N}$ the fraction the population that has contracted the disease before the epidemic collapses. Solving Eq. 5, we have: $R_0 = \frac{log(1-x)}{x}$, and R_0 estimates for different pandemics are shown in Fig. 10, see: https://www.the-scientist.com/features/why-r0-is-problematic-for-predicting-covid-19spread-67690ga=2.205136600.930086860.1594988120-662736184.1594988120.

2.4.1 Challenges and Issues in Estimating R_0

As above an estimate for R_0 is described for an SIR model, and has been called "arguably the most important quantity in the study of epidemics". Since it's playing a vital role as well as desiderata especially for public health professionals in their decision and policy making. Hence, it's very crucial and important to produce accurate and reliable estimates of this quantity R_0. This quantity precisely presents the whole outbreak of a disease, and it assess the magnitude and severity as well as helps to quantify the percentage of the population needed to be vaccinated to avoid the

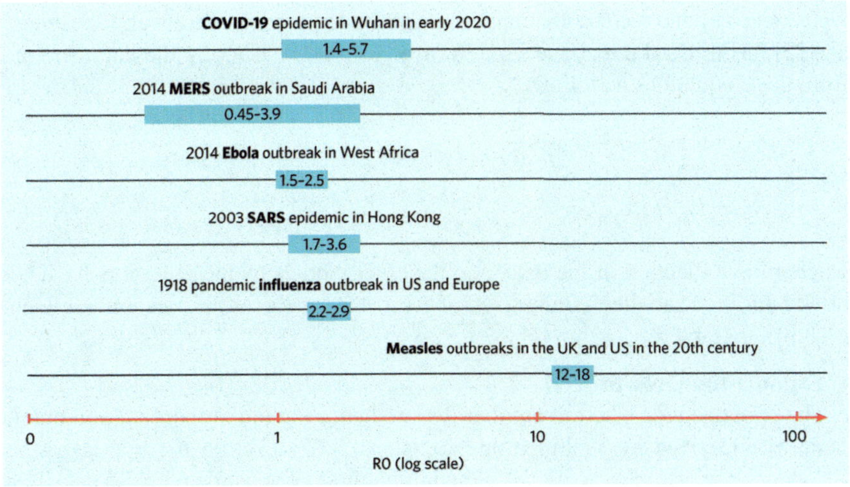

Fig. 10 R_0 estimates for different pandemic is shown adopted from The Scientist an article by Katarina Zimmer, July13, 2020

epidemic roughly as $1 - \frac{1}{R_0}$ is utilized to estimate final size of the total number of infected individuals; and is related to the probability of observing an outbreak under the same conditions (Anderson and May, 1992; Britton, 2010). Although there is an explicit definition of R_0, it is still difficult for an epidemiologists to standardize an estimator for R_0 (Hethcote 2000). An obvious issue in quantifying an estimate for R_0 is that it's solely depend on the property of the disease model apart from the commonly encountered noises inhibit in statistical models as well assumptions made by the researchers about the disease which had been transmitted in a population (Brown, Oleson, & Porter, 2016; Diekmann, Heesterbeek, & Roberts, 2009). To develop a good estimate for R_0 numerous research works had been done and the difficulties and nuances that's involved in estimating R0 can be found in Diekmann et al. (2009) [26], Heathcote [21], and Van den Driessche (2017), [27]. Based on eight different approaches Gallagher, et al. [25] had discussed the nuances pertaining in estimating R_0 for the 2009 pandemic influenza. The authors utilized the basic SIR model by adding the random into the model, and adding the noise the new compartment model as an stochastic model, and the expression with "hats" and without "hats" are distinguishes as stochastic and deterministic in equations (as observations were generated from the ODEs), are noises are given as below:

$$\hat{S(t)} = S(t) + \epsilon_{S,t} \tag{27}$$

$$\hat{I(t)} = N - \hat{S(t)} - \hat{R(t)} \tag{28}$$

$$\hat{R(t)} = \hat{R(t)} + \epsilon_{R,t} \tag{29}$$

where and $\epsilon_{S,t}$ and $\epsilon_{R,t}$ are the random noises in the model. Moreover, Gallagher, et al. [25] has utilized the above Eqs. 28-30 to estimate the R_0 by the data generated from these equations as follows:

$$Data = \left\{ \left(\hat{S(t)} = s(t), \hat{I(t)} = i(t), \hat{R(t)} = r(t) \right) : t = t_0, t_1, ..., t_T \right\} \tag{30}$$

$$\hat{R}_0 = m(Data) \tag{31}$$

where m is a function of the data, and the eight models by these authors have been briefly outlined and their comparison of estimates for R_0 for the pandemic influenza is shown in Table 2.

- **Exponential Growth(EG)**
  The effective reproduction number R0 and hence the initial reproduction number R_0, was derived by Wallinga and Lipsitch (2007) [31] on the hypothesis that "counts increase exponentially in the initial phase of an epidemic." So to estimate r, the per capita change in the number of new cases per unit of time and ω the serial interval, the distribution of time between a primary and secondary infection, then, $R_0 = e^{r\omega}$. This equation is based on the Lotka-Euler survival model, commonly utilized in demography, ecology as well as evolutionary biology. Expanding this equation $R_0 = e^{r\omega}$ by using Taylor series expansion up to first order to estimate R_0, whereas in Nishiura, Chowell, Safan, and Castillo-Chavez (2010) [32] had derived it's variant. This approach assumes an exponential growth during early phase as well as the occurrence of initial phase growth. The model has an advantage since it relies on estimates of the number of susceptible, how and when such a method should be used because of the initial growth assumption, Nishiura et al. (2010) [32] had given some guidelines. Moreover, there are several adjustments that could be done to this approach, for example: Wallinga and Lipsitch (2007) [31] describes to estimate R_0 by assuming ω a random variable, whereas Obadia, Haneef, & Boëlle, (2012) [33] assumed that r has it's own distribution.
- **Ratio Estimator (RE)**
  The second approach the Gallagher et al. applied to the SIR model is to minimize the joint mean square error for the data collected at each time point:

$$(\hat{\beta}, \hat{\gamma}) = argmin_{\beta,\gamma} \sum_t \left[(s(t) - S(t; \beta, \gamma))^2 + (i(t) - I(t; \beta, \gamma))^2 + (r(t) - R(t; \beta, \gamma))^2 \right] \tag{32}$$

  So the equation for the ratio estimator (RE) for R_0 will be as:

$$\hat{R}_0 = \frac{\hat{\beta}}{\hat{\gamma}} \tag{33}$$

  The above estimate could be found for the β and γ either with optimization algorithm or grid search methods.
- **Re-parameterized Ratio Estimator(rRE)**
  As the approach used to estimate β and γ to compute R_0 can also be estimated

by simply reparametrization of ODEs directly with R_0 via using the relationship $R_0 = \frac{\beta}{\gamma}$, and we have:

$$(\hat{R_0}, \hat{\gamma}) = argmin_{0,\gamma} \sum_t \left[(s(t) - S(t; R_0, \gamma))^2 + (i(t) - I(t; R_0, \gamma))^2 + (r(t) - R(t; R_0, \gamma))^2 \right] \tag{34}$$

The above estimate can again be found either grid search algorithm or optimization tools.

- **Log Linear (LL)**
  In Log-Linear model, the SIR model was reduced to ODEs by Harko, Lobo, and Mak(2014) [34] in two ODEs with one constraint for each equations as follows:

$$log\left(\frac{S(t)}{S(0)}\right) = -R_0 \frac{R(t)}{N} \tag{35}$$

  and estimated the R_0 as below:

$$\hat{R_0} = -\frac{\sum_{t_0}^{T} log\left(\frac{S(t)}{S(0)}\right)}{\sum_{t_0}^{T} \frac{R(t)}{N}} \tag{36}$$

- **Markov Chain (MC)**
  Based on Reed-Frost model Abbey(1952) [35] using the Reed-Frost Chain Binomial which as specific form of I(t), the number of infected individuals at time point t. So we have

$$S(\hat{t}) = \hat{S}(t-1) - I(\hat{t}) \tag{37}$$

$$\left(I(\hat{t}) | \hat{S}(t-1), \hat{I}(t-1)\right) \sim Binomial\left(\hat{S}(t-1), 1 - (1-\alpha)^{\hat{I}(t-1)}\right) \tag{38}$$

$$R(\hat{t}) = \hat{R}(t-1) + I(\hat{t}) \tag{39}$$

  Using the likelihood method and the optimization tools, $\hat{R}_0$ can be obtained as:

$$\hat{R}_0 = log\left(\frac{1}{1-\alpha}\right) \tag{40}$$

- **Likelihood-Based Estimation (LBE)**
  Using the likelihood based estimate the R_0 is given by see for detail Gallagher et al. [25]

$$R_0 = \frac{\hat{\beta}}{\hat{\gamma}} \tag{41}$$

- **Incidence to Prevalence (IPR)**
  The incidence to prevalence method was described by Nishiura and Chowell (2009) [32], the estimate for $\hat{R}_0$ is:

Table 2 Comparison of R_0 estimates for 2009 influenza, *Source* Exploring the nuances of R_0: eight estimates and application to 2009 pandemic influenza, by Shannon Gallagher, Andersen Chang, and William F. Eddy (a preprint), March 25, 2020

Estimation of R_0 using eight models: a comparison		
Methods	**SEIR R_0 (SE)**	**SIR R_0 (SE)**
EG	1.001 (<1e-04)	1.002 (2e-04)
RE	1.977 (0.0161)	1.767 (0.137)
rRE	1.977 (0.0162)	1.767 (0.0795)
LL	1.989 (0.021)	1.789 (0.0042)
MC	1.31 (0)	1.619 (0)
LBE	1.893 (0.0135)	1.742 (5.5501)
IPR	4.254 (0.8687)	1.177 (0.9889)
LMA	-0.645 (2.5491)	2.565 (0.175)

$$\hat{R}_0 = \frac{1}{\gamma} \cdot IPR(t^*) \tag{42}$$

- **Linear model approximation (LMA)**
  Chen and Li, 2009; and Hu, Teng, andLong (2014) [36] described method to estimate $\hat{R}_0$ by applying the linear approximation of the Kermack and McKendrick SIR model, this emthod is further extended by Gallagher et al. [25], so the estimate for R_0 is given as:

$$\hat{R}_0 = \frac{S'\hat{(0)}}{R'\hat{(0)}} \cdot \frac{N}{S\hat{(0)}} \tag{43}$$

2.4.2 Next Generation Method: R_0

As R_0 is the number of secondary infections in which a single individual subject is infected in a population. The issue is: how we deal if there were multiple types of infected subjects; for example malaria which is vector-borne disease or sexually transmitted disease (HIV). Such type pf problems can be handled using the structured epidemic models, the basic idea is simply average the expected number of new infections over all possible infected types. Now assuming that a system have multiple discrete type of infected individual subjects. Now introducing a 'next generation matrix' as square matrix G, and the elements of this matrix are denoted as g_{ij}, where i and j are the rows and columns of the matrix G. The g_{ij} gives the expected number of secondary infection type i, and it is caused by a single individual infected individual subjects of type j, whereas the population of type i completely susceptible. Hence all the elements in the matrix G are the reproduction number. The spectral radius of the matrix G gives the reproduction number, which is also known is the dominant eigenvalue. For example, consider G as a 2 by 2 matrix defined as:

$$G = \begin{bmatrix} a & b \\ c & d \end{bmatrix}$$

The eigenvalue of matrix G can be given as

$$\lambda_i = \frac{T}{2} \pm \sqrt{\left(\frac{T}{2}\right)^2 - D} \tag{44}$$

where T = a + d is the trace and D = ad - bc is the determinant of the matrix G.

The next generation matrix has a number of desirable properties such as it is a non-negative matrix and, it guarantees that there will be a single, unique eigenvalue which is positive, real, and strictly greater than all the others.

The estimation of reproduction number R_0 is discussed, and the next generation method is outlined in this subsection, a detail work can be found in [26–28].

2.5 *Stochastic Modeling*

Since with any modeling tools, there are always limitation, and it also exist with compartmental models. For example, the model may not able to describe the real or observed data. Due to the assumptions were not fully met namely: homogeneity assumption, not a close system, imbalance equations, where as in general with real world data compartments models fail to describe the system. These limitation could be avoided by extending the deterministic compartmental models into a stochastic model which incorporates the probabilistic theory. So it can be done by keeping time discrete and utilizes the stochastic processes. Another approach may be using continuous framework and time to infection as stochastic.

2.5.1 Reed-Frost Model

The Reed-Frost model is based on the *chain binomial model* since the infection spread dynamically through direct contact and assume that it's independent and have constant probability, and this model has the following characteristics [29, 30]:

- It is similar to compartmental model where each individuals are either susceptible, infectious or recovered.
- The population of the study population is closed and constant and have initial values such as: $s_0 \; and \; i_0 \in N$, where $s_0 = S_0$, and $i_0 = I_0$ are susceptible and infected individual subjects.
- The infection dynamic can be explained via discrete time Markov chain.

$$\begin{cases} I_{t+1} | \, S_t & = s_t, \; I_t = i_t \sim Bin\,(s_t, 1 - (1 - \omega)^{i_t})\,), \\ S_{t+1} & = S_t - I_{t+1} \end{cases} \tag{45}$$

where $t = 1, 2, \ldots$ are time steps and ω is the probability of an infectious individual who is a susceptible subjects in span of one time step.

- The epidemic final size is: $Z = \sum_{i=0}^{\infty} I_i$.

Now consider if ω is the probability of infection, then the probability of not infected subject will be $1 - \omega$, so the probability to escape from infection from contact will be $(1 - \omega)^i i$, hence the probability of infection will be $1 - (1 - \omega)^i$. The Reed-Frost model can be interpreted as an SIR model in which the incubation period and the recovery time is one unit time, whereas the basic reproduction number can be given as ωS_0. Moreover, the likelihood of the Reed-Frost model can be given as

$$L(\omega : \{i_0, i_1, , \ldots, i_T, s_0\}) = \prod_{i=0}^{T-1} \theta_t^{i_{t+1}} (1 - \theta_t)^{s_i - s_{i+1}}, \;\; \theta_t = 1 - (1 - \omega)_t^i \tag{46}$$

where T denotes the number of time steps.

2.5.2 Gillespie's Direct Method

The Gillespie's direct method asks two questions if the system is in a given state:

- When does the next event occur? The time to the next event (τ) is exponentially distributed and the rate equal to the sum of the rates over all possible events. The probability density function is given by

$$f(\tau) = (\sum_i a_i)e^{(-\tau \sum_i a_i)} \tag{47}$$

- Which event occurs next? We convert event rates into probabilities, and randomly select one of these events according

$$P(Event = v) = \frac{a_v}{\sum_i a_i} \tag{48}$$

where a_i are event rates.

Assuming the above distributions the algorithm is as follows:

1. Set initial population numbers $t \mapsto 0$.
2. Calculate the a_i for all i.
3. Choose τ from an exponential distribution with parameter $\sum_i a_i$ as in Eq. (30).
4. Choose the event v according to the distribution in Eq. (31).
5. Change the number of individuals to reflect the event, v. Set $t \mapsto t + \tau$.
6. Go to step 2.

The above algorithm simulates stochastic realizations of the exact process described by what's known as the master equation. Assume that $p_{SIR}(t)$ is the probability and it is in state (S,I,R) at a given time t, and N = S + I + R, then the master equation is given as follows describes as how this probability distribution evolves over the time:

$$\begin{aligned}\frac{dp_{SIR}(t)}{dt} =& p_{S-1,I,R}\,[\mu(N-1)\,] + p_{S+1,I,R}\,[\mu(S+1)\,]+ \\ & p_{S+1,I-1,R}\,[\beta\frac{(I-1)}{N}(S+1)\,] + p_{S,I+1,R-1}\,[\gamma(I+1)\,] \\ & + p_{S,I+1,R}\,[\mu(I+1)\,] + p_{S,I,R+1}\,[\mu(R+1)\,] \\ & - p_{S,I,R}\,[\mu N + \mu S + \beta\frac{I}{N}S + \gamma I + \mu I + \mu R\,]\end{aligned} \tag{49}$$

2.5.3 Example Based on SIR Model Using SimInf R-Package

The following example is based on the 'SimInf' an R-package https://cran.r-project.org/web/packages/SimInf/vignettes/SimInf.pdf.

Specification of the SIR model without scheduled events

This example is based on the predefined three compartments (SIR) model (susceptible: S, infected: R, and recovered: R). The mode of transmission of infection is to susceptible individuals is through direct contact between susceptible and infected individuals, this model has two transitions at each node i as follows:

$$S_i \xrightarrow{\beta S_i I_i/(S_+ I_i + R_i)} I_i$$

$$I_i \xrightarrow{\gamma I_i} R_i$$

where β, and γ are the transmission and recovery rates respectively. In order to create and SIR model object, define u0, a data.frame with the initial number of individuals in each compartment when the simulation starts, assume that a node has 999 susceptible with 1 infected and there are no recovered individuals. As the assumptions made in this example is that there are no interaction between nodes, so the stochastic model does not disturb any nodes in the model. So the R-code is as follows:

```
> install.packages('SimInf')
> library(SimInf)
> n <- 1000
> u0 <- data.frame(S = rep(999, n), I = rep(1, n), R = rep(0, n))
> tspan <- seq(from = 1, to = 180, by = 7)
> model <- SIR(u0 = u0, tspan = tspan, beta = 0.16, gamma = 0.077)
> model
> model
Model: SIR
Number of nodes: 1000
Number of transitions: 2
Number of scheduled events: 0

Local data
----------
 Parameter Value
 beta      0.160
 gamma     0.077

Compartments
------------
 - Empty, please run the model first
> set.seed(123)
> set_num_threads(1)
> result <- run(model = model)
> result
Model: SIR
Number of nodes: 1000
Number of transitions: 2
Number of scheduled events: 0

Local data
----------
 Parameter Value
 beta      0.160
 gamma     0.077

Compartments
------------
     Min. 1st Qu. Median  Mean 3rd Qu.  Max.
 S 108.0   368.0  993.0 755.4   999.0 999.0
 I   0.0     0.0    1.0  30.4    38.0 235.0
 R   0.0     1.0    5.0 214.2   484.0 891.0
> plot(result)
> plot(result, node = 1:10, range = FALSE)
> plot(result, node = 1:5, range = FALSE)
%%%%%
> head(trajectory(model = result, node = 1))
  node time   S  I  R
1    1    1 999  1  0
2    1    8 998  1  1
3    1   15 991  8  1
4    1   22 973 21  6
5    1   29 935 42 23
6    1   36 886 61 53
```

Specification of scheduled events in the SIR model Further continuing with predefined SIR model, and taking into account the demographic data. So specify each event as one column in the select matrix E using the select attribute of the event. The non-zero entries in the selected column in E specify the compartment involved, define E as

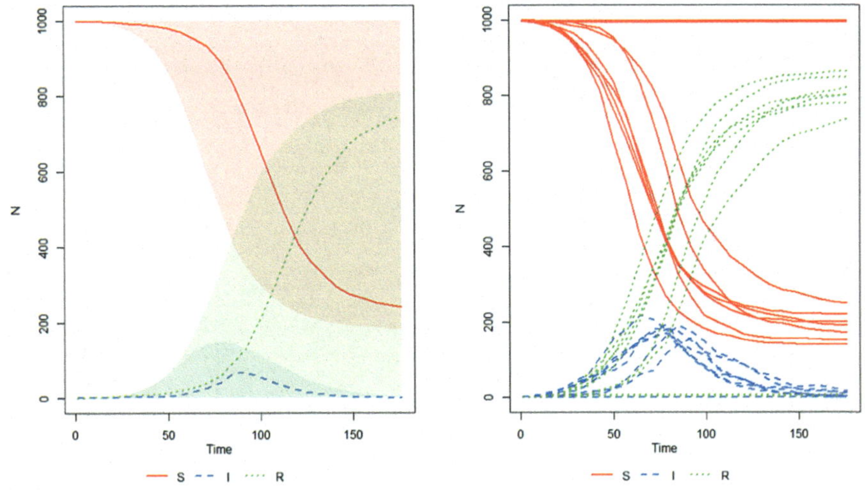

(a) 1a

(b) 1b

Fig. 11 The output result from a stochastic SIR model in 1000 nodes starting with 999 susceptible, 1 infected and 0 recovered individuals in each node ($\beta = 0.16$, $\gamma = 0.077$). There are no between-node interactions. Left (1a: The default plot shows the median and inter-quartile range of the count in each compartment through time across all nodes. Right 1b: Realizations from a subset of 10 nodes

$$\begin{array}{c} \begin{matrix} 1 & 2 & 3 & 4 \end{matrix} \\ \begin{pmatrix} 1 & 0 & 0 & 1 \\ 0 & 1 & 0 & 1 \\ 0 & 0 & 1 & 1 \end{pmatrix} \begin{matrix} S \\ I \\ R \end{matrix} \end{array}$$

In order to operate on a single compartment (S, I or R) as well as an event that involves all three compartment, we need to specify a scheduled event. When several compartments are involved in an event, the individuals affected by the event will be sampled without replacement from the specified compartments. The numerical solver performs an extensive error checking of the event before it is processed. And an error will be raised if the event is invalid, for example, if the event tries to move more individuals than exists in the specified compartments. Consider we have 4 scheduled events to include in a simulation. Below is a data.frame, that contains the events.

```
> u0 <- data.frame(S = rep(0, 5), I = rep(0, 5), R = rep(0, 5))
> add <- data.frame(event = "enter", time = rep(1:10, each = 5),
+                   node = 1:5, dest = 0, n = 1:5, proportion = 0, select = 1, shift = 0)
> infect <- data.frame(event = "enter", time = 25, node = 5,
+                      + dest = 0, n = 1, proportion = 0, select = 2, shift = 0)
> infect <- data.frame(event = "enter", time = 25, node = 5,
+                      dest = 0, n = 1, proportion = 0, select = 2, shift = 0)
> move <- data.frame(event = "extTrans", time = 35:45, node = c(5, 5, 5,
+                      5, 4, 4, 4, 3, 3, 2, 1), dest = c(4, 3, 3, 1, 3, 2, 1, 2, 1, 1, 2),
```

```
+                          n = 5, proportion = 0, select = 4, shift = 0)
> remove <- data.frame(event = "exit", time = c(70, 110),
+                          node = rep(1:5, each = 2), dest = 0, n = 0, proportion = 0.2,
+                          select = 4, shift = 0)
> model <- SIR(u0 = u0, tspan = 1:180, events = events, beta = 0.16,
+                    + gamma = 0.077)
> set.seed(3)
> set_num_threads(1)
> result <- run(model)
> plot(result, node = 1:5, range = FALSE)
> result
Model: SIR
Number of nodes: 1000
Number of transitions: 2
Number of scheduled events: 0

Local data
----------
 Parameter Value
 beta      0.160
 gamma     0.077

Compartments
------------
    Min. 1st Qu. Median  Mean 3rd Qu.  Max.
 S 103.0   337.0  992.0 744.5   999.0 999.0
 I   0.0     0.0    2.0  31.4    41.0 239.0
 R   0.0     1.0    5.0 224.1   528.0 896.0
```

3 Role of Reproduction Number and Growth Curve in Decision and Policy Making

The basic reproduction number plays a vital role in epidemiological sciences as well as in public health management, since it has been used to explain the dynamic of epidemics in population. For example Covid-19 (an infectious disease), R_0 is estimated between 2 and 2.5, whereas for measles it lies between 12 to 18. R_0 spread is order of exponential, for example if $R_0 = 2$, then a single person can generate new infections exponentially as 2^n, whereas if this number if less than 1 then it decays fast as well exponentially:

$$
\begin{aligned}
I\ generation &= 2\ new\ infections\\
II\ generation &= 4\ new\ infections\\
III\ generation &= 8\ new\ infections\\
IV\ generation &= 16\ new\ infections\\
V\ generation &= 32\ new\ infections
\end{aligned}
$$

Moreover in practice or real life $the\ effective\ reproduction\ number$ is utilized and denoted as R and defined as: the average number an infected person goes on to infect in a population where some people are immune (or some other interventions are in place). It related with R_0 as: $R = sR_0$, where is the proportion of susceptible

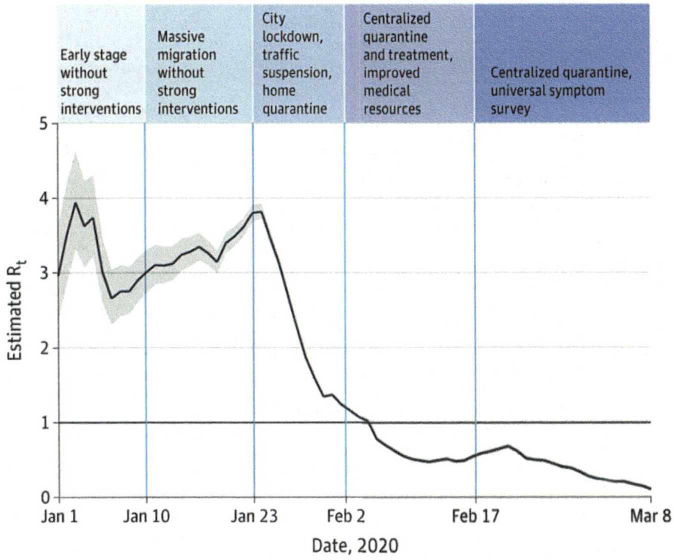

Fig. 12 The effective reproduction number based on laboratory-confirmed Corona virus (Covid-19) Cases in Wuhan, China (*Source* https://jamanetwork.com/journals/jama/fullarticle/2765665)

subjects for a population. As R is not a rate, and it cannot explain how fast the epidemic is growing in the population, and this can by quantified by using the *growth curve*, so the growth curve can be defined as exponential curve:

$$N(t) = constant\ e^{\lambda t} \tag{50}$$

where N is the number of cases and depends on time t in days and λ is the growth rate of of the disease per day. If the growth rate is positive this implies the rise in the epidemic cases whereas if sign of growth rate is negative means there are decrease in number of epidemic cases, and for growth rate zero gives number of cases constant. Now the question is: R or growth rate λ is better? The pros and cons as given in Table 3 below:

3.1 *Challenges and Issues in Modeling Infectious Diseases*

- Provide a systematic framework for when we should try to eradicate
- Develop quantitative models of the economics of control versus eradication
- Identify the most effective approaches to achieve eradication
- Quantify the landscape of susceptibility

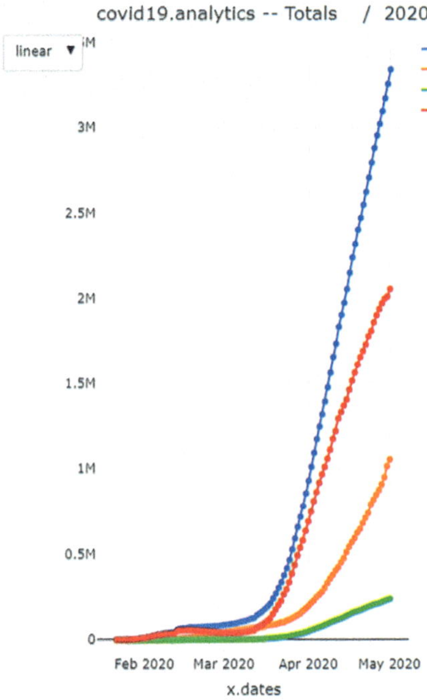

Fig. 13 Global growth rate of Corona virus: confirmed, recovered, deaths and active cases by using Covid-19analytics (R-package)

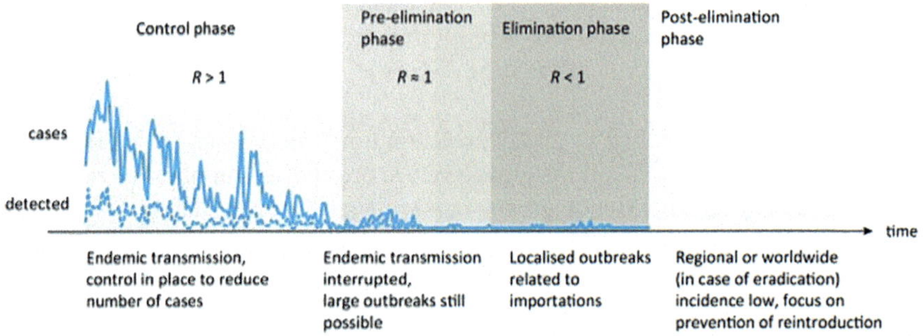

Fig. 14 Stages towards and after elimination in a given location and milestones on the path to elimination. Adapted from (Townsend et al., 2013b, World Health Organization, 2007). Shading illustrates control intensity (darker grey for heightened efforts), also see: https://www.sciencedirect.com/science/article/pii/S175543651400070X

Table 3 Comparing R and the growth rate, *Source* https://plus.maths.org/content/epidemic-growth-rate)

Comparison between reproduction number and the growth rate	
Reproduction ratio: R	**Growth rate per day:**
1. In planning to deal with the spread of epidemic using any intervention, then the reproduction number is most suitable in planning of the control measures such as: • if R=1.5 means then we need to plan for one third of reduction in transmission. • if R=2 means need to vaccinate half the susceptible people in the population; An intuitive way of predicting the strength of future interventions needed to stop an epidemic then consideration of R is a better choice. 2. if R>1 then exponential growth in epidemic cases if R=1 then the epidemic cases are constant or flat if R<1 then exponential decay in epidemic cases. 3. R a ratio of cases by infection generation. It is not a rate: there is no timescale involved. 4. R is not at all easy to measure in practice, but can be fitted using models if the timescales of infection are known. In principle it could be estimated by detailed epidemiological data on exactly who got infection from whom, but this is not usually feasible in typical settings.	1. Growth rate is more natural for thinking about how cases are oscillating over time. For example • $\lambda = 0.01$ per day means cases will increase by about 1% a day. • $\lambda = -0.02$ per day means cases will decrease by about 2% a day. The growth rate is a good description of what's happening now: if we have a certain number of cases today then we can work out how many to expect tomorrow, the day after, and so on. 2. if $\lambda > 0$ then exponential growth if $\lambda = 0$ then the growth is flat or constant if $\lambda < 0$ then growth curve is exponential decay 3. The growth rate λ is a rate, usually given in days for Covid-19. 4. The growth rate λ is relatively easy to estimate from time series data of cases or deaths (but see below about small numbers). A simple approach is just to find the gradient of the logged cases. More advanced approaches, which can take into account a time-varying growth rate, or heterogeneous population, again involve fitting epidemic models.

- Improve monitoring during and after the endgame
- Identify post-eradication opportunities and threats

4 Summary

The basic SIR, and stochastic models were outlined along with some notes on computational tools for these models. Briefly, the reproduction number R_0 was discussed based on different approaches. A famous quote by great mathematician Daniel Bernoulli:

> I simply wish that, in a matter which so closely concerns the well being of the human race, no decision shall be made without all the knowledge which a little analysis and calculation can provide." (Daniel Bernoulli,1760)

References

1. Kermack, W.O., McKendrick, A.G.: A contribution to the mathematical theory of epidemics. Proc. Roy. Soc. Lond. A **115**, 700–721, 192
2. Brauer, F.: The Kermack-McKendrick epidemic model revisited. Math Biosci. **198**(2), 119–31 (2005 Dec). Epub 2005 Aug 30
3. Jenness, S.M., Goodreau, S.M., Morris, M.: EpiModel: An R Package for mathematical modeling of infectious disease over networks. J. Stat. Softw. **84**(8) (2018)
4. Biomarkers Definition Working Group: Biomarkers and surrogate endpoints: preferred definitions and conceptual framework. Clin. Pharmacol. Therapeut. **69**, 89–95 (2001)
5. Simon, R.: Development and evaluation of therapeutically relevant predictive classifiers using gene expression profiling. J. Natl. Cancer Inst. **98**, 1169–1171 (2006)
6. World Health Organization (WHO). The World Health Report: Changing History [electronic resource], p. 2004. WHO, Geneva (2004)
7. WHO, Infuenza (seasonal). Fact sheet No. 211, March 2014., [online], http://www.who.int/mediacentre/factsheets/fs211/en/
8. Nair, H., Brooks, W.A., Katz, M., et al.: Global burden of respiratory infections due to seasonal influenza in young children: a systematic review and meta-analysis. The Lancet **378**(9807), 1917–1930. http://www.sciencedirect.com/science/article/pii/S0140673611610519
9. CDC, Influenza signs and symptoms and the role of laboratory diagnostics. http://www.cdc.gov/flu/professionals/diagnosis/labrolesprocedures.htm
10. CDC, People with heart disease and those who have had a stroke are at high risk of developing complications from influenza (the flu), http://www.cdc.gov/flu/heartdisease/
11. Berman S. Epidemiology of acute respiratory infections in children of developing countries. Rev. Infect. Dis. **13** Suppl 6, S454–462 (1991). http://www.ncbi.nlm.nih.gov/entrez/query.fcgicmd=Retrieve&db=PubMed&dopt=Citation&list_uids=1862276
12. Bernoulli, D.: Essai d'une nouvelle analyse de la mortalite causee par la petite verole. Mem Math Phy Acad Roy Sci Paris 1766. (English translation entitled 'An attempt at a new analysis of the mortality caused by smallpox and of the advantages of inoculation to prevent it' In Smallpox Inoculation: An Eighteenth Century Mathematical Controversy, Bradley L. Adult Education Department: Nottingham, 1971, 21)
13. Hamer, W.H.: Epidemic disease in England. Lancet **1**, 733–739 (1906)
14. Ross, R.: The Prevention of Malaria, 2nd edn. John Murray, London (1911)
15. Anderson, R.M. (ed.): Population Dynamics of Infectious Diseases. Chapman and Hall, London (1982)
16. Anderson, R.M., May, R.M. (eds.): Population Biology of Infectious Diseases. Springer Verlag, Berlin, Heidelberg, New York (1982)
17. Anderson, R.M., May, R.M. (eds.): Vaccination against rubella and measles: Quantitative investigations of different policies, J. Hyg. Camb. **90**, 259–325 (1983)
18. Anderson, R.M., May, R.M. (eds.): Infectious Diseases of Humans: Dynamics and Control, Oxford University Press, Oxford, UK, (1991)
19. Bailey, N.T.J.: The Mathematical Theory of Infectious Diseases, 2nd edn. Hafner, New York (1975)
20. Castillo-Chavez, C., Feng, Z., Huang, W.: On the computation of R0 and its role on global stability. In: Castillo-Chavez, C., Blower, S., van den Driessche, P., Kirschner, D., Yakubu, A.A. (eds.) Mathematical Approach for Emerging and Reemerging Infectious Diseases: An Introduction, Springer, (2002), p. 229
21. Hethcote, H.W.: The mathematics of infectious diseases. SIAM Soc. Ind. Appl. Math. **42**, 599–653 (2000)
22. Bokil, V.A.: Mathematical Modeling and Analysis of Infectious Disease Dynamics, Department of Mathematics Oregon State University, Corvallis, OR (USA)
23. Heesterbeek, J.A.P., Dietz, K.: The concept of R0 in epidemic theory. Statistica Neerlandica **50**(1), 89–110 (1996)

24. Heesterbeek, J.: A brief history of R0 and a recipe for its calculation. Acta Biotheoretica **50**, 189–204 (2002)
25. Notes On R_0 by James Holland Jones, Department of Anthropological Sciences, Stanford University
26. Diekmann, O., Heesterbeek, J.A.P., Metz, J.A.J.: On the definition and the computation of the basic reproduction ratio R0 in models for infectious diseases in heterogeneous populations. J. Math. Biol. **28**(4), 365–382 (1990). https://doi.org/10.1007/BF00178324. hdl:1874/8051. PMID 2117040
27. Van den Driessche, P., Watmough, J.: Reproduction numbers and sub-threshold endemic equilibria for compartmental models of disease transmission. Math. Biosci. **180** (1–2), 29–48. https://doi.org/10.1016/S0025-5564(02)00108-6. PMID 12387915
28. Hefferenan, J.M., Smith, R.J., Wahl, L.M.: Prospective on the basic reproductive ratio. J. R. Soc. Interface **2**(4), 281–93. https://doi.org/10.1098/rsif.2005.0042. PMC 1578275. PMID 16849186
29. Furrer, R.: Stochastic Modeling: An Excursion. Applied Statistics Group, July 10, 2018
30. Wearing, H.J.: Lecture Notes. Simple Stochastic Models for Epidemics, July 23, 2014
31. Wallinga, J., Lipsitch, M.: How generation intervals shape the relationship between growth rates and reproductive numbers. Proc. R. Soc. Lond. B: Biol. Sci. **274**(1609), 599–604 (2007)
32. Nishiura, H., Chowell, G., Safan, M., Castillo-Chavez, C.: Pros and cons of estimating the reproduction number from early epidemic growth rate of influenza a (h1n1) 2009. Theoret. Biol. Med. Modell. **7**(1), 1 (2010)
33. Obadia, T., Haneef, R., Boëlle, P.-Y.: The r0 package: a toolbox to estimate reproduction numbers for epidemic outbreaks. BMC Med. Inf. Decis. Making **12**(1), 147 (2012)
34. Harko, T., Lobo, F.S., Mak, M.: Exact analytical solutions of the susceptible-infected-recovered (sir) epidemic model and of the sir model with equal death and birth rates. Appl. Math. Comput. **236**, 184–194 (2014)
35. Abbey, H.: An examination of the Reed-Frost theory of epidemics. Hum. Biol. **24**(3), 201 (1952)
36. Chen, G., Li, T.: Stability of stochastic delayed sir model. Stochast. Dyn. **9**(2), 231–252 (2009)
37. Dietz, K., Heesterbeek, J.A.P.: Bernoulli was ahead of modern epidemiology. Nature **408**, 513–514 (2000)
38. Koopman, J.S.: Emerging objectives and methods in epidemiology. Am. J. Public Health **86**, 630–632 (1996)
39. Razvan, G.: Romanescu Rob Deardon. Fast Inference for Network Models of Infectious Disease Spread, Scandinavian J. Statist. Theory Appl. **44**(3), 666–683 (2017)
40. Hofmeyr, S.A., Forrest, S.: Architecture for an artificial immune system. Evol. Comput. **8**, 443–473 (2000). [PubMed]
41. Holland, J.H.: Hidden Order: How Adaptation Builds Complexity. Addison Wesley (1995)
42. Albert, R., Jeong, H., Barabasi, A.-L.: Error and attack tolerance of complex networks. Nature **406**, 378–382 (2000)
43. Pastor-Satorras, R., Vespignani, A.: Epidemic spreading in scale-free networks. Phys. Rev. Lett. **86**, 3200–3203 (2001)
44. Barabasi, A-L.: Linked: The new science of networks. (2002)
45. Lloyd, A.L., May, R.M.: Epidemiology: how viruses spread among computers and people. Science **292**, 1316–1317 (2001)
46. Watts, D.: Small worlds. The dynamics of networks between order and randomness (1999)
47. Rogers, D., Randoph, S., Snow, R.W., Hay, S.I.: Satellite imagery in the study and forecast of malaria. Nature **415**, 710–715 (2002)
48. Hay, S.I., Myers, M.F., Burke, D.S., et al.: Etiology of interepidemic periods of mosquito-borne disease. Proc. Natl. Acad. Sci. **97**, 9335–9339 (2000)
49. Grenfell, B.T., Bjornstad, O.N., Kappey, J.: Travelling waves and spatial hierarchies in measles epidemics. Nature **414**, 716–723 (2001)
50. Strebel, P.M., Cochi, S.L.: Waving goodbye to measles. Nature **414**, 695–696 (2001)

51. Burke, D.S., De Jong, K.A., Grefenstette, J.J., Ramsey, C.L., Wu, A.S.: Putting more genetics into genetic algorithms. Evol. Comput. **6**, 387–410 (1998)
52. Ray, T.S.: Evolution, ecology, and optimization of digital organisms. http://www.isd.atr.co.jp/ray/pubs/tierra (1995)
53. Wilke, C.O., Wang, J.L., Ofria, C., Lenski, R.E., Adami, C.: Evolution of digital organisms at high mutation rates leads to survival of the flattest
54. Radman, R., Matic, I., Taddei, F.: Evolution of evolvability. Ann. N Y Acad. Sci. **870**, 146–155 (1999)

Dynamics of Inter-community Spread of Covid-19

Emmanuel J. Dansu and Samuel T. Ogunjo

Abstract We developed a model for the spread of Covid-19 within a community, we paid attention to the sensitivity of the derived basic reproduction number to each model parameter. This model was extended to investigate the impact of migration between two communities on the spread of the disease. Three special cases: unidirectional migration, unrestricted bidirectional migration, and partial bidirectional migration, were considered. Covid-19 data for two Nigerian states, namely Lagos (high burden community) and Ogun (low burden community) were obtained from the website of the Nigeria Centre for Disease Control for parameter estimation and simulation. Our results show that the basic reproduction number of the original model is most sensitive to the recovery rate of symptomatic infectious individuals. From the inter-community spread model, we find that the rate of coupling plays a vital role in the control of the pandemic. Our results project the different possible scenarios based on different lockdown and infection rates in two different communities.

Keywords SEIR · Prediction · Stochastic modeling · Epidemic · Endemic · Reproduction number

1 Introduction

Mankind has always been plagued by pandemics which generally cause loss of human lives and negative economic impact across different regions of the world. The origin of many pandemic diseases have been traced to animals such as swine

E. J. Dansu (✉)
Department of Computer and Mathematical Sciences, Graduate School of Information Sciences, Tohoku University, Sendai, Japan

Department of Mathematical Sciences, Federal University of Technology, Akure, Ondo State, Nigeria
e-mail: ej.dansu@dc.tohoku.ac.jp; ejdansu@futa.edu.ng

S. T. Ogunjo
Department of Physics, Federal University of Technology, Akure, Nigeria
e-mail: stogunjo@futa.edu.ng

P. Agarwal et al. (eds.), *Analysis of Infectious Disease Problems (Covid-19) and Their Global Impact*, Infosys Science Foundation Series,
https://doi.org/10.1007/978-981-16-2450-6_18

(HIN1 Influenza), camels (Middle East Respiratory Syndrome Coronavirus- MERS-CoV) and bat (Severe Acute Respiratory Syndrome- SARS). Influenza pandemics were recorded in 1918 [23], 1957 [21], 1968 [46], and 2009 [45]. Other historical pandemics recorded include cholera in 1817 and 1961 [10], MERS-CoV in 2012 [7], SARS in 2002 [15], Acquired Immunodeficiency Syndrome (AIDS) in 1981 [43], and Ebola in 2013 [40]. The most recent global pandemic is the Severe Acute Respiratory Syndrome Coronavirus 2 (SARS-CoV-2).

SARS-CoV-2, officially known as coronavirus disease (Covid-19), began in Wuhan, Hubei Province of China in December 2019. It was said to have been caused by a family of animal viruses called Coronaviridae in the order and subfamily of Nidovirales and Coronavirina respectively. Coronaviridae are enveloped viruses with a positive sense, single-stranded RNA genome. The four subgroups of Coronaviridae are alpha (αCoV), beta (βCoV), gamma (γCoV), and delta (δCoV). δCoV and γCoV have avian genetic origin while the genetic origin of αCoV and βCoV have been found to be bats [30].

Covid-19 belongs to the βCoV group and it is transmitted through contact with droplets/aerosols or with infected individuals or surfaces. The response of the immune system to the virus attack on the respiratory system triggers mucus generation. Infected persons with underlying diseases such as diabetes can have their infection escalated [44]. Covid-19 has also been found to affect the nervous system [48]. The first confirmed case in Nigeria, and by extension, sub-Saharan Africa was declared on February 27, 2020. On March 11, 2020, the World Health Organization (WHO) officially declared Covid-19 a global pandemic [13].

The impact of Covid-19 extends to different facets of human existence. The pandemic has been found to severely affect transportation and tourism [20], health services [12], economy [6, 34] as well as the education/academic landscape [42]. As at June 28, 2020, a total of 9,843,073 persons had been infected with Covid-19 with 495,760 deaths worldwide [36]. The different attempts by governments around the world to reduce the spread of Covid-19 include local and international travel restrictions, isolation of infected persons, implementation of personal hygiene policies [27], among others. Being a novel disease with constantly evolving knowledge and little data to work with, it is imperative to use alternative approaches for the study, simulation and control of the pandemic.

Mathematical models offer a way to study the evolution, spread and impact of the pandemic using available data set. Mathematical models can be regarded as abstract realizations of physical events. They have been applied to several disciplines and subjects including population [24], neuronal dynamics [1], romantic love [47], alcoholism and drug abuse [9, 41], insurgency [26], and finance [25]. Mathematical models of pandemics and diseases can either be difference equations, ordinary differential equations, partial differential equations, stochastic differential equations, fractional order differential equations, etc. Due to their simplicity and accuracy, several diseases, infections and pandemics have been analysed using mathematical models such as Lassa fever [35], Ebola [8], West Nile virus [11], Influenza [32], Hepatitis B [50], Zika virus [3], and others [19, 39].

The need to understand the transmission of Covid-19 has led to different modelling approaches. The transmission dynamics of any pandemic is crucial in understanding and reducing its impact. A stochastic transmission dynamic model was designed for Covid-19 in the Wuhan region of China [28]. [18] developed a probabilistic cellular automata model for the spread of Covid-19, as well as the effectiveness of different control measures adopted by several countries. Macroscopic laws based on logistic growth models were developed to study the complex dynamics involved in the spread of Covid-19 [29]. The Susceptible Exposed Infectious Recovered (SEIR) model is the most common approach to describe disease epidemics. Since the beginning of the pandemic, several models for Covid-19 based on the SEIR idea has been proposed. The SEIR framework was extended to include insusceptible, quarantined and dead cases for Covid-19 by [38]. [37] proposed a fractional form of SEIR with vertical transmission to estimate infection rates of Covid-19. For better efficiency, [22] divided infected persons into "infected and detected" and "infected and undetected" in their model while new categories such as quarantined, hospitalized but fatal, dead, "recovered and detected", and "recovered but undetected" were also created. [33] modified the SEIR model to consider super-spreaders, infectious but asymptomatic, hospitalized, recovered, and fatal classes in a Covid-19 community. [31] accounted for latency of Covid-19 infections. The SEIR model with time delay was proposed by [4] for modelling of Covid-19.

Most of the developed Covid-19 models accounted for intra-community transmissions rather than inter-community spread. In this study, we propose a simple model for the propagation of Covid-19 infections and its transmission between two communities with sharply contrasting disease burdens. This is essential as travel restrictions are being lifted across communities globally. The results from this study will help to give an important perspective to policy makers on how to proceed with the fight against the raging Covid-19 pandemic.

2 Basic Model

The model used in this study is defined as

$$\begin{aligned}
\frac{dS}{dt} &= -\mathcal{B}_1\frac{E}{N}S - \mathcal{B}_2\frac{I}{N}S \\
\frac{dE}{dt} &= \mathcal{B}_1\frac{E}{N}S + \mathcal{B}_2\frac{I}{N}S - \mathcal{A}E - \Gamma_1 E \\
\frac{dI}{dt} &= \mathcal{A}E - \Gamma_2 I - \Phi I \\
\frac{dR}{dt} &= \Gamma_1 E + \Gamma_2 I
\end{aligned} \tag{1}$$

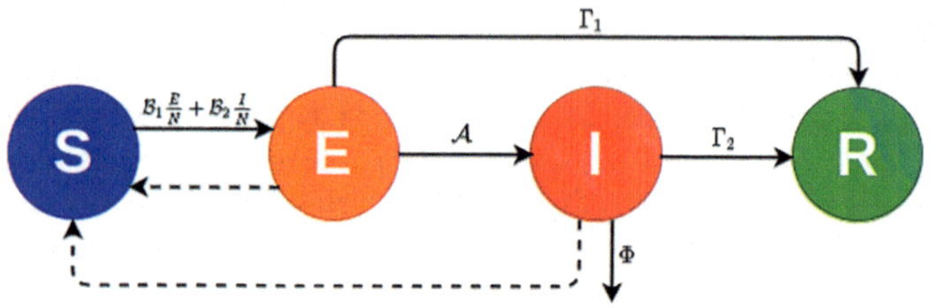

Fig. 1 Representation of the basic model

with initial condition $(S(0), E(0), I(0), R(0)) = (S_0, E_0, I_0, R_0)$ where $\mathcal{B}_1$ is the coefficient of transmission of infection from asymptomatic infectious people to susceptible people, $\mathcal{B}_2$ is the coefficient of transmission of infection from symptomatic infectious people to susceptible people, $\mathcal{A}$, Γ_1, Γ_2, Φ are the transition rate from asymptomatic to symptomatic infectious, recovery rate from the asymptomatic infectious state, recovery rate from the symptomatic infectious state, and death rate due to Covid-19 respectively. We see that $S + E + I + R = N$ and $dN/dt = -\Phi I$. It should be noted that dN/dt is solely dependent on the disease-induced death. The diagrammatic representation of the model and the temporal variation of the system are shown in Figs. 1 and 2 respectively.

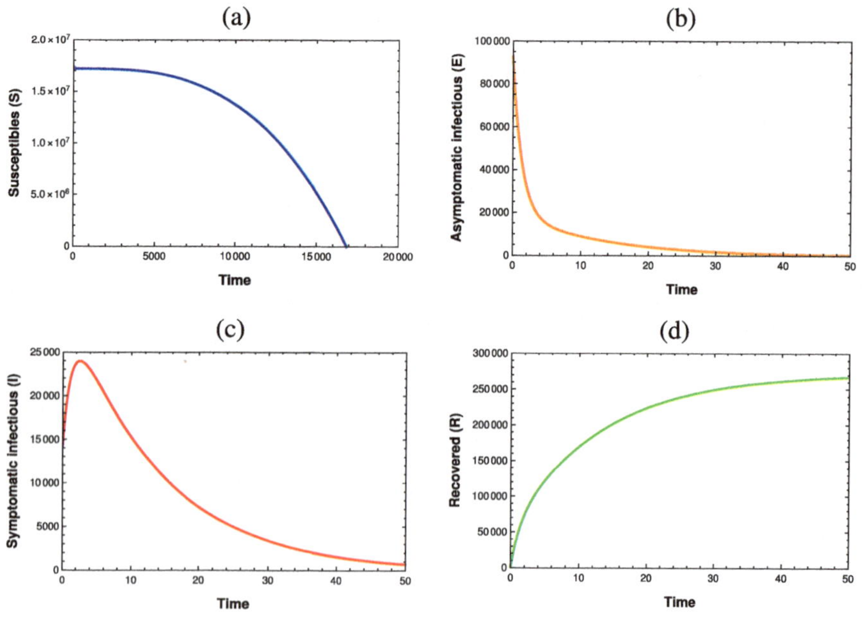

Fig. 2 Temporal variation of the system

2.1 Properties of Solution

Theorem 1 *The system* (1) *gives only positive solutions for positive initial conditions.*

Proof From $\frac{dS}{dt} = -\mathcal{B}_1 \frac{E(t)}{N(t)} S(t) - \mathcal{B}_2 \frac{I(t)}{N(t)} S(t)$, we have

$$\frac{1}{S(t)} \frac{dS(t)}{dt} dt = -\left(\mathcal{B}_1 \frac{E(t)}{N(t)} + \mathcal{B}_2 \frac{I(t)}{N(t)} \right)$$

$$S(t) = S(0) \exp \left[- \int_0^t \mathcal{B}_1 \frac{E(T)}{N(T)} + \mathcal{B}_2 \frac{I(T)}{N(T)} dT \right].$$

This result guarantees that the population size of susceptibles is always non-negative as required for our model. The same holds true for the other variables. □

Theorem 2 *The closed set* $\mathcal{D} = \{(S(t), E(t), I(t), R(t)) \in \mathbb{R}_+^4 : S(t) + E(t) + I(t) + R(t) \leq S_0\}$ *is positively invariant and attracts all solutions in* $\mathbb{R}_+^4$.

Proof We have

$$\begin{aligned} \frac{dN(t)}{dt} &= \frac{dS(t)}{dt} + \frac{dE(t)}{dt} + \frac{dI(t)}{dt} + \frac{dR(t)}{dt} \\ &= -\Phi I(t) \end{aligned}$$

$$N(t) = S_0 - \Phi \int_0^t I(T) dT.$$

At the disease-free equilibrium, $N(t) = S_0$. In the extreme situation that the whole population dies as a result of the pandemic, that is, $\Phi I(t) = S_0$, then $N(t) = 0$. By consequence,

$$N(t) \in [0, S_0]$$

and this completes the proof. □

2.2 Basic Reproduction Number

The basic reproduction number $\mathcal{R}_0$ is about the most important index that has been identified in quantitative epidemiology and it is defined as the expected number of secondary infections generated by a single infectious person in the midst of susceptible individuals. It helps to predict whether a disease will become an epidemic, will be endemic or it will be eliminated over time. Many methods have been developed for the derivation of $\mathcal{R}_0$ and the new generation matrix method is one of such approaches [14, 16]. We proceed with the method as follows.

We obtain the matrices T_m and T_s representing *transmissions* (occurrence of new infections) and *transitions* (changes in state) from the asymptomatic infectious and the symptomatic infectious compartments in model (1). We have

$$\begin{aligned} \frac{dE}{dt} &= \mathcal{B}_1 \frac{E}{N} S + \mathcal{B}_2 \frac{I}{N} S - \mathcal{A}E - \Gamma_1 E \\ \frac{dI}{dt} &= \mathcal{A}E - \Gamma_2 I - \Phi I \end{aligned} \tag{2}$$

such that

$$T_m = \begin{pmatrix} \mathcal{B}_1 \frac{S}{N} & \mathcal{B}_2 \frac{S}{N} \\ 0 & 0 \end{pmatrix} \rightarrow T_m = \begin{pmatrix} \mathcal{B}_1 & \mathcal{B}_2 \\ 0 & 0 \end{pmatrix} \tag{3}$$

at the disease free equilibrium $(S^*, E^*, I^*, R^*) = (N, 0, 0, 0)$ and

$$-T_s = \begin{pmatrix} -\mathcal{A} - \Gamma_1 & 0 \\ \mathcal{A} & -\Phi - \Gamma_2 \end{pmatrix} \rightarrow T_s = \begin{pmatrix} \mathcal{A} + \Gamma_1 & 0 \\ -\mathcal{A} & \Phi + \Gamma_2 \end{pmatrix}. \tag{4}$$

Next, we have

$$T_m T_s^{-1} = \begin{pmatrix} \frac{\mathcal{B}_1}{\mathcal{A} + \Gamma_1} + \frac{\mathcal{A}\mathcal{B}_2}{(\mathcal{A} + \Gamma_1)(\Phi + \Gamma_2)} & \frac{\mathcal{B}_2}{\Phi + \Gamma_1} \\ 0 & 0 \end{pmatrix}. \tag{5}$$

The basic reproduction number, being the spectral radius of $T_m T_s^{-1}$, is given as

$$\mathcal{R}_0 = \max \left\{ \frac{\mathcal{B}_1}{\mathcal{A} + \Gamma_1} + \frac{\mathcal{A}\mathcal{B}_2}{(\mathcal{A} + \Gamma_1)(\Phi + \Gamma_2)}, 0 \right\} \tag{6}$$

$$= \frac{\mathcal{B}_1}{\mathcal{A} + \Gamma_1} + \frac{\mathcal{A}\mathcal{B}_2}{(\mathcal{A} + \Gamma_1)(\Phi + \Gamma_2)} \tag{7}$$

$$= \mathcal{R}_{ai} + \mathcal{R}_{si}. \tag{8}$$

where $\mathcal{R}_{ai}$ and $\mathcal{R}_{si}$ are the basic reproduction numbers for the asymptomatic and symptomatic infectious respectively. The disease free equilibrium $(S(0), E(0), I(0),$

$R(0)) = (S_0, E_0, I_0, R_0) = (N, 0, 0, 0)$ is always locally asymptotically stable if $\mathcal{R}_0 < 1$. This guarantees that the disease dies out. However, it is unstable for $\mathcal{R}_0 > 1$ in which case the disease breaks out.

2.3 Sensitivity Analysis of $\mathcal{R}_0$

It is important to see how $\mathcal{R}_0$ responds when the parameters upon which it depends are tweaked. As such, the sensitivity analysis approach presented by [5] is quite helpful. The normalized sensitivity elasticity, $E_{(.)}$, which estimates the marginal change in the value of $\mathcal{R}_0$ due to a marginal change in the value of a certain parameter with other parameters kept constant is given by

$$E_{(.)} = \frac{(.)}{\mathcal{R}_0} \cdot \frac{\partial \mathcal{R}_0}{\partial (.)}. \tag{9}$$

For the parameters $\mathcal{A}$, $\mathcal{B}_1$, $\mathcal{B}_2$, Γ_1, Γ_2 and Φ, we have the following elasticities:

$$E_{\mathcal{A}} = \frac{\mathcal{A}}{\mathcal{R}_0} \cdot \frac{\partial \mathcal{R}_0}{\partial \mathcal{A}} = \frac{\mathcal{A}[\mathcal{B}_2\Gamma_1 - \mathcal{B}_1(\Phi + \Gamma_2)]}{(\mathcal{A} + \Gamma_1)[\mathcal{A}\mathcal{B}_2 + \mathcal{B}_1(\Phi + \Gamma_2)]}.$$
$$E_{\mathcal{B}_1} = \frac{\mathcal{B}_1}{\mathcal{R}_0} \cdot \frac{\partial \mathcal{R}_0}{\partial \mathcal{B}_1} = \frac{\mathcal{B}_1(\Phi + \Gamma_2)}{\mathcal{A}\mathcal{B}_2 + \mathcal{B}_1(\Phi + \Gamma_2)}.$$
$$E_{\mathcal{B}_2} = \frac{\mathcal{B}_2}{\mathcal{R}_0} \cdot \frac{\partial \mathcal{R}_0}{\partial \mathcal{B}_2} = \frac{\mathcal{A}\mathcal{B}_2}{\mathcal{A}\mathcal{B}_2 + \mathcal{B}_1(\Phi + \Gamma_2)}.$$
$$E_{\Gamma_1} = \frac{\Gamma_1}{\mathcal{R}_0} \cdot \frac{\partial \mathcal{R}_0}{\partial \Gamma_1} = -\frac{\Gamma_1}{\mathcal{A} + \Gamma_1}.$$
$$E_{\Gamma_2} = \frac{\Gamma_2}{\mathcal{R}_0} \cdot \frac{\partial \mathcal{R}_0}{\partial \Gamma_2} = -\frac{\Gamma_2(\mathcal{A} + \mathcal{B}_2)}{(\Phi + \Gamma_2)[\mathcal{A} + \mathcal{B}_1(\Phi + \Gamma_2) + \mathcal{B}_2]}.$$
$$E_{\Phi} = \frac{\Phi}{\mathcal{R}_0} \cdot \frac{\partial \mathcal{R}_0}{\partial \Phi} = -\frac{\Phi(\mathcal{A} + \mathcal{B}_2)}{(\Phi + \Gamma_2)[\mathcal{A} + \mathcal{B}_1(\Phi + \Gamma_2) + \mathcal{B}_2]}.$$

The signs indicate that $\mathcal{R}_0$ increase with $\mathcal{A}$, $\mathcal{B}_1$, $\mathcal{B}_2$ and decrease with Γ_1, Γ_2 and Φ. As such, strategies to eradicate the disease should be about reducing $\mathcal{A}$, $\mathcal{B}_1$, $\mathcal{B}_2$ and increasing Γ_1, Γ_2 and Φ such that $\mathcal{R}_0$ goes below unity.

3 Inter-community Transmission Model

3.1 Assumptions

The inter-community transmission model between community 1 and community 2 is developed based on the following assumptions.

- There are two communities, community 1 with a significantly heavier burden of Covid-19 infections compared to community 2.

- In each community, there are susceptible people (S), asymptomatic infectious/exposed people (E), symptomatic infectious people (I) and recovered people (R).
- Susceptible and asymptomatic infectious people tend to move freely between the communities while symptomatic infectious and recovered people don't get to move that freely due to restrictions based on their health conditions and awareness of the reality of the disease respectively.
- Population change due to natural causes is negligible.

3.2 Model

The bidirectional coupling approach proposed by [49] is used to study the dynamics of two communities under Covid-19 infection.

Community 1 is defined by

$$\begin{aligned}
\frac{dS_1}{dt} &= -\mathcal{B}_1\frac{E_1}{N_1}S_1 - \mathcal{B}_2\frac{I_1}{N_1}S_1 + d_{11}(S_2 - S_1)\\
\frac{dE_1}{dt} &= \mathcal{B}_1\frac{E_1}{N_1}S_1 + \mathcal{B}_2\frac{I_1}{N_1}S_1 - \mathcal{A}E_1 - \Gamma_1 E_1 + d_{12}(E_2 - E_1)\\
\frac{dI_1}{dt} &= \mathcal{A}E_1 - \Gamma_2 I_1 - \Phi I_1 + d_{13}(I_2 - I_1)\\
\frac{dR_1}{dt} &= \Gamma_1 E_1 + \Gamma_2 I_1 + d_{14}(R_2 - R_1)
\end{aligned} \tag{10}$$

and community 2 by

$$\begin{aligned}
\frac{dS_2}{dt} &= -\beta_1\frac{E_2}{N_2}S_2 - \beta_2\frac{I_2}{N_2}S_2 + d_{21}(S_1 - S_2)\\
\frac{dE_2}{dt} &= \beta_1\frac{E_2}{N_2}S_2 + \beta_2\frac{I_2}{N_2}S_2 - \alpha E_2 - \gamma_1 E_2 + d_{22}(E_1 - E_2)\\
\frac{dI_2}{dt} &= \alpha E_2 - \gamma_2 I_2 - \phi I_2 + d_{23}(I_1 - I_2)\\
\frac{dR_2}{dt} &= \gamma_1 E_2 + \gamma_2 I_2 + d_{24}(R_1 - R_2)
\end{aligned} \tag{11}$$

where the d_{ij}'s represent net migration rates between the communities. The initial condition is

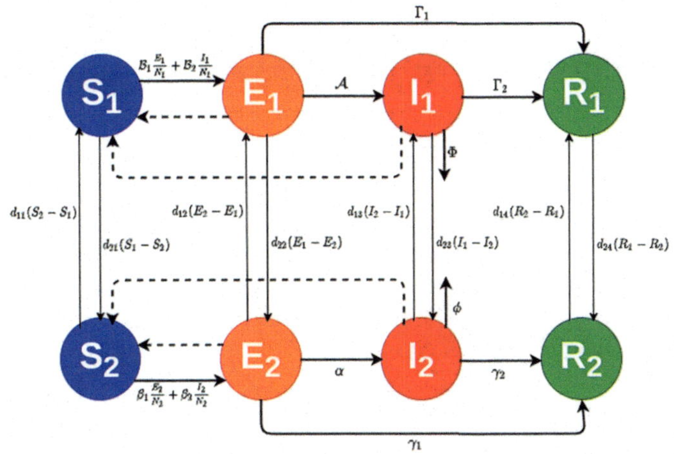

Fig. 3 Representation of the coupled model

$$(S_1(0), E_1(0), I_1(0), R_1(0), S_2(0), E_2(0), I_2(0), R_2(0))$$
$$= (S_{10}, E_{10}, I_{10}, R_{10}, S_{20}, E_{20}, I_{20}, R_{20})$$

and $N(t) = N_1(t) + N_2(t)$. Furthermore, we have $\mathcal{B}_i$ (transmission coefficients in community 1), $\mathcal{A}$ (transition rate from asymptomatic to symptomatic infectious in community 1), Γ_i (recovery rates in community 1), Φ (mortality rate due to Covid-19 in community 1), β_i (transmission coefficients in community 2), α (transition rate from asymptomatic to symptomatic infectious in community 2), γ_i (recovery rates in community 2) and ϕ (mortality rate due to Covid-19 in community 2). The schematic diagram of the coupled model is shown in Fig. 3.

The new generation matrix for the system inter-community model, based on the disease-free equilibrium $(S_1^*, E_1^*, I_1^*, R_1^*, S_2^*, E_2^*, I_2^*, R_2^*) = (N_1, 0, 0, 0, N_2, 0, 0, 0)$, is given as

$$\mathcal{M} = \begin{pmatrix} \dfrac{\mathcal{B}_1 - d_{12}}{\mathcal{A} + \Gamma_1} & \dfrac{d_{12}}{\alpha + \gamma_1} \\ \dfrac{d_{22}}{\mathcal{A} + \Gamma_1} & \dfrac{\beta_1 - d_{22}}{\alpha + \gamma_1} \end{pmatrix} \tag{12}$$

with characteristic polynomial

$$\lambda^2 - (\textbf{Trace } \mathcal{M})\lambda + (\textbf{Determinant } \mathcal{M}) = 0 \tag{13}$$

where

$$\textbf{Trace } \mathcal{M} = \frac{\mathcal{B}_1 - d_{12}}{\mathcal{A} + \Gamma_1} + \frac{\beta_1 - d_{22}}{\alpha + \gamma_1}$$

and

$$\textbf{Determinant } \mathcal{M} = \frac{(\mathcal{B}_1 - d_{12})}{(\mathcal{A} + \Gamma_1)}\frac{(\beta_1 - d_{22})}{(\alpha + \gamma_1)} - \frac{d_{12}d_{22}}{(\alpha + \gamma_1)(\mathcal{A} + \Gamma_1)}.$$

The basic reproduction number in this case is then given as

$$\mathcal{R}_0 = \frac{1}{2}\left[\textbf{Trace } \mathcal{M} + \sqrt{(\textbf{Trace } \mathcal{M})^2 - 4(\textbf{Determinant } \mathcal{M})}\right]. \tag{14}$$

3.3 *Stability of Coupled System*

Let community 1 and community 2 be denoted by X and Y respectively. The state vectors can then be represented as

$$\begin{aligned} \dot{X} &= AX + g(X) + D_1(Y - X) \\ \dot{Y} &= AY + g(Y) + D_2(X - Y) \end{aligned} \tag{15}$$

where D_1, D_2 are $n \times n$ diagonal matrices which control the rate of migration between the two communities. If we define the error between system (10) and system (11) as $e = x - y$, then the error dynamics can be expressed as

$$\dot{e} = (A + M_{X,Y} - (D_1 + D_2))e \tag{16}$$

where $M_{X,Y} = g(X) - g(Y)$.

Theorem 3 *([49]) If there exists a positive definite symmetric constant matrix P and a constant $\epsilon > 0$, such that*

$$(A + M_{X,Y} - (D_1 + D_2))^T P + P(A + M_{X,Y} - (D_1 + D_2)) \leq -\epsilon I \tag{17}$$

where I is an identity matrix, then the error between system (10) and system (11) is stable.

Using the above theorem, we obtained for the systems (10) and (11)

$$A = \begin{pmatrix} -\frac{\mathcal{B}_1+\mathcal{B}_2}{N} & -\frac{\mathcal{B}_1}{N} & -\frac{\mathcal{B}_2}{N} & 0 \\ \frac{\mathcal{B}_1+\mathcal{B}_2}{N} & \frac{\mathcal{B}_1}{N} - \Gamma_1 - \mathcal{A} & \frac{\mathcal{B}_2}{N} & 0 \\ 0 & \mathcal{A} & -\Gamma_2 - \phi & 0 \\ 0 & \Gamma_1 & \Gamma_2 & 0 \end{pmatrix} \tag{18}$$

and

$$M = \begin{pmatrix} -E_1 - I_1 & S_2 & S_2 & 0 \\ E_1 + I_1 & S_2 & S_2 & 0 \\ 0 & 0 & 0 & 0 \\ 0 & 0 & 0 & 0 \end{pmatrix} \tag{19}$$

$D_1 = diag(d_{11}, d_{12}, d_{13}, d_{14})$, and $D_2 = diag(d_{21}, d_{22}, d_{23}, d_{24})$. We chose a positive definite symmetric constant matrix $P = diag(p_1, p_2, p_3, p_4)$ with $p\{i = 1, 2, 3, 4\} > 0$. Then,

$$(A + M_{X,Y} - (D_1 + D_2))^T P + P(A + M_{X,Y} - (D_1 + D_2)) + \epsilon I$$

$$= \begin{pmatrix} 2p_1\left(g_1 - \frac{\epsilon}{2p_1}\right) & p_2g_2 - p_1\left(\frac{B_1}{N} + S_2\right) & -p_1\left(\frac{B_2}{N} - S_2\right) & -p_4\left(d_{14} + d_{24}\right) \\ p_2g_2 - p_2\left(\frac{B_1}{N} - S_2\right) & 2p_2\left(g_2 - \frac{\epsilon}{2p_2}\right) & Ap_3 + p_2\left(\frac{B_2}{N} + S_2\right) & 0 \\ -p_1\left(\frac{B_2}{N} - S_2\right) & Ap_3 + p_2\left(\frac{B_2}{N} + S_2\right) & 2p_3\left(g_4 - \frac{\epsilon}{2p_3}\right) & 0 \\ 0 & 0 & 0 & -2p_4\left(d_{14} + d_{24} - \frac{\epsilon}{2p_4}\right) \end{pmatrix} \tag{20}$$

where $g_1 = -k_1 - E_1 - I_1 - d_{11} - d_{21}$, $g_2 = \frac{B_1+B_2}{N} + E_1 + I_1$, $g_3 = \frac{B_1}{N} - \Gamma_1 - A + S_2 - d_{12} - d_{22}$, and $g_4 = -\Gamma_2 - \phi - d_{13} - d_{23}$.

Matrix (20) is negative definite, if and only if, $D_1 < 0$, $D_2 > 0$, $D_3 < 0$, and $D_4 > 0$. This condition is fulfilled if and only if it is observed that all positive values of d_{ij}, $i = 1, 2;\ j = 1, 2, 3, 4$ satisfy the inequalities in Eqs. (21)–(24).

$$D_1 = -2p_1\left(k_1 + E_1 + I_1 + d_{11} + d_{21} - \frac{\epsilon}{2p_1}\right) < 0 \tag{21}$$

$$D_2 = 4p_1p_2\left(g_1 - \frac{\epsilon}{2p_1}\right)\left(g_2 - \frac{\epsilon}{2p_2}\right) - \left[p_2g_2 - p_1\left(\frac{B_1}{N} + S_2\right)\right] \left[p_2g_2 - p_2\left(\frac{B_1}{N} - S_2\right)\right] > 0 \tag{22}$$

$$D_3 = 2p_3\left(g_4 - \frac{\epsilon}{2p_3}\right)D_2 - \left(Ap_3 + p_2\left(\frac{B_2}{N} + S_2\right)\right)\left[D_1\left(Ap_3 + p_2\left(\frac{B_2}{N} + S_2\right)\right)\right] + p_1\left(\frac{B_2}{N} - S_2\right)\left(p_2g_2 - p_2\left(\frac{B_1}{N} - S_2\right)\right) - p_1\left(\frac{B_2}{N} - S_2\right)[\left(p_2g_2 - p_1\left(\frac{B_1}{N} + S_2\right)\right) \left(Ap_3 + p_2\left(\frac{B_2}{N} + S_2\right)\right) + 2p_1p_2\left(g_2 - \frac{\epsilon}{2p_2}\right)\left(\frac{B_2}{N} - S_2\right)] < 0 \tag{23}$$

$$D_4 = -2p_4\left(d_{14} + d_{24} - \frac{\epsilon}{2p_4}\right)D_3 > 0 \tag{24}$$

It was observed that all positive values of d_{ij}, $i = 1, 2;\ j = 1, 2, 3, 4$ satisfy the inequalities in Eqs. (21)–(24).

Table 1 Sensitivity of $\mathcal{R}_0$ to model parameters

Parameter	Elasticity	Value
$\mathcal{A}$	$E_{\mathcal{A}}$	0.6218
$\mathcal{B}_1$	$E_{\mathcal{B}_1}$	0.1835
$\mathcal{B}_2$	$E_{\mathcal{B}_2}$	0.8165
Γ_1	E_{Γ_1}	-0.8047
Γ_2	E_{Γ_2}	-0.8954
Φ	E_{Φ}	-0.0821

4 Numerical Simulation

For our simulation, we estimated model parameters and initial values based on data from the Nigeria Centre for Disease Control website (https://covid19.ncdc.gov.ng/) as at Saturday, 26th July 2020. We took Lagos and Ogun States of Nigeria as communities 1 and 2 respectively. The population of each community is estimated based on the total tested samples. The estimation approaches by [2] and [17] are quite instructive in this regard.

For community 1 ($N_1 = 17500000$), we have parameters $\mathcal{B}_1 = 0.0714$, $\mathcal{B}_2 = 0.3572$, $\mathcal{A} = 0.1429$, $\Gamma_1 = 0.5888$, $\Gamma_2 = 0.1472$, $\Phi = 0.0135$. For community 2 ($N_2 = 5900000$), we have $\beta_1 = 0.0305$, $\beta_2 = 0.1524$, $\alpha = 0.1429$, $\gamma_1 = 3.1360$, $\gamma_2 = 0.7840$, $\phi = 0.0185$.

Based on sensitivity analyses in Subsection 2.3 and the estimated parameters, we have the numerical estimates of the elasticities of each parameter in Table 1.

The coupled system was solved using the fifth order Dormand-Prince method with a time step of 1×10^4. The initial conditions were chosen as [17390783, 92830, 14300, 2087] and [5889674, 8075, 1244, 1007] for community 1 and community 2 respectively. To quantify the relationship between the trajectory of the two communities, we define a parameter, δ as

$$\delta = \max I_1 - \max I_2. \tag{25}$$

Three distinct scenarios of the general case were considered. This quantity will give an indication of differences between the total number of infected persons in the two communities. A lower value of δ means the total infected persons in the two communities are very close.

4.1 Unidirectional Migration

We consider the case where susceptible, exposed, infected, and recovered people are free to move from community 1 to community 2 with varying degrees of restriction.

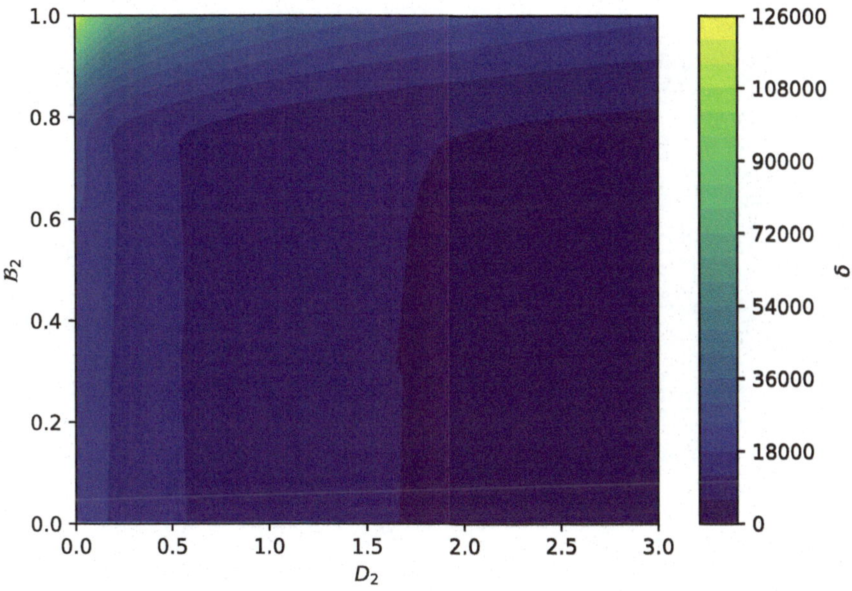

Fig. 4 Unidirectional case with $d_{11} = d_{12} = d_{13} = d_{14} = 0$

However, movement of all categories of people from community 2 to community 1 are restricted totally. In this case, we set $d_{11} = d_{12} = d_{13} = d_{14} = 0$, $d_{21} = d_{22} = d_{23} = d_{24} = D_2$ and studied the variation of δ in the range $0 < d_{22} < 3$ and $0 < \mathcal{B}_2 < 1$. The resulting spatial plot is shown in Fig. 4. The maximum number of infected persons in the two communities become very close as the coupling strength D_2 increases. This implies that individual communities need to take proactive actions to limit transmission of the virus. Unrestricted movement from a high risk community to a low risk community will drive the number of infected persons to the level in high risk community. This is more pronounced at high values of $\mathcal{B}_2$.

4.2 Unrestricted Bidirectional Migration

There exist situations where two neighbouring communities do not enforce control measures such as lock-down of borders. In this case, there is free movement of all categories of people from community 1 to community 2 and vice versa. For ease of computation, we set $d_{11} = d_{12} = d_{13} = d_{14} = D_1$ and $d_{21} = d_{22} = d_{23} = d_{24} = D_2$. The coupling strengths are considered in the range $0 < D_1, D_2 < 3$. A graphical representation of the scenario is shown in Figure 5. It is noted that the highest difference between maximum number of infected persons in the two communities are maximum when lock-down is enforced ($D_1 = 0$ and $D_2 = 0$). The change in δ

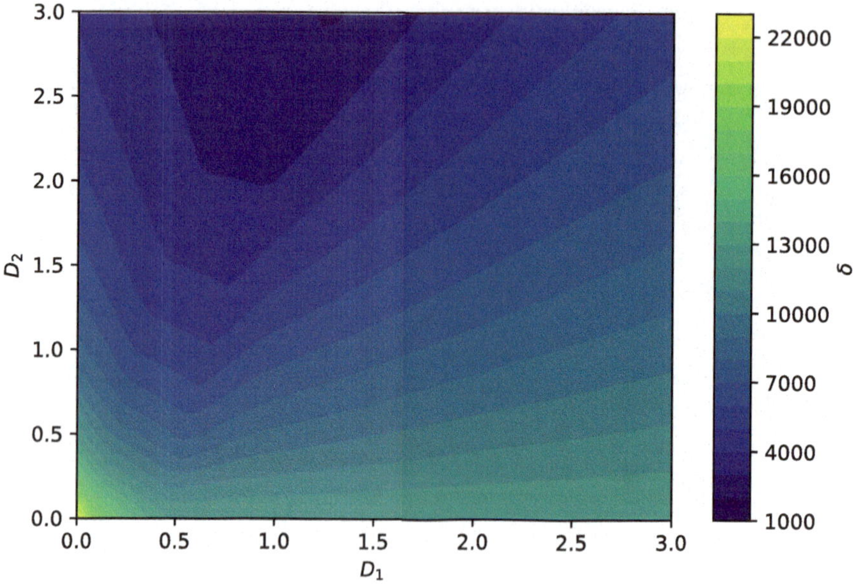

Fig. 5 Case of unrestricted bidirectional migration between an high risk community and a low risk community

is not strongly influenced by migration rate from community 1. However, the value of δ reduces as migration rate from community 2 increases.

4.3 *Partial Bidirectional Migration*

In this case, we consider the possibility of migrations of only exposed people between the two communities. Thus, we set $d_{11} = d_{13} = d_{14} = 0$ and $d_{21} = d_{23} = d_{24} = 0$. The migration rates are then considered in the range $0 < D_{12}, D_{22} < 2$. Figure 5 shows the variation of δ values with changing values of D_1 and D_2. In this case, we consider the possibility of migrations of only exposed people between the two communities. Thus, we set $d_{11} = d_{13} = d_{14} = 0$ and $d_{21} = d_{23} = d_{24} = 0$. The migration rates are then considered in the range $0 < D_{12}, D_{22} < 2$. Figure 6 shows the variation of δ values with changing values of D_1 and D_2. As the number of exposed persons moving from community 1 to community 2 increases, the difference between the infected persons of the two communities reduces. This implies that the movement of exposed persons alone is sufficient to increase the number of infected persons in community 2.

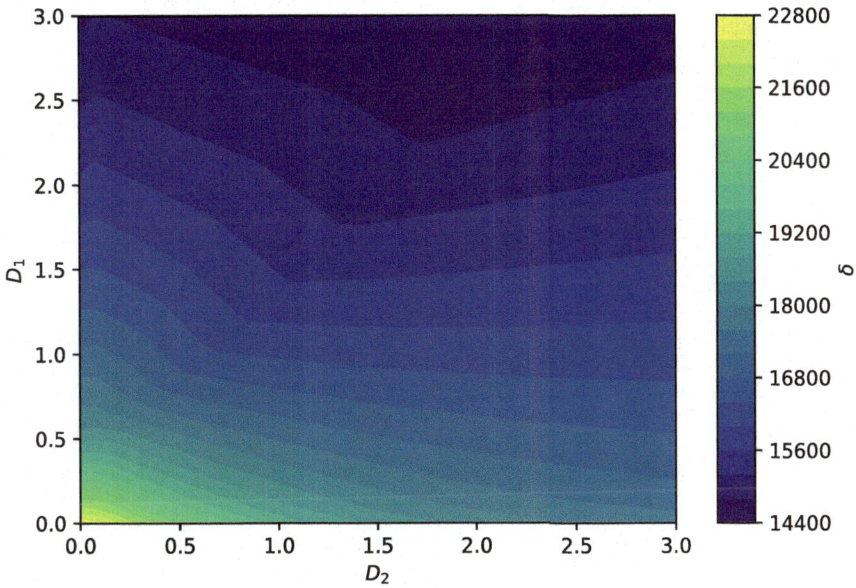

Fig. 6 Partial migration from community 1 to community 2

5 Conclusion

In this study, we have developed a simple SEIR model for the spread of Covid-19 within a community. We established the properties of the solution of the system, investigated the sensitivity of the basic reproduction number of the basic model to the parameters on which it depends. We also considered the stability of the system. From the sensitivity analysis, it can be inferred that the basic reproduction number for the one-community model is most sensitive to the recovery rate of symptomatic infectious individuals followed by the transmission coefficient from symptomatic infectious, recovery rate of asymptomatic infectious, rate of incubation (rate of transition from asymptomatic to symptomatic infectious), transmission coefficient from asymptomatic infectious, and the death rate.

The basic model was extended to study the interaction between two communities with respect to Covid-19 transmissions. This was done by bidirectional coupling which represents the role of movement between the two communities. Our results showed that, with very low coupling between the two communities, rate of infections are reduced. As coupling strengths between the two communities increases, so does the number of infected persons in them. We considered the case where one community limits the movement of persons into her region while the other community does not. Our results indicate that to reduce the spread of Covid-19, all communities have roles to play.

The simple model we have studied can be extended to higher order SEIR models to consider more peculiarities of Covid-19. It can also be extended to consider the spread of Covid-19 in a network of interconnected communities. Furthermore, the roles of both bidirectional coupling and environmental coupling could be considered in future studies.

References

1. Abbott, L., Kepler, T.B.: Model neurons: from Hodgkin-Huxley to Hopfield. In: Statistical Mechanics of Neural Networks, pp. 5–18. Springer (1990)
2. Adeniyi, M., Ekum, M., Iluno, C., Ogunsanya, A., Akinyemi, J., Oke, S., Matadi, M.: Dynamic model of COVID-19 disease with exploratory data analysis. Sci. African **000**(e00477), 1–21 (2020)
3. Agusto, F.B., Bewick, S., Fagan, W.: Mathematical model of Zika virus with vertical transmission. Infect. Dis. Modell. **2**(2), 244–267 (2017)
4. Anastassopoulou, C., Russo, L., Tsakris, A., Siettos, C.: Data-based analysis, modelling and forecasting of the COVID-19 outbreak. PloS One **15**(3), e0230405 (2020)
5. Arriola, L., Hyman, J.M.: Sensitivity analysis for uncertainty quantification in mathematical models. In: Hyman, J.M., Bettencourt, L.M.A., Castillo-Chavez, C. (eds.) Chowell G. Mathematical and Statistical Estimation Approaches in Epidemiology Springer, Dordrecht (2009)
6. Atkeson, A.: What will be the economic impact of COVID-19 in the us? Rough estimates of disease scenarios. Tech. rep, National Bureau of Economic Research (2020)
7. Bauch, C.T., Oraby, T.: Assessing the pandemic potential of MERS-COV. The Lancet **382**(9893), 662–664 (2013)
8. Berge, T., Lubuma, J.S., Moremedi, G., Morris, N., Kondera-Shava, R.: a simple mathematical model for Ebola in Africa. J. Biol. Dyn. **11**(1), 42–74 (2017)
9. Bhunu, C.P.: A mathematical analysis of alcoholism. World J. Model. Simul. **8**(2), 124–134 (2012)
10. Blake, P.A.: Historical perspectives on pandemic cholera. In: Vibrio cholerae and Cholera, American Society of Microbiology, pp. 293–295 (1994)
11. Bowman, C., Gumel, A., Van den Driessche, P., Wu, J., Zhu, H.: A mathematical model for assessing control strategies against West Nile virus. Bull. Math. Biol. **67**(5), 1107–1133 (2005)
12. Chatterjee, K., Chatterjee, K., Kumar, A., Shankar, S.: Healthcare impact of COVID-19 epidemic in India: A stochastic mathematical model. Medical Journal Armed Forces India (2020)
13. Cucinotta, D., Vanelli, M.: Who declares COVID-19 a pandemic. Acta bio-medica: Atenei Parmensis **91**(1), 157–160 (2020)
14. Dansu, E.J., Seno, H.: A model for epidemic dynamics in a community with visitor subpopulation. J. Theoret. Biol. **478**, 115–127 (2019)
15. De Wit, E., Van Doremalen, N., Falzarano, D., Munster, V.J.: SARS and MERS: recent insights into emerging coronaviruses. Nat. Rev. Microbiol. **14**(8), 523 (2016)
16. Diekmann, O., Heesterbeek, J.A.P., Roberts, M.G.: The construction of next-generation matrices for compartmental epidemic models. J. R. Soc. Interface **7**, 873–885 (2010)
17. Gatto, M., Bertuzzo, E., Mari, L., Miccoli, S., Carraro, L., Casagrandi, R., Rinaldo, A.: Spread and dynamics of the COVID-19 epidemic in Italy: effects of emergency containment measures. PNAS **117**(19), 10484–10491 (2020)
18. Ghosh, S., Bhattacharya, S.: Computational model on COVID-19 pandemic using probabilistic cellular automata (2020) 2006.11270
19. Glass, K.: Ecological mechanisms that promote arbovirus survival: a mathematical model of Ross River virus transmission. Trans. R. Soc. Trop. Med. Hygiene **99**(4), 252–260 (2005)

20. Gössling, S., Scott, D., Hall, C.M.: Pandemics, tourism and global change: a rapid assessment of COVID-19. J. Sustain. Tourism **1–20**,(2020)
21. Housworth, J., Langmuir, A.D.: Excess mortality from epidemic influenza, 1957–1966. Am. J. Epidemiol. **100**(1), 40–48 (1974)
22. Ivorra, B., Ferrández, M.R., Vela-Pérez, M., Ramos, A.: Mathematical modeling of the spread of the coronavirus disease 2019 (COVID-19) taking into account the undetected infections. the case of china. Commun. Nonlinear Sci. Numer. Simul. 105303 (2020)
23. Johnson, N.P., Mueller, J.: Updating the accounts: global mortality of the 1918–1920 "Spanish" influenza pandemic. Bull. Hist. Med. **105–115**, (2002)
24. Kapitza, S.P.: A mathematical model for global population growth. Matematicheskoe modelirovanie **4**(6), 65–79 (1992)
25. Kareem, S.O., Ojo, K., Njah, A.: Function projective synchronization of identical and non-identical modified finance and Shimizu-Morioka systems. Pramana **79**(1), 71–79 (2012)
26. Kolebaje, O., Popoola, O., Khan, M.A., Oyewande, O.: An epidemiological approach to insurgent population modeling with the Atangana-Baleanu fractional derivative. Chaos, Solit. Fractals 139, 109970 (2020)
27. Kraemer, M.U., Yang, C.H., Gutierrez, B., Wu, C.H., Klein, B., Pigott, D.M., Du Plessis, L., Faria, N.R., Li, R., Hanage, W.P., et al.: The effect of human mobility and control measures on the COVID-19 epidemic in China. Science **368**(6490), 493–497 (2020)
28. Kucharski, A.J., Russell, T.W., Diamond, C., Liu, Y., Edmunds, J., Funk, S., Eggo, R.M., Sun, F., Jit, M., Munday, J.D., et al.: Early dynamics of transmission and control of COVID-19: a mathematical modelling study. The Lancet Infect, Dis (2020)
29. Lanteri, D., Carco, D., Castorina, P.: How macroscopic laws describe complex dynamics: asymptomatic population and COVID-19 spreading. arXiv preprint arXiv:200312457 (2020)
30. Lau, S.K., Li, K.S., Tsang, A.K., Lam, C.S., Ahmed, S., Chen, H., Chan, K.H., Woo, P.C., Yuen, K.Y.: Genetic characterization of betacoronavirus lineage C viruses in bats reveals marked sequence divergence in the spike protein of pipistrellus bat coronavirus HKU5 in japanese pipistrelle: implications for the origin of the novel Middle East Respiratory Syndrome coronavirus. J. Virol. **87**(15), 8638–8650 (2013)
31. Liu, Z., Magal, P., Seydi, O., Webb, G.: A covid-19 epidemic model with latency period. Infectious Disease Modelling **5**, 323–337 (2020). https://doi.org/10.1016/j.idm.2020.03.003
32. Möhler, L., Flockerzi, D., Sann, H., Reichl, U.: Mathematical model of influenza a virus production in large-scale microcarrier culture. Biotech. Bioeng. **90**(1), 46–58 (2005)
33. Ndairou F, Area I, Nieto JJ, Torres DF (2020) Mathematical modeling of COVID-19 transmission dynamics with a case study of Wuhan. Chaos, Solitons & Fractals p 109846
34. Nicola, M., Alsafi, Z., Sohrabi, C., Kerwan, A., Al-Jabir, A., Iosifidis, C., Agha, M., Agha, R.: The socio-economic implications of the coronavirus and COVID-19 pandemic: a review. International Journal of Surgery (2020)
35. Okuonghae, D., Okuonghae, R.: A mathematical model for Lassa fever. J. Nigerian Assoc. Math. Phys. **10**(1), (2006)
36. Organization WH, et al. (2020) Coronavirus disease 2019 (covid-19): situation report, 160
37. ÖZalp N, Demirci E, : A fractional order SEIR model with vertical transmission. Math. Comp. Model. **54**(1–2), 1–6 (2011)
38. Peng L, Yang W, Zhang D, Zhuge C, Hong L (2020) Epidemic analysis of COVID-19 in china by dynamical modeling. arXiv preprint arXiv:200206563
39. Pongsumpun, P.: Mathematical model of Dengue disease with the incubation period of virus. World Acad. Sci. Eng. Technol. **44**, 328–332 (2008)
40. Richardson, E.T., Barrie, M.B., Kelly, J.D., Dibba, Y., Koedoyoma, S., Farmer, P.E.: Biosocial approaches to the 2013–2016 Ebola pandemic. Health Human Rights **18**(1), 115 (2016)
41. Rossi C (2002) The role of dynamic modelling in drug abuse epidemiology. Bull. Narc. **54**(1 and 2):33–44
42. Sahu, P.: Closure of universities due to coronavirus disease 2019 (COVID-19): impact on education and mental health of students and academic staff. Cureus **12**(4), (2020)

43. Sharp, P.M., Hahn, B.H.: Origins of HIV and the AIDS pandemic. Cold Spring Harbor Perspect. Med. **1**(1), a006841 (2011)
44. Shim, E., Tariq, A., Choi, W., Lee, Y., Chowell, G.: Transmission potential and severity of COVID-19 in South Korea. Int. J. Infect. Dis. (2020)
45. Vaillant, L., La Ruche, G., Tarantola, A., Barboza, P., et al.: Epidemiology of fatal cases associated with pandemic H1N1 influenza 2009. Eurosurveillance **14**(33), 19309 (2009)
46. Viboud, C., Grais, R.F., Lafont, B.A., Miller, M.A., Simonsen, L.: Multinational impact of the 1968 Hong Kong influenza pandemic: evidence for a smoldering pandemic. J. Infect. Dis. **192**(2), 233–248 (2005)
47. Wauer, J., Schwarzer, D., Cai, G., Lin, Y.: Dynamical models of love with time-varying fluctuations. Appl. Math. Comput. **188**(2), 1535–1548 (2007)
48. Wu Y, Xu X, Chen Z, Duan J, Hashimoto K, Yang L, Liu C, Yang C (2020) Nervous system involvement after infection with COVID-19 and other coronaviruses. Brain, Behavior, and Immunity
49. Yu, Y., Zhang, S.: The synchronization of linearly bidirectional coupled chaotic systems. Chaos, Solitons & Fractals **22**(1), 189–197 (2004)
50. Zhao, S., Xu, Z., Lu, Y.: A mathematical model of Hepatitis B virus transmission and its application for vaccination strategy in China. Int. J. Epidemiol. **29**(4), 744–752 (2000)

Similarity Measure of q-Rung Orthopair Fuzzy Soft Sets and Its Application in Covid-19 Problem

Manash Jyoti Borah and Bipan Hazarika

Abstract In this chapter, we introduce q-rung orthopair fuzzy soft sets (q-ROFSSs) and some basic properties. Also we define a similarity measure of q-ROFSSs and their properties are studied. Finally, we provide an application of q-ROFSSs in Covid-19.

Keywords 34-XX Ordinary differential equations · 37N25 Dynamical systems in biology · 92D25 Population dynamics (general) · 92D30 Epidemiology · 93A30 Mathematical modeling

1 Introduction

Zadeh [35], in 1965 was the first to come up theory of fuzzy set for dealing with uncertainties problems in our daily life, where conventional mathematical tools fail. In 1986, Atanassov [2] extended the fuzzy set to intuitionistic fuzzy set (IFS) by adding the non-membership degree. Yager [30] generalized the IFS and introduced the Pythagorean fuzzy set (PFS) $P =< x_i, (\mu_P(x_i), \nu_P(x_i)); x_i \in X >$, where $0 \leq \mu_P^2(x_i) + \nu_P^2(x_i) \leq 1$. The PFS has been widely studied and applied in many fields, one can see [8, 28, 31] related to PFS. Yager [32, 33] introduced a new form of fuzzy set known as q-rung orthopair fuzzy set ($q - ROFS$), which can be described as $Q =< x_i, (\mu_Q(x_i), \nu_Q(x_i))_q; x_i \in X >$, where $0 \leq \mu_Q^q(x_i) + \nu_Q^q(x_i) \leq 1$. When $q = 1$ and 2, we can see that the IFS and PFS are special cases of q-ROFS, respectively. The cosine similarity measures and distance measures between q-rung orthopair fuzzy sets was studied by Liu et al. [14] in 2019.

M. J. Borah
Department of Mathematics, Bahona College, Jorhat 785 101, Assam, India

B. Hazarika (✉)
Department of Mathematics, Gauhati University, Guwahati 781014, Assam, India
e-mail: bh_rgu@yahoo.co.in; bh_gu@gauhati.ac.in

P. Agarwal et al. (eds.), *Analysis of Infectious Disease Problems (Covid-19) and Their Global Impact*, Infosys Science Foundation Series,
https://doi.org/10.1007/978-981-16-2450-6_19

In 1999, Molodtsov [24] initiated fuzzy soft set theory, which is developed and applied Maji et al. [16–18]. Afterwards many researchers have worked several directions of fuzzy soft sets e.g. intuionistic fuzzy soft sets [2, 3, 19], interval-valued fuzzy soft sets [34], interval-valued intuionistic fuzzy soft sets [11], generalized fuzzy soft sets [13, 21] and references therein. The q-rung orthopair fuzzy soft set and their basic operators were discussed by Hussain et al. [10] in the year 2020.

Similarity measure play a vital role in fuzzy soft sets. Chen [5–7], Li and Xu [15], Hong and Kim [9], Pappis [27], Majumdar and Samanta [20, 22], Karaaslan [12] and many other researchers have studied the problem of similarity measurement between fuzzy sets, fuzzy numbers, vague sets, fuzzy soft sets and possibility neutrosophic soft sets. This paper is an extension work of similarity measure of soft sets initiated by Majumdar and Samanta [20, 22].

The whole world is fight against Covid-19 more than one year from end of 2019. The first case was detected in the city of Wuhan China which is the capital of Hubei province on end of 2019. There are currently several research directions work by researchers [1, 23, 29, 36] on Covid-19. On March 11, 2020, the World Health Organization (WHO) formally declared the outbreak of novel corona virus as a Global panedemic. As of March 18, 2021 a total of 122,149,402 cases are confirmed in more than 219 countries. There are 20,974,059 active cases, 98,478,189 recovered and 2,697,154 deaths. Now India has become largest affected countries in Asia. As of March 18, 2021 a total of 11,513,524 cases are confirmed in India. There are 2,52,364 active cases, 11,081,335 recovered and 1,59,402 deaths., against the global 1.39. Total number of vaccinated people are 3,71,43,255 on March 18, 2021 in India.

The Government of India is proposing multiple lockdowns to prevent the spread of this virus. Initially, in lockdown 1.0 (March 25, 2020, to April 14, 2020), the entire nation was under complete lockdown except for essential services and lockdown 2.0 (April 15, 2020, to May 3, 2020) was implemented with relaxation in areas where the virus was contained and lockdown 3.0 (May 4, 2020, to May 17, 2020) with more relaxations in areas where there were fewer number of coronavirus cases. Due to these lockdowns, there has been a decrease in the number of cases. Lockdown 4.0 (May 18, 2020 to 31 May 2020)and lockdown 5.0 (1st June, 2020 to ongoing) only for containment zones.

The remainder of this chapter organized as follows. In Sect. 2, some basic concepts of Intuitionistic fuzzy sets, Pythagorean fuzzy sets, q-ROFSs, fuzzy soft sets and q-ROFSSs are briefly reviewed, which will be used in the analysis throughout this chapter. In Sect. 3, similarity measures between q-ROFSSs and q-rung orthopair fuzzy soft points(q-ROFSPs) are proposed and proved. In Sect. 4, weighted similarity measures between q-ROFSSs and q-ROFSPs are proposed and proved. In Sect. 5, we give one application of similarity of q-ROFSSs in Covid-19. In Sect. 6, we give another application of weighted similarity of q-ROFSSs in Covid-19. The chapter is concluded in Sect. 7.

2 Preliminary Definitions

In this section we recall some basic concepts and definitions fuzzy soft sets, q-ROFSs and q-ROFSSs.

Definition 1 [33] Let $X = \{x_1, x_2, ..., x_n\}$ be a fixed set; then the q-Rung orthopair fuzzy set (q-ROFS) Q on X is defined as

$$Q = \{< x_i, (\mu_Q(x_i), \nu_Q(x_i)) >; x_i \in X\},$$

where $\mu_Q(x_i) : X \longrightarrow [0, 1]$ and $\nu_Q(x_i) : X \longrightarrow [0, 1]$ represent the membership and non-membership degrees of $x_i \in X$, respectively. For each $x_i \in X$, they satisfy with $0 \leq \mu_Q^q(x_i) + \nu_Q^q(x_i) \leq 1$, and the hesitancy degree $\pi_Q(x_i) = 1 - \mu_Q(x_i) - \nu_Q(x_i)$. Obviously, $0 \leq \pi_Q(x_i) \leq 1$.

If the set $X = \{x_1, x_2, ..., x_n\}$ has only one element, that is, $X = \{x_i\}$, then the q-ROFS Q is reduced to $Q = (\mu_Q(x_i), \nu_Q(x_i)) = (\mu_i, \nu_i)$. For convenience, we call $Q = (\mu_i, \nu_i)$ an q-Rung orthopair fuzzy number (q-ROFN).

Definition 2 [33] Let $Q_1 = (\mu_{Q_1}, \nu_{Q_1})_q$, and $Q_2 = (\mu_{Q_2}, \nu_{Q_2})_q$, be any two q-ROFNs; then the operation laws between them can be defined as:

(i) $Q_1 \bigcup Q_2 = (\max\{\mu_{Q_1}, \mu_{Q_2}\}, \min\{\nu_{Q_1}, \nu_{Q_2}\})_q$.
(ii) $Q_1 \bigcap Q_2 = (\min\{\mu_{Q_1}, \mu_{Q_2}\}, \max\{\nu_{Q_1}, \nu_{Q_2}\})_q$.
(iii) $Q_1 \leq Q_2$if and only if $\mu_{Q_1} \leq \mu_{Q_2}, \nu_{Q_1} \geq \nu_{Q_2}$.

Definition 3 [18] Let U be an initial universe and F be a set of parameters. Let $\tilde{P}(U)$ denote the power set of U and A be a non-empty subset of F. Then F_A is called a fuzzy soft set over U where $F : A \rightarrow \tilde{P}(U)$ is a mapping from A into $\tilde{P}(U)$.

Definition 4 [10] Let U be an initial universe and F be a set of parameters. Let A be a non-empty subset of F. Then F_A^Q is called a q-rung orthopair fuzzy soft set over U, where $F : A \rightarrow q - ROFS$, which is defined as

$$F_A^Q = \left\{< x_i, (\mu^q_{e_i(F_A^Q)}, \nu^q_{e_i(F_A^Q)})_q >; x_i \in U \text{ and } q \geq 1\right\},$$

where q-ROFS represent the collection of all q-ROFSs of U. Here $\mu^q_{e_i(F_A^Q)}$ and $\nu^q_{e_i(F_A^Q)}$, denotes the membership and non-membership degrees of an object $x_i \in U$ and satisfying the condition that $0 \leq \mu^q_{e_i(F_A^Q)} + \nu^q_{e_i(F_A^Q)} \leq 1$ and $q \geq 1$. Moreover, the degree of hesitancy for q-ROFS number is defined as $\pi^q_{e_i(F_A^Q)} = \sqrt{1 - \left(\mu^q_{e_i(F_A^Q)} + \nu^q_{e_i(F_A^Q)}\right)}$.

Definition 5 [10] Let $F_A^q = (\mu^q_{e_i(F_A^Q)}, \nu^q_{e_i(F_A^Q)})_q$, and $G_B^q = (\mu^q_{e_i(G_B^Q)}, \nu^q_{e_i(G_B^Q)})_q$, be any two q-ROFNs; then the operation laws between them can be defined as:

(i) $F_A^q \bigcup G_B^q = \left(\max\left\{\mu^q_{e_i(F_A^Q)}, \mu^q_{e_i(G_B^Q)}\right\}, \min\left\{\mu^q_{e_i(F_A^Q)}, \mu^q_{e_i(G_B^Q)}\right\}\right).$

(ii) $F_A^q \bigcap G_B^q = \left(\min\left\{\mu^q_{e_i(F_A^Q)}, \mu^q_{e_i(G_B^Q)}\right\}, \max\left\{\mu^q_{e_i(F_A^Q)}, \mu^q_{e_i(G_B^Q)}\right\}\right).$

Definition 6 [22] Let F_E and G_E be two fuzzy soft sets over U. Then the similarity between them, denoted by $\tilde{S}(F_E, G_E)$ is defined by

$$\tilde{S}(F_E, G_E) = \frac{\sum_{i=1}^{n} \{\mathbf{F}(e_i) \bullet \mathbf{G}(e_i)\}}{\sum_{i=1}^{n} \left\{(\mathbf{F}(e_i))^2 \vee (\mathbf{G}(e_i))^2\right\}}.$$

Definition 7 [22] We denote $\tilde{M}(F_E, G_E)$ the similarity between the soft sets F_E and G_E, and $\tilde{M}_i(F_E, G_E)$ the similarity between the two e_i approximations $F(e_i)$ and $G(e_i)$. Then

$$\tilde{M}_i(F_E, G_E) = \frac{\sum_{i=1}^{n} (F_{ij} \wedge G_{ij})}{\sum_{i=1}^{n} \left(F_{ij} \vee G_{ij}\right)}$$

and

$$\tilde{M}(F_E, G_E) = \max_i \tilde{M}_i(F_E, G_E).$$

Definition 8 [20] Let F_A and G_B be two fuzzy soft sets over the same universe U. We call the two soft sets significantly similar if $\tilde{S}(F_A, G_B) \tilde{\geq} 0.5$.

3 Similarity Measures Between Q-ROFSSs and Q-ROFSPs

In this section, define similarity measure between two q-rung orthopair fuzzy soft sets (q-ROFSSs) and q-rung orthopair fuzzy soft points (q-ROFSPs). Also some of its examples and properties are studied.

Definition 9 Let F_A^Q and G_B^Q be two q-rung orthopair fuzzy soft sets. Then the similarity between them, denoted by $\tilde{S}(F_A^Q, G_B^Q)$ is defined by

$$\tilde{S}(F_A^Q, G_B^Q) = \frac{\sum_{t=1}^{n} \left\{\mu^q_{e_i(F_A^Q)}(h_t) \bullet \mu^q_{e_i(G_B^Q)}(h_t) + \nu^q_{e_i(F_A^Q)}(h_t) \bullet \nu^q_{e_i(G_B^Q)}(h_t)\right\}}{\max\left[\sum_{t=1}^{n} \left(\mu^{2q}_{e_i(F_A^Q)}(h_t) + \nu^{2q}_{e_i(F_A^Q)}(h_t)\right), \sum_{t=1}^{n} \left(\mu^{2q}_{e_i(G_B^Q)}(h_t) + \nu^{2q}_{e_i(G_B^Q)}(h_t)\right)\right]},$$

where $i = 1, 2, 3, \ldots, m$.

Problem 1 Let $F_A^Q = \{F(e_1) = \{< h_1, (0.9, 0.5) >, < h_2, (0.8, 0.2) >, < h_3, (0.9, 0.2) >\}$, $F(e_2) = \{< h_1, (0.8, 0.4) >, < h_2, (0.5, 0.1) >, < h_3, (0.7, 0.3) >\}\}$

$G_A^Q = \{G(e_1) = \{< h_1, (0.6, 0.3) >, < h_2, (0.7, 0.6) >, < h_3, (0.5, 0.4) >\},$
$G(e_2) = \{< h_1, (0.9, 0.4) >, < h_2, (0.8, 0.3) >, < h_3, (0.7, 0.2) >\}\}.$

Now we have expressed F_A^Q and G_A^Q in tabular form as given below.

F_A^Q	e_1	e_2
h_1	$(0.9, 0.5)_q$	$(0.8, 0.4)_q$
h_2	$(0.8, 0.2)_q$	$(0.5, 0.1)_q$
h_3	$(0.9, 0.2)_q$	$(0.7, 0.3)_q$
G_A^Q	e_1	e_2
h_1	$(0.6, 0.3)_q$	$(0.9, 0.4)_q$
h_2	$(0.7, 0.6)_q$	$(0.8, 0.3)_q$
h_3	$(0.5, 0.4)_q$	$(0.7, 0.2)_q$

Now if we consider $q = 3$, then we have expressed q-rung orthopair fuzzy soft sets F_A^Q and G_A^Q in tabular form as given below.

F_A^Q	e_1	e_2
h_1	$(0.729, 0.125)_3$	$(0.512, 0.064)_3$
h_2	$(0.512, 0.008)_3$	$(0.125, 0.001)_3$
h_3	$(0.729, 0.008)_3$	$(0.343, 0.027)_3$
G_A^Q	e_1	e_2
h_1	$(0.216, 0.027)_3$	$(0.729, 0.064)_3$
h_2	$(0.343, 0.216)_3$	$(0.512, 0.027)_3$
h_3	$(0.125, 0.064)_3$	$(0.343, 0.008)_3$

Therefore similarity measure of q-rung orthopair fuzzy soft sets F_A^Q and G_A^Q, for $q = 3$ is $\tilde{S}(F_A^Q, G_B^Q) = 0.5680$.

Proposition 1 *Let F_A^Q and G_B^Q be two q-rung orthopair fuzzy soft sets. Then*

(i) $\tilde{S}(F_A^Q, G_B^Q) = \tilde{S}(F_A^Q, G_B^Q)$.
(ii) $0 \lesssim \tilde{S}(F_A^Q, G_B^Q) \lesssim 1$.
(iii) $\tilde{S}(F_A^Q, G_B^Q) = 1$, *if* $F_A^Q = G_B^Q$.

Proof (i) For $i = 1, 2, 3, ..., m$, we get

$$\tilde{S}(F_A^Q, G_B^Q) = \frac{\sum_{t=1}^{n}\left\{\mu^q_{e_i(F_A^Q)}(h_t) \bullet \mu^q_{e_i(G_B^Q)}(h_t) + \nu^q_{e_i(F_A^Q)}(h_t) \bullet \nu^q_{e_i(G_B^Q)}(h_t)\right\}}{\max\left[\sum_{t=1}^{n}\left(\mu^{2q}_{e_i(F_A^Q)}(h_t) + \nu^{2q}_{e_i(F_A^Q)}(h_t)\right), \sum_{t=1}^{n}\left(\mu^{2q}_{e_i(G_B^Q)}(h_t) + \nu^{2q}_{e_i(G_B^Q)}(h_t)\right)\right]}$$

$$= \frac{\sum_{t=1}^{n}\left\{\mu^q_{e_i(G_B^Q)}(h_t) \bullet \mu^q_{e_i(F_A^Q)}(h_t) + \nu^q_{e_i(G_B^Q)}(h_t) \bullet \nu^q_{e_i(F_A^Q)}(h_t)\right\}}{\max\left[\sum_{t=1}^{n}\left(\mu^{2q}_{e_i(G_B^Q)}(h_t) + \nu^{2q}_{e_i(G_B^Q)}(h_t)\right), \sum_{t=1}^{n}\left(\mu^{2q}_{e_i(F_A^Q)}(h_t) + \nu^{2q}_{e_i(F_A^Q)}(h_t)\right)\right]}$$

$$= \tilde{S}(G_B^Q, F_A^Q).$$

(ii) obvious.
(iii) Let $F_A^Q = G_B^Q$ and for $i = 1, 2, 3, ..., m$, we have

$$\tilde{S}(F_A^Q, G_B^Q) = \frac{\sum_{t=1}^{n}\left\{\mu^q_{e_i(F_A^Q)}(h_t)\bullet\mu^q_{e_i(G_B^Q)}(h_t)+\nu^q_{e_i(F_A^Q)}(h_t)\bullet\nu^q_{e_i(G_B^Q)}(h_t)\right\}}{\max\left[\sum_{t=1}^{n}\left(\mu^{2q}_{e_i(F_A^Q)}(h_t)+\nu^{2q}_{e_i(F_A^Q)}(h_t)\right),\sum_{t=1}^{n}\left(\mu^{2q}_{e_i(G_B^Q)}(h_t)+\nu^{2q}_{e_i(G_B^Q)}(h_t)\right)\right]}$$

$$= \frac{\sum_{t=1}^{n}\left\{\mu^{2q}_{e_i(F_A^Q)}(h_t)+\nu^{2q}_{e_i(F_A^Q)}(h_t)\right\}}{\max\left[\sum_{t=1}^{n}\left(\mu^{2q}_{e_i(F_A^Q)}(h_t)+\nu^{2q}_{e_i(F_A^Q)}(h_t)\right),\sum_{t=1}^{n}\left(\mu^{2q}_{e_i(F_A^Q)}(h_t)+\nu^{2q}_{e_i(F_A^Q)}(h_t)\right)\right]}$$

$$= \frac{\sum_{t=1}^{n}\left\{\mu^{2q}_{e_i(F_A^Q)}(h_t)+\nu^{2q}_{e_i(F_A^Q)}(h_t)\right\}}{\sum_{t=1}^{n}\left(\mu^{2q}_{e_i(F_A^Q)}(h_t)+\nu^{2q}_{e_i(F_A^Q)}(h_t)\right)}$$

$$= 1.$$

□

Definition 10 Let $e_i(F_A^Q)$ and $e_j(G_B^Q)$ be two q-rung orthopair fuzzy soft sets. Then the similarity between them, denoted by $\tilde{S}(e_i(F_A^Q), e_j(G_B^Q))$ is defined by

$$\tilde{S}(e_i(F_A^Q), e_j(G_B^Q)) = \frac{\sum_{t=1}^{n}\left\{\mu^q_{e_i(F_A^Q)}(h_t)\bullet\mu^q_{e_j(G_B^Q)}(h_t)+\nu^q_{e_i(F_A^Q)}(h_t)\bullet\nu^q_{e_j(G_B^Q)}(h_t)\right\}}{\max\left[\sum_{t=1}^{n}\left(\mu^{2q}_{e_i(F_A^Q)}(h_t)+\nu^{2q}_{e_i(F_A^Q)}(h_t)\right),\sum_{t=1}^{n}\left(\mu^{2q}_{e_j(G_B^Q)}(h_t)+\nu^{2q}_{e_j(G_B^Q)}(h_t)\right)\right]},$$

where $i = 1$ or 2 or $\ldots$ or m; $j = 1$ or 2 or $\ldots$ or m.

Problem 2 From Problem 1. Let $e_1(F_A^Q) = \{< h_1, (0.9, 0.5) >, < h_2, (0.8, 0.2) >, < h_3, (0.9, 0.2) >\}$; $e_2(G_A^Q) = \{< h_1, (0.9, 0.4) >, < h_2, (0.8, 0.3) >, < h_3, (0.7, 0.2) >\}\}$.

Now we have expressed $e_1(F_A^Q)$ and $e_2(G_A^Q)$ in tabular form as given below.

$e_1(F_A^Q)$	e_1
h_1	$(0.9, 0.5)_q$
h_2	$(0.8, 0.2)_q$
h_3	$(0.9, 0.2)_q$
$e_2(G_A^Q)$	e_2
h_1	$(0.9, 0.4)_q$
h_2	$(0.8, 0.3)_q$
h_3	$(0.7, 0.2)_q$

Now if we consider $q = 3$, then we have expressed q-rung orthopair fuzzy soft points $e_1(F_A^Q)$ and $e_2(G_A^Q)$ in tabular form as given below.

$e_1(F_A^Q)$	e_1
h_1	$(0.729, 0.125)_3$
h_2	$(0.512, 0.008)_3$
h_3	$(0.729, 0.008)_3$
$e_2(G_A^Q)$	e_2
h_1	$(0.729, 0.064)_3$
h_2	$(0.512, 0.027)_3$
h_3	$(0.343, 0.008)_3$

Therefore similarity measure of q-rung orthopair fuzzy soft points $e_1(F_A^Q)$ and $e_2(G_A^Q)$, for $q = 3$ is $\tilde{S}(e_i(F_A^Q), e_2(G_A^Q)) = 0.784$.

Proposition 2 *Let $e_i(F_A^Q)$ and $e_j(G_B^Q)$ be two q-rung orthopair fuzzy soft sets. Then*

(i) $\tilde{S}(e_i(F_A^Q), e_j(G_B^Q)) = \tilde{S}(e_j(G_B^Q), e_i(F_A^Q))$.
(ii) $0 \tilde{\leq} \tilde{S}(e_i(F_A^Q), e_j(G_B^Q)) \tilde{\leq} 1$.
(iii) $\tilde{S}(e_i(F_A^Q), e_j(G_B^Q)) = 1$, *if* $e_i(F_A^Q) = e_j(G_B^Q)$.

Proof Obvious. □

4 Weighted Similarity Measures Between Q-ROFSSs and Q-ROFSPs

In this section, definitions and examples of weighted similarity measures between q-ROFSSs and q-ROFSPs are studied. Further some of its properties are introduced.

Definition 11 Let $E = \{e_1, e_2, ..., e_m\}$ be the set of parameters and w_i be the weight of e_i, and $w_i \in [0, 1]$, but not all zero. Let F_A^Q and G_B^Q be two q-rung orthopair fuzzy soft sets over (U, E). Then their weighted similarity between them, denoted by $\tilde{WS}(F_A^Q, G_B^Q)$ is defined by

$$\tilde{WS}(F_A^Q, G_B^Q) = \frac{\sum_{t=1}^{n} w_i . \left\{ \mu^q_{e_i(F_A^Q)}(h_t) \bullet \mu^q_{e_i(G_B^Q)}(h_t) + \nu^q_{e_i(F_A^Q)}(h_t) \bullet \nu^q_{e_i(G_B^Q)}(h_t) \right\}}{\max\left[\sum_{t=1}^{n} \left(\mu^{2q}_{e_i(F_A^Q)}(h_t) + \nu^{2q}_{e_i(F_A^Q)}(h_t) \right), \sum_{t=1}^{n} \left(\mu^{2q}_{e_i(G_B^Q)}(h_t) + \nu^{2q}_{e_i(G_B^Q)}(h_t) \right) \right]} / \sum_{=1}^{m} w_i,$$

where $i = 1, 2, 3, ..., m$.

Problem 3 From Problem 1. We have expressed F_A^Q and G_A^Q in tabular form (for q=3) as given below.

F_A^Q	e_1	e_2
h_1	$(0.729, 0.125)_3$	$(0.512, 0.064)_3$
h_2	$(0.512, 0.008)_3$	$(0.125, 0.001)_3$
h_3	$(0.729, 0.008)_3$	$(0.343, 0.027)_3$
G_A^Q	e_1	e_2
h_1	$(0.216, 0.027)_3$	$(0.729, 0.064)_3$
h_2	$(0.343, 0.216)_3$	$(0.512, 0.027)_3$
h_3	$(0.125, 0.064)_3$	$(0.343, 0.008)_3$

Now we consider 0.3 and 0.6 are the weight of e_1 and e_2 respectively. Then q-rung orthopair fuzzy soft sets F_A^Q and G_A^Q in tabular form (for q=3) as given below.

F_A^Q	$e_1(0.3)$	$e_2(0.6)$
h_1	$(0.219, 0.037)_3$	$(0.307, 0.038)_3$
h_2	$(0.154, 0.002)_3$	$(0.075, 0.001)_3$
h_3	$(0.219, 0.002)_3$	$(0.206, 0.016)_3$
G_A^Q	$e_1(0.3)$	$e_2(0.6)$
h_1	$(0.065, 0.008)_3$	$(0.437, 0.038)_3$
h_2	$(0.103, 0.065)_3$	$(0.307, 0.016)_3$
h_3	$(0.038, 0.019)_3$	$(0.206, 0.005)_3$

Therefore weighted similarity measure of q-rung orthopair fuzzy soft sets F_A^Q and G_A^Q, for $q = 3$ is $\tilde{WS}(F_A^Q, G_B^Q) = 0.076$.

Proposition 3 *Let F_A^Q and G_B^Q be two q-rung orthopair fuzzy soft sets. Then*

(i) $\tilde{WS}(F_A^Q, G_B^Q) = \tilde{WS}(G_B^Q, F_A^Q)$.
(ii) $0 \tilde{\leq} \tilde{WS}(F_A^Q, G_B^Q) \tilde{\leq} 1$.
(iii) $\tilde{WS}(F_A^Q, G_B^Q) = 1$, *if* $F_A^Q = G_B^Q$.

Proof (i) For $i = 1, 2, 3, ..., m$, we obtain

$$\tilde{WS}(F_A^Q, G_B^Q) = \frac{\sum_{t=1}^{n} w_i \cdot \left\{ \mu^q_{e_i(F_A^Q)}(h_t) \bullet \mu^q_{e_i(G_B^Q)}(h_t) + \nu^q_{e_i(F_A^Q)}(h_t) \bullet \nu^q_{e_i(G_B^Q)}(h_t) \right\}}{\max\left[\sum_{t=1}^{n} \left(\mu^{2q}_{e_i(F_A^Q)}(h_t) + \nu^{2q}_{e_i(F_A^Q)}(h_t) \right), \sum_{t=1}^{n} \left(\mu^{2q}_{e_i(G_B^Q)}(h_t) + \nu^{2q}_{e_i(G_B^Q)}(h_t) \right) \right]} \Big/ \sum_{=1}^{m} w_i$$

$$= \frac{\sum_{t=1}^{n} w_i \cdot \left\{ \mu^q_{e_i(G_B^Q)}(h_t) \bullet \mu^q_{e_i(F_A^Q)}(h_t) + \nu^q_{e_i(G_B^Q)}(h_t) \bullet \nu^q_{e_i(F_A^Q)}(h_t) \right\}}{\max\left[\sum_{t=1}^{n} \left(\mu^{2q}_{e_i(G_B^Q)}(h_t) + \nu^{2q}_{e_i(G_B^Q)}(h_t) \right), \sum_{t=1}^{n} \left(\mu^{2q}_{e_i(F_A^Q)}(h_t) + \nu^{2q}_{e_i(F_A^Q)}(h_t) \right) \right]} \Big/ \sum_{=1}^{m} w_i$$

$$= \tilde{WS}(G_B^Q, F_A^Q).$$

(ii) obvious.
(iii) Let $F_A^Q = G_B^Q$, and for $i = 1, 2, 3, ..., m$, we get

$$\tilde{WS}(F_A^Q, G_B^Q) = \frac{\sum_{t=1}^{n} w_i \cdot \left\{ \mu^q_{e_i(F_A^Q)}(h_t) \bullet \mu^q_{e_i(G_B^Q)}(h_t) + \nu^q_{e_i(F_A^Q)}(h_t) \bullet \nu^q_{e_i(G_B^Q)}(h_t) \right\}}{\max\left[\sum_{t=1}^{n} \left(\mu^{2q}_{e_i(F_A^Q)}(h_t) + \nu^{2q}_{e_i(F_A^Q)}(h_t) \right), \sum_{t=1}^{n} \left(\mu^{2q}_{e_i(G_B^Q)}(h_t) + \nu^{2q}_{e_i(G_B^Q)}(h_t) \right) \right]} / \sum_{=1}^{m} w_i$$

$$= \frac{\sum_{t=1}^{n} w_i \cdot \left\{ \mu^{2q}_{e_i(F_A^Q)}(h_t) + \nu^{2q}_{e_i(F_A^Q)}(h_t) \right\}}{\max\left[\sum_{t=1}^{n} \left(\mu^{2q}_{e_i(F_A^Q)}(h_t) + \nu^{2q}_{e_i(F_A^Q)}(h_t) \right), \sum_{t=1}^{n} \left(\mu^{2q}_{e_i(F_A^Q)}(h_t) + \nu^{2q}_{e_i(F_A^Q)}(h_t) \right) \right]} / \sum_{=1}^{m} w_i$$

$$= \frac{\sum_{t=1}^{n} w_i \cdot \left\{ \mu^{2q}_{e_i(F_A^Q)}(h_t) + \nu^{2q}_{e_i(F_A^Q)}(h_t) \right\}}{\sum_{t=1}^{n} \left(\mu^{2q}_{e_i(F_A^Q)}(h_t) + \nu^{2q}_{e_i(F_A^Q)}(h_t) \right)} / \sum_{=1}^{m} w_i$$

$$= 1.$$

□

Definition 12 Let $E = \{e_1, e_2, ..., e_m\}$ be the set of parameters and w_i be the weight of e_i and $w_i \in [0, 1]$, but not all zero. Let F_A^Q and G_B^Q be two q-rung orthopair fuzzy soft sets over (U, E), and $\sum_{=1}^{m} w_i = 1$. Then their weighted similarity between them, denoted by $\tilde{WS}(F_A^Q, G_B^Q)$ is defined by

$$\tilde{WS}(F_A^Q, G_B^Q) = \frac{\sum_{t=1}^{n} w_i \cdot \left\{ \mu^q_{e_i(F_A^Q)}(h_t) \bullet \mu^q_{e_i(G_B^Q)}(h_t) + \nu^q_{e_i(F_A^Q)}(h_t) \bullet \nu^q_{e_i(G_B^Q)}(h_t) \right\}}{\max\left[\sum_{t=1}^{n} \left(\mu^{2q}_{e_i(F_A^Q)}(h_t) + \nu^{2q}_{e_i(F_A^Q)}(h_t) \right), \sum_{t=1}^{n} \left(\mu^{2q}_{e_i(G_B^Q)}(h_t) + \nu^{2q}_{e_i(G_B^Q)}(h_t) \right) \right]},$$

where $i = 1, 2, 3, ..., m$.

Definition 13 Let $E = \{e_1, e_2, ..., e_m\}$ be the set of parameters and w_i be the weight of e_i, and $w_i \in [0, 1]$, but not all zero. Let $e_i(F_A^Q)$, and $e_j(G_B^Q)$ be two q-rung orthopair fuzzy soft points. Then the weighted similarity between them, denoted by $\tilde{WS}(e_i(F_A^Q), e_j(G_B^Q))$ is defined by

$$\tilde{WS}(e_i(F_A^Q), e_j(G_B^Q)) = \frac{\sum_{t=1}^{n} w_i \cdot \left\{ \mu^q_{e_i(F_A^Q)}(h_t) \bullet \mu^q_{e_j(G_B^Q)}(h_t) + \nu^q_{e_i(F_A^Q)}(h_t) \bullet \nu^q_{e_j(G_B^Q)}(h_t) \right\}}{\max\left[\sum_{t=1}^{n} \left(\mu^{2q}_{e_i(F_A^Q)}(h_t) + \nu^{2q}_{e_i(F_A^Q)}(h_t) \right), \sum_{t=1}^{n} \left(\mu^{2q}_{e_j(G_B^Q)}(h_t) + \nu^{2q}_{e_j(G_B^Q)}(h_t) \right) \right]} / \sum_{i=1}^{m} w_i,$$

where $i = 1$ or 2 or $\ldots$ or m; $j = 1$ or 2 or $\ldots$ or m.

Problem 4 From Problem 3. We have expressed $e_1(F_A^Q)$ and $e_2(G_A^Q)$ in tabular form as given below.

F_A^Q	$e_1(0.3)$
h_1	$(0.219, 0.037)_3$
h_2	$(0.154, 0.002)_3$
h_3	$(0.219, 0.002)_3$
G_A^Q	$e_2(0.6)$
h_1	$(0.437, 0.038)_3$
h_2	$(0.307, 0.016)_3$
h_3	$(0.206, 0.005)_3$

Therefore weighted similarity measure of q-rung orthopair fuzzy soft points $e_1(F_A^Q)$ and $e_2(G_B^Q)$, for $q = 3$ is $\tilde{W}S(e_1(F_A^Q), e_2(G_B^Q)) = 0.157$.

Proposition 4 *Let $e_i(F_A^Q)$ and $e_j(G_B^Q)$ be two q-rung orthopair fuzzy soft points. Then*

(i) $\tilde{W}S(e_i(F_A^Q), e_j(G_B^Q)) = \tilde{W}S(e_j(G_B^Q), e_i(F_A^Q))$.
(ii) $0 \tilde{\leq} \tilde{W}S(e_i(F_A^Q), e_j(G_B^Q)) \tilde{\leq} 1$.
(iii) $\tilde{W}S(e_i(F_A^Q), e_j(G_B^Q)) = 1$, *if* $e_i(F_A^Q) = e_j(G_B^Q)$.

Proof Obvious. □

5 Application of Similarity of Q-ROFSSs in Covid-19

Now India has become largest affected countries of Covid-19 in Asia. It can be easily seen that the virus has spread to entire country with the worst hit states being Maharashtra (74,761 cases), Gujarat (32,643), Tamil Nadu (90,167) and Karnataka (15,242) on 30th Jun, 2020. Figure 1, show the total cases in these states on Jun 30, 2020.

In this section, we have tried to find similarity between two region of India being with the help of q-rung orthopair fuzzy soft set. We consider Two states Maharashtra and Gujarat of West region and Tamil Nadu and Karnataka of south region of India. Based on the data available from crowdsourced database of Covid-19 India dot org [36], four states details(Confirmed, Active and Recovered cases) created.Here only 20th April, 20th May and 20th July 2020 data were collected.

In our model universal set contain three elements i.e. $U = \{h_1, h_2, h_3\}$, where $h_1 =$ 20th April, $h_2 =$ 20th May, $h_3 =$ 20th Jun. Different States of regions of India is considered as a parameter set E. Let $E = \{e_1(\text{Maharashtra}), e_2(\text{Gujarat}), e_3(\text{Tamilnadu}), e_4(\text{Karnataka})\}$. Here we have used the following algorithms.

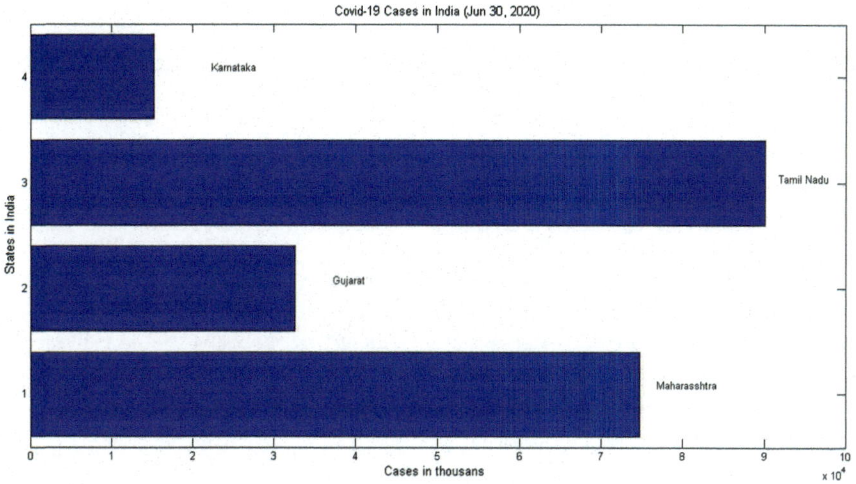

Fig. 1 Covid-19 cases in India (Jun 30, 2020)

Algorithms:
Step (i): To Collect data from crowdsourced database of Covid-19 India dot org [36] in tabular form.
Step (ii): To convert Step(i) data to decimal form with the help of confirmed cases.
Step (iii): To express step(ii) data q-RFSSs model F_A^Q and G_B^Q in tabular form.
Step (iv): To Express q-RFSSs model F_A^Q and G_B^Q for q=3,in tabular form.
Step (v): Find the similarity measures between q-RFSSs model F_A^Q and G_B^Q for q=3.
Step (vi): Find the similarity measures between q-rung orthopair fuzzy soft points of q-RFSSs model F_A^Q and G_B^Q for q=3.
Step (vii): If similarity values of Step(v) and Step(vi) are greater than 0.5 [20], then we conclude that the regions and states are possibly spread of Covid-19 similar.

Table 1 Date wise collected data

Date	Regions	State	Confirmed	Active	Recovered
20th April, 2020	West India	Maharashtra	4,666	3,862	572
20th April, 2020	West India	Gujarat	1,939	1,737	131
20th April, 2020	South India	Tamil Nadu	1,520	1,046	457
20th April, 2020	South India	Karnataka	408	280	112
20th May, 2020	West India	Maharashtra	39,297	27,589	10,318
20th May, 2020	West India	Gujarat	12,539	6,571	5,219
20th May, 2020	South India	Tamil Nadu	13,191	7,221	5,882
20th May, 2020	South India	Karnataka	1,462	864	556
20th Jun, 2020	West India	Maharashtra	1,28,205	58,054	64,153
20th Jun, 2020	West India	Gujarat	26,737	6,396	18,702
20th Jun, 2020	South India	Tamil Nadu	56,845	24,825	31,316
20th Jun, 2020	South India	Karnataka	8,697	3,168	5,393

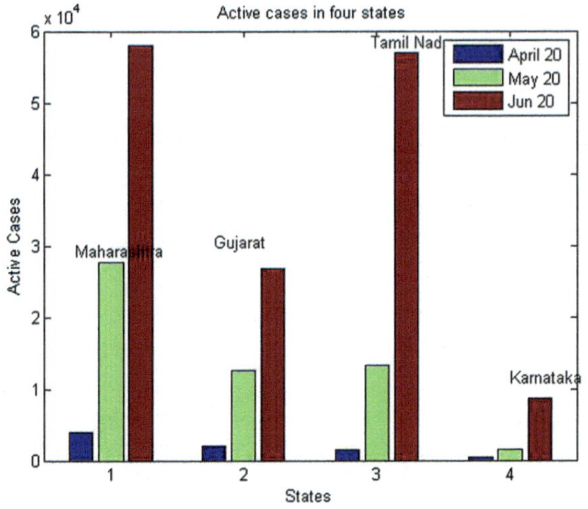

Fig. 2 Active cases in four states

We express active and recover cases in bar diagram from Table 1 in Figs. 2 and 3. Now we have express data (Table-2) q-ROFSSs F_A^Q and G_B^Q in Table-3. After this, we have convert q-ROFSSs F_A^Q and G_B^Q in Table-4 for q=3.

From Table 4 we have draw F_A^Q and G_B^Q with the help of Matlab in Graph 1, Graph 2 and Graph 3 as follows:

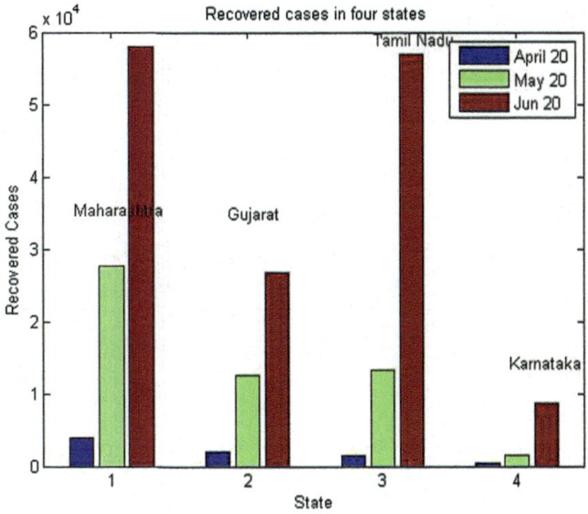

Fig. 3 Recovered cases in four states

Table 2 Date wise converted Data

Date	Regions	State	Active	Recovered
20th April, 2020	West India	Maharashtra	0.828	0.122
20th April, 2020	West India	Gujarat	0.895	0.068
20th April, 2020	South India	Tamil Nadu	0.688	0.301
20th April, 2020	South India	Karnataka	0.686	0.275
20th May, 2020	West India	Maharashtra	0.702	0.263
20th May, 2020	West India	Gujarat	0.524	0.416
20th May, 2020	South India	Tamil Nadu	0.547	0.446
20th May, 2020	South India	Karnataka	0.591	0.380
20th Jun, 2020	West India	Maharashtra	0.453	0.500
20th Jun, 2020	West India	Gujarat	0.239	0.699
20th Jun, 2020	South India	Tamil Nadu	0.437	0.551
20th Jun, 2020	South India	Karnataka	0.364	0.620

Table 3 Tabular form of F_A^Q and G_B^Q

F_A^Q	e_1	e_2
h_1	$(0.828, 0.122)_q$	$(0.895, 0.068)_q$
h_2	$(0.702, 0.263)_q$	$(0.524, 0.416)_q$
h_3	$(0.453, 0.500)_q$	$(0.239, 0.699)_q$
G_B^Q	e_3	e_4
h_1	$(0.688, 0.301)_q$	$(0.686, 0.275)_q$
h_2	$(0.547, 0.446)_q$	$(0.591, 0.380)_q$
h_3	$(0.437, 0.551)_q$	$(0.364, 0.620)_q$

Table 4 Tabular form of F_A^Q and G_B^Q for q = 3

F_A^Q	e_1	e_2
h_1	$(0.5677, 0.0018)_3$	$(0.7169, 0.0003)_3$
h_2	$(0.3459, 0.0182)_3$	$(0.1439, 0.0720)_3$
h_3	$(0.0930, 0.1250)_3$	$(0.0137, 0.3415)_3$
G_B^Q	e_3	e_4
h_1	$(0.3257, 0.0273)_3$	$(0.3228, 0.0208)_3$
h_2	$(0.1637, 0.0887)_3$	$(0.2064, 0.0549)_3$
h_3	$(0.0835, 0.1673)_3$	$(0.0482, 0.2383)_3$

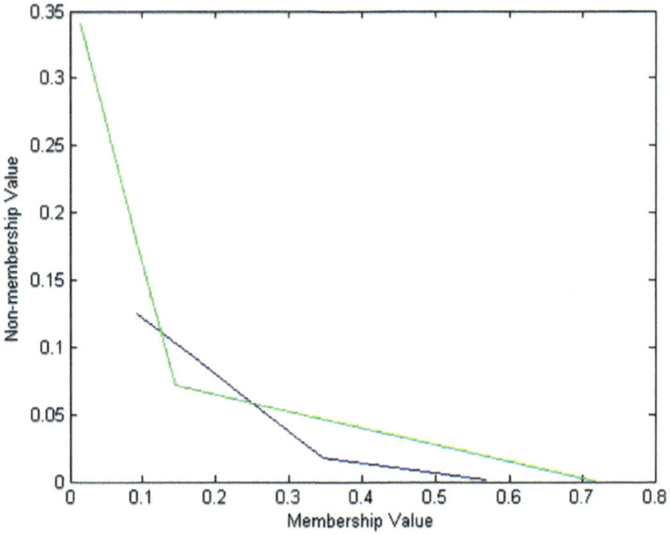

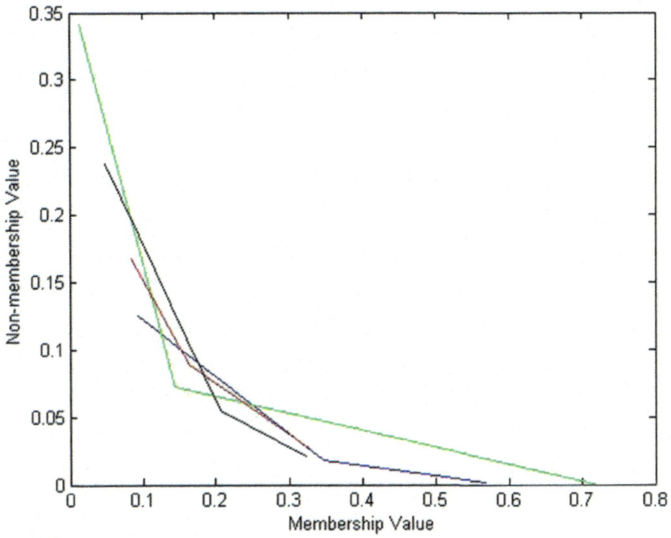

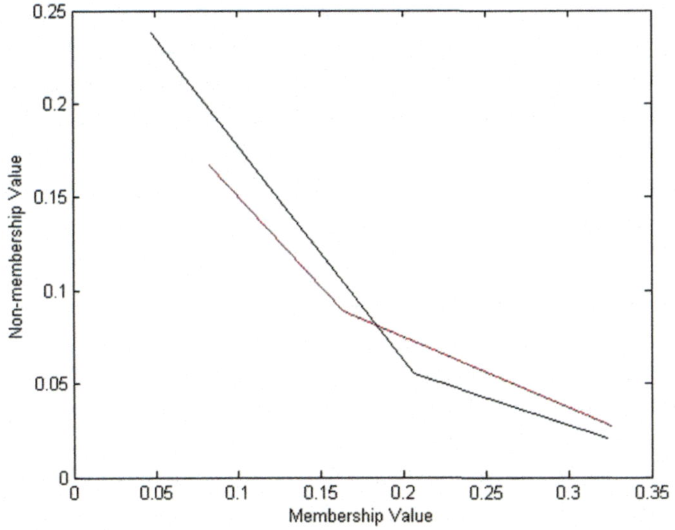

Finally, we have find the following values.

From the Table 5, we have seen that all the values greater than 0.5 except $\tilde{S}(e_2(F_A^Q), e_3(G_B^Q))$. Therefore both North and South region, and all states spread similarly Covid-19 except the states Gujarat and Tamil Nadu.

Table 5 Similarity in tabular form

$\tilde{S}(F_A^q, G_B^q) = 0.550. > 0.5.$	
Similarity between States	Values
$\tilde{S}(e_1(F_A^Q), e_3(G_B^Q))$	$0.5828 > 0.5.$
$\tilde{S}(e_1(F_A^Q), e_4(G_B^Q))$	$0.6214 > 0.5.$
$\tilde{S}(e_2(F_A^Q), e_3(G_B^Q))$	$0.4899 \cong 0.5.$
$\tilde{S}(e_2(F_A^Q), e_4(G_B^Q))$	$0.5286 > 0.5.$

6 Application of Weighted Similarity of Q-ROFSSs in Covid-19

In this section, we have been applying weight similarity measure of q-ROFSSs in Covid-19. Aim of the this section, to reduce to spread of the Covid-19 virus in the mention regions and states. Based on the number of tested samples of particular state, we have applied weight . Maharashtra, Gujarat, Tamil Nadu and Karnataka are completed 1.3M, 449.3K, 1.5M and 798.4K sample test on Jun 10, 2020. On basis of this data we find the weight 0.32, 0.11, 0.37 and 0.20 of the given states. Therefore weight of $\{e_1(\text{Maharashtra}) = 0.32, e_2(\text{Gujarat}) = 0.11, e_3(\text{Tamilnadu}) = 0.37 \text{ and } e_4(\text{Karnataka}) = 0.20\}$.

Here we have used the following algorithms.

Algorithms:
Step (i): To consider all the collected data of Sect. 5.
Step (ii): To multiplying the data(Table 4) by corresponding weight of parameters.
Step (iii): Find the weighted similarity measures between q-RFSSs model F_A^Q and G_B^Q for q=3.
Step (iv): Find the weighted similarity measures between q-rung orthopair fuzzy soft points of q-RFSSs model F_A^Q and G_B^Q for q=3.
Step (v): If similarity values of Step(iii) and Step(iv) are near to zero, then we conclude that the regions and states are reduce to spread of Covid-19 virus.

We have consider the data from Sect. 5 and implement of weight of the corresponding parameters, the Table 4 convert to Table 6 as

Table 6 Tabular form of $e_1(F_A^Q)$ and $e_2(G_B^Q)$ for q=3

F_A^Q	$e_1(0.32)$	$e_2(0.11)$
h_1	$(0.18166, 0.00058)_3$	$(0.07886, 0.00003)_3$
h_2	$(0.11069, 0.00580)_3$	$(0.01583, 0.00792)_3$
h_3	$(0.02976, 0.04000)_3$	$(0.00151, 0.03757)_3$
G_B^Q	$e_3(0.37)$	$e_4(0.20)$
h_1	$(0.12051, 0.01010)_3$	$(0.06456, 0..00416)_3$
h_2	$(0.06057, 0.03282)_3$	$(0.04128, 0.01098)_3$
h_3	$(0.03090, 0.06190)_3$	$(0.00964, 0.04766)_3$

Finally, we have find the following values.

Table 7 Weighted similarity in tabular form

$\tilde{W}S(F_A^Q, G_B^Q) = 0.03$	
Weighted similarity between States	Values
$\tilde{W}S(e_1(F_A^Q), e_3(G_B^Q))$	0.06.
$\tilde{W}S(e_1(F_A^Q), e_4(G_B^Q))$	0.03.
$\tilde{W}S(e_2(F_A^Q), e_3(G_B^Q))$	0.11.
$\tilde{W}S(e_2(F_A^Q), e_4(G_B^Q))$	0.06.

From the Table 7, we have seen that all the values of weighted similarity nearest to zero.

7 Conclusion

In this chapter, a new similarity measure and a weighted similarity measure for q-RFSSs and q-RFSPs are presented and some of its basic properties are being discussed. Moreover, we provide an application of q-ROFSSs in Covid-19 virus. we have proposed deep learning models for predicting the number of Covid-19 confirm cases in Indian states. Based on the number of active and recovered cases of Covid-19 of the states, we have prepared the algorithm. A control-theoretic approach is used to develop an epidemic model to find similarity of four most effected states of two regions of India. Results depict a rapid increase in the number of cases in the coming days. However, it is pertinent to mention that the future estimation provide is subjected to certain system parameters and can vary based on the external inputs like lock-down measures, social-distancing, vaccine/drug development, rapid testing, etc. This approach will be useful to handle several realistic uncertainty problems such as problems in pattern recognition, image processing, coding theory, economic system etc.

References

1. Arora, P., Kumar, H., Panigrahi, B.K.: Prediction and analysis of COVID-19 positive cases using deep learning models: A descriptive case study of India. Chaos, Solit. Fractals **139**, 110017 (2020)
2. Atanassov, K.T.: Intuitionistic fuzzy sets. Fuzzy Sets Syst. **20**(1), 87–96 (1986)
3. Bustince, H., Burillo, P.: Vague sets are intuitionistic fuzzy sets. Fuzzy Sets Syst. **79**(3), 403–405 (1996)
4. Çaman, N., Enginolu, N.S.: Soft Set theory and Uni-int decision making. Euro. J. Oper. Res. **207**, 848–855 (2010)
5. Chen, S.M.: Measures of similarity between vague sets. Fuzzy Sets Syst. **74**, 217–223 (1995)
6. Chen, S.M., Yeh, M.S., Hsaio, P.Y.: A comparison of similarity measures of fuzzy values. Fuzzy Sets Syst. **72**(1), 79–89 (1995)
7. Chen, S.M.: Similarity measures between vague sets and between elements. IEEE Trans. Syst. Man. Cybern. (Part B) **27(1)**, 153–158. (1997)
8. Garg, H.: A novel correlation coefficients between Pythagorean fuzzy sets and its applications to decision making processes. Int. J. Intell. Syst. **31**(12), 1234–1252 (2016)
9. Hong, D.H., Kim, C.A.: Note on similarity measure between vague sets and elements. Inf. Sci. **115**, 83–96 (1999)
10. Hussain, A., Ali, M.I., Mahmood, T., Munir, M.: q-Rung orthopair fuzzy soft average aggregation operators and their application in multicriteria decision making. Int. J. Intell. Syst. **35**(4), 571–599 (2020)
11. Jiang, Y., Tang, Y., Chen, Q., Liu, H., Tang, J.: Interval-valued intuitionistic fuzzy soft sets and their properties. Comput. Math. Appl. **60**(3), 906–918 (2010)

12. Karaaslan1, F.: Similarity measure between possibility neutrosophic soft sets and its applications. U.P.B. Sci. Bull. Series A **78(3)** (2016) https://doi.org/10.5281/ZENODO.32275
13. Kharal, A., Ahmad, B.: Mapping on fuzzy soft classes. Adv. Fuzzy Syst. Article ID 407890, 6 pages, (2009) doi.org/10.1155/2009/407890
14. Liu, D., Chen, X., Peng, S.D.: Some cosine similarity measures and distance measures between q-rung orthopair fuzzy sets. Int. J. Intell. Syst. **34**, 1572–1587 (2019)
15. Li, F., XU, Z.Y.: Similarity measure between vague sets. Chinese J. Softw. **12(6)**, 922–927 (2001)
16. Maji, P.K., Roy, R., Biswas, R.: An application of soft sets in a decision making problem. Comput. Math. Appl. **44**, 1077–1083 (2002)
17. Maji, P.K., Biswas, R., Roy, A.R.: Soft set theory. Comput. Math. Appl. **45**, 555–562 (2003)
18. Maji, P.K., Biswas, R., Roy, A.R.: Fuzzy soft sets. J. Fuzzy Math. **9**(3), 589–602 (2001)
19. Maji, P.K., Biswas, R., Roy, A.R.: Intuitionistic fuzzy soft sets. J. Fuzzy Math. **9**(3), 677–692 (2001)
20. Majumdar, P., Samanta, S.K.: Similarity measure of soft sets. New Math. Natural Comput. **4**(1), 1–12 (2008)
21. Majumdar, P., Samanta, S.K.: Generalised fuzzy soft sets. Comput. Math. Appl. **59**(4), 1425–1432 (2010)
22. Majumdar, P., Samanta, S.K.: On Similarity measures of fuzzy soft sets. Int. J. Adv. Soft Comput. Appl. **3**(2), 1–8 (2011)
23. Melin, P., Monica, J.C., Sanchez, D., Castillo, O.: Analysis of spatial spread relationships of Coronavirus (COVID-19) pandemic in the world using self organizing maps. Chaos, Solit. Fractals **138**, 109917 (2020)
24. Molodstov, D.A.: Soft set theory-first result. Comput. Math. Appl. **37**, 19–31 (1999)
25. Molodtsov, D.A., Leonov, V.Y., Kovkov, D.V.: Soft sets technique and its application. Nechetkie Sistemy i Myagkie Vychisleniya **1**(1), 8–39 (2006)
26. Neog, T.J., Sut, D.K., Hazarika, G.C.: Fuzzy soft topological spaces. Inter. J. Latest Trends Math. **2**(1), 54–67 (2012)
27. Pappis, C.P., Karacapilidis, N.I.: A comparative assessment of measures of similarity of fuzzy values. Fuzzy Sets Syst. **56**, 171–174 (1993)
28. Peng, X., Yang, Y.: Some results for Pythagorean fuzzy sets. Int J. Intell Syst. **30**(11), 1133–1160 (2015)
29. Rafiqa, D., Suhaila, S.A., Bazaza, M.A: Evaluation and prediction of COVID-19 in India: a case study of worst hit states. Chaos, Solit. Fractals (2020) https://doi.org/10.1016/j.chaos.2020.110014.
30. Yager, R.R.: Pythagorean fuzzy subsets. In: Proceedings of the Joint IFSA World Congress and NAFIPS Annual Meeting. Edmonton, Canada, 57–6 (2013)
31. Yager, R.R.: Pythagorean membership grades in multicriteria decision making. IEEE Trans Fuzzy Syst. **22**, 958–965 (2014)
32. Yager, R.R., Alajlan, N.: Approximate reasoning with generalized orthopair fuzzy sets. Inf Fusion. **38**, 65–73 (2017)
33. Yager, R.R., Alajlan, N., Bazi, Y.: Aspects of generalized orthopair fuzzy sets. Int J Intell Syst. **33**(11), 2154–2174 (2018)
34. Yang, X., Lin, T.Y., Yang, J., Li, Y., Yu, D.: Combination of interval-valued fuzzy set and soft set. Comput Math. Appl. **58**(3), 521–527 (2009)
35. Zadeh, L.A.: Fuzzy sets. Inf. Control **8**, 338–353 (1965)
36. Govt. of India updates about Coronavirus link www.covid19india.org

Local Fractional Calculus to Design the Growth System of Covid-19 Using Measure of Non-compactness

Hemant Kumar Nashine and Rabha W. Ibrahim

Abstract In this chapter, we use the concept of local fractional calculus and measure of non-compactness to design the growth system of Covid-19. To achieve this, we establish a fixed point and coupled fixed point theorems for new μ-set contraction condition in partially ordered Banach spaces, whose positive cone $\mathbb{K}$ is normal. We provide adequate examples to validate the epidemic dynamics with graphical presentations. We also use present available data to validate it.

Keywords Fractional calculus · Epidemic model · SIR system · Partial ordered Banach spaces · Fixed point · Measures of noncompactness

1 Introduction

The application of mathematical representations to designate infectious disease changing aspects is a methodical approach of converting molds and information (statistical, numerical info) concerning disease diffusion into quantitative approximations of how an epidemic progresses through time and space. Alike methods are utilized in traditional physics to calculate the movement of a body by transforming inactivity and gravity and the force and direction at which a body is thrown (the information) into the curve of the body (the prediction). Epidemics of infectious diseases between persons are motivated by diffusion of the infectious mediator among persons directly, either by fomites (items or materials which are likely to carry infection, such as clothes, utensils, and furniture.) in the environment or by animal paths. Dis-

H. K. Nashine (✉)
Department of Mathematics, School of Advanced Sciences, Vellore Institute of Technology, Vellore 632014, TN, India

Department of Pure and Applied Mathematics, Faculty of science, University of Johannesburg, P O Box 524, Auckland Park, 2006, South Africa
e-mail: drhknashine@gmail.com; hemant.nashine@vit.ac.in

R. W. Ibrahim (✉)
Nonlinear Dynamics Research Center (NDRC), Ajman University, 346, Ajman, UAE
e-mail: rabhaibrahim@yahoo.com

P. Agarwal et al. (eds.), *Analysis of Infectious Disease Problems (Covid-19) and Their Global Impact*, Infosys Science Foundation Series,
https://doi.org/10.1007/978-981-16-2450-6_20

ease diffusion can similarly depend on biological features of both the pathogen and the host, as well as shared, communication and environmental factors. It is promising to definite these dynamics in expressions of mathematical equations. While the dynamics of infectious diseases can be exceedingly complex, in numerous suitcases comparatively parsimonious simulations can be utilized to designate the necessary properties of epidemic dynamics.

The outcome Susceptible-Infectious-Recovered (SIR) system can be utilized to refer to the number of persons in each class on time t, ($\varsigma(t)$, $\Upsilon(t)$ and $\rho(t)$) based on two supplementary molds. Originally, the rate at which predisposed persons become infected through any interval of fractal time Δ^γ (see [35]) is expected to be related to the frequency of infectious persons. Secondly, infected persons recover with lifelong immunity after an average infectious period. These conventions can be interpreted into the following fractal equations labeling the epidemic dynamics:

$$\begin{aligned} \Delta^\gamma \varsigma(t) &= -B\Upsilon(t)\varsigma(t) \\ \Delta^\gamma \Upsilon(t) &= B\Upsilon(t)\varsigma(t) - A\Upsilon(t), \end{aligned} \tag{1}$$

where

$$\Delta^\gamma \varsigma(t) = \frac{\Gamma(\gamma+1)[\varsigma(t) - \varsigma(t_0)]}{(t-t_0)^\gamma}, \quad \gamma \in (0, 1]$$

similarly,

$$\Delta^\gamma \Upsilon(t) = \frac{\Gamma(\gamma+1)[\Upsilon(t) - \Upsilon(t_0)]}{(t-t_0)^\gamma}, \quad \gamma \in (0, 1]$$

and A and B are the connection constants. Basically, theses constant are defined the reproductive number $\varrho := \frac{BN}{A}$, where $N = \varsigma + \Upsilon$ at time t. This rate is indicated as the regular number of secondary cases created by an index instance when an epidemic arises in a entirely inclined people. If $\varrho < 1$, then an amount will die, out devoid of producing extensive infections. For a given $\varrho > 1$, the epidemic could yield an epidemic and a smaller generation time would be related with higher growth rate.

In 1930, Kuratowski [15] discussed a new direction of research with the notion of MNC that combines with some algebraic arguments are useful for studying the mathematical formulations, particularly for solving the existence of solutions of some nonlinear problems under certain conditions. The Kuratowskii and Hausdorff MNC in a metric space are well-known in the literature. Fixed point theory has two main branches: Constructive fixed point theorems in the line of Banach Contraction Principle, and nonconstructive fixed point theorems, where results are obtained by using topological properties in the direction of Brouwer's/ Schauder's/ Darbo's fixed point theorem. Schauder discussed the convexity of domains and the compactness of operators. Darbo relaxed the strong condition of compactness of operators with the use of MNC and defined appropriate classes of operators [8] which is extended and generalized by many authors [1, 2, 4, 5, 14, 16–22, 32].

On the other hand, Ran and Reurings [31] was the first who extended the Banach contraction principle to partially ordered sets with applications to linear and nonlinear matrix equations. Subsequently, Nieto and Rodríguez-López [28, 29], Nashine and Samet [25] and many others extended the results [31] and given application to ordinary differential equation and integral equation. The combination of MNC with partially ordered normed and Banach spaces are discussed in the literature [9, 10, 23, 24, 26, 27, 30, 33, 34].

With above discussion in mind, an attempt has been made to give monotone version with the relaxed conditions of domain of underlying operator into partially ordered Banach spaces. To achieve the proposed results in partially ordered Banach spaces, we define a notion of MNC. Then we use this notion to prove some FPTs for $\mu-$set contraction condition in partially ordered Banach spaces whose positive cone $\mathbb{K}$ is norm. We will relaxed the conditions of bounds, closed and convexity of the domain of operator at the expense that the operator is monotone and bounded. Further we apply the coupled fixed point result to get solution of epidemic dynamic system for $\gamma = 1$. Finally we illustrate some examples to validate the epidemic dynamics with graphical presentations. We also use present WHO available data to verify it.

2 Preliminaries

Let $(\mathcal{X}, \|\cdot\|)$ is an infinite dimensional Banach space and θ be its zero element. $\mathcal{B}(\vartheta, \varsigma)$ will denote the closed ball with center ϑ are radius ς and $\mathcal{B}_\varsigma$ will stand for $\mathcal{B}(\theta, \varsigma)$. Moreover, $\mathcal{M}_\mathcal{X}$ will denote the family of nonempty bounded subsets of $\mathcal{X}$ and $\mathcal{N}_\mathcal{X}$ its subfamily consisting of all relatively compact sets.

Definition 1 [6] A mapping $\mu : \mathcal{M}_\mathcal{X} \to \mathbb{R}^+$ is said to be a measure of noncompactness (MNC, for short) in $\mathcal{X}$ if it satisfies the following conditions ($\mathcal{Y}, \mathcal{Y}_1, \mathcal{Y}_2 \in \mathcal{M}_\mathcal{X}$):

(1°) $\ker \mu := \{\mathcal{Y} \in \mathcal{M}_\mathcal{X} : \mu(\mathcal{Y}) = 0\} \neq \emptyset$ and $\ker \mu \subset \mathcal{N}_\mathcal{X}$,
(2°) $\mathcal{Y}_1 \subseteq \mathcal{Y}_2 \Rightarrow \mu(\mathcal{Y}_1) \leq \mu(\mathcal{Y}_2)$,
(3°) $\mu(\overline{\mathcal{Y}}) = \mu(\mathcal{Y})$,
(4°) $\mu(\text{conv}\, \mathcal{Y}) = \mu(\mathcal{Y})$,
(5°) $\mu(\lambda\mathcal{Y}_1 + (1-\lambda)\mathcal{Y}_2) \leq \lambda\mu(\mathcal{Y}_1) + (1-\lambda)\mu(\mathcal{Y}_2)$ for $\lambda \in [0, 1]$,
(6°) $\mu(\mathcal{Y}_1 \cup \mathcal{Y}_2) = \max\{\mu(\mathcal{Y}_1), \mu(\mathcal{Y}_2)\}$,
(7°) If $(\mathcal{Y}_n)$ is a decreasing sequence of non-empty closed sets in $\mathcal{M}_\mathcal{X}$ and if $\lim_{n\to\infty} \mu(\mathcal{Y}_n) = 0$, then the set $\mathcal{Y}_\infty = \bigcap_{n=1}^{\infty} \mathcal{Y}_n$ is non-empty and compact.

A map $\alpha : \mathcal{M}_\mathcal{X} \to \mathbb{R}^+$ is said to be a Kuratowski MNC [15] if

$$\alpha(\mathcal{Y}) = \inf\left\{\epsilon > 0 : \mathcal{Y} \subset \bigcup_{k=1}^{n} \mathcal{S}_k, \mathcal{S}_k \subset \mathcal{X}, \text{diam}(\mathcal{S}_k) < \epsilon \ (k \in \mathbb{N})\right\}. \tag{2}$$

We denote $\Lambda(\mathcal{X})$ a nonempty, bounded, closed and convex set on Banach space $\mathcal{X}$. The following extensions of topological Schauder fixed point theorem and classical Banach fixed point theorem were proved by Darbo (DFPT, in short) in 1955.

Theorem 1 *[6] Let $\mathcal{X}$ be a Banach space, $\mathcal{Y} \in \Lambda(\mathcal{X})$ and $\mathcal{T} : \mathcal{Y} \to \mathcal{Y}$ be a continuous operator such that there exists a $\lambda \in [0, 1)$ with*

$$\mu(\mathcal{T}(\mathcal{A})) \leq \lambda\, \mu(\mathcal{A})$$

for any $\emptyset \neq \mathcal{A} \subset \mathcal{Y}$, here μ is the Kuratowski MNC on $\mathcal{X}$. Then we can conclude that $\mathcal{T}$ has a fixed point.

3 Fixed Point Results

Let $\mathcal{X}$ be a Banach space with the norm $\|\cdot\|$ whose positive cone is defined by $\mathbb{K} = \{x \in \mathcal{X} : x \geq 0\}$. We have $(\mathcal{X}, \|\cdot\|)$ is a partially ordered Banach space with the order relation $\sqsubseteq$ induced by cone $\mathbb{K}$.

Definition 2 [7] A continuous mapping $F : \mathbb{R}_+^2 \to \mathbb{R}$ is called a C-class function if it is satisfies

(1) $F(s, t) \leq s$,
(2) $F(s, t) = s$ implies that either $s = 0$ or $t = 0$, for all $s, t \in \mathbb{R}_+$.

Definition 3 [7] A C-class function has a property C_F, if there exists a $C_F \geq 0$ such that

(1) $F(s, t) > C_F \Rightarrow s > t$,
(2) $F(t, t) \leq C_F$, for all $s, t \in \mathbb{R}_+$.

Definition 4 [7]. Let $\Delta(\Theta, C_F)$ be the family of extended C_F-simulation functions $\Theta : \mathbb{R}_+^2 \to \mathbb{R}$ satisfying following conditions:

(Δ_1) $\Theta(s, t) < F(t, s)$ for all $s, t > 0$, where $F \in C$ with property C_F;
(Δ_2) if $\{s_n\}, \{t_n\} \in (0, +\infty)$ such that $\lim_{n\to\infty} s_n = \lim_{n\to\infty} t_n = \ell$, where $\ell \in (0, +\infty)$ and $t_n > \ell$ for all $n \in \mathbb{N}$, then $\limsup_{n\to\infty} \Theta(s_n, t_n) < C_F$;
(Δ_3) if $\{s_n\} \in (0, +\infty)$ such that $\lim_{n\to\infty} s_n = \ell \in (0, +\infty)$, $\Theta(s_n, \ell) \geq C_F$ implies $\ell = 0$.

We denote Geraghty function [12] as family of functions,
$\Omega := \{\beta : [0, +\infty) \to (0, 1)|$ for $\{\zeta_n\} \subset [0, +\infty)$ and $\lim_{n\to+\infty} \beta(\zeta_n) = 1^-$ implies $\zeta_n \to 0^+$ as $n \to +\infty\}$.

We now discuss our results in partially ordered Banach spaces.

Theorem 2 *Let $(\mathcal{X}, \|\cdot\|, \sqsubseteq)$ be a partially ordered Banach space, whose positive cone $\mathbb{K}$ is normal. Suppose that $\mathcal{T} : \mathcal{X} \to \mathcal{X}$ is a continuous, nondecreasing and bounded mapping satisfying the following contraction:*

$$\Theta(\mu(\mathcal{T}\mathcal{V}), \beta(\mu(\mathcal{V}))\mu(\mathcal{V})) \geq C_F \tag{3}$$

for all nonempty bounded subset $\mathcal{V}$ in $\mathcal{X}$, where μ denotes the arbitrary MNC, $\Theta \in \Delta(\Theta, C_F)$ and $\beta \in \Omega$.

If there exists an element $\varsigma_0 \in \mathcal{X}$ such that $\varsigma_0 \sqsubseteq \mathcal{T}\varsigma_0$, then $\mathcal{T}$ has a fixed point ϱ^* and the sequence $\{\mathcal{T}^n \varsigma_0\}$ of successive iterations converges monotonically to ϱ^*.

Proof Assume $\varsigma_0 \in \mathcal{X}$ and define a sequence $\{\varsigma_n\} \subset \mathcal{X}$ by

$$\varsigma_{n+1} = \mathcal{T}\varsigma_n, n \in \mathbb{N}^* = \mathbb{N} \cup \{0\} \tag{4}$$

Since $\mathcal{T}$ is nondecreasing and $\varsigma_0 \sqsubseteq \mathcal{T}\varsigma_0$, we have

$$\varsigma_0 \sqsubseteq \varsigma_1 \sqsubseteq \varsigma_2 \sqsubseteq \ldots \sqsubseteq \varsigma_n \sqsubseteq \ldots \tag{5}$$

Denote $\mathcal{U}_n = \overline{conv}\{\varsigma_n, \varsigma_{n+1}, \ldots\}$ for $n \in \mathbb{N}^*$. By (4) and (5), each $\mathcal{U}_n$ is a bounded and closed subset in $\mathcal{X}$ and

$$\mathcal{U}_0 \supset \mathcal{U}_1 \supset \ldots \supset \mathcal{U}_n \supset \ldots. \tag{6}$$

Following (3), we obtain

$$\begin{aligned}\Theta(\mu(\mathcal{U}_{n+1}), \beta(\mu(\mathcal{U}_n))\mu(\mathcal{U}_n)) &= \Theta(\mu(\overline{\text{Conv}}(\mathcal{T}\mathcal{U}_n)), \beta(\mu(\mathcal{U}_n))\mu(\mathcal{U}_n))\\ &= \Theta(\mu(\mathcal{T}\mathcal{U}_n), \beta(\mu(\mathcal{U}_n))\mu(\mathcal{U}_n))\\ &\geq C_F,\end{aligned}$$

that is,

$$\begin{aligned}C_F &\leq \Theta(\mu(\mathcal{U}_{n+1}), \beta(\mu(\mathcal{U}_n))\mu(\mathcal{U}_n))\\ &\leq F(\beta(\mu(\mathcal{U}_n))\mu(\mathcal{U}_n), \mu(\mathcal{U}_{n+1}))\\ \beta(\mu(\mathcal{U}_n))\mu(\mathcal{U}_n) &> \mu(\mathcal{U}_{n+1})\\ \mu(\mathcal{U}_n) &> \mu(\mathcal{U}_{n+1})\end{aligned} \tag{7}$$

for all $n \in \mathbb{N}$.

By the construction of $\mathcal{U}_n$, it is clear that $\mathcal{U}_{n+1} \subset \mathcal{U}_n$ and so by the Definition 1.1, the sequence $\{\mathcal{U}_n\}$ is nonincreasing and nonnegative. Thus, there exists $\varrho \to 0$ such that $\mu(\mathcal{U}_n) \to \varrho$ when $n \to \infty$.

Suppose, to the contrary, that $\varrho \neq 0$. Therefore from (7) we have

$$\frac{\mu(\mathcal{U}_{n+1})}{\mu(\mathcal{U}_n)} \leq \beta(\mu(\mathcal{U}_n)) < 1.$$

This yields

$$\beta(\mu(\mathcal{U}_n)) \to 1 \text{ as } n \to \infty.$$

Since $\beta \in \Omega$, we get $\varrho = 0$, and hence

$$\mu(\mathcal{U}_n) \to 0, \text{ as } n \to \infty.$$

Since $\mathcal{U}_n \subset \mathcal{U}_{n-1}$, we have

$$\overline{\mathcal{U}_\infty} = \bigcap_{n=1}^{\infty} \mathcal{U}_n \neq \emptyset \text{ and } \mathcal{U}_\infty \in Ker\mu.$$

Hence, for every $\epsilon > 0$ there exists an $n_0 \in \mathbb{N}$ such that

$$\mu(\mathcal{U}_n) < \epsilon \ \forall n \geq n_0.$$

This concluded that $\overline{\mathcal{U}_{n_0}}$ and consequently $\mathcal{U}_0$ is a compact chain in $\mathcal{X}$. Hence, $\{\varsigma_n\}$ has a convergent subsequence. Applying the monotone property of $\mathcal{T}$ and the normality of cone $\mathbb{K}$, the whole sequence $\{\varsigma_n\} = \{\mathcal{T}^n \varsigma_0\}$ converges monotonically to a point, say $\varrho^* \in \mathcal{U}_0$. Finally, from the continuity of $\mathcal{T}$, we get

$$\mathcal{T}\varrho^* = \mathcal{T}(\lim_{n\to\infty} \varsigma_n) = \lim_{n\to\infty} \mathcal{T}\varsigma_n = \lim_{n\to\infty} \varsigma_{n+1} = \varrho^*.$$

□

On different setting of functions $\Theta \in \Delta(\Theta, C_F)$ and $\beta \in \Omega$ satisfying the condition (3) in Theorem 2, we can get some new fixed point results.

Theorem 3 *Let $(\mathcal{X}, \|\cdot\|, \sqsubseteq)$ be a partially ordered Banach space, whose positive cone $\mathbb{K}$ is normal. Suppose that $\mathcal{T} : \mathcal{X} \to \mathcal{X}$ is a continuous, nondecreasing and bounded mapping satisfying the following contraction:*

$$\Theta(\mu(\mathcal{T}\mathcal{V}), \beta(\mu(\mathcal{V}))\mu(\mathcal{V})) \geq 0 \tag{8}$$

for all nonempty bounded subset $\mathcal{V}$ in $\mathcal{X}$, where μ denotes the arbitrary MNC, $\Theta \in \Delta(\Theta, C_F)$ and $\beta \in \Omega$.

If there exists an element $\varsigma_0 \in \mathcal{X}$ such that $\varsigma_0 \sqsubseteq \mathcal{T}\varsigma_0$, then $\mathcal{T}$ has a fixed point ϱ^* and the sequence $\{\mathcal{T}^n\varsigma_0\}$ converges monotonically to ϱ^*.

Proof If we set $\Delta(\Theta, C_F)$ with $C_F = 0$ in Theorem 2, we get the result. □

If we set

$$\psi(\zeta) = \begin{cases} \varphi(\zeta), & \text{for } 0 \leq \zeta \leq \mu(\mathcal{X}), \\ \varphi(\beta(\mathcal{X})), & \text{for } \zeta > \mu(\mathcal{X}) \end{cases} \tag{9}$$

and $\beta(\zeta) = \frac{\psi(\zeta)}{\zeta}$ for $\zeta > 0$ and $\beta(0) = \frac{1}{2}$.

Theorem 4 *Let $(\mathcal{X}, \|\cdot\|, \sqsubseteq)$ be a partially ordered Banach space, whose positive cone $\mathbb{K}$ is normal. Suppose that $\mathcal{T} : \mathcal{X} \to \mathcal{X}$ is a continuous, non-decreasing and bounded mapping satisfying the following contraction:*

$$\Theta(\mu(\mathcal{T}\mathcal{V}), \varphi(\mu(\mathcal{V}))) \geq C_F \tag{10}$$

for all nonempty bounded subset $\mathcal{V}$ *in* $\mathcal{X}$*, where* μ *denotes the arbitrary MNC,* $\Theta \in \Delta(\Theta, C_F)$ *and* $\varphi : \mathbb{R}_+ \to \mathbb{R}_+$ *is a nondecreasing and upper semi-continuous function such that* $\varphi(\zeta) < \zeta$ *for all* $\zeta > 0$.

If $\exists$ *an element* $\varsigma_0 \in \mathcal{X}$ *such that* $\varsigma_0 \sqsubseteq \mathcal{T}\varsigma_0$*, then* $\mathcal{T}$ *has a fixed point* ϱ^* *and the sequence* $\{\mathcal{T}^n\varsigma_0\}$ *of successive iterations converges monotonically to* ϱ^*.

Proof The proof follows of Theorem 2 and Corollary 2.2 in [1], with φ given in (9). □

Theorem 5 *Let* $(\mathcal{X}, \|\cdot\|, \sqsubseteq)$ *be a partially ordered Banach space, whose positive cone* $\mathbb{K}$ *is normal. Suppose that* $\mathcal{T} : \mathcal{X} \to \mathcal{X}$ *is a continuous, nondecreasing and bounded mapping satisfying the following contraction:*

$$\Theta(\mu(\mathcal{T}\mathcal{V}), \lambda\, \mu(\mathcal{V})) \geq 0 \tag{11}$$

for all nonempty bounded subset $\mathcal{V}$ *in* $\mathcal{X}$*, where* μ *denotes the arbitrary MNC,* $\Theta \in \Delta(\Theta, C_F)$ *and* $\lambda \in [0, 1)$.

If there exists an element $\varsigma_0 \in \mathcal{X}$ *such that* $\varsigma_0 \sqsubseteq \mathcal{T}\varsigma_0$*, then* $\mathcal{T}$ *has a fixed point* ϱ^* *and the sequence* $\{\mathcal{T}^n\varsigma_0\}$ *of successive iterations converges monotonically to* ϱ^*.

If we take $diam(\mathcal{U}) = diameter\ of\ \mathcal{U}$, then we have

Proposition 1 *Let* $(\mathcal{X}, \|\cdot\|, \sqsubseteq)$ *be a partially ordered Banach space, whose positive cone* $\mathbb{K}$ *is normal. Suppose that* $\mathcal{T} : \mathcal{X} \to \mathcal{X}$ *is a continuous, nondecreasing and bounded mapping satisfying the following contraction:*

$$\Theta(diam(\mathcal{T}(\mathcal{V})), \lambda\, diam(\mathcal{V})) \geq C_F \tag{12}$$

for all nonempty bounded subset $\mathcal{V}$ *in* $\mathcal{X}$*, where* $\Theta \in \Delta(\Theta, C_F)$ *and* $\lambda \in [0, 1)$.

If there exists an element $\varsigma_0 \in \mathcal{X}$ *such that* $\varsigma_0 \sqsubseteq \mathcal{T}\varsigma_0$*, then* $\mathcal{T}$ *has a fixed point* ϱ^* *and the sequence* $\{\mathcal{T}^n\varsigma_0\}$ *of successive iterations converges monotonically to* ϱ^*.

Proof Theorem 2 and Proposition 3.2 [11] claim the existence of a $\mathcal{T}$-invariant nonempty closed convex subset $\mathcal{V}$ with $\text{diam}(\mathcal{V}_\infty) = 0$, that is, $\mathcal{V}_\infty$ has singleton element, hence fixed point of $\mathcal{T} \neq \emptyset$.

To prove uniqueness, we suppose that there exist two distinct fixed points $\zeta, \xi \in \mathcal{V}$, then we may define the set $\mathcal{U} := \{\zeta, \xi\}$. In this case $\text{diam}(\mathcal{U}) = \text{diam}(\mathcal{T}(\mathcal{U})) = \|\xi - \zeta\| > 0$. Then using (12), we get

$$\begin{aligned} C_F &\leq \Theta(\text{diam}(\mathcal{T}(\mathcal{U})), \lambda\, \text{diam}(\mathcal{U})) \\ &\leq F(\text{diam}(\mathcal{U}), \lambda\, \text{diam}(\mathcal{U})), \end{aligned}$$

a contradiction from Definition 3 and hence the result. □

Following is the generalized classical fixed point result derived from Theorem 4.

Theorem 6 *Let $(\mathcal{X}, \|\cdot\|, \sqsubseteq)$ be a partially ordered Banach space, whose positive cone $\mathbb{K}$ is normal. Suppose that $\mathcal{T} : \mathcal{X} \to \mathcal{X}$ is a continuous, nondecreasing and bounded mapping satisfying the following contraction:*

$$\Theta(\|\mathcal{T}\zeta - \mathcal{T}\xi\|, \lambda \|\zeta - \xi\|) \geq C_F \tag{13}$$

for all $\zeta, \xi \in \mathcal{X}$, where $\Theta \in \Delta(\Theta, C_F)$ and $\lambda \in [0, 1)$. If there exists an element $\varsigma_0 \in \mathcal{X}$ such that $\varsigma_0 \sqsubseteq \mathcal{T}\varsigma_0$, then $\mathcal{T}$ has a unique fixed point ϱ^* and the sequence $\{\mathcal{T}^n \varsigma_0\}$ of successive iterations converges monotonically to ϱ^*.

Proof Let $\mu : \mathcal{M}_{\mathcal{X}} \to \mathbb{R}^+$ be a set quantity defined by the formula $\mu(\mathcal{X}) = diam\mathcal{X}$, where $diam\mathcal{X} = \sup\{\|\zeta - \xi\| : \zeta, \xi \in \mathcal{X}\}$ stands for the diameter of $\mathcal{X}$. It is easily seen that μ is a MNC in a space $\mathcal{X}$ in the sense of Definition 1. Therefore from (13) we have

$$\begin{aligned} C_F &\leq \sup_{\zeta,\xi\in\mathcal{U}} \Theta(\|\mathcal{T}\zeta - \mathcal{T}\xi\|, \lambda \|\zeta - \xi\|) \\ &\leq \Theta(\sup_{\zeta,\xi\in\mathcal{U}} \|\mathcal{T}\zeta - \mathcal{T}\xi\|, \lambda \sup_{\zeta,\xi\in\mathcal{U}} \|\zeta - \xi\|) \\ &= \Theta(diam(\mathcal{T}(\mathcal{U})), \lambda\, diam(\mathcal{U})) \end{aligned}$$

which implies that

$$\Theta(diam(\mathcal{T}(\mathcal{U})), \lambda\, diam(\mathcal{U})) \geq C_F.$$

Thus following Theorem 4, $\mathcal{T}$ has an unique fixed point. □

Definition 5 [13] An element $(u^*, v^*) \in \mathcal{X}^2$ is called a coupled fixed point of a mapping $\mathcal{G} : \mathcal{X}^2 \to \mathcal{X}$ if $\mathcal{G}(u^*, v^*) = u^*$ and $\mathcal{G}(v^*, u^*) = v^*$.

Definition 6 Let $(\mathcal{X}, \|\cdot\|, \sqsubseteq)$ be a partially ordered Banach space and let $\mathcal{G} : \mathcal{X}^2 \to \mathcal{X}$ be a mapping. A map $\mathcal{G}$ is said to have the monotone property if $\mathcal{G}(u, v)$ is monotone nondecreasing in both variables u and v, that is, for any $u, v \in \mathcal{X}$,

$$u_1, u_2 \in \mathcal{X},\ u_1 \sqsubseteq u_2 \Rightarrow \mathcal{G}(u_1, v) \sqsubseteq \mathcal{G}(u_2, v)$$

and

$$v_1, v_2 \in \mathcal{X},\ v_1 \sqsubseteq v_2 \Rightarrow \mathcal{G}(u, v_1) \sqsubseteq \mathcal{G}(u, v_2).$$

Lemma 1 *[3] Suppose that $\mu_1, \mu_2, \ldots, \mu_n$ are MNCs (in Banach spaces $\mathcal{X}_1, \mathcal{X}_2, \ldots, \mathcal{X}_n$), respectively. We assume that the function $\mathcal{G} : \mathbb{R}^n_+ \to \mathbb{R}_+$ is convex and $\mathcal{G}(\zeta_1, \zeta_2, \ldots, \zeta_n) = 0$ if and only if $\zeta_i = 0$ for $i = 1, 2, 3, \ldots, n$. Then*

$$\mu(\mathfrak{B}) = \mathcal{G}(\mu_1(\mathfrak{B}_1), \mu_2(\mathfrak{B}_2), \ldots, \mu_n(\mathfrak{B}_n)),$$

defines a MNCs in $\mathcal{X}_1 \times \mathcal{X}_2 \times \mathcal{X}_3 \times \ldots \times \mathcal{X}_n$ where $\mathfrak{B}_i$ denotes the natural projection of $\mathfrak{B}$ into $\mathcal{X}_i$, for $i = 1, 2, 3, \ldots, n$.

Theorem 7 *Let $(\mathcal{X}, \|\cdot\|, \sqsubseteq)$ be a partially ordered Banach space whose positive cone $\mathbb{K}$ is normal. Suppose that $\mathcal{G} : \mathcal{X}^2 \to \mathcal{X}$ is a continuous and bounded mapping, having monotone property and satisfying*

$$\Theta(\mu(\mathcal{G}(\mathfrak{B}_1 \times \mathfrak{B}_2)), \beta(\max\{\mu(\mathfrak{B}_1), \mu(\mathfrak{B}_2)\}) \max\{\mu(\mathfrak{B}_1), \mu(\mathfrak{B}_2)\}) \leq C_F \quad (14)$$

for all bounded subsets $\mathfrak{B}_1, \mathfrak{B}_2$ in $\mathcal{X}$, where μ denotes the MNC in $\mathcal{X}^2$, $\Theta \in \Delta(\Theta, C_F)$ and $\beta \in \Omega$. If there exist elements $u_0, v_0 \in \mathcal{X}$ such that $u_0 \sqsubseteq \mathcal{G}(u_0, v)$ for any $v \in \mathcal{X}$ and $v_0 \sqsubseteq \mathcal{G}(v_0, u)$ for any $u \in \mathcal{X}$, then $\mathcal{G}$ has at least a coupled fixed point (u^*, v^*).

Proof We consider the map $\widehat{\mathcal{G}} : \mathcal{X}^2 \to \mathcal{X}^2$ defined by

$$\widehat{\mathcal{G}}(u, v) = (\mathcal{G}(u, v), \mathcal{G}(v, u)).$$

Then $\widehat{\mathcal{G}}$ is a continuous and bounded mapping, having monotone property.

For any $\mathfrak{B} = \mathfrak{B}_1 \times \mathfrak{B}_2$, we define a new MNC in the space $\mathcal{X}^2$ as

$$\widehat{\mu}(\mathfrak{B}) = \max\{\mu(\mathfrak{B}_1), \mu(\mathfrak{B}_2)\}$$

where $\mathfrak{B}_i$, $i = 1, 2$ denote the natural projections of $\mathfrak{B}$. Now let $\mathfrak{B} \subset \mathcal{X}^2$ with $\mathfrak{B} = \mathfrak{B}_1 \times \mathfrak{B}_2$ be a nonempty bounded subset. We can conclude

$$\begin{aligned}
&\Theta(\widehat{\mu}(\widehat{\mathcal{G}}(\mathfrak{B})), \beta(\widehat{\mu}(\mathfrak{B}))\widehat{\mu}(\mathfrak{B})) \\
&\leq \Theta(\widehat{\mu}(\mathcal{G}(\mathfrak{B}_1 \times \mathfrak{B}_2) \times \mathcal{G}(\mathfrak{B}_2 \times \mathfrak{B}_1)), \beta(\max\{\mu(\mathfrak{B}_1), \mu(\mathfrak{B}_2)\}) \max\{\mu(\mathfrak{B}_1), \mu(\mathfrak{B}_2)\}) \\
&= \Theta(\max\{\mu(\mathcal{G}(\mathfrak{B}_1 \times \mathfrak{B}_2)), \mu(\mathcal{G}(\mathfrak{B}_2 \times \mathfrak{B}_1))\}, \beta(\max\{\mu(\mathfrak{B}_1), \mu(\mathfrak{B}_2)\}) \max\{\mu(\mathfrak{B}_1), \mu(\mathfrak{B}_2)\}) \\
&= \max\left\{ \begin{array}{l} \Theta(\mu(\mathcal{G}(\mathfrak{B}_1 \times \mathfrak{B}_2)), \beta(\max\{\mu(\mathfrak{B}_1), \mu(\mathfrak{B}_2)\}) \max\{\mu(\mathfrak{B}_1), \mu(\mathfrak{B}_2)\}), \\ \Theta(\mu(\mathcal{G}(\mathfrak{B}_2 \times \mathfrak{B}_1)), \beta(\max\{\mu(\mathfrak{B}_2), \mu(\mathfrak{B}_1)\}) \max\{\mu(\mathfrak{B}_2), \mu(\mathfrak{B}_1)\}) \end{array} \right\} \\
&\geq C_F.
\end{aligned}$$

That is,

$$\Theta(\widehat{\mu}(\widehat{\mathcal{G}}(\mathfrak{B})), \beta(\widehat{\mu}(\mathfrak{B}))\widehat{\mu}(\mathfrak{B})) \geq C_F.$$

Next, we show that there is a $\widehat{u}_0 \in \mathfrak{B}$ such that $\widehat{u}_0 \sqsubseteq \widehat{\mathcal{G}}(\widehat{u}_0)$. Since there exist elements $u_0, v_0 \in \mathcal{X}$ such that $u_0 \sqsubseteq \mathcal{G}(u_0, v)$ for any $v \in \mathcal{X}$ and $v_0 \sqsubseteq \mathcal{G}(v_0, u)$ for any $u \in \mathcal{X}$, set $\widehat{u}_0 = (u_0, v_0)$. Then by the definition of $\widehat{\mathcal{G}}$, we have

$$\begin{aligned}
\widehat{u}_0 = (u_0, v_0) &\sqsubseteq (\mathcal{G}(u_0, v_0), \mathcal{G}(v_0, u_0)) = \widehat{\mathcal{G}}(u_0, v_0) \\
&= \widehat{\mathcal{G}}(\widehat{u}_0)
\end{aligned}$$

Theorem 2 implies that $\widehat{\mathcal{G}}$ has a fixed point, and hence $\mathcal{G}$ has a coupled fixed point. □

4 Application

In this section, we aim to discuss the most recent issue in the world, which is Covid-19 mathematically. When $\gamma = 1$, we have the well-known SIR system [36]. To proceed to investigate the existence and uniqueness of (1) by using Theorem 7, we put the system in the formula

$$\begin{aligned} \Delta^{\gamma}\varsigma(t) &= \sigma_1(t, \varsigma, \Upsilon) \\ \Delta^{\gamma}\Upsilon(t) &= \sigma_2(t, \varsigma, \Upsilon), \end{aligned} \tag{15}$$

where $\sigma_1(t, \varsigma, \Upsilon) := -B\Upsilon(t)\varsigma(t)$ and $\sigma_2(t, \varsigma, \Upsilon) := B\Upsilon(t)\varsigma(t) - A\Upsilon(t)$ are local fractal continuous on an interval $J := [a, b]$. We denote this space by $C_\gamma(J)$; that is for all $\epsilon > 0$ there is $\delta > 0$ such that

$$|\sigma_1(t, \varsigma, \Upsilon) - \sigma_1(t_0, \varsigma, \Upsilon)| \le \epsilon^{\gamma}$$

when $|t - t_0| \le \delta$. Similarly for σ_2. The fractal integral system corresponding to (15) is formulated as follows for $t \in [a, b]$:

$$\begin{aligned} \varsigma(t) &= \frac{1}{\Gamma(1+\gamma)} \int_a^b \sigma_1(t, \varsigma, \Upsilon)(dt)^{\gamma} \\ \Upsilon(t) &= \frac{1}{\Gamma(1+\gamma)} \int_a^b \sigma_2(t, \varsigma, \Upsilon)(dt)^{\gamma}, \end{aligned} \tag{16}$$

where $(dt)^{\gamma} = \frac{t^{1-\gamma}}{\Gamma(2-\gamma)} dt^{\gamma}$. The variation of σ_1 and σ_2 can be indicated by ς and Υ to be autonomous of frequency that is there exists positive constants c_1 and c_2 such that $c_2 \ge c_1$ and

$$c_1 \le \sup_{t\in[a,b]} |\sigma_1(t, \varsigma, \Upsilon)| \le c_1 \left(\|\varsigma\| \|\Upsilon\|\right), \quad c_1 \in (0, \infty)$$

and

$$c_2 \le \sup_{t\in[a,b]} |\sigma_2(t, \varsigma, \Upsilon)| \le c_2 \left(\|\varsigma\| \|\Upsilon\|\right), \quad c_2 \in (0, \infty).$$

Moreover, since σ_1 and σ_2 are fractal continuous functions then by the mean value theorem for local fractional integrals

$$I^{\gamma}\sigma_1(\varsigma, \Upsilon) := \frac{1}{\Gamma(1+\gamma)} \int_a^b \sigma_1(t, \varsigma, \Upsilon)(dt)^{\gamma} = \sigma_1(\zeta) \frac{(b-a)^{\gamma}}{\Gamma(1+\gamma)}, \quad \zeta \in (a, b)$$

and

$$I^{\gamma}\sigma_2(\varsigma, \Upsilon) := \frac{1}{\Gamma(1+\gamma)} \int_a^b \sigma_2(t, \varsigma, \Upsilon)(dt)^{\gamma} = \sigma_2(\zeta) \frac{(b-a)^{\gamma}}{\Gamma(1+\gamma)}, \quad \zeta \in (a, b).$$

Therefore, for $i = 1, 2$, we have

$$I^{\gamma}\sigma_i \in [\underline{\sigma}_i \frac{(b-a)^{\gamma}}{\Gamma(1+\gamma)}, \bar{\sigma}_i \frac{(b-a)^{\gamma}}{\Gamma(1+\gamma)}],$$

where $\underline{\sigma}_i, \bar{\sigma}_i$ indicate the lower and upper bounds of σ_i respectively. Consequently, a non-decreasing sequence $(\eta_n) \subset [\underline{\sigma}_i \frac{(b-a)^{\gamma}}{\Gamma(1+\gamma)}, \bar{\sigma}_i \frac{(b-a)^{\gamma}}{\Gamma(1+\gamma)}]$ converges to $\eta^* := \bar{\sigma}_i \frac{(b-a)^{\gamma}}{\Gamma(1+\gamma)}$. Based on the properties of $\sigma_1(J) \subseteq \sigma_2(J)$, it is sufficient to consider $\sigma_2 := \sigma$ to obtain our result, where

$$c \leq \sup_{t\in[a,b]} |\sigma(t, \varsigma, \Upsilon)| \leq c\,(\|\varsigma\|\|\Upsilon\|), \quad c \in (0, \infty).$$

Moreover, we can define a positive fractal cone on a fractal continuous set $C_{\gamma} := \mathcal{X}$ as follows: $\mathbb{K}_{\gamma} := \{\chi \in \mathcal{X} : \chi \geq 0\}$.

We have the following outcome:

Theorem 8 *Let* $(\mathcal{X} := C_{\gamma}[0, b], \|\cdot\|, \sqsubseteq)$ *be a partially ordered Banach space whose positive fractal cone* $\mathbb{K}_{\gamma} = \{\chi \in \mathcal{X} : \chi \geq 0\}$ *is normal. Define the mapping* $G : \mathcal{X}^2 \to \mathcal{X}$ *achieving the assumptions*

$$G(\varsigma, \Upsilon) = \frac{1}{\Gamma(1+\gamma)} \int_0^b \sigma(t, \varsigma, \Upsilon)(dt)^{\gamma} \tag{17}$$

If $\frac{b^{\gamma}c}{\Gamma(1+\gamma)}(\|\varsigma\|\|\Upsilon\|) \in [1, \infty)$ *then* G *admits a couple fixed point.*

Proof It is clear that

$$\begin{aligned} |G(\varsigma, \Upsilon)| &= |\frac{1}{\Gamma(1+\gamma)} \int_0^b \sigma(t, \varsigma, \Upsilon)(dt)^{\gamma}| \\ &\leq \frac{b^{\gamma}c}{\Gamma(1+\gamma)}(\|\varsigma\|\|\Upsilon\|). \end{aligned} \tag{18}$$

Thus, G is bounded. Moreover, since σ is nondecreasing function, then

$$\varsigma_1 \sqsubseteq \varsigma_2 \Rightarrow \|\varsigma_1\| \leq \|\varsigma_2\| \Rightarrow G(\varsigma_1, \Upsilon) \sqsubseteq G(\varsigma_2, \Upsilon);$$

and

$$\Upsilon_1 \sqsubseteq \Upsilon_2 \Rightarrow \|\Upsilon_1\| \leq \|\Upsilon_2\| \Rightarrow G(\varsigma, \Upsilon_1) \sqsubseteq G(\varsigma, \Upsilon_2).$$

Hence, G admits the monotone nondecreasing property. Now, we proceed to achieve all the conditions in Theorem 7. Now by letting $\beta(\max\{.\}) = (0, 1)$, we have

$$\begin{aligned}&\Theta\Big(\max\{\|G(\varsigma,\Upsilon)\|,\|G(\Upsilon,\varsigma)\|\},\beta\,(\max\{\|\varsigma\|,\|\Upsilon\|\})\times\max\{\|\varsigma\|,\|\Upsilon\|\}\Big)\\&\leq\Theta\Big(\max\{\|G(\varsigma,\Upsilon)\|,\|G(\Upsilon,\varsigma)\|\},\max\{\|\varsigma\|,\|\Upsilon\|\}\Big)\\&=\Theta\Big(\max\{\|G(\varsigma,\Upsilon)\|,\|G(\Upsilon,\varsigma)\|\},\max\{\|\varsigma\|,\|\Upsilon\|\}\Big)>0.\end{aligned} \tag{19}$$

By using the condition $\frac{b^\gamma c}{\Gamma(1+\gamma)}\,(\|\varsigma\|\|\Upsilon\|)\in[1,\infty)$, it remains to show the following assertion: it is clear that

$$\|\varsigma_0\|\leq\frac{b^\gamma c}{\Gamma(1+\gamma)}\,(\|\varsigma_0\|\|\Upsilon\|),\quad \|\Upsilon_0\|\leq\frac{b^\gamma c}{\Gamma(1+\gamma)}\,(\|\varsigma\|\|\Upsilon_0\|)$$

which imply that $\varsigma_0\sqsubseteq G(\varsigma_0,\Upsilon)$ and $\Upsilon_0\sqsubseteq G(\varsigma,\Upsilon_0)$. Combining the above facts, we obtain

$$(\varsigma_0,\Upsilon_0)\sqsubseteq\Big(G(\varsigma_0,\Upsilon),G(\varsigma,\Upsilon_0)\Big).$$

Hence, G admits a couple fixed point. □

4.1 Numerical Examples

In this part, we shall use Theorem 8 to exam the solution of fractal SIR system (1) for different values of $\gamma\in(0,1]$ and $X=C_\gamma[0,1]$.

Example 1 Consider the system

$$\begin{aligned}&\Delta^{0.9}\varsigma(t)=-0.3\Upsilon(t)\varsigma(t)\\&\Delta^{0.9}\Upsilon(t)=0.3\Upsilon(t)\varsigma(t)-1.4\Upsilon(t),.\end{aligned} \tag{20}$$

subject to the initial condition (0.6, 0.2). In this case, one can take $A=1.4$ and $B=0.3$ which imply the Lyapunov exponent: $\lambda=0.4\approx\varrho<1$ after two iterations. It is clear that $0<\lambda=0.4\leq max\{A,B\}:=c$ and

$$\frac{b^\gamma c}{\Gamma(1+\gamma)}\,(\|\varsigma\|\|\Upsilon\|)=\frac{1.4}{0.88}=1.6>1.$$

This implies that the system has a solution (by Theorem 8) taking the fractal value

$$(\varsigma,\Upsilon)=\left(\frac{0.12411}{\Gamma(1+\gamma)},\frac{0.25688}{\Gamma(1+\gamma)}\right)=\left(\frac{0.12411}{0.88},\frac{0.25688}{0.88}\right)\approx(0.14,0.29).$$

Figure 1 shows the behavior of the solution, where the system has no limit cycle.

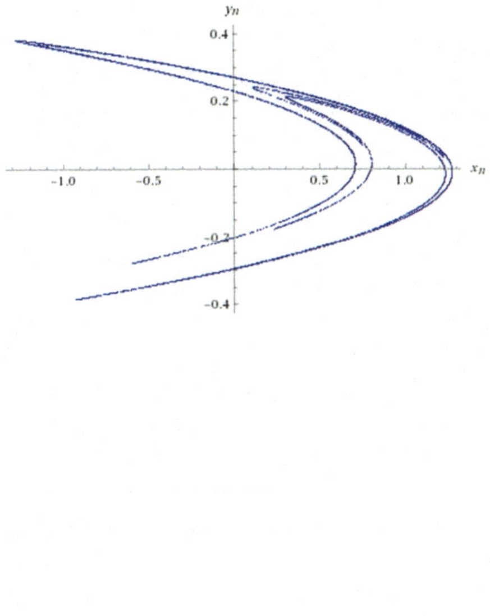

Fig. 1 Bifurcation diagrams of System (20), when $A = 1.4$, $B = 0.3$ and $\lambda = 0.4$ The left graph represents the attraction solution while the right indicates the Bifurcation diagrams (iterations and chaotic)

Example 2 Consider the system

$$\begin{aligned} \Delta^{0.5}\varsigma(t) &= -0.2\Upsilon(t)\varsigma(t) \\ \Delta^{0.5}\Upsilon(t) &= 0.2\Upsilon(t)\varsigma(t) - 1.1\Upsilon(t), . \end{aligned} \tag{21}$$

subject to the initial condition (0.4, 0.2). In this case, we select take $A = 1.1$ and $B = 0.3$ which give the Lyapunov exponent: $|\lambda| \approx 0.1$, while $\varrho = \frac{0.2\times 1}{1.1} = 0.18 < 1$ in the first iteration. It is clear that $0 < \lambda = 0.18 \leq \max\{A, B\} := c$ and

$$\frac{b^{\gamma} c}{\Gamma(1+\gamma)}(\|\varsigma\|\|\Upsilon\|) = \frac{c}{\Gamma(1.9)} = \frac{1.1}{0.96} = 1.1 > 1.$$

This implies that the system has a couple solution (by Theorem 8) having the formal

$$(\varsigma, \Upsilon) = \left(\frac{1.0240}{\Gamma(1+\gamma)}, \frac{0.0800}{\Gamma(1+\gamma)}\right) = \left(\frac{1.0240}{0.96}, \frac{0.0800}{0.96}\right) \approx (1, 0.01).$$

Figure 2 represents the behavior of the solution, where the system has a limit cycle of iteration 4.

Table 1 shows the simulation of Example 2. The value of ϱ is closed to the value of λ (Lyapunov exponent) and λ in Theorem 8. Also, it indicates the infection fatality rate (IFR) which is the ration between death and infection numbers. The data of the

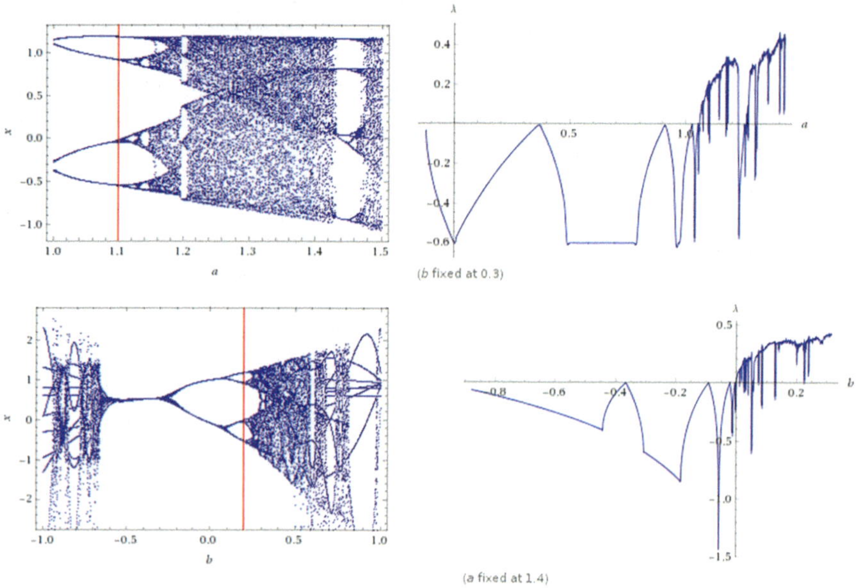

Fig. 2 Bifurcation diagrams of System (21), when $A = 1.1$, $B = 0.2$ and $\lambda = 0.18$. The limit cycle of iteration four

Table 1 Simulated data of Covid-19 in Jun (see [37]) by (1)

Country Name	Total (N)	Infected number (I)	Death	IFR
USA	2,983,155	1,560,897	132,571	10%
Brazil	1,604,585	561,070	64,900	11%
Russia	687,862	223,237	10,296	5%
Spain	297,625	196,958	28,385	14%

system are: $|\lambda| = 0.11 \approx$ IFR, $A = 0.96$, $B = 0.2$ with the initial condition $(0, 0)$ (see Fig. 3). Note that

$$\frac{b^{\gamma} c}{\Gamma(1+\gamma)} (\|\varsigma\| \|\Upsilon\|) = \frac{0.96}{0.96} = 1$$

and the solution formulated by

$$(\varsigma, \Upsilon) = \left(\frac{1.985}{\Gamma(1+\gamma)}, \frac{0.00800}{\Gamma(1+\gamma)} \right) = \left(\frac{1.985}{0.96}, \frac{0.00800}{0.96} \right) \approx (2, 0.01).$$

In this case, the solution is defined in $X = C_{\gamma}[0, 2]$.

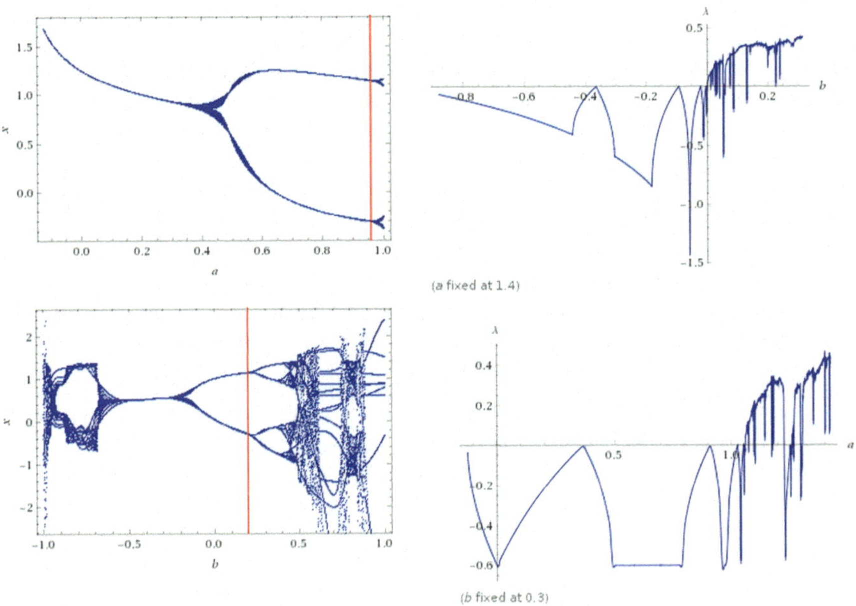

Fig. 3 Bifurcation diagrams of System (21), when $A = 0.96$, $B = 0.2$ and $\lambda = 0.11$ The limit cycle of iteration two

Acknowledgements We are grateful to the learned referee for useful suggestions which helped us to improve the text.

References

1. Aghajani, A., Allahyari, R., Mursaleen, M.: A generalization of Darbo's theorem with application to the solvability of systems of integral equations. J. Comput. Appl. Math. **260**, 68–77 (2014)
2. Aghajani, A., Banas, J., Sabzali, N.: Some generalizations of Darbofixed point theorem and applications. Bull. Belg. Math. Soc. Simon Stevin **20**, 345–358 (2013)
3. Akmerov, R., Kamenski, M., Potapov, A., Rodkina, A., Sadovskii, B.: Measures of Noncompactness and Condensing Operators. Birkhauser-Verlag, Basel (1992)
4. Arab, R.: Some fixed point theorems in generalized Darbo fixed point theorem and the existence of solutions for system of integral equations. J. Korean Math. Soc. **52**(1), 125–139 (2015)
5. Banaei, Sh., Mursaleen, M., Parvaneh, V.: Some fixed point theorems via measure of noncompactness with applications to differential equations. Comput. Appl. Math. **39**, 139 (2020)
6. Banas, J., Goebel, K.: Measures of noncompactness in Banach Spaces. LectureNotes in Pure and Applied Mathematics, p. 60. Dekker, New York (1980)
7. Chanda, A., Ansari, A.H., Dey, L.K., Damjanović, B.: On non-linear contractions via extended CF-simulation functions. Filomat **32**(10), 3731–3750 (2018)
8. Darbo, G.: Punti uniti in transformazioni a codominio non compatto (Italian). Rend. Sem. Math. Univ. Padova **24**, 84–92 (1955)

9. Dhage, B.: Hybrid fixed point theory in partially ordered normed linear spaces and applications to fractional integral equations. J. Differ. Equ. Appl. **2**, 155–184 (2013)
10. Dhage, B.: Partially continuous mappings in partially ordered normed linear spaces and applications to functional integral equations. Tamkang J. Math. **45**, 397–426 (2014)
11. Falset, J.G., Latrach, K.: On Darbo-Sadovskii's fixed point theorems type for abstract measures of (weak) noncompactness. Bull. Belg. Math. Soc. Simon Stevin **22**, 797–812 (2015)
12. Geraghty, M.: On contractive mappings. Proc. Amer. Math. Soc. **40**(2), 604–608 (1973)
13. Guo, D., Lakshmikantham, V., Liu, X.: Nonlinear Integral Equations in Abstract Spaces. Mathematics and Its Applications, vol. 373. Kluwer Academic Publishers, Dordrecht, The Netherlands (1996)
14. Khanehgir, M., Allahyari, R., Mursaleen, M., Kayvanloo H.A.: On infinite system of Caputo fractional differential inclusions with boundary conditions for convex-compact multivalued mappings. Alexandria Eng. J. https://doi.org/10.1016/j.aej.2020.08.030
15. Kuratowski, K.: Sur les espaces completes. Fund. Math. **15**, 301–309 (1930)
16. Mursaleen, M., Mohiuddine, S.A.: Applications of measures of noncompactness to the infinite system of differential equations in l_p spaces. Nolinear Anal. (TMA) **75**, 2111–2115 (2012)
17. Mursaleen, M., Alotaibi, A.: Infinite system of differential equations in some spaces. Abstr. Appl. Anal. **2012**, Special Issue (2012), Article ID 863483, 20 pages (2012). https://doi.org/10.1155/2012/863483
18. Mursaleen, M., Rizvi, S.M.H.: Solvability of infinite system of second order differential equations in c_0 and ℓ_1 by Meir-Keeler condensing operator. Proc. Amer. Math. Soc. **144**(10), 4279–4289 (2016)
19. Mursaleen, M., Bilalov, B., Rizvi, S.M.H.: Applications of measures of noncompactness to infinite system of fractional differential equations. Filomat **31**(11), 3421–3432 (2017)
20. Nashine, H.K., Arab, R.: Existence of solutions to nonlinear functional-integral equations via the measure of noncompactness. J. Fixed Point Theory Appl. **20**(6), (2018). https://doi.org/10.1007/s11784-018-0546-1
21. Nashine, H.K., Arab, R., Agarwal, R.P.: Ali Shole Haghighi, Darbo type fixed and coupled fixed point results and its application to integral equation. Period Math. Hung. **77**, 94–107 (2018)
22. Nashine, H.K., Arab, R., Agarwal, R.P., De la Sen, M.: Positive solutions of fractional integral equations by the technique of measure of noncompactness. J. Inequalities Appl. **2017**, 225 (2017)
23. Nashine, H.K., Ibrahim, R.W.: Monotone solutions of iterative fractional equations found by modified Darbo-type fixed-point theorems. J. Fixed Point Theory Appl. **19**(14), 3217–3229 (2017)
24. Nashine, H.K., Ibrahim, R.W., Agarwal, R.P.: Moments solution of fractional evolution equation found by new krasnoselskii type fixed point theorems. Fixed Point Theory (2019)
25. Nashine, H.K., Samet, B.: Fixed point results for mappings satisfying (ψ, φ)-weakly contractive conditions in partially orderen metric spaces. Nonlinear Anal. (TMA) **74**, 2201–2209 (2011)
26. Nashine, H.K., Yang, H., Agarwal, R.P.: Fixed point theorems via MNC in ordered Banach space with application to fractional integro-differential evolution equations. Taiwanees J. Math. **22**(2), 421–438 (2018)
27. Nashine, H.K., Yang, H., Agarwal, R.P.: Fractional evolution equations with nonlocal conditions in partially ordered Banach space. Carpathian J. Math. **34**(3), 379–390 (2018)
28. Nieto, J., Rodríguez-López, R.: Contractive mapping theorems in partially ordered sets and applications to ordinary differential equations. Order **22**, 223–239 (2005)
29. Nieto, J., Rodríguez-López, R.: Existence and uniqueness of fixed point in partially ordered sets and applications to ordinary differential equations. Acta. Math. Sinica, English Series. **23**, 2205–2212 (2007)
30. Pathak, H.K., Rodríguez-López, R.: Existence and approximation of solutions to nonlinear hybrid ordinary differential equations. Appl. Math. Lett. **39**, 101–106 (2015)
31. Ran, A., Reurings, M.: A fixed point theorem in partially ordered sets and some applications to matrix equations. Proc. Amer. Math. Soc. **132**, 1435–1443 (2004)

32. Samadi, A., Avini, M.M., Mursaleen, M.: Solutions of an infinite system of integral equations of Volterra-Stieltjes type in the sequence spaces ℓ_p $(1<p<1)$ and c_0. AIMS Math. **5**(4), 3791–3808 (2020)
33. Yang, H., Agarwal, R.P., Nashine, H.K.: Coupled fixed point theorems with applications to fractional evolution equations. Adv. Diff. Equ. **2017**, 239 (2017). https://doi.org/10.1186/s13662-017-1279-y
34. Yang, H., Agarwal, R.P., Nashine, H.K., Liang, Y.: Fixed point theorems in partially ordered Banach spaces with applications to nonlinear fractional evolution equations. J. Fixed Point Theory Appl. **19**, 1661–1678 (2017)
35. Xiao-Jun, Y., Baleanu, D., Srivastava, H.M.: Local Fractional Integral Transforms and Their Applications. Academic Press (2015)
36. Wu, Joseph T., Cowling, Benjamin J.: The use of mathematical models to inform influenza pandemic preparedness and response. Exp. Biol. Med. **236**(8), 955–961 (2011)
37. https://covid19.who.int/

Social Opinion Influence on Epidemic Scenarios

Alejandro Carballosa, Mariamo Mussa-Juane, and Alberto P. Muñuzuri

Abstract The current global health situation has forced governments all over the world to rule policies to control the expansion of the Covid-19 pandemic. One conclusion coming out from these events is the necessity to have a realistic mathematical model to predict the evolution and avoid uncontrollable situations. Confinement of drastic reduction of the population mobility has become one of the most popular policies established by governments. Under these circumstances, it has been observed that the population behavior (the human factor) is critical in order to achieve the desired goal. We considered different scenarios describing the eagerness of the population to accept the confinement policies and propose a way to directly include this information into an epidemic model.

Keywords Social networks · Social opinion influence in epidemiology · SIR epidemic model · Control · Complex networks

1 Introduction

The coronavirus pandemic has dramatically changed the way people relate to each other. It is well known that social interactions are carriers of diseases [6, 13]. For instance, the Black Death (The Plague) in the 1300 s killed up to 25–200 million people in Eurasia and North Africa. The population was, then, decimated by a 30 to 60% of Europe's total population. As mobility in that time was through short-range movements (walking, carts pulled by animals, horses, ...), the spreading of the pandemic may be considered to be diffusive [7, 15], and the total epidemic event could take several decades. As time goes by, transport evolved and so did the infection timing. Think about the First Industrial Revolution and the onset of the rail transport. This new technology enabled the transference of goods and passengers

A. Carballosa · M. Mussa-Juane · A. P. Muñuzuri (✉)
Group of Nonlinear Physics. Fac. Physics, University of Santiago de Compostela, 15782 Santiago de Compostela, Spain
e-mail: alberto.perez.munuzuri@usc.es

P. Agarwal et al. (eds.), *Analysis of Infectious Disease Problems (Covid-19) and Their Global Impact*, Infosys Science Foundation Series,
https://doi.org/10.1007/978-981-16-2450-6_21

through longer distances in shorter times. Pandemics could move even faster and reach locations inaccessible before.

This is what happened in the late XIX century with the Third Plague. This pandemic was initiated in China in 1894. However, it was not as severe as the first one, in Europe victims could be counted by thousands, the geographical hot spots being pretty similar to those in the actual coronavirus epidemic. Not so its timing. The pace was much slower. And, again, it strongly depended on human mobility. This plague traveled through cargo ships from the busy port of Hong Kong. The plague bacteria could spend years till reaching the most remote places. In 1896, it arrived to Bombay (now Mumbai), India's leading port and a central node of the British colonies and from there to the world aided by ships and the railway. With the passage of time and the emergence of the airplane, this lapse of years turns into days as in the coronavirus scenario, where the smaller innermost village is not free of infection. The important lesson we infer from the previous pandemics is that the mobility is crucial in the spatial spreading of the infection [8]. The trade network, that constitutes an important type of social interaction, is behind the advance of a pandemic.

In addition, we can find similarities if we analyze the phenomena going from local to global mobility. Diffusive networks operate in a local scale. Think about families, villages or urban neighborhoods where face-to-face interactions dominate. As the scale increases, that diffusive network turns into a small world network where certain long-range interactions appear [1]. This could be the case of cities or mobility among a district of cities and villages interacting. Richer network structures emerge analyzing wider territories like countries or continents: Capital cities provide services and functions as strong sources and sinks of people and occupy central locations of the network. Meanwhile, villages occupy the peripheries of the network pointing to cities but also between them, resulting in short-range networks.

Thus, historical context and geography are of relevance to determine the propagation of a pandemic. These are environmental factors that, individually, we cannot change so easily. We cannot change neither the transportation nor the era we are living in. However, we can change the social predisposition to establish or not contact. During the medium age plagues, cities locked their walls in order to control or even avoid the epidemic. Nowadays, we continue using similar measurements adapted to our never-stopping frenetic way of life. Thus, social distancing and quarantines appear back. Today, as many centuries ago, the population faces the same dilemma, either accept the policies imposed by the ruling class or try to avoid the restrictions and continue interacting with the rest of the population. The evolution of the pandemic curves will strongly depend on this decision. In fact, the positioning of the population with respect to this dilemma produces a polarized spectrum of opinion, basically a bimodal distribution. Along this manuscript, we consider different scenarios describing the spectrum of approaches of the population to the social distancing measurements. This information is introduced in the classical epidemic models, and the results are analyzed.

The text is organized as follows. First, we present the model used to describe the evolution of the pandemic. Here we also describe how the mobility restrictions can be incorporated in such models and the different opinion spectra that we will consider. In the next section, the results of intensive numerical simulations are presented analyzing the different scenarios considered. We finish with the discussion and conclusions.

2 Coupling an Opinion Distribution with the SIR Model

Along this section, we present the epidemic model used for our simulations and the way to couple it with opinion distributions. The opinion distributions describe theoretical scenarios of population response to confinement and social distance policies.

2.1 *SIR Model in Extended Systems*

In order to incorporate the opinion distribution into epidemic models, first we need to introduce the model itself and how this model can be interpreted and adapted in an extended system. We choose to consider a simple model that still preserves the basic features of a pandemic spread. In particular, we consider the classical SIR model [4] named by the initials of the three compartments, and the population is considered to be (susceptible, infected and recovered or death) as we will explain in more details below. More complicated models have been implemented in the literature in order to accurately predict the coronavirus expansion [11]. As we are trying to illustrate how the effect of the opinion can modify the infection curves, we chose a basic generic model for the propagation of a pandemic. Nevertheless, our way to introduce the opinion distribution is generic and could be similarly implemented in different models. The SIR model contemplates three epidemiological classes: susceptible (S), the group of people that are prone to get infected; infected (I), already carrying the infection; recovered (R), this group describes both the recovered population that are supposed to be immune (at least for the considered timescale) and the death. See Fig. 1 for a scheme of the mechanism.

In the scheme of Fig. 1, β and μ are the probabilities of infection and recovery, respectively. β measures the chance of the susceptible group to get infected. In this context, β measures the rate of the pandemic spreading. Once a susceptible individual

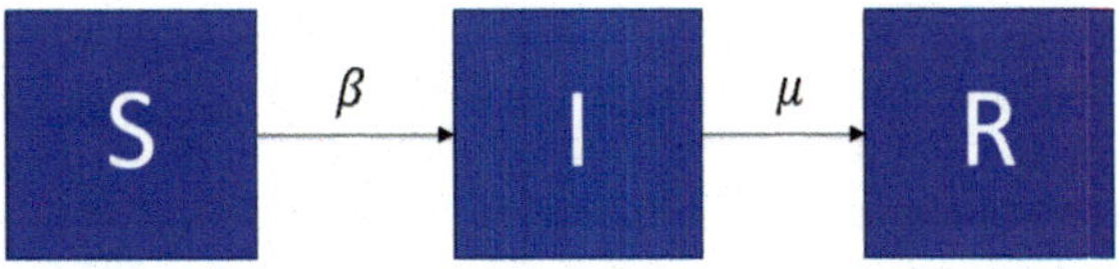

Fig. 1 Scheme of the SIR model

is infected, the individual moves to the infected class. Once in the infected class, they have a chance μ to get recovered. The recovered class gains immunity and cannot get infected again.

We consider that all individuals interrelate with each other as they are part of a complex network of connections. Depending on the structure of the network, interactions between the individuals from the different groups may happen and, thus, induce a change from an epidemiological class to another. The topology of the network of connections may change completely the output of the model and the infection curves. For the present study, we consider that such a network follows a Watts–Strogatz topology [17]. This is a paradigm for a small world network configuration. As we briefly discussed in the introduction, the kind of interaction among individuals of our population and during a period of disease spreading is probably confined to interactions with physically close individuals with the exception of a limited number of interactions with distant individuals. A small world network mainly structures itself with short-range connections, and some long-range ones, thus, accurately describes the situation we aim to investigate. This type of network is characterized by a quite homogeneous connectivity (number of connections of a specific node) with small deviations, meaning that almost all individuals within the network have the same degree. This allows to describe societies with simple internal structures such as families, neighborhoods and villages. In this context, thus, each node of the network represents one of the aforementioned social units (i.e., families, neighborhoods, etc.). This is just an extension of the SIR model to extended systems described by a complex network whose nodes are described above.

In order to build a Watts–Strogatz network, we consider that the individuals are interconnected forming a ring of N nodes with k initial neighbors and a probability p of rewiring or establishing new connections. The higher is p, the closer the graph is to a fully random network with the characteristics of a Erdos–Renyi graph [5]. If we relate this ring-shaped network with a spatial distribution of individuals, when p tends to 0, random interactions far from our neighborhood are prohibited, alike a confinement situation with strictly reduced mobility. This makes the Watts–Strogatz network a suitable one to study our concerned case where a restricted mobility can be mimicked reducing the rewiring probability p. Note that the choice of the network is important because its topology may result in completely different behaviors as analyzed in [9].

Once the Watts–Strogatz network is generated, all nodes are set to the susceptible state except for a given amount of randomly chosen nodes that are infected. Simulations are run as follows. At each time step, the chance that each infected individual spreads the disease to each of its susceptible connections is evaluated by means of a Monte Carlo method [2] with a probability given by β. Then, the chance of each infected individual being recovered is evaluated at the end of the time step in the same manner. This process is repeated until reaching the stationary state where infected individuals disappear.

Each simulation presented along this manuscript was run at least 1000 times in order to have some statistical significance of the results. The dynamic equations were integrated using a fourth-order Runge–Kutta method [12].

2.2 Opinion-Biased SIR Model

So far we have introduced several notions about why measuring the social state of a population can be of use to different dynamic processes and especially the modeling of an epidemic spread. This section intends to give the reader a practical example of how to implement these ideas from a theoretical point of view, although the method could be extrapolated to real data sets obtained through statistical polls, social media, etc. We also explore and analyze a few statistics of interest that can be exploited to extract information on how the different control parameters of the model could affect the evolution of the disease. For that purpose, we have carried out a series of simulations based on the mechanisms explained in the previous sections and show here the results. The parameters used on the epidemic model, namely the infection and recovery parameters β and μ are not chosen to fit any data but to highlight the impact of the opinion on the epidemic. The same criterion is applied to the parameters of the synthetic network in which the disease propagates, i.e., the mean connectivity of the network and its size.

In this manuscript, we create an imaginary society with a more or less polarized spectrum of opinion. Social polarization can be implemented as a bimodal distribution ($\{u_i\}$) [18] where two distinct opinions depict the centers of two Gaussian distributions with standard deviation σ. This bimodal distribution ensembles two populations: N_0 and N_1. Population N_0 has an opinion closer to 0. We consider that this population does not follow the recommendations of the government and disobeys the confinement policies of staying home or social distancing. Population N_1, closer to the opinion 1, follows the social restrictions. The opinion distribution considered here is a simplified image of an actual society as certainly several sensibilities are not reflected here, nevertheless we consider it as a good approach still preserving the main features we want to outline. The distribution of opinions is given by $\{u_i\}$ where u_i is the opinion of individual i that lays between 0 and 1 being 0 complete disagreement with mobility restrictions and 1 complete agreement.

In this context, if two individuals, one susceptible and another one infected, are within the population N_0, meaning that they do not follow the confinement policies, then they are more prone to get infected. In order to incorporate this into the epidemic model, we consider the infection rate parameter β to be dependent on the two nodes interacting, thus β_{ij}. We define

$$\beta_{ij} = \beta \overline{u_i} \cdot \overline{u_j} \quad (1)$$

which accounts for the effective susceptibility of infection between an infected node i and a susceptible node j. Here $\overline{u_i}$ quantifies the mobility of node i that ranges from 0 (no mobility and full adhesion to confinement policies) to 1 (normal mobility and total neglect of mobility restrictions). We define this mobility factor as the complementary to the opinion of such node, $1 - u_i$. $\overline{u_j}$ is the equivalent magnitude for individual j. Note that if both individuals (nodes) are likely to follow the social distance rules, their opinion will be close to 1 and, thus, their mobility factor, $\overline{u_i}$ will approach 0. In

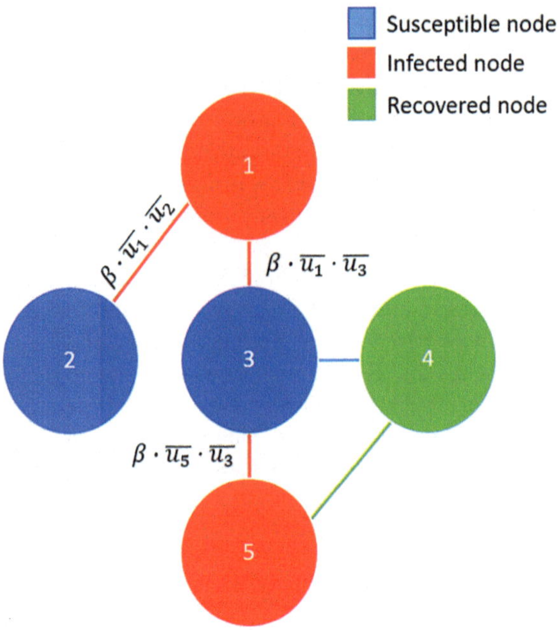

Fig. 2 Susceptibility to get infected taking into account a spectrum of opinion. Red links interconnect infected and susceptible individuals and trace the possible spreading path of the pandemic

this case, the probability to get infected diminishes dramatically approaching zero. Figure 2 exemplifies the process through a network diagram, where blue, red and green nodes represent susceptible, infected and recovered individuals, respectively. Red connections account for possible infections with chance β_{ij}.

Along the manuscript, we will be comparing the different opinion scenarios with the situation described as *free mobility*, where all infection rates β_{ij} approach the constant value β as all mobility factors equal 1 (all the opinions lay down to 0). We want to know how the opinions of the individuals within this social network with a bimodal spectrum of opinion interfere with the basic disease's model propagation, the SIR, described in the previous section.

In order to generate a bimodal distribution, we have two main free parameters, namely the width σ of the Gaussian distributions and the amount of counts that compose each Gaussian distribution. If we sample a higher number of counts on the Gaussian centered on zero, we shall say that the generated distribution represents a set of opinions that tends to disagree with the external given opinion, while if a higher number of counts are sampled on the Gaussian located on one, our opinion distribution will tend to agree with the external opinion. Following the previous notation, we shall refer to the counts located around the zero value as N_0 and to the counts located around the value of one as N_1, so we can specify if a opinion distribution tends to one of the extreme values accordingly to the ratio:

$$\nu = \frac{N_1}{N_0} \tag{2}$$

Note that if $\nu \simeq 0$, the general trend of the distribution will be to disagree with the rulers' opinion and vice versa ($\nu \simeq 1$). Thus, in summary, with σ and ν, we can tune how much distributed our opinions are and which one is the trend of these opinions. In general, measuring the social state of a group of citizens or a whole population is a difficult task since real data obtained through statistical polls or social media is usually hugely heterogeneous. Being in either complete agreement or disagreement with an idea (values 1 and 0, respectively) is less common than being in an intermediate state or even has an intermediate opinion (value of 0.5) describing people that are likely to follow or not the social distancing policies with equal probability (depending on the circumstances one may say) [3]. Therefore, trying to model opinions through mathematical means can be a little naive because of the richness of the data and the susceptibility to the topic: The distribution of opinions would probably be strongly different if one is to choose between his or her favorite food rather than his or her political affiliation, for example. Describing how a social state is measured or modeled would require a whole book for itself to be covered properly, and it is beyond the scope of this chapter. Nevertheless, considering some theoretical clearly differentiated scenarios may help understanding the main configurations that can be present in a more complex and real situations.

Here, for the sake of focusing on how these opinions can be implemented in the epidemic dynamics, we will center our efforts in proposing different theoretical scenarios, and we will use the parameter σ, which marks the full width at half maximum of the Gaussian distributions, as a measure of the dispersion on the opinions. We are mainly interested in studying polarized cases, and this are topics where the population either tends to have an either high affinity with the opinion at hand or a very low one and see how the different trends affect to the global evolution of the epidemic. On the other hand, a state where all opinions are approximately uniformly distributed is easy to model, and we shall study this case too. These examples of distributions that will lately be used are found on Fig. 3, for three different values of σ and three different trends for each of the ν values.

3 Results

3.1 Generating the SIR Dynamics in a Network

As previously mentioned, complex networks offer a nice and suitable framework for epidemic models, allowing for the possibility of scaling down to the individual interactions if one considers a multi-agent-based simulation [14], where each node represents an individual of a population, or spatial distribution if one considers a metapopulation model [16], where each node represents a population itself where the disease is transmitted locally. Besides, complex networks accommodate easily the combination of the epidemic model with the opinion distributions, since we can extrapolate the latter to assign to each individual node an opinion value. In this

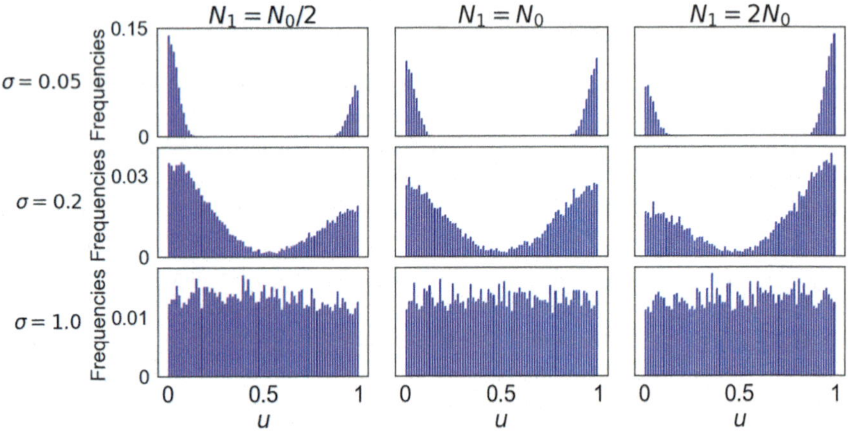

Fig. 3 Normalized opinion distributions generated accordingly to a bimodal distribution, for different values of the dispersion parameter σ. Panels on the left show scenarios where opinions tend to be in total disagreement with the external given opinion, panels on the middle scenarios where around the same amount of population have opposite opinions and panels on the right where opinions tend to be in high agreement. Each row belongs to a different value of the dispersion parameter, being, respectively, σ =0.05, 0.2, 1.0. Note that the lower row represents an approximately uniform distribution of opinions

subsection, we will see the different outcomes of including the opinion distributions of Fig. 3 to the SIR model as we explained in the previous sections.

Let us recapitulate now what exactly the external given opinion meant and how it can affect the dynamics of the epidemic. If this external opinion is, for example, to stay at home and isolate from society, we are imposing a restriction to the population in terms of mobility. This translates in the complex network as a rupture of edges and isolation of nodes, reducing drastically the connectivity and the possibility that an infectious node can transmit the disease to its connections or "nearest neighbors". Thus, if all opinions tend to 0, the connectivity of the network remains unaltered, while in the opposite case all nodes become isolated and the disease dies out in the infected nodes. For the implementation in the epidemic model, it is important to remember that we do not use the value of the opinion u directly, but that of its inverse value $\overline{u} = 1 - u$ (the mobility) and it is this new variable which then multiplies the infection parameter β. In this way, an opinion of $u = 1$ would become a mobility factor $\overline{u} = 0$ that when multiplied by β would cancel the probability of infection (this is equivalent to removing all the edges of this node, leaving it isolated).

The effect that the opinion induces on the dynamics of the epidemic is clear with the behavior of the curves as shown in Fig. 4. All figures represent the evolution of the total number of infected individuals in the network with time. Each curve represents the averaged behavior observed over more that a 1000 simulations of each case (note the colored shadow of each curve meaning the dispersion of the simulated cases).

Figure 4a corresponds with simulations with $\sigma = 0.05$, the population described is very polarized, and almost only two opinions are considered (namely adhesion to the

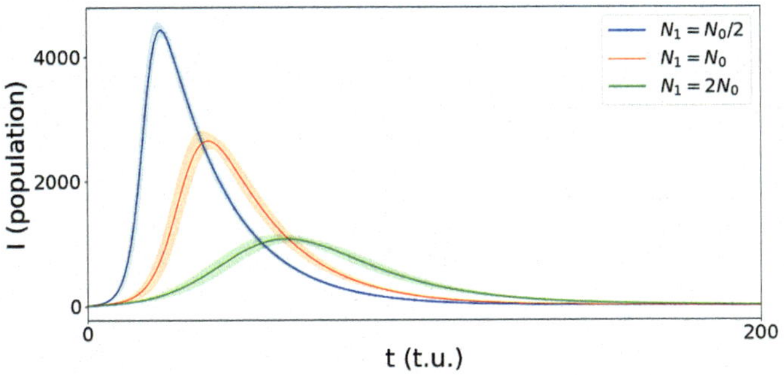

(a) $\sigma = 0.05$

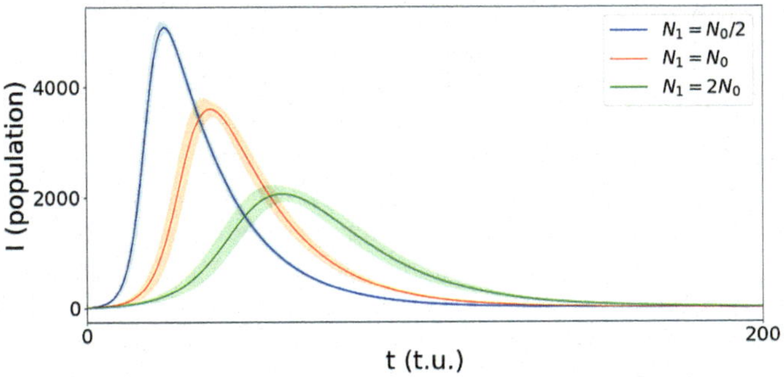

(b) $\sigma = 0.2$

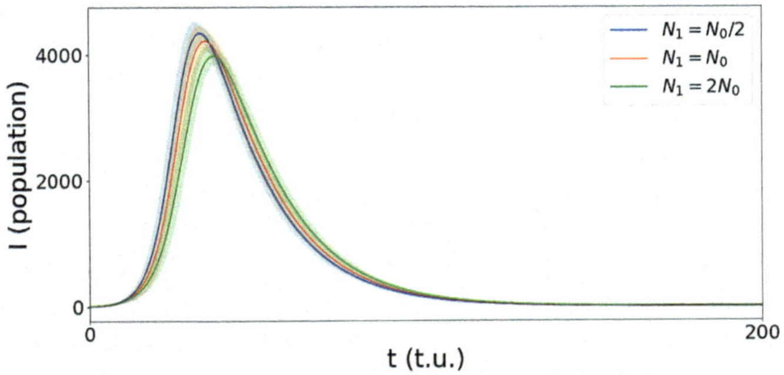

(c) $\sigma = 1.0$

Fig. 4 Time evolution of new infected cases according to the SIR model biased with the opinion distributions shown in Fig. 3

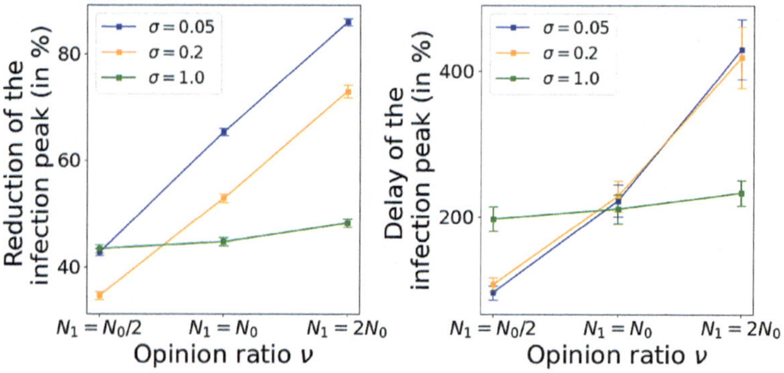

Fig. 5 Peak statistics for the scenarios presented on Fig. 4

confinement policies or not). Here, three infection curves are presented corresponding to different ratios of N_1/N_2. As this ratio becomes larger, more and more individuals accept mobility restrictions and the peak of the curve is delayed as well as its intensity is decreased (meaning in a practical case that the health system does not saturate). The higher the agreement with the confinement restrictions, the more flattened is the curve of new infected cases over time. As the value of σ is increased (Fig. 4b) to $\sigma = 0.2$, the infection curves present, roughly, the same behavior as in the previous case. The last of the cases considered in this figure (Fig. 4c) corresponds with a value of $\sigma = 1.0$. In this case, the distribution of opinions is homogeneous, and so it is the mobility factors distribution. All opinions have the same representation in this distribution. Changes in the ratio N_1/N_2 do not introduce any significant difference in the final infection curve. Just note that the intensity and location of the peak almost coincide with the least favorable case in the previous two figures.

Although the visualizations are clear enough, it would be desirable to quantify these effects and explore how the tuning of the parameters impacts on the main statistic that we have here: the peak of infection and the time it happens. Accurately quantifying these parameters is usually one of the main goals of epidemiology, since there are limits to the hospitalization of patients on the healthcare system of a nation. We present all our results comparing them with a simulation of the SIR model (same parameters for infection and recovery, β and γ) without opinion factor included. With this comparison, we can extract two sources of information: On one hand we have the reduction of the number of absolute cases on the peak, and on the other hand, the temporal delay of the peak. We shall express these new statistics in a relative fashion and refer to them as peak statistics.

Let us focus our attention now to Fig. 5, in which we summarize the peak statistics of the curves of Fig. 4. Figure 5a presents the variation of the intensity of the peak for the different scenarios considered (varying σ and the opinion ratio N_1/N_0). Figure 5b plots the values of the induced time delay in the infection peak for the different scenarios. Regarding the reduction of the number of new infected cases on the peak, breaking down the network mobility carries out at least a 40% reduction

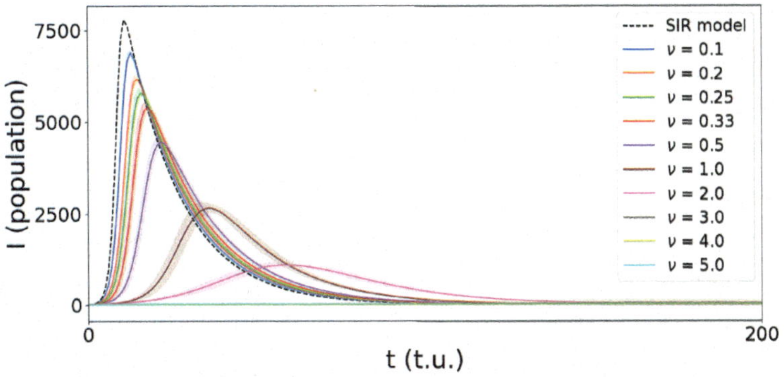

Fig. 6 Time evolution of new infected cases for a range of values of the parameter ν, for $\sigma = 0.05$. The rewiring probability was fixed to $p = 0.25$

for every scenario contemplated, which scales up to an 85% reduction in the most optimistic scenario, this is, low dispersion of the opinions ($\sigma = 0.05$) with a marked tendency to agree with the external opinion ($\nu = 2$). The latter case, as one could have expected, is the one which outcomes the higher reductions on the infections, since it is the one with higher restrictions on the mobility (remember that the higher the value of the opinion, the more likely it is the node to be isolated). Now, with respect to the time delay of the peak, incorporating the opinion distribution to the network delays at least a 100% the timing of the peak, which makes sense considering that if the connections between nodes are largely broken, the outbreak of the epidemic will take far longer to reach its tipping point. This delay is exaggerated again in the most optimistic scenario, obtaining delays of almost a 400% of the original timing. An interesting point that this second figure highlights is that of the behavior of the statistic with the dispersion parameter, which is telling us that no further delay is achieved by increasing it, or at least for $\sigma < 0.2$. For the uniform opinion distribution, we have found that similar values are obtained in the three cases, although this was already pointed out by Fig. 4c.

Now that we have introduced the main concepts and statistics; let us explore more in detail how a wider sweep of the parameters affects the peak statistics. We commented earlier at the beginning of this section that the opinion distribution responds mainly to two parameters: the ratio ν between counts on both extremes of the distribution, and the dispersion of the distributions σ. Let us introduce now another control parameter regarding the topology of the network that was previously mentioned in this chapter: the probability of random rewiring between nodes of the Watts–Strogatz model. Remembering that, if this probability is set to 0 or near zero, the outcome is a highly clustered population in which the epidemic has a lot of difficulties to percolate [10]. Values of this rewiring probability close to 1 mean that the network stops being a small world network and becomes a random one. These three parameters will be considered in the following section.

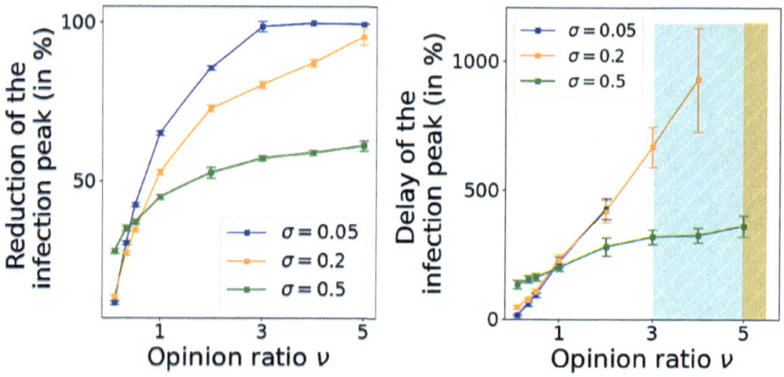

Fig. 7 Peak statistics for a range of values of the parameter ν, for $\sigma = 0.05$, $\sigma = 0.2$ and $\sigma = 0.5$. The rewiring probability was fixed to $p = 0.25$

The time evolution of the infection curves for different values of the opinion ratio ν is represented on Fig. 6. Note that for comparison purposes, the temporal evolution of the infected individuals in the SIR model without opinion is plotted in a dashed black line. It can easily grasp the two asymptotic behaviors of the parameter, for $\nu \to 0$ almost all opinions tend to completely disagree with the external given opinion (government opinion imposing social distancing measures), and the dynamics of the usual SIR model are recovered. On the other hand, for $\nu > 2$ the outbreak of the epidemic dies out or it never really happens. In Fig. 7, these two asymptotic behaviors can be grasped from the peak statistics. Again, we are plotting the intensity of the peak reduction as well as the time delayed induced by the opinion effect. The dashed blue and orange bars in Fig. 7b represent the absence of a clear peak of infection. For larger values of the dispersion parameter σ, namely $\sigma = 0.2$ and $\sigma = 0.5$, although the same tendency is observed, larger values of ν are required for the epidemic outbreak to die out. Note how for $\nu = 3$ and $\nu = 4$ there is still a peak of infection with dispersion $\sigma = 0.2$, although it is heavily delayed (7 to 10 times the original peak predicted by the SIR model). For a higher value of the dispersion parameter, $\sigma = 0.5$, the slope of the trend is significantly reduced with increasing ν, until this slope becomes practically zero as we saw on Fig. 5 with the dispersion parameter $\sigma = 1.0$. For values of $\sigma > 0.5$, the distribution begins to become more uniform each time, which tends to homogenize the number of counts of the opinion spectrum. This effect is responsible for the higher values on the statistics obtained for $\sigma = 0.5$ when ν is smaller than 0.5.

Let us move on now to the dispersion parameter σ, fixing ν at 0.5 to represent a more pessimistic scenario where the trend is to disagree the given opinion and break the social distancing policies. Our intention is to grasp in this scenario how a lower or higher dispersion could improve or worsen the evolution of the disease. According to the peak statistics in Fig. 8, it is curious to find that low to none dispersion produces a further reduction on the number of absolute cases on the peak of infection. This can be understood as follows: With $\sigma \simeq 0$, the counts are located either at 0 or at

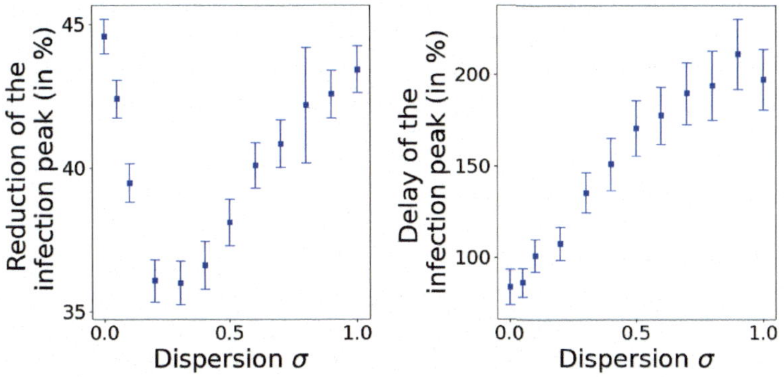

Fig. 8 Infection peak statistics for different values of the parameter σ, with $\nu = 0.5$ and the probability of rewiring set to $p = 0.25$

1. Counts very close to one are isolated and thus cannot be infected by any means, while counts on 0 are all susceptible to the disease with its original connectivity. As σ increases, counts with a precise value of 1 decrease and become vulnerable, while the opposite process occurs with those with a precise value of 0. In this balance between counts that are increasingly isolated and others that are increasingly more vulnerable, the effects of the latter predominate for lower values of σ since there are now more nodes susceptible to infection, while the former have still plenty of mobility. A point of equilibrium seems to be found around $\sigma = 0.2$, point from which the net reduction of the infection peak starts to increase due to the wider spread of opinions. On the other hand, regarding the delay of the peak, we see that this statistic grows slightly but monotonically with the dispersion parameter.

Finally, another parameter of interest is the grade of clustering in our synthetic society, controlled by the rewiring parameter of the Watts–Strogatz network model, p. As previous studies with small world-type networks have shown [10], the phenomena of clustering in a complex network affect the percolation of the disease, as the panels on Fig. 9 show. For increasing values of the rewiring probability, both reduction and delay of the infection are decreased to the point of saturating around a 30% and a 100%, respectively, existing barely no differences for values of the rewiring probability $p \geq 0.3$ This can be understood in terms of the average shortest path of the network [1], which is a measure of the network topology that tells the average minimum number of steps required to travel between any two nodes of the network. The rewiring of edges starting from a ring topology where only the nearest neighbors are connected introduces in the network a series of shortcuts between long-distance nodes, which decreases the average shortest path exponentially fast. Thus, it makes sense that the epidemic is able to propagate faster through the network on the presence of these shortcuts. These saturation points can also be understood in terms of a percolation process, as p increases, the clustering of the network decreases and the probability of global infection becomes 1. From the data in Fig. 9, this percolation threshold takes place at $p \simeq 0.3$.

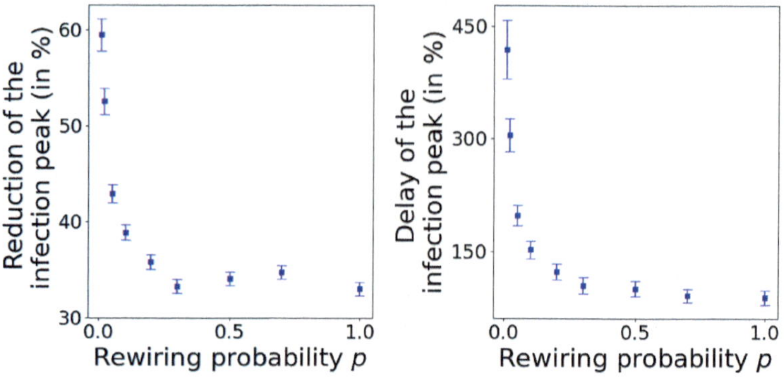

Fig. 9 Peak statistics for different values of the rewiring probability p of the Watts–Strogatz network model, with $\sigma = 0.2$ and $\nu = 0.5$

3.2 Adding More Complexity to the Model: Trimodal Opinion Distributions

So far we have considered the case where we have two opposite opinions, 0 and 1, and the most intermediate case consisted of a uniform distribution. But, as we pointed out before, another plausible situation involves the existence of a third mayor opinion that, basically, decides to keep the social distance or not with equal probability. This opinion corresponds with people that behaves differently depending on the occasion or simply reduces their interactions but not dramatically. This is an state in which they do not have a formed opinion, want to remain skeptical or are not concerned with the topic, to figure out some possibilities. Let us picture, for example, the case in which the government recommends to wear a facial mask in order to help with the constraining of a virus. Experience has told us that population is divided between concerned people (opinion 1) who wear it at all times, skeptical ones that are suffocated by the breathing restriction or see their free will cropped and refuse to wear it (opinion 0), and another group who although are slightly concerned and neither want to catch the disease nor propagate it, and they wear it only occasionally due to its uncomfortability or any other reason (opinion 0.5 approximately).

This trimode scenario could be modeled following the current reasoning of this chapter by introducing a third Gaussian distribution in the middle of the spectrum: $u = 0.5$, obtaining a trimodal distribution which obeys the same parameters that we have already explored. Again, note that this scenario is a purely theoretical one and real experimental data on the proposed example could completely differ, but let us cope with it for the time being and for the sake of simplicity. We intend not to redo a complete sweep of the parameters, since adding a new distribution to the model involves plenty of new realizations of the system, but to show further possibilities with the proposed model. In particular, let us propose the scenarios presented in Fig. 10. Here we consider three different opinion distributions clearly showing three different opinions in each case. We have once more that one of the opinions predominates

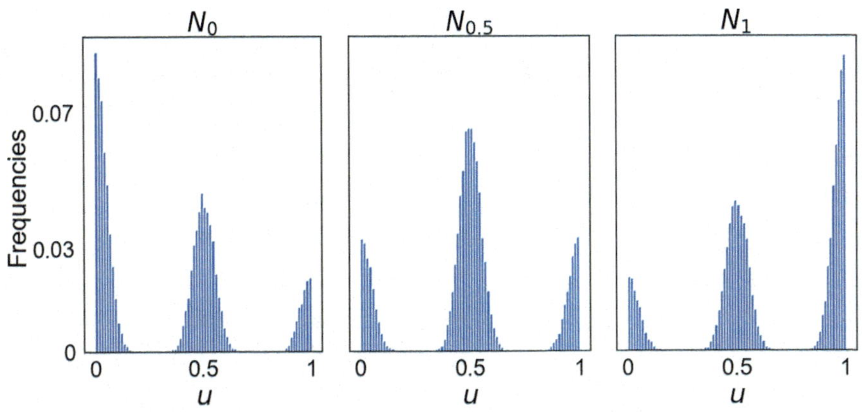

Fig. 10 Three possible opinion distributions (normalized) generated with a trimodal distribution model, with the dispersion parameter set to $\sigma = 0.05$

clearly. We will refer to N_0 as the one where opinion 0 predominates (Fig. 10a), $N_{0.5}$ the one with a peak on $u = 0.5$ (Fig. 10b) and N_1 where the trend is to follow the government opinion (Fig. 10c). The dispersion parameter was set to $\sigma = 0.05$ so the three Gaussians would not overlap, and the three peaks were clearly distinguishable. We have chosen this specific configuration in order to compare the outcome of this model with the results from Fig. 3. What if instead of a nicely and smooth distribution of opinions across the whole spectrum they grouped themselves into three clear clusters? That is what we intend to show briefly with this subsection.

Figure 11 shows the comparison between the bimodal and the trimodal distributions according to the peak statistics of the infection curves. Note that in the bimodal distributions, N_0 refers to the scenario with $\nu = 0.5$ and N_1 to that with $\nu = 2.0$, and we have obviated the case with $\nu = 1.0$. Instead, we have chosen the scenario with an uniform distribution ($\sigma = 1.0$) to compare with the trimodal case where there is a peak on $u = 0.5$ ($N_0.5$). For the chosen σ of the trimodal distribution, we see that the outcome for both statistics is practically identical to that of the uniform distribution, which could point out that these two distributions are equivalent when applied to the epidemic model. On the other hand, for the scenarios in which one of the opposite opinions predominates, we see that the difference lies mainly in the chosen value of the dispersion parameter. In the N_0 scenario, the bimodal distribution outcomes a further reduction of the infection peak for both values of σ, although in N_1 the trimodal distribution returns a further reduction than the bimodal distribution with $\sigma = 0.2$, but still does not reach the one yielded by $\sigma = 0.05$. Regarding the time delay of the peak, while for N_0 and $N_{0.5}$ all distributions outcome similar results, and a clear difference is found for N_1, where the trimodal distribution yields a significant further delay of the infection peak. In other words, although the number of infected individuals on the peak remains practically the same for both models, the timing of this peak is strongly delayed with the trimodal distribution. A loss of counts with opinion values near 1 in favor of those with opinion around 0.5 results in a far more

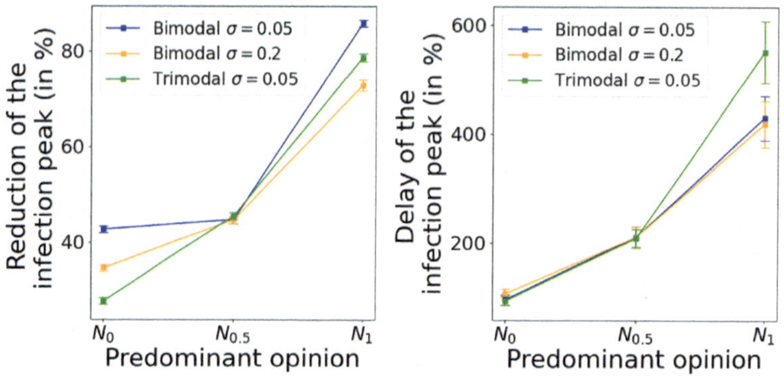

Fig. 11 Peak statistics for the trimodal opinion distributions vs the bimodal distributions. N_0 represents the case where the opinion 0 predominates, N_1 the case where opinion 1 predominates and $N_{0.5}$ represents the case with a peak on $u = 0.5$ of the trimodal distribution and the uniform distribution of the bimodal case

optimal control of the disease, giving actual importance to the opinionless individuals. This can be understood in terms of the population that remains in an skeptical attitude with opinion near 0 in the bimodal distribution. In the trimodal distributions, those counts are now distributed not only around 0 but around 0.5 as well, leaving a significant amount of vulnerable nodes that are protected from other infected nodes $\simeq 50\%$ of the time. In this scenario, although these nodes can be equally infected and contribute to the amount of infected individuals on the peak, at each time step, there are less active nodes and the disease has it more difficult to percolate, decreasing the speed of the outbreak. In this sense, this could indicate that a policy of confinement that leaves in circulation half of the nodes at each time step (in the sense that the nodes are being intercalated) could be more effective on the control of the disease than a policy that confines a huge part of the population and leaves a significant percentage of the population circulating during the outbreak of the disease. However, to confirm this premise further, more exhaustive studies on the topic should be carried out.

4 Discussion and Conclusions

Along this manuscript, we present a systematic way to include the state of opinion of a society into the evolution of an epidemic. We considered some theoretical scenarios in order to identify the more important parameters and features of this model. Once the opinion distribution is built (either from experimental observations or from theoretical considerations such as in the present case), we know how the population intends to react when facing mobility restrictions imposed by the ruling class. This opinion distribution is directly translated into a mobility factor for each node in the network that reduces or increases its risk or probability of infection.

The results presented here are clear and confirm the experimental evidence, the spread of an epidemic can be controlled by the people suffering it. The decision of the population to adhere to social distancing policies can induce dramatic reductions in the infection peak intensity (up to 100%) and significantly delay its occurrence. For some cases, the peak can even be completely suppressed or inhibited only due to the appropriate decisions of the population.

One first conclusion of the present work is the need to raise the awareness of the importance of social distancing policies. The more aware the population is, the larger the value of ν is and, thus, the infection peak is lowered and delayed significantly. Another parameter that was analyzed is the dispersion of the opinions in the distributions considered. It plays an important role that depending on the parameter ν can help to control the epidemic or otherwise. The case shown in Fig. 8 constitutes an example where the dispersion of opinions helps preventing the spread of the epidemic. Large values of σ significantly decrease the amplitude of the infection peak and induce large delays. Figure 7 shows both behaviors at the same time. For lower values of $\nu < 0.5$ (corresponding with a majority of the population opposing the confinement restrictions), the increase of the opinion dispersion plays a positive role to constrain the epidemic spread. On the other hand, for values of $\nu > 0.5$, the behavior is the opposite; an increase in the opinion dispersion (σ) results in worse conditions and a steeper infection curve that happens early in time.

Another parameter that was analyzed along the manuscript is the so-called rewiring probability that controls the number of distant connections for each node. In practical applications, it determines how clustered the network is. During its analysis, we observe the importance of keeping the connection of each node local and low, avoiding distant connections. In this way, the number of individuals connected with each node remains low (small hub), and the epidemic finds more difficult to propagate. It is important to maintain the network clustered and avoid reaching the percolation threshold that triggers the infection peak.

More complexity can be added into the opinion models and distributions, but the main features remain basically the same. We believe the method deployed here to include opinion factors into infection curves is crucial as we demonstrate that can dramatically change the outcome of the model and completely influence the evolution of the epidemic.

Acknowledgements This research is supported by the Spanish Ministerio de Economa y Competitividad and European Regional Development Fund, research grant No. COV20/00617 and RTI2018-097063-B-I00 AEI/FEDER, UE; by Xunta de Galicia, Research Grant No. 2018-PG082, and the CRETUS Strategic Partnership, AGRUP2015/02, supported by Xunta de Galicia. All these programs are co-funded by FEDER (UE). We also acknowledge support from the Portuguese Foundation for Science and Technology (FCT) within the Project n. 147. A substantial portion of the simulations was run at the Centro de Supercomputacion de Galicia (Spain), and we acknowledge their support.

References

1. Albert, R., Barabási, A.-L.: Statistical mechanics of complex networks. Rev. Mod. Phys. **74**(1), 47 (2002)
2. Anderson, H.L.: Metropolis, Monte Carlo and the MANIAC. Los Alamos Sci. **14**, 96–108 (1986)
3. Carballosa, A., Mussa-Juane, M., & Muñuzuri, A. P.: Incorporating social opinion in the evolution of an epidemic spread (2020). arXiv preprint arXiv:2007.04619
4. Diekmann, O., Heesterbeek, J.: Mathematical Epidemiology of Infectious Diseases: Model Building, Analysis and Interpretation. John Wiley & Sons (2000)
5. Erdös, P., Rényi, A.: On random graphs I. Math. debrecen **6**, 290–297 (1959)
6. Eubank, S., Guclu, H., Kumar, V.A., Marathe, M.V., Srinivasan, A., Toroczkai, Z., Wang, N.: Modelling disease outbreaks in realistic urban social networks. Nature **429**(6988), 180–184 (2004)
7. Gaudart, J., Ghassani, M., Mintsa, J., Rachdi, M., Waku, J., Demongeot, J.: Demography and diffusion in epidemics: malaria and black death spread. Acta. Biotheor. **58**(2–3), 277–305 (2010)
8. Jeger, M.J., Pautasso, M., Holdenrieder, O., Shaw, M.W.: Modelling disease spread and control in networks: implications for plant sciences. New Phytol. **174**(2), 279–297 (2007)
9. Mimar, S., Juane, M.M., Park, J., Munuzuri, A.P., Ghoshal, G.: Turing patterns mediated by network topology in homogeneous active systems. Phys. Rev. E **99**(6), 062303 (2019)
10. Moore, C., & Newman, M.E.J.: Epidemics and percolation in small-world networks. Phys. Rev. E **61**, 5678–5682 (2000). https://doi.org/10.1103/Phys-RevE.61.5678
11. Ndairou, F., Area, I., Nieto, J.J., Torres, D.F.: Mathematical modeling of COVID-19 transmission dynamics with a case study of Wuhan. Chaos, Solitons Fractals **135**, 109846 (2020). https://doi.org/10.1016/j.chaos.2020.109846
12. Press, W., Flannery, B., Teukolsky, S., Vetterling, W.: Numerical Recipes in C the Art of Scientific Computing. Cambridge University Press (1988)
13. Read, J.M., Eames, K.T., Edmunds, W.J.: Dynamic social networks and the implications for the spread of infectious disease. J. R. Soc. Interface **5**(26), 1001–1007 (2008)
14. Siebers, P., Aickelin, U.: Introduction to multi-agent simulation (2008). arXiv preprint abs:0803.3905
15. Sun, G.-Q.: Pattern formation of an epidemic model with diffusion. Nonlinear Dyn. **69**(3), 1097–1104 (2012)
16. Watts, D.J., Muhamad, R., Medina, D.C., Dodds, P.S.: Multiscale, resurgent epidemics in a hierarchical metapopulation model. Proc. Natl. Acad. Sci. **102**(32), 11157–11162 (2005)
17. Watts, D.J.,& Strogatz, S.H. : Collective dynamics of small-world networks. Nature **393**, 440–442 (1998)
18. Wu, Y., Shen, F.: Negativity makes us polarized: a longitudinal study of media tone and opinion polarization in Hong Kong. Asian J. Commun. **30**(3–4), 199–200 (2020). https://doi.org/10.1080/01292986.2020.1784968

Modelling the Significant Effect of Public Health Interventions on Covid-19 Transmission

Abhineshwary Bhalraj and Amirah Azmi

Abstract A major Coronavirus outbreak, which was first identified in Wuhan, China in December 2019, has rapidly spread all over the world. On 11 March 2020, the World Health Organization (WHO) has declared the novel Coronavirus Disease 2019 (Covid-19) outbreak a global pandemic. The increase in the number of reported infections and deaths due to Coronavirus outbreak inspired many countries to implement intervention measures. In this work, we use Susceptible-Exposed-Infected-Recovered (SEIR) model to predict the outbreak of the disease. SEIR model was chosen compared to SIR model because exposed individuals whom are asymptomatic or having mild symptoms contribute to the increase of number of infections. We also work on modelling the transmission dynamics of Covid-19 in the presence of three intervention measures. The proposed model describes the evolution of the disease in the population when preventive measures, active case-finding and hospitalization interventions are implemented as strategies to control and eradicate the disease. Variation in the effectiveness of combined interventions for infectious individuals are observed and analyzed by simulating the Covid-19 model with interventions. Our simulation results shows that more rigorous and stringent public health interventions would reduce the risk of Covid-19 spreading. It is of great importance and practical significance to ensure early prevention, early detection and early treatment to combat Covid-19.

Keywords Public Health Interventions · Modelling · SEIR Covid-19 model

1 Introduction

The World Health Organization (WHO) China Country Office was informed of a total of 44 cases of pneumonia detected in Wuhan City, Hubei Province of China on 31 December 2019 [1]. Majority of these cases were exposed to Huanan South

A. Bhalraj · A. Azmi (✉)
School of Mathematical Sciences, Universiti Sains Malaysia, 11800 Penang, Malaysia
e-mail: amirahazmi@usm.my

P. Agarwal et al. (eds.), *Analysis of Infectious Disease Problems (Covid-19) and Their Global Impact*, Infosys Science Foundation Series,
https://doi.org/10.1007/978-981-16-2450-6_22

China Seafood Market in Wuhan city [2]. After a series of investigation, a novel type of Coronavirus was isolated from a patient on 7 January 2020 [3]. The virus was named as the 2019-novel Coronavirus (2019-nCoV) temporarily on 12 January 2020 and later, on 11 February 2020, the virus was officially named as Coronavirus disease 2019 (Covid-19) by the WHO [4]. The Covid-19 outbreak caused by Severe Acute Respiratory Syndrome Coronavirus 2 (SARS-CoV-2) was declared as a Public Health Emergency of International Concern on 30 January 2020 and it was proclaimed as a pandemic by the WHO on 11 March 2020 [5].

Coronavirus are a large family of viruses that cause illness ranging from the common cold to more severe illnesses like SARS, Middle East Respiratory Syndrome (MERS) and Covid-19 [6]. Coronavirus is confirmed to be human to human transmission as soon as it was brought into the crowd from the seafood market. For example, when one infected person returned home, six out of seven of the family members whom have not visited the seafood market got infected [7]. When an infected person coughs or sneezes, SARS-CoV-2 virus spread mainly through close contact from person-to-person in respiratory droplets [8]. The most common symptoms of Covid-19 are fever, cough, shortness of breath, muscle ache, confusion, headache, sore throat, rhinorrhea, chest pain, diarrhea, nausea and vomiting [9]. The incubation period (time from exposure to the development of symptoms) of the virus is estimated to be between 2 and 14 days [10]. The average time from onset of symptoms to clinical recovery for mild cases is approximately 2 weeks whereas for patients with severe or critical disease, the mean time is 3–6 weeks [11].

As of 23 July 2020, Covid-19 has been affecting 213 countries and territories around the world, with a total of 15, 405, 273 confirmed cases, 631, 021 deaths and 9, 381, 496 recovered cases. Among them, a total of 2, 726, 918 confirmed cases were reported in Europe, 4, 806, 569 in North America, 3, 618, 687 in Asia, 3, 463, 246 in South America and 774, 134 in Africa [10]. In this work, we restrict our study area to five countries in Asia. India, Bangladesh, Iraq, Indonesia and Philippines have been selected for analysis purposes because these are some of the countries in Asia that are still in the acceleration stage of Covid-19 outbreak.

With the outbreak of Covid-19, it is essential for us to forecast the trend and peak of the infection so that effective strategies can be carried out for every country. The number of infected people is expanding and the effect of containment measures are being assessed on an empirical basis due to the incomprehensible of the mechanisms for the propagation of Covid-19. These circumstances raised many questions. When will the spread of the pandemic reaches the peak or turn to stabilize? How many people will be at the risk of being infected? How do interventions curtail Covid-19 and to what extent interventions help in managing the pandemic? Therefore, it would be much more interesting if more quantitative analysis can be done on the pandemic spreading.

There have been several mathematical models developed by various researchers to forecast the dynamics of Covid-19 since the outbreak of the pandemic in Wuhan [6, 8, 12–25]. However, most of the models ignored birth and death rate of the population. Although the number of paediatric cases remains small, it is vital to make sure everyone is counted in the model.

From analysis point of view, a number of studies analyzed the effects of particular intervention in order to combat Covid-19. Falco et al. [26] investigated the consequences of variations in the social distancing level on the evolution over time of Covid-19 spreading in Italy by optimizing SEIR model. Li et al. [27] built a modified SEIR model to assess quarantine measures based on current clinical and epidemiological data in China. Read et al. [3] explored the effectiveness of travel restrictions from and to Wuhan by considering air travel only. As far as we know, no previous research has evaluated the effect of combined interventions such as implementing preventive measures, active case-finding and hospitalization.

The objective of the current study is to implement SEIR mathematical model to forecast the future of Covid-19 in terms of the number of days it will take to reach the peak and also to contain the outbreak. The study also aims to analyze the impact of combined interventions on the spread of the pandemic. The scope of this study is limited to estimate the trend of Covid-19 for India, Bangladesh, Iraq, Indonesia and Philippines and uses ordinary differential equations (ODEs) based forecasting methods which are easy to build, easy to describe our nature of problem and the solutions can be obtained efficiently.

The research is organized as follows. Section 2 briefly discusses the mathematical model of Covid-19 with the absence and presence of interventions. The mathematical analysis of the models with the absence and presence of interventions are carried out in Sect. 3. In Sect. 4, we present the numerical simulations and analysis of the proposed model for each of the countries stated above. Finally, we conclude our work in the closure section.

2 Covid-19 Mathematical Model

In this section, we describe the transmission of Covid-19 by an SEIR model. SEIR refers to Susceptible, Exposed, Infected and Recovered individuals respectively. The total population for humans is denoted by N, where we assume that initially all individuals are susceptible to Covid-19. Figure 1 below shows the compartment diagram of SEIR Covid-19 model. When Covid-19 is introduced to a population, it splits the human population from Susceptible compartment to Exposed compartment by the transmission rate, β and then to Infected compartment by infectious rate, ε. When individuals reach Recovered compartment by recovery rate, γ, we assume that they either survived the disease and are now immune or succumbed to the illness and are out of the population. We also assume that the population is closed, which means the increase or decrease of population is only caused by birth and death while the increase and reduction caused by other factors is ignored. Besides, death caused by factors other than Covid-19 infection is considered a natural death.

The population of susceptible individuals is increased by birth rate (which is assumed susceptible), at the rate of b. The susceptible human population decreased by following the effective contact with the SARS-CoV-2 virus at the rate β. The population of susceptible human is further decreased with the natural death rate of

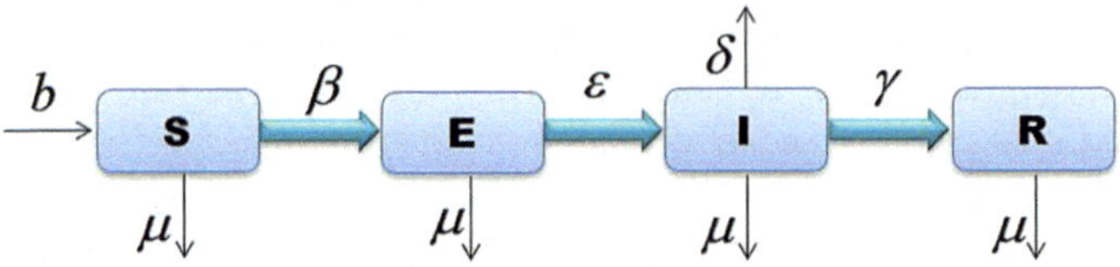

Fig. 1 Compartment diagram of SEIR Covid-19 model

human, μ. So, we can write, the rate of change of the susceptible human population is given by

$$\frac{dS}{dt} = b - \beta SI - \mu S.$$

The population of exposed individuals is generated by the transmission rate, β. The population of exposed human is decreased by the infectious rate, ε, where the exposed individuals develop symptoms of Covid-19. The exposed human population is further decreased by the natural death rate of human, μ. So, we can write, the rate of change for exposed human population is given by

$$\frac{dE}{dt} = \beta SI - (\varepsilon + \mu)E.$$

The population of infected individuals is increased by infectious rate, ε. The population of infected human is decreased by the natural death rate of human, μ. Infected individuals can either recover at a rate γ or they die from Covid-19 at the rate δ. So, we can write, the rate of change for infected human population is given by

$$\frac{dI}{dt} = \varepsilon E - (\gamma + \mu + \delta)I.$$

The population of recovered individuals is generated by the recovery rate of human, γ while decreased by the natural death rate of human, μ. Thus, the rate of change for recovered human population can be expressed as follows

$$\frac{dR}{dt} = \gamma I - \mu R.$$

We assume that all the parameters stated in Fig. 1 are non-negative. The transmission of Covid-19 pandemic is described by the following system of nonlinear ODEs:

$$\left.\begin{aligned}
\frac{dS}{dt} &= b - \beta SI - \mu S, && S(0)\geq 0,\\
\frac{dE}{dt} &= \beta SI - (\varepsilon + \mu)E, && E(0)\geq 0,\\
\frac{dI}{dt} &= \varepsilon E - (\gamma + \mu + \delta)I, && I(0)\geq 0,\\
\frac{dR}{dt} &= \gamma I - \mu R, && R(0)\geq 0.
\end{aligned}\right\} \tag{1}$$

Next, we discuss the transmission of Covid-19 model by incorporating three intervention strategies into System (1). The implementation of these strategies is motivated by the idea of the Ebola virus disease (EVD) article [28]. Figure 2 below depicts the compartment diagram of SEIR Covid-19 model with interventions. The main strategy to halt further spread of the disease is through interventions, which we include them as parameters into System (1). This can be done through preventive measures, u_1 which encourage behavioral changes like the use of hand sanitizer regularly, the use of face mask whenever being in public especially for sick person or close contact with people, maintain social distancing in crowded area and the best option is to stay at home.

The second strategy that we are proposing is to gain more information on possible infections in the population through active case-finding or detection, u_2 which consists of searching for and recording cases in the community by talking to local leaders, families or any possible informants. It significantly helps in limiting further contamination of Covid-19 infection.

The final strategy is considering the case when an individual is infected by Covid-19, his chances of recovery can be increased through hospitalization, u_3 which consist of providing essential medical equipment for infected individual as well as personal protective equipment (PPE) for medical frontliners. The reason we chose the interventions mentioned above is because, as we are all aware, the three key to a healthier lifestyle during this hard situation of the Covid-19 pandemic are early prevention, early detection and early treatment in order to reduce the risk of Covid-19 infection.

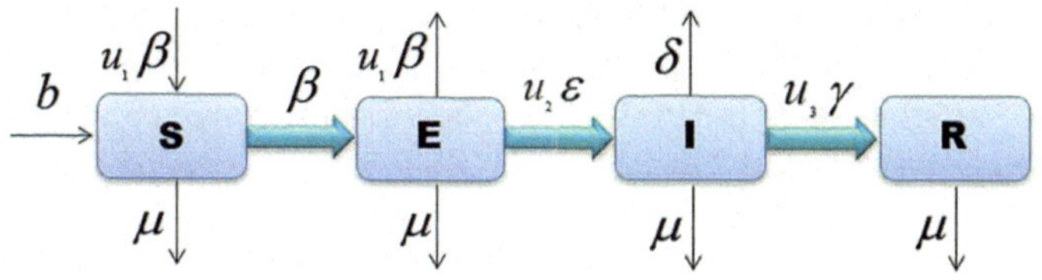

Fig. 2 Compartment diagram of SEIR Covid-19 model with interventions

We assume that all the parameters stated in Fig. 2 are non-negative. The parameters involved in Systems (1) and (2) are described below in Table 1. The transmission of Covid-19 pandemic with interventions is described by the following system of nonlinear ODEs :

$$\left.\begin{aligned}
\frac{dS}{dt} &= b - (1-u_1)\beta SI - \mu S, && S(0)\geq 0,\\
\frac{dE}{dt} &= (1-u_1)\beta SI - (u_2\varepsilon + \mu)E, && E(0)\geq 0,\\
\frac{dI}{dt} &= u_2\varepsilon E - (u_3\gamma + \mu + \delta)I, && I(0)\geq 0,\\
\frac{dR}{dt} &= u_3\gamma I - \mu R, && R(0)\geq 0.
\end{aligned}\right\} \quad (2)$$

Table 1 Description of parameters used in systems (1) and (2)

Parameter	Description
β	Transmission rate
ε	Infectious rate
γ	Recovery rate
δ	Death rate due to Covid-19
b	Birth rate
μ	Natural death rate
u_1	Level of preventive measures
u_2	Level of active case-finding
u_3	Level of hospitalization

3 Mathematical Analysis

In this section, the Covid-19 models with the absence and presence of interventions are analyzed by determining the equilibrium points and the basic reproduction number. Then, we investigate the local stability analysis of the equilibrium points obtained from Systems (1) and (2). By setting the left hand side of each of the systems equal to zero and solving them simultaneously, we obtain the equilibrium points in which they can be classified into two categories; disease free equilibrium point (DFEP) and pandemic equilibrium point (PEP). Through some algebraic manipulation, we obtain the solutions given in Tables 2 and 3.

Table 2 Equilibrium points for system (1)

Variable	DFEP (E_{01})	PEP (E_{11})
S	$\frac{b}{\mu}$	$\frac{(\varepsilon+\mu)(\gamma+\mu+\delta)}{\beta\varepsilon}$
E	0	$\frac{b}{\varepsilon+\mu} - \frac{\mu(\gamma+\mu+\delta)}{\beta\varepsilon}$
I	0	$-\frac{\mu}{\beta} + \frac{b\varepsilon}{(\varepsilon+\mu)(\gamma+\mu+\delta)}$
R	0	$-\frac{\gamma}{\beta} + \frac{b\varepsilon\gamma}{\mu(\varepsilon+\mu)(\gamma+\mu+\delta)}$

Table 3 Equilibrium points for system (2)

Variable	DFEP (E_{02})	PEP (E_{12})
S	$\frac{b}{\mu}$	$\frac{(\mu+\varepsilon u_2)(\mu+\delta+\gamma u_3)}{\beta\varepsilon(-1+u_1)u_2}$
E	0	$\frac{\mu^3+b\beta\varepsilon(-1+u_1)u_2+\varepsilon\mu u_2(\delta+\gamma u_3)+\mu^2(\delta+\varepsilon u_2+\gamma u_3)}{\beta\varepsilon(-1+u_1)u_2(\mu+\varepsilon u_2)}$
I	0	$\frac{\mu^3+b\beta\varepsilon(-1+u_1)u_2+\varepsilon\mu u_2(\delta+\gamma u_3)+\mu^2(\delta+\varepsilon u_2+\gamma u_3)}{\beta(-1+u_1)(\mu+\varepsilon u_2)(\mu+\delta+\gamma u_3)}$
R	0	$\frac{\gamma u_3(\mu^3+b\beta\varepsilon(-1+u_1)u_2+\varepsilon\mu u_2(\delta+\gamma u_3)+\mu^2(\delta+\varepsilon u_2+\gamma u_3))}{\beta\mu(-1+u_1)(\mu+\varepsilon u_2)(\mu+\delta+\gamma u_3)}$

The basic reproduction number, R_0, which represents the expected number of secondary infections per infected individual in a totally susceptible population. If $R_0 > 1$, the number of infected people will increase, if $R_0 = 1$, the disease becomes pandemic and when $R_0 < 1$, the number of infected people is likely to decline [29]. This can be calculated by employing the next generation matrix approach [30]. The basic reproduction number of Systems (1) and (2) are given respectively as follows:

$$R_{01} = \frac{b\beta\varepsilon}{\mu(\varepsilon+\mu)(\gamma+\mu+\delta)}, \tag{3}$$

$$R_{02} = \frac{b\beta(1-u_1)(u_2\varepsilon)}{\mu(\varepsilon u_2+\mu)(\gamma u_3+\mu+\delta)}. \tag{4}$$

Next, we examine the local stability analysis of DFEP and PEP of each of the Systems (1) and (2) by the theorem below:

Theorem 1 *The disease free equilibrium point, E_{01} is locally asymptotically stable if $R_{01} < 1$ and unstable if $R_{01} > 1$ [31].*

Proof First, we compute the Jacobian matrix, J of the System (1) by taking partial derivatives with respect to S, E, I and R. The Jacobian matrix, J is then evaluated at the disease free equilibrium, E_{01} as follows:

$$J(E_{01}) = \begin{bmatrix} -\mu & 0 & -\beta\frac{b}{\mu} & 0 \\ 0 & -(\varepsilon+\mu) & \beta\frac{b}{\mu} & 0 \\ 0 & \varepsilon & -(\gamma+\mu+\delta) & 0 \\ 0 & 0 & \gamma & -\mu \end{bmatrix}.$$

By performing elementary row operations, the characteristic equation of the above matrix can be written as

$$(\mu+\lambda)(\mu+\lambda)(\lambda^2+a_1\lambda+a_0) = 0, \tag{5}$$

where

$$a_1 = (2\mu + \delta + \gamma + \varepsilon)$$
$$a_0 = (\mu + \delta + \gamma)(\varepsilon + \mu)(1 - R_{01})$$

It is easy to see that the roots of the characteristic equation (5) are $-\mu$ and $-\mu$ (which is the same root repeated) have negative real parts. The other two roots can be obtained from the second order polynomial of the characteristic equation (5). The Routh-Hurwitz stability criterion for quadratic polynomial is satisfied as $a_1 > 0$ and $a_0 > 0$ if $R_{01} < 1$. Thus, all the eigenvalues of the characteristic equation (5) have negative real parts. Therefore, the disease free equilibrium point, E_{01} is locally asymptotically stable if $R_{01} < 1$. .

Theorem 2 *The pandemic equilibrium point,* E_{11} *is locally asymptotically stable if* $R_{01} > 1$ *and unstable if* $R_{01} < 1$. *[31]*

Proof First, we compute the Jacobian matrix, J of the System (1) by taking partial derivatives with respect to S, E, I and R. The Jacobian matrix, J is then evaluated at the pandemic equilibrium, E_{11} as follows:

$$J(E_{11}) = \begin{bmatrix} -\beta I^* - \mu & 0 & -\beta S^* & 0 \\ \beta I^* & -(\varepsilon + \mu) & \beta S^* & 0 \\ 0 & \varepsilon & -(\gamma + \mu + \delta) & 0 \\ 0 & 0 & \gamma & -\mu \end{bmatrix},$$

where $S^* = \frac{(\varepsilon+\mu)(\gamma+\mu+\delta)}{\beta\varepsilon}$, and $I^* = \frac{\mu}{\beta}(R_{01} - 1)$.

By performing elementary row operations, the characteristic equation of the above matrix can be written as

$$\lambda^4 + a_3\lambda^3 + a_2\lambda^2 + a_1\lambda + a_0, \tag{6}$$

where

$$\begin{aligned} a_0 &= (\varepsilon\mu^3 + \mu^4 + \varepsilon\mu^2\gamma + \mu^3\gamma + \varepsilon\mu^2\delta + \{\mu^3\delta - \beta\varepsilon\mu^2 S^*\} + \beta\varepsilon\mu^2 I^* + \beta\mu^3 I^* \\ &\quad + \beta\varepsilon\mu\gamma I^* + \beta\mu^2\gamma I^* + \beta\varepsilon\mu\delta I^* + \beta\mu^2\delta I^*), \\ a_1 &= (3\varepsilon\mu^2 + 4\mu^3 + 2\varepsilon\mu\gamma + 3\mu^2\gamma + 2\varepsilon\mu\delta + \{3\mu^2\delta - 2\beta\varepsilon\mu S^*\} + 2\beta\varepsilon\mu I^* + 3\beta\mu^2 I^* \\ &\quad + \beta\varepsilon\gamma I^* + 2\beta\mu\gamma I^* + 2\beta\mu\delta I^*), \\ a_2 &= (3\varepsilon\mu + 6\mu^2 + \varepsilon\gamma + 3\mu\gamma + \varepsilon\delta + \{3\mu\delta - \beta\varepsilon S^*\} + \beta\varepsilon I^* + 3\beta\mu I^* + \beta\gamma I^* + \beta\delta I^*), \\ a_3 &= (\varepsilon + 4\mu + \gamma + \delta + \beta I^*). \end{aligned}$$

The Routh-Hurwitz stability criterion for quartic polynomial is satisfied as $a_0 > 0$, $a_1 > 0$, $a_2 > 0$, $a_3 > 0$ and $a_1a_2a_3 - a_1^2 - a_0a_3^2 > 0$ if $R_{01} > 1$ and the terms under braces are positive. Thus, all the eigenvalues of the characteristic equation (6) have negative real parts. Therefore, the pandemic equilibrium point, E_{11} is locally asymptotically stable if $R_{01} > 1$ and the terms under braces are positive.

Theorem 3 *The disease free equilibrium point,* E_{02} *is locally asymptotically stable if* $R_{02} < 1$ *and unstable if* $R_{02} > 1$*. [31]*

Proof First, we compute the Jacobian matrix, J of the System (2) by taking partial derivatives with respect to S, E, I and R. The Jacobian matrix, J is then evaluated at the disease free equilibrium, E_{02} as follows:

$$J(E_{02}) = \begin{bmatrix} -\mu & 0 & -(1-u_1)\beta\frac{b}{\mu} & 0 \\ 0 & -(u_2\varepsilon+\mu) & (1-u_1)\beta\frac{b}{\mu} & 0 \\ 0 & u_2\varepsilon & -(u_3\gamma+\mu+\delta) & 0 \\ 0 & 0 & u_3\gamma & -\mu \end{bmatrix}.$$

By performing elementary row operations, the characteristic equation of the above matrix can be written as

$$(\mu+\lambda)(\mu+\lambda)(\lambda^2+a_1\lambda+a_0)=0, \tag{7}$$

where

$$\begin{aligned} a_1 &= (2\mu+\delta+\gamma u_3+\varepsilon u_2), \\ a_0 &= (\mu^2+\varepsilon u_2(\delta+\gamma u_3)+\mu(\delta+\varepsilon u_2+\gamma u_3))(1-R_{02}). \end{aligned}$$

It is easy to see that the roots of the characteristic equation (7) are $-\mu$ and $-\mu$ (which is the same root repeated) have negative real parts. The other two roots can be obtained from the second order polynomial of the characteristic equation (7). The Routh-Hurwitz stability criterion for quadratic polynomial is satisfied as $a_1 > 0$ and $a_0 > 0$ if $R_{02} < 1$. Thus, all the eigenvalues of the characteristic equation (7) have negative real parts. Therefore, the disease free equilibrium point, E_{02} is locally asymptotically stable if $R_{02} < 1$.

Theorem 4 *The pandemic equilibrium point,* E_{12} *is locally asymptotically stable if* $R_{02} > 1$ *and unstable if* $R_{02} < 1$*. [31]*

Proof First, we compute the Jacobian matrix, J of the System (2) by taking partial derivatives with respect to S, E, I and R. The Jacobian matrix, J is then evaluated at the pandemic equilibrium, E_{12} as follows:

$$J(E_{12}) = \begin{bmatrix} -(1-u_1)\beta I^*-\mu & 0 & -(1-u_1)\beta S^* & 0 \\ (1-u_1)\beta I^* & -(u_2\varepsilon+\mu) & (1-u_1)\beta S^* & 0 \\ 0 & u_2\varepsilon & -(u_3\gamma+\mu+\delta) & 0 \\ 0 & 0 & u_3\gamma & -\mu \end{bmatrix},$$

where

$$S^* = \frac{(\mu + \varepsilon u_2)(\mu + \delta + \gamma u_3)}{\beta\varepsilon(-1 + u_1)u_2},$$
$$I^* = \frac{\mu^3 + \varepsilon\mu u_2(\delta + \gamma u_3) + \mu^2(\delta + \varepsilon u_2 + \gamma u_3)}{\beta(1 - u_1)(\mu + \varepsilon u_2)(\mu + \delta + \gamma u_3)}(R_{02} - 1).$$

By performing elementary row operations, the characteristic equation of the above matrix can be written as

$$\lambda^4 + a_3\lambda^3 + a_2\lambda^2 + a_1\lambda + a_0 = 0, \tag{8}$$

where

$$\begin{aligned}
a_0 = {} & (\mu^4 + \delta\mu^3 + \beta\mu^3 I^* + \{\beta\mu^2\delta I^* - \beta\varepsilon\mu\gamma u_1u_2u_3 I^* - \beta\mu^3 u_1 I^* - \beta\mu^2\delta u_1 I^* \\
& - \beta\varepsilon\mu^2 u_2 S^* - \beta\varepsilon\mu^2 u_1u_2 I^* - \beta\varepsilon\mu\delta u_1u_2 I^* - \beta\mu^2\gamma u_1u_3 I^*\} + \varepsilon\mu^3 u_2 + \varepsilon\mu^2\delta u_2 \\
& + \beta\varepsilon\mu^2 u_2 I^* + \beta\varepsilon\mu\delta u_2 I^* + \beta\varepsilon\mu^2 u_1u_2 S^* + \mu^3\gamma u_3 + \beta\mu^2\gamma u_3 I^* + \varepsilon\mu^2\gamma u_2u_3 \\
& + \beta\varepsilon\mu\gamma u_2u_3 I^*), \\
a_1 = {} & (3\delta\mu^2 + 4\mu^3 + 3\beta\mu^2 I^* + \{2\beta\mu\delta I^* - 3\beta\mu^2 u_1 I^* - 2\beta\mu\delta u_1 I^* - 2\beta\varepsilon\mu u_2 S^* \\
& - 2\beta\varepsilon\mu u_1u_2 I^* - \beta\varepsilon\delta u_1u_2 I^* - 2\beta\mu\gamma u_1u_3 I^* - \beta\varepsilon\gamma u_1u_2u_3 I^*\} + 3\varepsilon\mu^2 u_2 \\
& + 2\varepsilon\mu\delta u_2 + 2\beta\varepsilon\mu u_2 I^* + \beta\varepsilon\delta u_2 I^* + 2\beta\varepsilon\mu u_1u_2 S^* + 3\mu^2\delta u_3 + 2\beta\mu\gamma u_3 I^* \\
& + 2\varepsilon\mu\gamma u_2u_3 + \beta\varepsilon\gamma u_2u_3 I^*), \\
a_2 = {} & (3\delta\mu + 6\mu^2 + 3\beta\mu I^* + \{\beta\delta I^* - 3\beta\mu u_1 I^* - \beta\varepsilon u_2 S^* - \beta\delta u_1 I^* - \beta\gamma u_1u_3 I^* \\
& - \beta\varepsilon u_1u_2 I^*\} + 3\varepsilon\mu u_2 + \varepsilon\delta u_2 + \beta\varepsilon u_2 I^* + \beta\varepsilon u_1u_2 S^* + 3\mu\gamma u_3 + \beta\gamma u_3 I^* \\
& + \varepsilon\gamma u_2u_3), \\
a_3 = {} & (\varepsilon u_2 + 4\mu + \gamma u_3 + \delta + \{\beta I^* - \beta u_1 I^*\}).
\end{aligned}$$

The Routh-Hurwitz stability criterion for quartic polynomial is satisfied as $a_0 > 0$, $a_1 > 0$, $a_2 > 0$, $a_3 > 0$ and $a_1a_2a_3 - a_1^2 - a_0a_3^2 > 0$ if $R_{02} > 1$ and the terms under braces are positive. Thus, all the eigenvalues of the characteristic equation (8) have negative real parts. Therefore, the pandemic equilibrium point, E_{12} is locally asymptotically stable if $R_{02} > 1$ and the terms under braces are positive.

4 Numerical Analysis

In this section, we present the numerical solution of the Systems (1) and (2) for India, Bangladesh, Iraq, Indonesia and Philippines. Since our main goal is to forecast the trend of Covid-19 outbreak for the said countries, so our discussion will focus on the number of infected people only. Thus, only infected compartment curves are plotted throughout this section. Then, we compare the predicted number of infected individuals without interventions and predicted number of infected individuals with interventions with the real dataset from Worldometer [10] for each of the country stated above. In addition, we also vary the effectiveness of combined interventions for infected cases from 50 to 90%. The given systems of equations are solved numerically by using the built-in function, called NDSolve in MATHEMATICA. We obtained the data of birth rate and death rate from the Countrymeters [32], number of infected individuals, infectious rate and death rate due to Covid-19 from the Worldometer [10], recovery rate from WHO report [11] and the transmission rate is estimated based on real-world data. We also assumed level of preventive measures, level of active case-finding and level of hospitalization to be 90% or equal to 0.9.

4.1 India

The parameter values used in the numerical solution are $b = 0.000056$, $\beta = 0.000062$, $\mu = 0.00002$, $\varepsilon = 0.142857$, $\gamma = 0.0714286$, $\delta = 0.0246$, $u_1 = 0.9$, $u_2 = 0.9$, and $u_3 = 0.9$. The initial conditions $S(0) = 5,000,000$, $E(0) = 1$, $I(0) = 0$ and $R(0) = 0$ are used in Fig. 3.

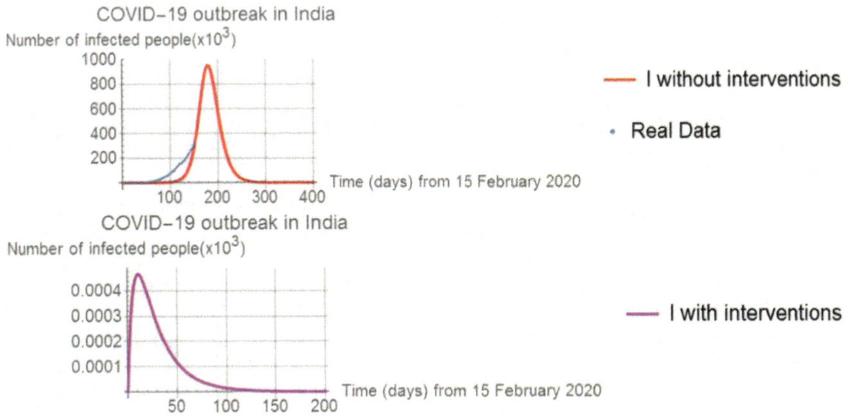

Fig. 3 Comparison of forecasted number of infected individuals without interventions (red curve) and forecasted number of infected individuals with interventions (pink curve) with real data (blue dots) of Covid-19 outbreak in India

The top of Fig. 3 shows the forecasted trend of Covid-19 pandemic in the absence of interventions whereas the bottom figure shows the forecasted trend of the pandemic in the presence of interventions up to 90% in India with respect to time in days. Day 0 in each of the figures above corresponds to 17th day since the first pandemic case was reported in India, that is on 15 February 2020. It can be seen from Fig. 3 that, without any interventons, the number of infected people will reach its peak in about 180 days with a total of approximately 950, 000 people. Then, this number tends to decrease and will eventually approaches zero around 1 December 2020. Considering the prediction on the number of cases when combined interventions is introduced, it is shown that the number of infected people may reach a maximum of one person only in 10 day and will eventually come to an end after 150 day from the period of initial consideration. We can also see that the data plotted by System (1) are in good accordance with the real-word data as shown in graph without any interventions strategies applied.

4.2 *Bangladesh*

The parameter values used in the numerical solution are $b = 0.000055$, $\beta = 0.000444$, $\mu = 0.000015$, $\varepsilon = 0.142857$, $\gamma = 0.0714286$, $\delta = 0.013$, $u_1 = 0.9$, $u_2 = 0.9$, and $u_3 = 0.9$. The initial conditions $S(0) = 600, 000$, $E(0) = 1$, $I(0) = 0$ and $R(0) = 0$ are used in Fig. 4.

Referring to Fig. 4, the top curves show the forecasted and real trend of Covid-19 pandemic in the absence of interventions whereas the bottom figure shows the forecasted trend of the pandemic in the presence of interventions up to 90% in Bangladesh with respect to time in days. Day 0 in each of the figures above cor-

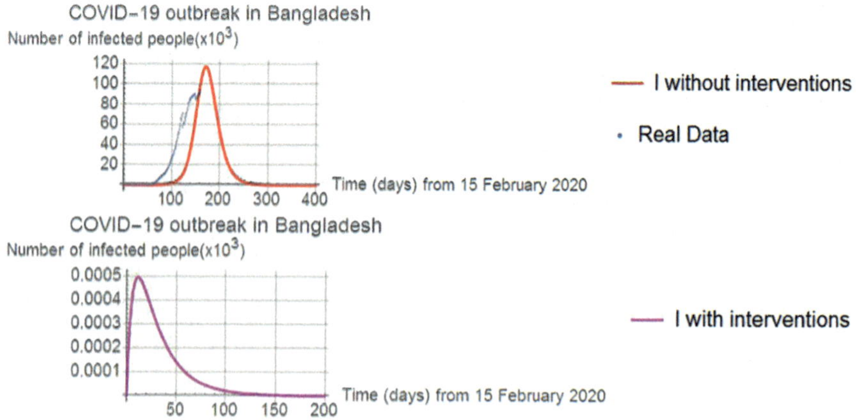

Fig. 4 Comparison of forecasted number of infected individuals without interventions (red curve) and forecasted number of infected individuals with interventions (pink curve) with real data (blue dots) of Covid-19 outbreak in Bangladesh

responds to 15 February 2020, that is 23 days before the first pandemic case was reported in Bangladesh. Without any interventions, we expects the peak of the infection to take place around 5 August 2020 with the number of infectious individuals equal to approximately 116, 900 people. The curve alo tells us that the pandemic cases would gradually disappear by the end of November 2020. On the other hand, adapting maximum intervention strategies depicts that the outbreak in Bangladesh will only reach its peak of the number of infected cases with one person in 12 d. The results also shows that, Bangladesh is expected to have no new cases or the infected cases gradually being close to zero by the middle of July 2020. The data plotted from System (1) whereby no interventions are taking into account is in good accordance with the real-world data as shown in the without any interventions graph. Comparing the real-word data in Figs. 3 and 4, it is clear that India reported higher number of cases compared to Bangladesh in approximately 150 days since 15 February 2020.

4.3 *Iraq*

The parameter values used in the numerical solution are $b = 0.000094$, $\beta = 0.000466$, $\mu = 0.000014$, $\varepsilon = 0.142857$, $\gamma = 0.0714286$, $\delta = 0.0402$, $u_1 = 0.9$, $u_2 = 0.9$, and $u_3 = 0.9$. The initial conditions $S(0) = 600, 000$, $E(0) = 1$, $I(0) = 0$ and $R(0) = 0$ are used in Fig. 5.

Moving on to Fig. 5, the top curves display the forecasted trend of Covid-19 pandemic in the absence of interventions whereas the bottom curve displays the forecasted trend of the pandemic in the presence of interventions up to 90% in

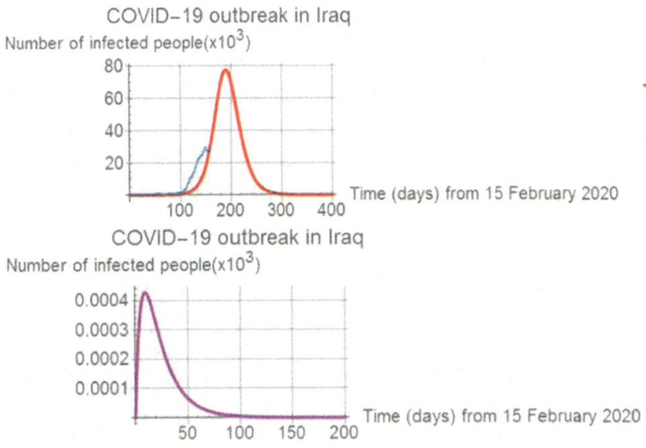

Fig. 5 Comparison of forecasted number of infected individuals without interventions (red curve) and forecasted number of infected individuals with interventions (pink curve) with real data (blue dots) of Covid-19 outbreak in Iraq

Iraq with respect to time in days. Day 0 in each of the figures above corresponds to 15 February 2020, that is 8 days before the first pandemic case was reported in Bangladesh. System (1) placed the peak time of infection in Iraq as 189 days after its initiate date 15 February 2020, with a maximum number of about 77, 220 infected individuals. The figure also shows that the number of infected people declines steadily and then stabilizes at zero in December 2020. On the contrary, the bottom pink curve portrays that with interventions, Iraq will reach its turning point of infection in 9 days with an estimated number of one people infected. It will then decelerate and finally leveled off in 118 days to the value of zero. The data provided by System (1) without interventions are in good accordance with the real-word data as it can be seen in the top curves. It can be furthermore observe by comparing real-world data in Figs. 3, 4 and 5 that India reported higher number of cases compared to Bangladesh and Iraq whereas Bangladesh reported higher number of cases compared to Iraq in approximately 150 days since 15 February 2020.

4.4 Indonesia

The parameter values used in the numerical solution are $b = 0.000056$, $\beta = 0.0.00044$, $\mu = 0.00002$, $\varepsilon = 0.142857$, $\gamma = 0.0714286$, $\delta = 0.0486$, $u_1 = 0.9$, $u_2 = 0.9$, and $u_3 = 0.9$. The initial conditions $S(0) = 700,000$, $E(0) = 1$, $I(0) = 0$ and $R(0) = 0$ are used in Fig. 6.

Correspondingly, the numerical analysis for Indonesia without any interventions is illustrated by the red curve in the top of Fig. 6. Whereas, the bottom pink curve illustrates the forecasted trend of the pandemic in the presence of interventions up to

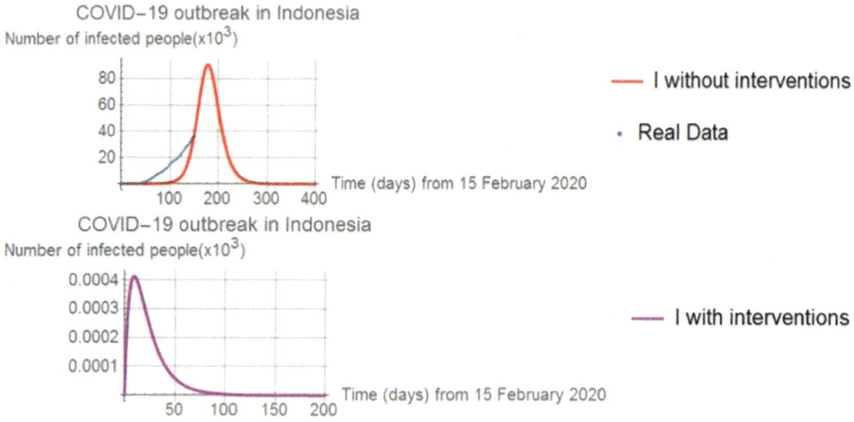

Fig. 6 Comparison of forecasted number of infected individuals without interventions (red curve) and forecasted number of infected individuals with interventions (pink curve) with real data (blue dots) of Covid-19 outbreak in Indonesia

90% with respect to time in days. Day 0 in each of the figures above corresponds to 15 February 2020, that is 17 days before the first pandemic case was reported in Indonesia. The estimated number of infections would reach the peak in early April, with roughly 90, 000 people as evidenced in the red curve and this pandemic is expected to completely disappear by early of December 2020. Undoubtedly, only if the country is equipped with maximum combined interventions, the pink curve shows that number of infected people will reach a maximum of one people in 9 days and then drop to zero in early of June 2020. The data provided by System (1) without interventions are in good accordance with the real-word data as shown by the blue dots compared to the red curve. On top of that, comparing real-world data in Figs. 3, 4, 5 and 6, it is easily seen that India reported higher number of cases compared to Bangladesh, Iraq and Indonesia whereas Iraq reported higher number of cases compared to Indonesia in approximately 150 days since 15 February 2020.

4.5 *Philippines*

The parameter values used in the numerical solution are $b = 0.000065$, $\beta = 0.00038$, $\mu = 0.0000182$, $\varepsilon = 0.142857$, $\gamma = 0.0714286$, $\delta = 0.0255$, $u_1 = 0.9$, $u_2 = 0.9$, and $u_3 = 0.9$. The initial conditions $S(0) = 700,000$, $E(0) = 1$, $I(0) = 0$ and $R(0) = 0$ are used in Fig. 7.

Similarly, as observed from the curves at the top of Fig. 7, the graph displays the forecasted trend of Covid-19 pandemic in the absence of interventions whereas the bottom pink curve displays the forecasted trend of the pandemic in the presence of interventions up to 90% in Philippines with respect to time in days. Day 0 in each of the figures above corresponds to 17th day since the first pandemic case was

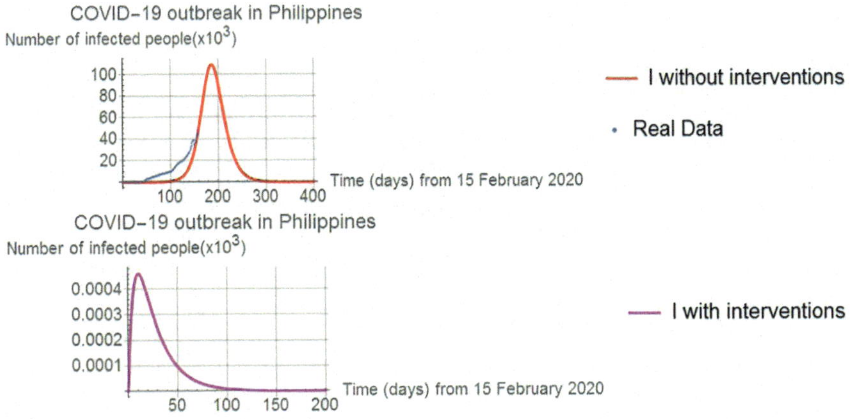

Fig. 7 Comparison of forecasted number of infected individuals without interventions (red curve) and forecasted number of infected individuals with interventions (pink curve) with real data (blue dots) of Covid-19 outbreak in Philippines

reported in Philippines, that is 15 February 2020 . System (1) placed the peak time of infection in Philippines as 186 days after its initiate date 15 February 2020, with a maximum number of infected individuals of about 108, 800 people as demonstrated in red curve. The number of infected people declines steadily and stabilizes at zero in December 2020. The pink curve portrays that with interventions, Philippines will reach its turning point of infection in 10 days with an estimated number of one people infected. It will then decelerate and finally leveled off in 130 days to the value of zero. The data provided by the model without interventions are in good accordance with the real-word data as it can be seen in the top of Fig. 7. A comparison is made between real-word data in Figs. 3, 4, 5, 6 and 7, we can see that India reported higher number of cases compared to Bangladesh, Iraq, Indonesia and Philippines whereas Indonesia reported higher number of cases compared to Philippines in approximately 150 days since 15 February 2020. Among all of the countries in Figs. 3 , 4, 5, 6 and 7 without interventions, India has the highest number of infected people followed by Bangladesh, Iraq, Indonesia and Philippines. In contrast, with interventions, India, Bangladesh, Iraq, Indonesia and Philippines reach their peak of infection in approximately 9 to 12 days.

4.6 Variation Intervention Level

In this section, we will be looking at the variation of the combined interventions levels of infectious individuals.

Combined interventions mentioned throughout this section includes all kind of preventive measures, active case-finding and hospitalization. Although most of the countries stated above have began to carry out some of the interventions to prevent transmission of the pandemic, the number of infected people still rising. Due to insufficient interventions which was assumed to be below 50%, so we estimate the trend of number of infected people in each of the countries shown from Figs. 8, 9, 10, 11 and 12 with the effect of combined interventions ranging from 50 to 90%. We do not consider the effect of combined interventions up to 100% because we assume that it is impossible for each of the individuals to obey and practice the preventive measures and as well as, it is difficult to obtain the essential medical equipment in a shorter time. It is obvious from Fig. 8, 9, 10, 11 and 12 that, flattening of the curve of infection cases occur as the implementation of combined interventions increases. The main aim of flattening the curve is to prevent a sharp peak of cases and spread out the infection over a longer period of time so that the healthcare system will not be overwhelmed.

As can be observed from Figs. 8, 9, 10, 11 and 12, the peak of Covid-19 infections will be 640, 000 in India, 92, 600 in Bangladesh, 35, 615 in Iraq, 37, 888 in Indonesia and 66, 770 in Philippines with enforcement of interventions up to 50%. When enforcement of interventions is raised up to 60%, the peak of infection cases will be 334, 900 in India, 48, 360 in Bangladesh, 10, 280 in Iraq, 11, 110 in Indonesia and 26, 940 in Philippines. If the enforcement of interventions is raised further up to 90%,

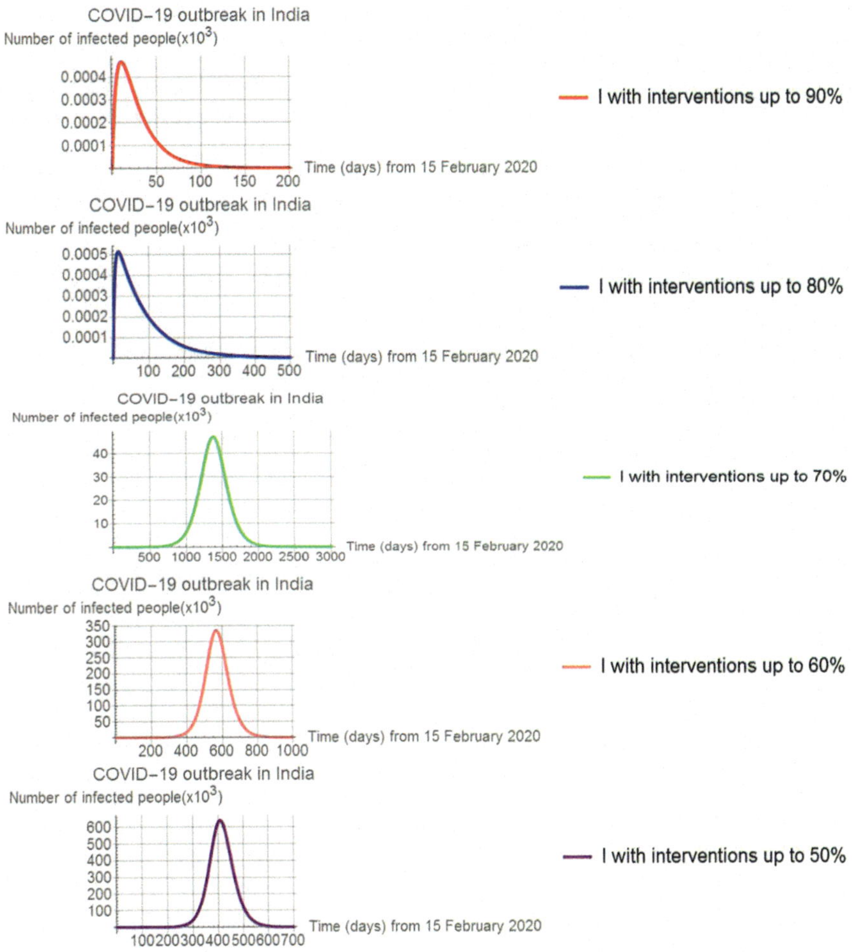

Fig. 8 Effectiveness of combined interventions levels for infectious individuals in India

the number of infected people finally become manageable, reducing from thousands to tens or merely a single digit as was discussed in previous parts of this section. We can see the effectiveness of combined interventions for infectious individuals as summarized below in Table 4. Table 4 outlines the forecasted maximum size of Covid-19 outbreak without interventions and also with interventions ranging from 50% to 90% as has been observed in Figs. 3, 4, 5, 6, 7, 8, 9, 10, 11 and 12 for each of the respective countries

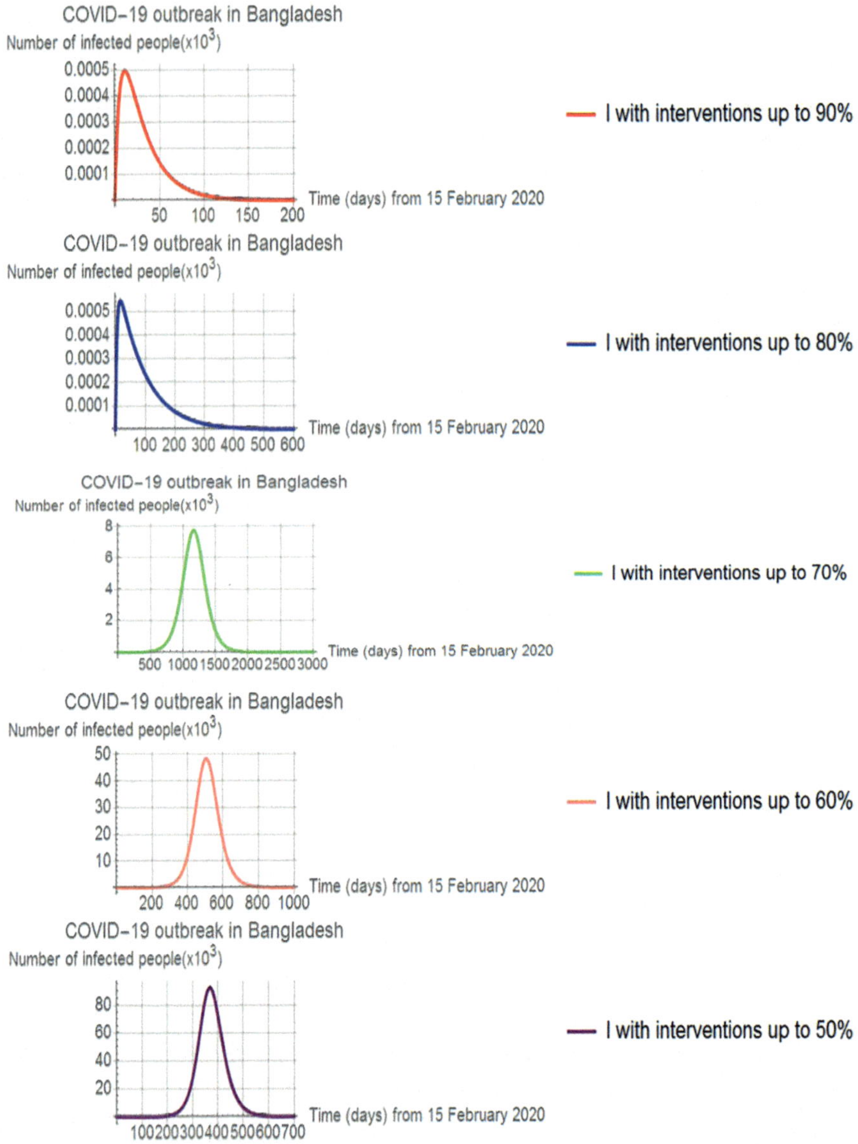

Fig. 9 Effectiveness of combined interventions levels for infectious individuals in Bangladesh

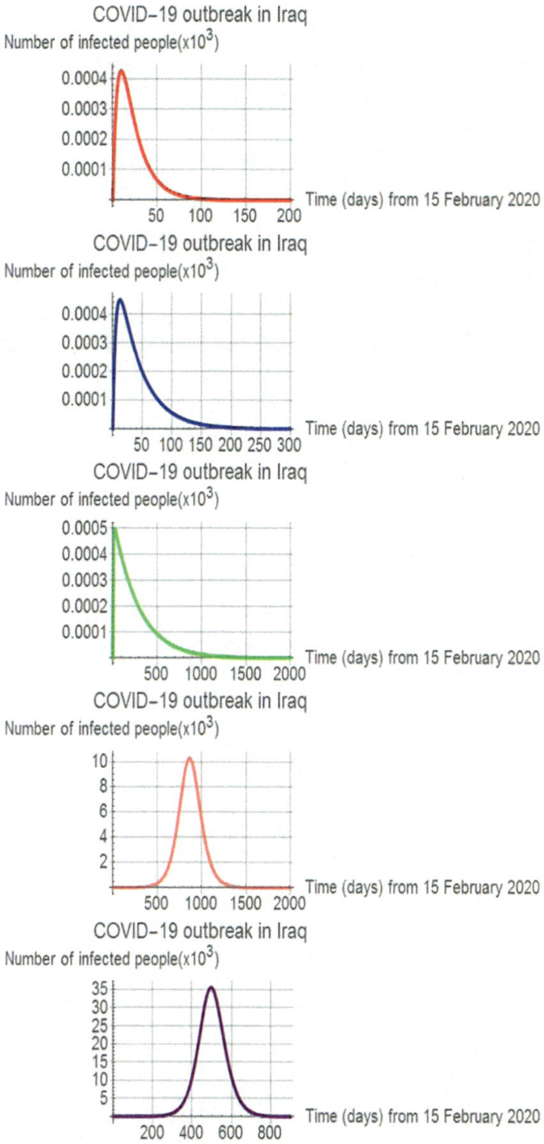

Fig. 10 Effectiveness of combined interventions levels for infectious individuals in Iraq

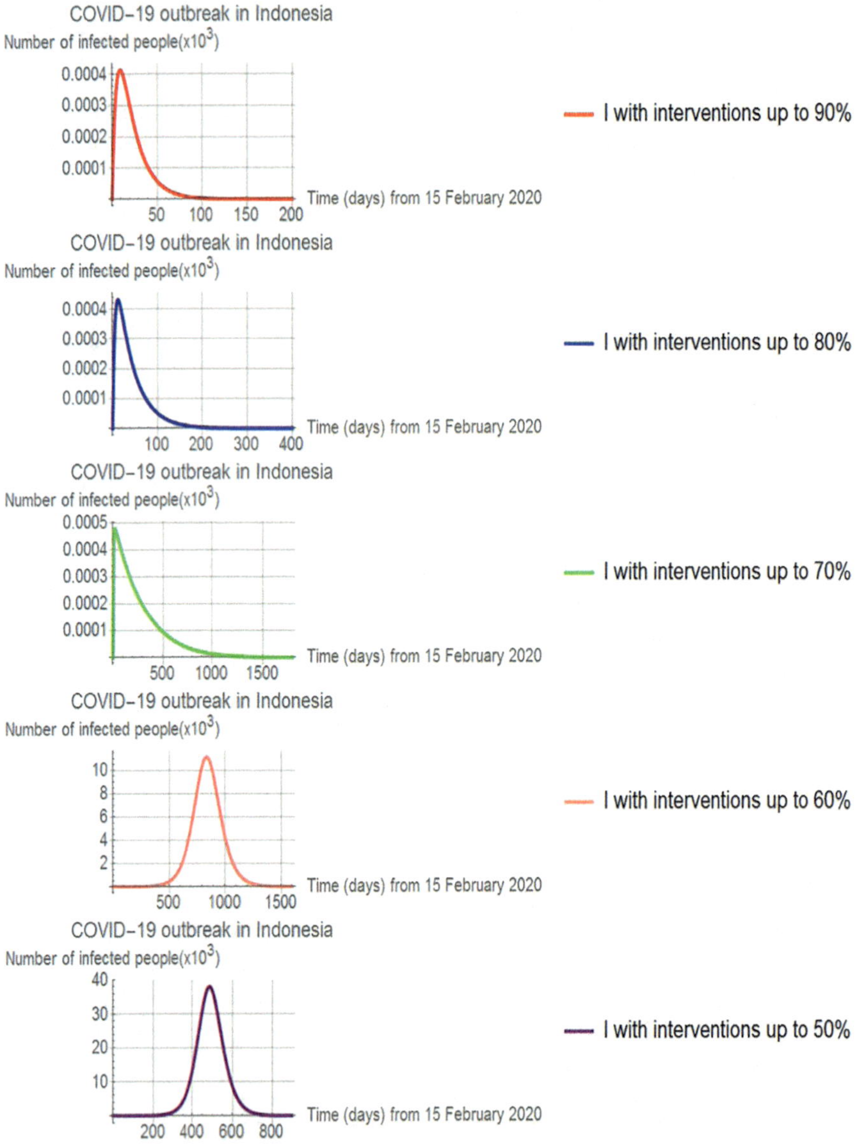

Fig. 11 Effectiveness of combined interventions levels for infectious individuals in Indonesia

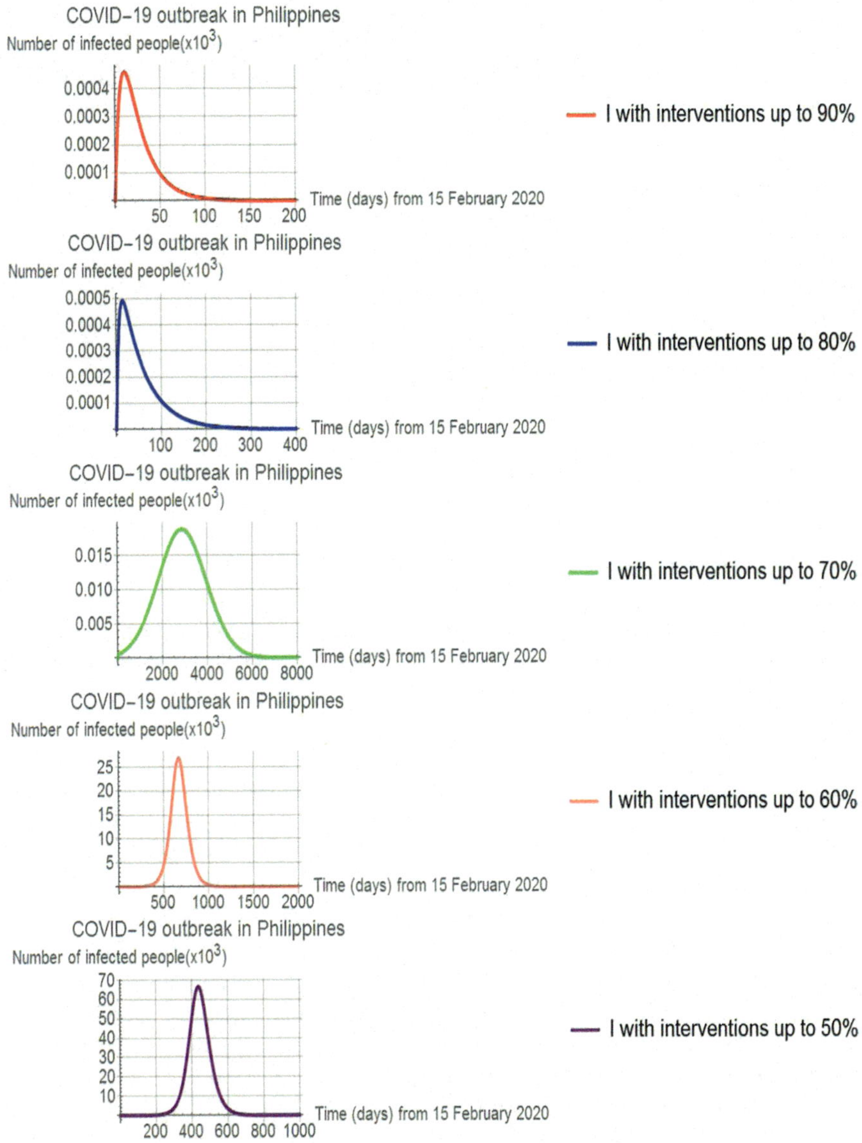

Fig. 12 Effectiveness of combined interventions levels for infectious individuals in Philippines

Table 4 The forecasted peak (maximum number) of the outbreak without interventions and with interventions ranging from 50% to 90%

Intervention Level	India	Bangladesh	Iraq	Indonesia	Philippines
Without interventions	950, 000	116, 900	77, 220	90, 000	108, 800
50% intervention	640, 000	92, 600	35, 615	37, 888	66, 770
60% intervention	334, 900	48, 360	10, 280	11, 110	26, 940
70% intervention	47, 190	7, 750	1	1	18
80% intervention	1	1	1	1	1
90% intervention	1	1	1	1	1

5 Conclusion

In this research, a compartmental SEIR model is constructed to describe the transmission of Covid-19 in human population. In order to curb Covid-19 outbreak, combined interventions are crucial and hence, we incorporate three interventions strategies as parameters into our SEIR model. These combined interventions include all kind of preventive measures, active case-finding and hospitalization such as enforcement of wearing masks, using hand sanitizer regularly, maintain social distancing, in-home quarantine, minimizing outdoor activities, obeying lockdown and movement control order, conducting active case-detection, providing essential medical equipment for infected individual and as well as personal protective equipment for medical frontliners. Then, we compare the forecasted simulation of the outbreak with the absence and presence of interventions in India, Bangladesh, Iraq, Indonesia and Philippines. In addition, variation in the effectiveness of combined interventions for infectious individuals ranging from 50% to 90% are observed and examined graphically by simulating the Covid-19 model incorporating interventions strategies. Numerical simulation of the model reflects that by implementing combined interventions, it could lead to flattening of the curve of infected cases. This indicates that increasing the enactment of combined interventions up to 90% is of great significance for the pandemic eradication, which means not only reduces the peak of infected human, but also helping the healthcare management team to be under control. We hope this study can serve as a useful guideline to Indian, Bangladeshi, Iraqi, Indonesian and Philippines government as well as to the government of any other countries in which Covid-19 spreading is occurring. From a purely scientific standpoint, putting in place a combination of interventions as early as possible is the best way to alleviate the transmission risk and reduce the size of the Covid-19 outbreak.

Acknowledgements The authors acknowledge financial support from the School of Mathematical Sciences, Universiti Sains Malaysia, Penang and the enormous support provided throughout the research.

References

1. World Health Organization: Novel Coronavirus (2019-nCoV) Situation Report (Report No. 1) (2020)
2. Massoonnaud, C., Roux, J., Crepey, P.: COVID-19: Forecasting short term hospital needs in France. medRxiv 1–11 (2020)
3. Read, J. M., Bridgen, J. R. E., Cummings, D. A. T., Ho, A. Jewell, C. P.: Novel coronavirus 2019-nCoV: early estimation of epidemiological parameters and epidemic predictions. medRxiv 1–11 (2020)
4. Fang, Y., Nie, Y., Penny, M.: Transmission dynamics of the COVID-19 outbreak and effectiveness of government interventions: a data-driven analysis. J. Med. Virol. 1–15 (2020)
5. Pedersen, M. G., Meneghini, M.: Quantifying undetected COVID-19 cases and effects of containment measures in Italy: predicting phase 2 dynamics 1–8 (2020)
6. Traini, M.C., Caponi, C., Socio, G.V.D.: Modelling the epidemic 2019-nCoV event in Italy: a preliminary note. medRxiv 1–5 (2020)
7. Chen, Y., Wang, B., Sun, Z.: A novel SEIR model based on the data of quarantined, suspected, hospitalized, identified and recovered cases to forecast the trend of 2019-nCov epidemics after February 12, 2020, 1–26 (2020)
8. Zhou, X., Hong, N., Ma, Y., He, J., Jiang, H., Liu, C., Shan, G., Su, L., Zhu, W., Long, Y.: Forecasting the worldwide spread of COVID-19 based on logistic model and SEIR model. medRxiv 1–15 (2020)
9. Wang, H., Wang, Z., Dong, Y., Chang, R., Xu, C., Yu, X., Zhang, S., Tsamlag, L., Shang, M., Huang, J., Wang, Y., Xu, G., Shen, T., Zhang, X., Cai, Y.: Phase-adjusted estimation of the number of Coronavirus Disease 2019 cases in Wuhan. China Cell Discov. **6**(10), 1–8 (2020)
10. Worldometer: COVID-19 coronavirus pandemic (2020). Retrieved from https://www.worldometers.info/coronavirus/
11. World Health Organization: WHO-China joint mission on coronavirus disease 2019 (COVID-19) (2020)
12. Labadin, J., Hong, B.H.: Transmission dynamics of 2019-nCoV in Malaysia. medRxiv 1–5 (2020)
13. Nesteruk, I.: Estimations of the coronavirus epidemic dynamics in South Korea with the use of SIR model **1–6** (2020)
14. Peng, L., Yang, W., Zhang, D., Zhuge, C., Hong, L.: Epidemic analysis of COVID-19 in China by dynamical modeling 1–10 (2020)
15. Zhang, Y., You, C., Cai, Z., Sun, J., Hu, W., Zhou, X.H.: Prediction of the COVID-19 outbreak based on a realistic stochastic model. medRxiv 1–38 (2020)
16. Tang, Z., Li, X., Li, H.: Prediction of new coronavirus infection based on a modified SEIR model. medRxiv 1–9 (2020)
17. Tang, K., Huang, Y., Chen, M.: Novel Coronavirus 2019 (Covid-19) epidemic scale estimation: topological network-based infection dynamics model. medRxiv 1–15 (2020)
18. Sun, H., Qiu, Y., Yan, H., Huang, Y., Zhu, Y., Chen, S. X.: Tracking and predicting COVID-19 epidemic in China mainland. medRxiv 1–20 (2020)
19. Nesteruk, I.: Statistics-based predictions of Coronavirus epidemic spreading in mainland China. Innov. Biosyst. Bioeng. **4**(1), 13–18 (2020)
20. Li, X., Zhou, X., Sun, Y.: The lockdown of Hubei Province causing different transmission 2 dynamics of the novel coronavirus (2019-nCoV) in Wuhan and 3 Being 1–13 (2020)

21. Hamzah, F.A., Lau, C.H., Nazri, H., Ligot, L., Tan, C.L., Shaib, M.K.M., Zaidon, U.H., Abdullah, A., Chung, M.H., Ong, C.H., Chew, P.Y., Salunga, R.E.: CoronaTracker: world-wide COVID-19 outbreak data analysis and prediction. WHO Bull. 1 - 32 (2020)
22. Rabajan, Q., Liu, Z., Liu, J., Zhu, Y., Zhu, D., Li, Z., Gao, L., Zhou, J., Yang, Wang, Q.: Insights from early mathematical models of 2019-nCoV acute respiratory disease (COVID-19) dynamics. medRxiv, 1–15, 2–20 (2020)
23. Liu, Q., Liu, Z., Zhu, J., Zhu, Y., Li, D., Gao, Z., Zhou, L., Yang, J., Wang, Q.: Assessing the global tendency of COVID-19 Outbreak. medRxiv 1–15 (2020)
24. Zhou, T., Liu, Q., Yang, Z., Liao, K., Yang, J., Bai, W., Lu, X., Zhang, W.: Preliminary prediction of the basic reproduction number of the Wuhan novel coronavirus 2019-nCoV. J. Evid. Based Med. **13**(1), 3–7 (2020)
25. Ayubali, A.A., Satheesh, S.R.: On predicting the novel COVID-19 human infections by using Infectious Disease modelling method in the Indian State of Tamil Nadu during 2020. medRxiv 1–14 (2020)
26. Falco, I.D., Cioppa, A.D., Scafuri, U., Tarantino, E.: Coronavirus Covid-19 spreading in Italy: optimizing an epidemiological model with dynamic social distancing through differential evolution 1– 8 (2020)
27. Li, R., Lu, W., Yang, X., Feng, P., Muqimova, O., Chen, X., Wei, G.: Prediction of the Epidemic of COVID-19 based on quarantined surveillance in China. medRxiv 1–10 (2020)
28. Njankou, S.D.D., Nyabadza, F.: An optimal control model for Ebola virus disease. J. Biol. Syst. **24**(1), 29–49 (2016)
29. Sardar, T., Nadim, S.S., Rana, S., Chattopadhyay, J.: Assessment of 21 Days lockdown effect in some states and overall India: a predictive mathematical study on COVID-19. Outbreak Chaos Soliton Fract 1–31,(2020)
30. Li, J., Blakeley, D., Smith, R.J.: The Failure of R_0. Comput. Math. Methods Med. **2011**(1), 1–17 (2011)
31. Bhalraj, A., Azmi, A.: Mathematical modelling of the spread of Leptospirosis. In: Proceedings of the International Conference on Mathematical Sciences and Technology 2018 (MathTech 2018), AIP Conference Proceedings 2184, (American Institute of Physics, Penang, Malaysia, 2018), pp. 060031-1–060031-10
32. Countrymeters: Population Change Rates in 2020 (2020). Retrieved from https://countrymeters.info/en

Country Specific Analysis

Optimal Control of Vaccination and Plasma Transfusion with Potential Usefulness for Covid-19

Juliana Couras, Iván Area, Juan J. Nieto, Cristiana J. Silva, and Delfim F. M. Torres

Abstract The SEIR model is a compartmental model used to simulate the dynamics of an epidemic. In this chapter, we introduce two control functions in the compartmental SEIR model representing vaccination and plasma transfusion. Optimal control problems are proposed to study the effects of these two control measures, on the reduction of infected individuals and increase of recovered ones, with minimal costs. Up to our knowledge, the plasma transfusion treatment has never been considered as a control strategy for epidemics mitigation. The proposed vaccination and treatment strategies may have a real application in the challenging and hard problem of controlling the Covid-19 pandemic.

Keywords SEIR model · Optimal control problems · Ordinary differential equations

J. Couras
University of Aveiro, 3810-193 Aveiro, Portugal
e-mail: julianacouras@ua.pt

I. Area
CITMAGA, Universidade de Vigo, Departamento de Matematica Aplicada II, E. E. Aeronaautica e do Espazo, Campus de Ourense, 32004 Ourense, Spain
e-mail: area@uvigo.es

J. J. Nieto
CITMAGA, Instituto de Matemáticas, Universidade de Santiago de Compostela, 15782 Santiago de Compostela, Spain
e-mail: juanjose.nieto.roig@usc.es

C. J. Silva · D. F. M. Torres (✉)
Center for Research and Development in Mathematics and Applications (CIDMA), Department of Mathematics, University of Aveiro, 3810-193 Aveiro, Portugal
e-mail: delfim@ua.pt

C. J. Silva
e-mail: cjoaosilva@ua.pt

P. Agarwal et al. (eds.), *Analysis of Infectious Disease Problems (Covid-19) and Their Global Impact*, Infosys Science Foundation Series,
https://doi.org/10.1007/978-981-16-2450-6_23

1 Introduction

Like many other physical and biological processes, epidemics can be modelled mathematically. Epidemic mathematical modelling is important, not only to understand the disease progression, but also to provide predictions about the epidemics evolution and insights about the dynamics of the transmission rate and the effectiveness of control measures. There are several compartmental models in epidemiology, like the SI, SIR, $SICA$ and the $SEIR$ model, see, e.g., [1–3] and references cited therein. In this chapter, we consider the SEIR model, where the human population is divided into four mutually exclusive compartments: susceptible S, latent E, infected I, and a recovered or removed (dead) R. We assume that the population is homogeneous and the various classes are uniformly mixed. We consider the case of constant total population N, that is, $S(t) + E(t) + I(t) + R(t) = N$ for every time t in the time window $t \in [0, T]$ under study. In this case, the fraction of individuals in each compartment is defined as $s = S/N$, $e = E/N$, $i = I/N$ and $r = R/N$. The balance condition becomes $s + e + i + r = 1$. The assumptions made about the transmission of the infection and incubation period are reflected in the equations and parameters [2] and are explained below. We consider the following parameters:

- transmission coefficient—β;
- infectious rate—γ;
- recovery rate—μ.

Then the *seir* model is given by the following system of ordinary differential equations:

$$\begin{cases} \frac{ds}{dt}(t) = -\beta\, s(t)\, i(t), \\ \frac{de}{dt}(t) = \beta\, s(t)\, i(t) - \gamma e(t), \\ \frac{di}{dt}(t) = \gamma\, e(t) - \mu\, i(t), \\ \frac{dr}{dt}(t) = \mu\, i(t)\,, \end{cases} \tag{1}$$

represented graphically in the diagram of Fig. 1. The term $\beta\, s\, i$ represents the gain in the exposed class, which is proportional to the fraction of infective (and infectious) and susceptible individuals, where the transmission coefficient $\beta > 0$ is a constant parameter. Individuals are transferred from the susceptible class s to the exposed e at this rate $\beta\, s\, i$. The incubation period is of $1/\gamma$ days, with $\gamma > 0$, and after that time exposed individuals become infectious. The rate of removal of infective to the removed class is proportional to the number of infective, $\mu\, i$, with $\mu > 0$, where $1/\mu$ is a measure of the time spent in the infectious state [2].

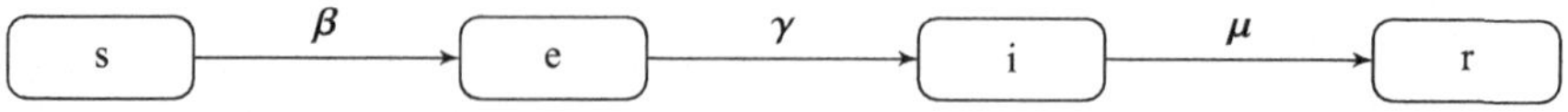

Fig. 1 Diagram of the compartmental model (1)

The *seir* model (1) is an extension of the classical Kermack–McKendrick 1927 model [4, 5], where the class of exposed (latent) individuals is considered. SEIR type compartmental models have been extensively used to model the Covid-19 pandemic, see, e.g., [6, 7], and researchers have shown that it can describe the spread of Covid-19 in different countries: see [8] for a simulation of the Covid-19 spread in Lombardy (Italy) and also modifications of the SEIR model in [9–11]. Namely, in [9] three classes are added for confined, under quarantine and Covid-19 induced deaths. The model in [10] considers the age of the population, time delay on the development of the pandemic, and resusceptibility to Covid-19 with temporal immune response. An age-structured SEIR model is proposed in [11] considering 5-year bands until the age of 70 years and a single category aged 75 and older (resulting in 16 age categories for each class of individuals).

Optimal control theory is a branch of mathematics that involves finding optimal ways of controlling a dynamic system [12, 13]. Optimal control has been applied to epidemiological models for many different infectious diseases, such as HIV/AIDS, malaria, Ebola, tuberculosis and cholera [14–17], and also non communicable diseases like cancer: see [18] and references cited therein.

Optimal control theory allows the study of the most cost-effective intervention strategy that changes the dynamics of a controlled system while minimizing a so-called objective function. In this chapter, we introduce two control functions in the *seir* model (1) that represent vaccination and plasma transfusion. Although vaccination has been widely studied from an optimal control point of view applied to epidemiological models, up to our knowledge, the plasma transfusion treatment has never been considered before. Plasma transfusion has been considered as a possible treatment for Covid-19, although it is still under study [19].

We propose five objective cost functionals and five corresponding optimal control problems for the three control systems that correspond to vaccination only, plasma transfusion treatment only, and combination of vaccination and plasma transfusion.

This chapter is organized as follows. In Sect. 2, the vaccination and plasma transfusion are introduced in the *seir* model, isolated and in combination, giving rise to three control systems that will be part of the optimal control problems proposed in Sect. 3. In Sect. 4, the solutions of the optimal control problems are compared numerically. We end with Sect. 5 of discussion and conclusions.

2 Control System: *seir* Model with Vaccination and Plasma Transfusion

In this section, in order to control the spread of the infection, two types of interventions are introduced into the *seir* model (1): vaccination u and plasma transfusion p. Instead of representing the vaccination and plasma transfusion by constant positive parameters, we assume that vaccination and plasma transfusion are given by two functions $u(\cdot)$ and $p(\cdot)$, respectively, that change in time and that modify the dynamical behavior of model (1). In optimal control theory, functions $u(\cdot)$ and $p(\cdot)$ are usually called *controls*.

Starting by the vaccine, we introduce a control $u(\cdot)$ that represents the vaccination rate. By definition, it only makes sense to vaccinate people if they are susceptible to the disease. After being vaccinated, these people would become immune to the disease. In terms of the $seir$ model states, this means that an individual in the s state would jump to the r state after being vaccinated. Thus, the model must be rewritten in the following way:

$$[\textit{vaccination based control}] \quad \begin{cases} \frac{ds}{dt}(t) = -\beta\, s(t)\, i(t) - u(t)\, s(t), \\ \frac{de}{dt}(t) = \beta\, s(t)\, i(t) - \gamma\, e(t), \\ \frac{di}{dt}(t) = \gamma\, e(t) - \mu\, i(t), \\ \frac{dr}{dt}(t) = \mu\, i(t) + u(t)\, s(t), \end{cases} \tag{2}$$

where the control function $u(\cdot)$ is bounded between 0 and $u_{\max} \leq 1$.

Regarding treatment, the aim is to emulate a serological treatment, that is, a plasma transfusion. A plasma transfusion consists on infusing sick individuals with the blood plasma harvested from the immune individuals. Thus, in terms of the model, it requires that a recovered individual r donates plasma to an infectious individual i. The control is the rate at which this transfusion happens. Let the control be $p(\cdot)$. Then, the $seir$ model (1) is rewritten in the following way:

$$[\textit{plasma transfusion based control}] \quad \begin{cases} \frac{ds}{dt}(t) = -\beta\, s(t)\, i(t), \\ \frac{de}{dt}(t) = \beta\, s(t)\, i(t) - \gamma\, e(t), \\ \frac{di}{dt}(t) = \gamma\, e(t) - \mu\, i(t) - p(t)\, r(t)\, i(t), \\ \frac{dr}{dt}(t) = \mu\, i(t) + p(t)\, r(t)\, i(t), \end{cases} \tag{3}$$

where the control $p(\cdot)$ satisfies the control constraint $0 \leq p(\cdot) \leq p_{\max} \leq 1$.

Finally, the two previous controls are considered simultaneously, being the resulting model the following:

$$[\textit{vaccination and plasma transfusion}] \quad \begin{cases} \frac{ds}{dt}(t) = -\beta\, s(t)\, i(t) - u(t)\, s(t), \\ \frac{de}{dt}(t) = \beta\, s(t)\, i(t) - \gamma\, e(t), \\ \frac{di}{dt}(t) = \gamma\, e(t) - \mu\, i(t) - p(t)\, r(t)\, i(t), \\ \frac{dr}{dt}(t) = \mu\, i(t) + p(t)\, r(t)\, i(t) + u(t)\, s(t). \end{cases} \tag{4}$$

The set of admissible controls functions is given by

$$\Omega = \left\{ (u(\cdot), p(\cdot)) \in \left(L^{\infty}(0, T)\right)^2 \mid 0 \leq u(t) \leq u_{\max}, 0 \leq p(t) \leq p_{\max}, \forall t \in [0, T] \right\}. \tag{5}$$

3 Optimal Control

Consider non-negative initial conditions for the state variables $(s, e, i, r) \in \left(R_0^+\right)^4$:

$$s(0) \geq 0\,, \quad e(0) \geq 0\,, \quad i(0) \geq 0\,, \quad r(0) \geq 0\,, \tag{6}$$

where the state variables satisfy $s(t) + e(t) + i(t) + r(t) = 1$, for all $t \in [0, T]$. In order to formulate an optimal control problem, a cost functional needs to be proposed, which in our case we intend to maximize. We propose an optimal control problem for the control systems given by (2), (3) or (4), with five different L^2 objective functionals, denoted for simplicity by J_i, $i = 1, \ldots, 5$. All of them are obtained from

$$\mathcal{J}_\eta = \int_0^T \left(\eta_1 r(t) - \eta_2 i(t) - \eta_3 u^2(t) - \eta_4 p^2(t)\right) dt$$

as follows: $J_1 = \mathcal{J}_{(0,1,1,0)}$, $J_2 = \mathcal{J}_{(1,1,1,0)}$, $J_3 = \mathcal{J}_{(0,1,0,1)}$, $J_4 = \mathcal{J}_{(1,1,0,1)}$, and $J_5 = \mathcal{J}_{(0,1,1,1)}$. Other cases of cost functionals are obviously possible, but we found these five to be the most interesting. We also do not consider all possible combinations between the three control systems and the five costs to be maximized, restricting ourselves to five optimal control problems. Regarding the vaccination based control (2), we consider the two objective functionals

$$J_1(u(\cdot)) = \int_0^T \left(-i(t) - u^2(t)\right) dt \tag{7}$$

and

$$J_2(u(\cdot)) = \int_0^T \left(r(t) - i(t) - u^2(t)\right) dt\,. \tag{8}$$

When the cost functional is considered to be J_1, the main goal of maximizing the functional is to minimize the fraction of infected individuals and, at the same time, the vaccination costs. We compare the solution to this optimal control problem with the one that maximizes J_2, that is, the one that maximize the fraction of recovered (immune) individuals and, simultaneously, minimizes the fraction of infected individuals and the vaccination costs. The numerical solutions are compared in Sect. 4.

When only the treatment by plasma transfusion is considered, that is, when we focus ourselves on the control system (3), we use the objective functionals J_3 and J_4:

$$J_3(p(\cdot)) = \int_0^T \left(-i(t) - p^2(t)\right) dt\,, \tag{9}$$

$$J_4(p(\cdot)) = \int_0^T \left(r(t) - i(t) - p^2(t)\right) dt\,, \tag{10}$$

where maximizing J_3 corresponds to minimizing the fraction of infected individuals and the costs associated with plasma transfusion treatment, and for maximizing J_4 the main goal is to maximize the fraction of recovered individuals, by treatment, and, at the same time, minimize the fraction of infected individuals with less treatment cost as possible.

Finally, when both controls are considered simultaneously, modelled by the vaccination and plasma transfusion based control system (4), the objective functional considered to be maximized was J_5:

$$J_5(u(\cdot), p(\cdot)) = \int_0^T \left(-i(t) - u^2(t) - p^2(t)\right) dt \tag{11}$$

with the main goal to minimize the fraction of infected individuals and the costs associated with vaccination and plasma transfusion treatment.

Associated to each of the cost functionals J_i, $i = 1, \ldots, 5$, we propose an optimal control problem of determining the state trajectories $(s^*(\cdot), e^*(\cdot), i^*(\cdot), r^*(\cdot))$, associated to an admissible control $u^*(\cdot) \in \Omega$ and/or $p^*(\cdot) \in \Omega$ on the time interval $[0, T]$, satisfying one of the control systems (2)–(4), as explained, the initial conditions (6), and maximizing the corresponding functional. The five optimal control problems are denoted by (OC_i), $i = 1, \ldots 5$, and are now summarized.
Vaccination based control system (2) and maximizing the cost functional J_1:

$$J_1(u^*(\cdot)) = \max_{\Omega} \int_0^T \left(-i(t) - u^2(t)\right) dt. \tag{OC_1}$$

Vaccination based control system (2) and maximizing the cost functional J_2:

$$J_2(u^*(\cdot)) = \max_{\Omega} \int_0^T \left(r(t) - i(t) - u^2(t)\right) dt. \tag{OC_2}$$

Plasma transfusion based control system (3) and maximizing the cost functional J_3:

$$J_3(p^*(\cdot)) = \max_{\Omega} \int_0^T \left(-i(t) - p^2(t)\right) dt. \tag{OC_3}$$

Plasma transfusion based control system (3) and maximizing the cost functional J_4:

$$J_4(p^*(\cdot)) = \max_{\Omega} \int_0^T \left(r(t) - i(t) - p^2(t)\right) dt. \tag{OC_4}$$

Vaccination and plasma transfusion control system (4) and maximizing the cost functional J_5:

$$J_5(u^*(\cdot), p^*(\cdot)) = \max_{\Omega} \int_0^T \left(-i(t) - p^2(t) - u^2(t)\right) dt. \tag{OC_5}$$

Note that all optimal control problems have a L^2-cost functional, in other words, the integrand of the cost J_i, $i = 1, \ldots, 5$, is always convex with respect to the controls u and p. Moreover, the control systems (2)–(4) are Lipschitz with respect to the state variables (s, e, i, r). These properties ensure the existence of an optimal control $(u^*(\cdot), p^*(\cdot))$ for the optimal control problems (OC_1)–(OC_5). Moreover, we apply the Pontryagin Maximum Principle (see, e.g., [13]), which is a first order necessary optimality condition. The obtained result, here formulated and proved for the optimal control problem (OC_1), can be trivially extended to the other optimal control problems (OC_i), $i = 2, \ldots, 5$.

Theorem 1 *The optimal control problem (OC_1) with fixed final time T admits a unique optimal solution $(s^*(\cdot), e^*(\cdot), i^*(\cdot), r^*(\cdot))$ associated to the optimal control $u^*(\cdot)$ given by*

$$u^*(t) = \min\left\{\max\left\{0, \frac{(\lambda_4(t) - \lambda_1(t))\, s(t)}{2}\right\}, u_{\max}\right\} \tag{12}$$

on $[0, T]$, where the adjoint functions λ_i satisfy

$$\begin{cases} \dot{\lambda}_1(t) = -\lambda_1(t)\,(-i(t)\,\beta - u(t)) - \lambda_2(t)\, i\,\beta - \lambda_4(t)\, u(t), \\ \dot{\lambda}_2(t) = \lambda_2(t)\,\gamma - \lambda_3(t)\,\gamma, \\ \dot{\lambda}_3(t) = 1 + \lambda_1(t)\,\beta\, s(t) - \lambda_2(t)\,\beta\, s(t) + \lambda_3(t)\,\mu - \lambda_4(t)\,\mu, \\ \dot{\lambda}_4(t) = 0, \end{cases} \tag{13}$$

with the transversality conditions $\lambda_i(T) = 0$, $i = 1, \ldots, 4$.

Proof The existence of an optimal control $u^*(\cdot)$ of the optimal control problem (OC_1) is due to the convexity of the L^2-cost functional J_1 and to the fact that the vaccinated based control system (2) is Lipschitz with respect to the state variables (s, e, i, r): see, e.g., [12]. The uniqueness of the optimal control u^* comes from the boundedness of the state and adjoint functions and the Lipschitz property of system (2) (see [20, 21] and references cited therein). According to the Pontryagin Maximum Principle, if $u^*(\cdot)$ is optimal for the problem (OC_1) with fixed final time T, then there exists a nontrivial absolutely continuous mapping $\Lambda : [0, T] \to \mathbb{R}^4$, $\Lambda(t) = (\lambda_1(t), \lambda_2(t), \lambda_3(t), \lambda_4(t))$, called the *adjoint vector*, such that

$$\dot{s} = \frac{\partial H}{\partial \lambda_1}, \quad \dot{e} = \frac{\partial H}{\partial \lambda_2}, \quad \dot{i} = \frac{\partial H}{\partial \lambda_3}, \quad \dot{r} = \frac{\partial H}{\partial \lambda_4}$$

and

$$\dot{\lambda}_1 = -\frac{\partial H}{\partial s}, \quad \dot{\lambda}_2 = -\frac{\partial H}{\partial e}, \quad \dot{\lambda}_3 = -\frac{\partial H}{\partial i}, \quad \dot{\lambda}_4 = -\frac{\partial H}{\partial r},$$

where

$$
\begin{aligned}
H = H(s(t), i(t), c(t), a(t)) &= -i(t) - u^2(t) \\
&+ \lambda_1(t)\,(-\beta\, s(t)\, i(t) - u(t)\, s(t)) \\
&+ \lambda_2(t)\,(\beta\, s(t)\, i(t) - \gamma\, e(t)) \\
&+ \lambda_3(t)\,(\gamma\, e(t) - \mu\, i(t)) \\
&+ \lambda_4(t)\,(\mu\, i(t) + u(t)\, s(t))
\end{aligned}
$$

is the *Hamiltonian*, and the maximality condition

$$
\begin{aligned}
&H(s^*(t), e^*(t), i^*(t), r^*(t), \lambda^*(t), u^*(t)) \\
&\qquad = \max_{0 \le u \le u_{\max}} H(s^*(t), e^*(t), i^*(t), r^*(t), \lambda^*(t), u(t))
\end{aligned}
$$

holds almost everywhere on $[0, T]$. Moreover, the transversality conditions

$$
\lambda_i(T) = 0\,, \qquad i = 1, \ldots, 4,
$$

hold. Furthermore, from the maximality condition, we have

$$
u^*(t) = \min\left\{\max\left\{0, \frac{(\lambda_4(t) - \lambda_1(t))\, s(t)}{2}\right\}, u_{\max}\right\}.
$$

The proof is concluded.

To solve optimal control problems numerically, two approaches are possible: direct and indirect. Indirect methods are based on Pontryagin's Maximum Principle but not very much widespread since they are not immediately available by software packages. We refer the reader to [22] for the implementation of Pontryagin's Maximum Principle using Octave/MATLAB. Direct methods consist in the discretization of the optimal control problem, reducing it to a nonlinear programming problem [23, 24]. In the next section, we use the Applied Modeling Programming Language AMPL [25] to discretize the optimal control problems $(OC_i), i = 1, \ldots, 5$. Then, the resulting nonlinear programming problems are solved using the Interior-Point optimization solver developed by Wächter and Biegler [26], through the NEOS Server [27]. For more details on the numerical aspects see [28].

4 Numerical Simulations and Results

In this section, we provide numerical simulations for the solutions of the optimal control problems $(OC_i), i = 1, \ldots, 5$, proposed in Sect. 3. The following values for the initial conditions are considered:

$$s(0) = 0.88\,, \quad e(0) = 0.07\,, \quad i(0) = 0.05\,, \quad r(0) = 0\,, \tag{14}$$

and the parameter values

$$\beta = 0.3\,, \quad \gamma = 0.1887\,, \quad \mu = 0.1\,. \tag{15}$$

The initial conditions (14) were chosen arbitrarily, considering an hypothetical situation where 88% of the total population is susceptible to the disease and there is a relatively small percentage of infected population and no recovered individuals. The parameter values are chosen in such a way that model (1) simulates an epidemic outbreak, caused by a communicable disease. Moreover, we consider the control constraints with $u_{\max} = 0.5$ and $p_{\max} = 0.3$, that is, the admissible controls $(u, p) \in \Omega$ must satisfy $0 \leq u(t) \leq 0.5$ and $0 \leq p(t) \leq 0.3$ for all $t \in [0, T]$.

All computations have been performed with an Intel i7-4720HQ 2.60GHz processor, 8 GB of RAM, and an SSD disk of 128 GB under Windows 10, Home Edition of 64 bits.

4.1 The *seir* Model Without Controls

The *seir* model differential equations were integrated using the ode45 MATLAB routine, which is based on an explicit Runge–Kutta method [29]. For the parameter values (15), the dynamic evolution of the uncontrolled system (1) is described in Fig. 2.

These results were obtained in "real time" under MATLAB.

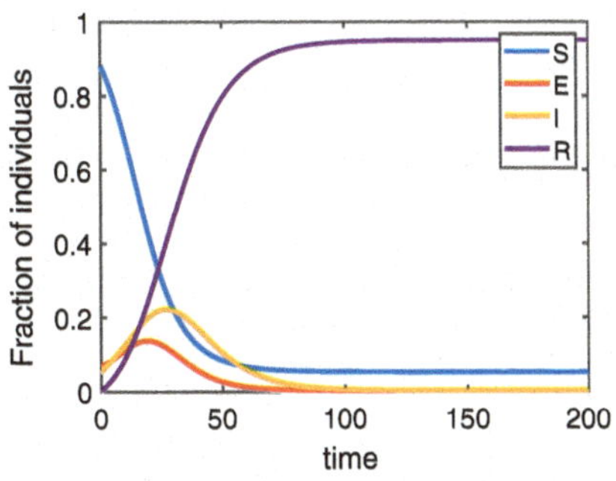

Fig. 2 Joint evolution of the state variables s, e, i and r of the uncontrolled model (1), during 200 time units

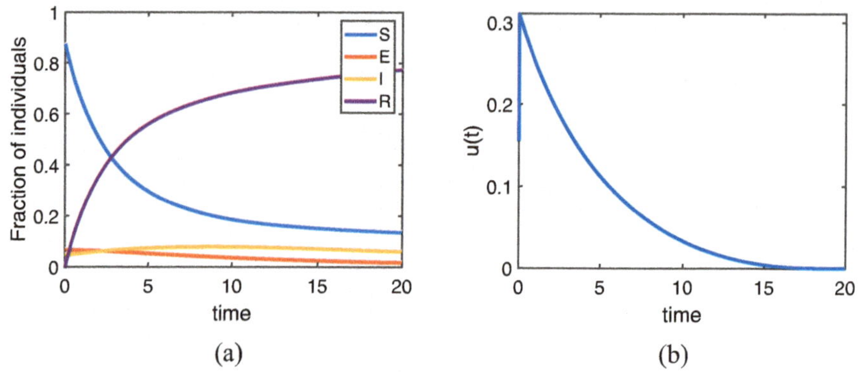

Fig. 3 Effect of vaccinating the population during 20 time units considering (OC_1). **a** $seir$ state variables applying vaccination. **b** Vaccination control $u(\cdot)$

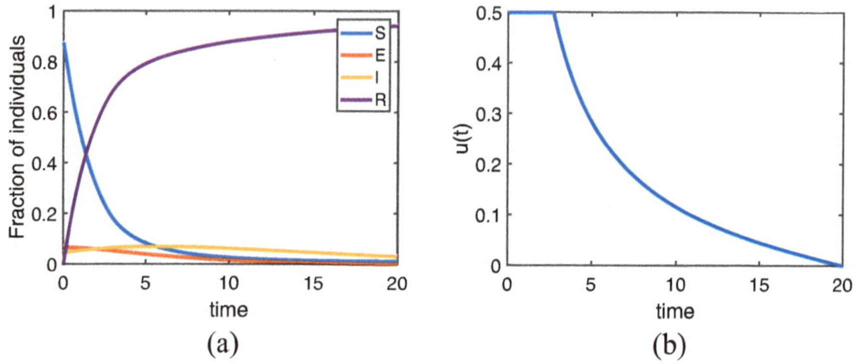

Fig. 4 Effect of vaccinating the population during 20 time units considering (OC_2). **a** $seir$ state variables applying vaccination. **b** Vaccination control $u(\cdot)$

4.2 *The $seir$ Model with Controls*

It is desirable to minimize the fraction of infected individuals that get infected by the disease with minimal costs.

4.2.1 Optimal Control Problems (OC_1) and (OC_2)

Firstly, we consider the effect of vaccinating the population at the first 20 time units, aiming at maximizing J_1 subject to the vaccination based control system (2), the initial conditions (14), and the control constraint $0 \leq u(t) \leq 0.5$. The results obtained are given in Figs. 3 and 4.

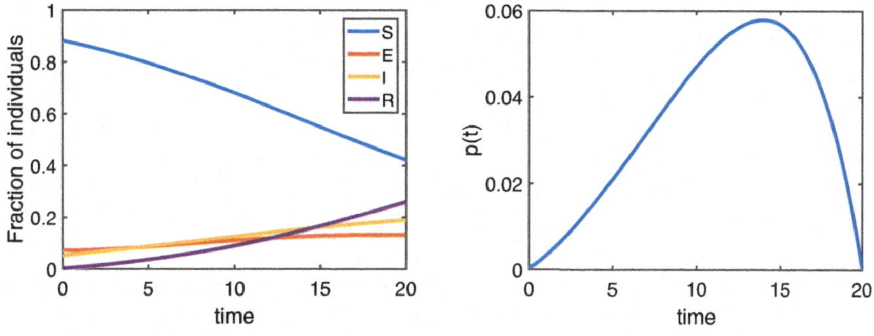

(a) (b)

Fig. 5 Effect of infusing infectious individuals with plasma, during 20 time units, considering (OC_3). **a** $seir$ state variables applying plasma transfusion. **b** Plasma transfusion control $p(\cdot)$

We see that in both $seir$ evolutions, the susceptible s and recovered r states seem to interchange, as expected by the vaccination based control system (2). Further, looking at the vaccination control $u(\cdot)$ evolution, it is possible to see that in both Figs. 3 and 4 its value starts at a maximum and then decays as time passes. This makes sense, since at the beginning of the epidemic there are more susceptible individuals s. Thus, it is expected that the rate of vaccination is larger at this time in order to try to vaccinate the most susceptible individuals s as possible before they start getting infected. Further, comparing the vaccination control of Figs. 3 and 4, one can see that applying the condition of maximizing the fraction of recovered individuals r with the cost functional J_2 translates into keeping the rate of vaccination at its maximum for 3 units of time before starting to decay with a less steeper slope than its analogue in J_1.

4.2.2 Optimal Control Problems (OC_3) and (OC_4)

Regarding the plasma transfusion treatment, one can see that, in contrast to the vaccine control, here the control $p(\cdot)$ peaks later in time (see Figs. 5 and 6). Again, this is something that makes sense since, in order for the treatment to be applied, there must be not only individuals in the infected i state, that are able to received the plasma, but also individuals in the recovered r state, that are able to donate the plasma. Evidently, these recovered individuals r must have been in the infected state i before.

Because this is an intervention that presupposes that the disease has evolved for some time, then a larger time window could allow one to visualize a stronger impact in the fractions of the i and r states. That said, a simulation for optimal control problems (OC_3) and (OC_4) is performed using $T = 100$.

The simulation that made the control increase the most with the time change was the one for the optimal control problem (OC_3) (Fig. 7). Further, the control peak

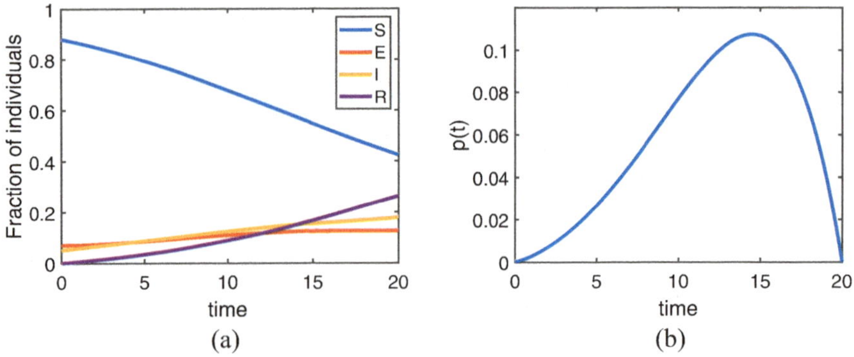

Fig. 6 Effect of infusing infectious individuals with plasma, during 20 time units, considering (OC_4). **a** *seir* state variables applying plasma transfusion. **b** Plasma transfusion control $p(\cdot)$

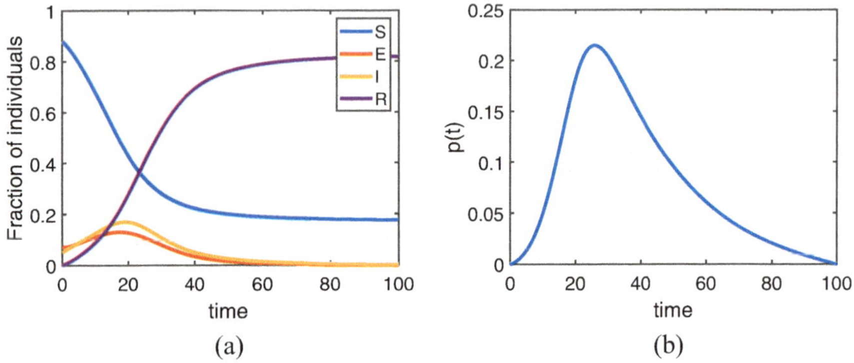

Fig. 7 Effect of infusing infectious individuals with plasma, during 100 time units, considering the cost functional J_3. **a** *seir* state variables, applying plasma transfusion. **b** Plasma transfusion control $p(\cdot)$

at Fig. 7 also occurs before the control peak at Fig. 8. This is expected since (OC_4) requires maximizing the r state, which implies again that more individuals must get into the i state so that they can get into the r state after recovering. It is also interesting to note that, according to the (OC_4) optimal control problem, one should not proceed with plasma transfusion to any infected individual during the beginning of the epidemic, in order to obtain the optimal control.

4.2.3 Optimal Control Problem (OC_5)

Finally, the combined effect of the two controls for the optimal control problem (OC_5) is presented in Fig. 9. As expected, the peak of the vaccination rate occurs before the peak of the plasma transfusion rate. Apparently, the results in minimizing

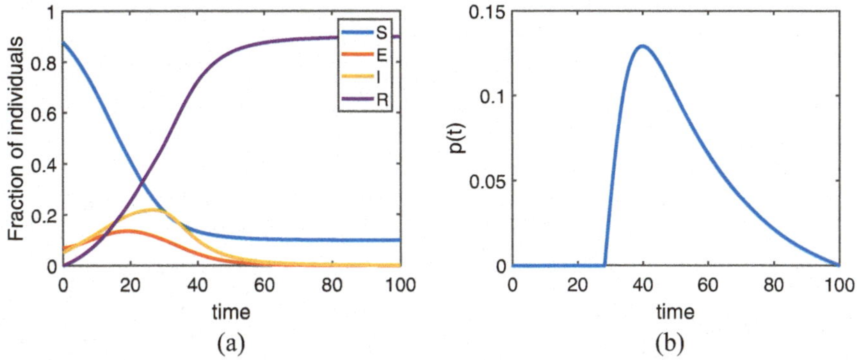

Fig. 8 Effect of infusing infectious individuals with plasma, during 100 time units, considering the cost functional J_4. **a** *seir* state variables applying plasma transfusion. **b** Plasma transfusion control $p(\cdot)$

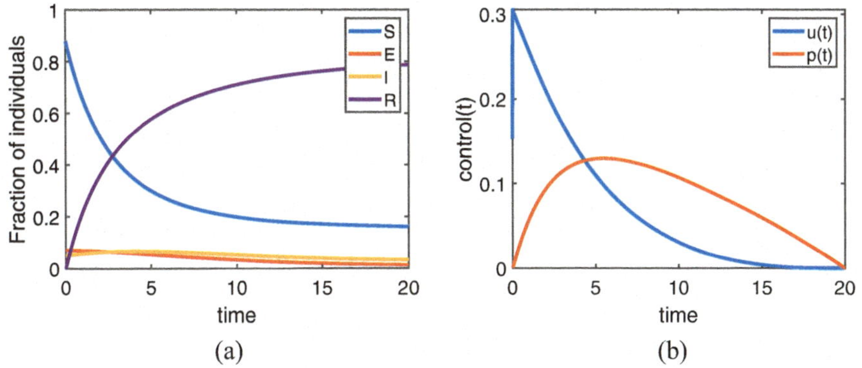

Fig. 9 Effect of both vaccinating susceptible individuals and infusing infectious individuals with plasma during 20 time units considering J_5. **a** *seir* states applying vaccination and plasma transfusion. **b** Controls $u(t)$ and $p(t)$

the fraction of individuals in the infected state i are better, when comparing Fig. 9a with Figs. 3a and 5a, but Fig. 10 gives us a better understanding of the controls effects in the *seir* dynamics. Figure 10 shows the effect of the controls in the individual s, e, i, r states. Since the main objective of the control functionals is to minimize the number of individuals in the infected state i, then, by looking at Fig. 10c, one can see that the control that minimizes the i fraction the most is the conjugation of both vaccination and plasma transfusion. This is also an intuitive result, since the vaccination makes more people jumping into the r state, which is the pool of individuals from where the plasma comes. On the other hand, the plasma transfusion by itself seems to be the less effective control in minimizing the infected fraction i (Fig. 10c). This is expected since, as explained above, the plasma transfusion control needs more time to kick in the absence of a larger pool of recovered individuals r.

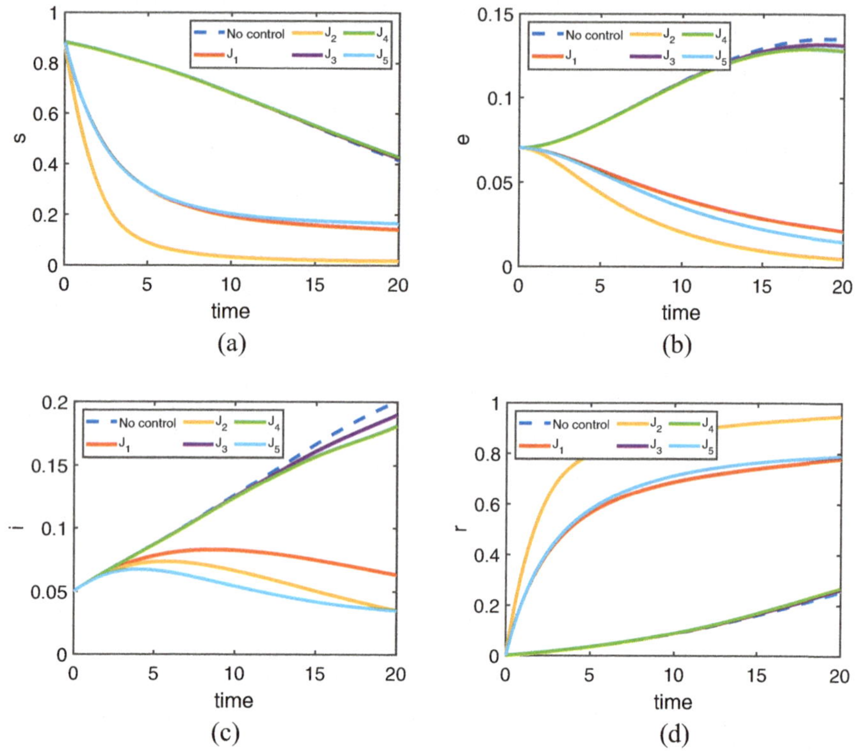

Fig. 10 Individual evolution of the controlled and uncontrolled states $s\ e\ i\ r$, during 20 time units. **a** susceptible state s. **b** exposed state e. **c** infected state i. **d** removed state r

Furthermore, if the aim is to maximize the recovered state r or to minimize the susceptible s and exposed e states, then the vaccination is the best control (Fig. 10d), a result also predicted by system (2). By analysing the control comparison at Fig. 11, one can see that the control that benefits the most with the combined approach of both vaccination and plasma transfusion is the plasma control. This can be explained since one can think that if we apply vaccination in the beginning of the epidemics, then the fraction of recovered individuals r increases faster, providing a bigger substract to do plasma transfusion sooner and at a higher rate.

All the optimal control simulations were carried out using NEOS Server 6.0, their duration varying between 0.508 and 1.149 s, for 20 units of time, and between 24.431 and 30.702 s, for 100 units of time.

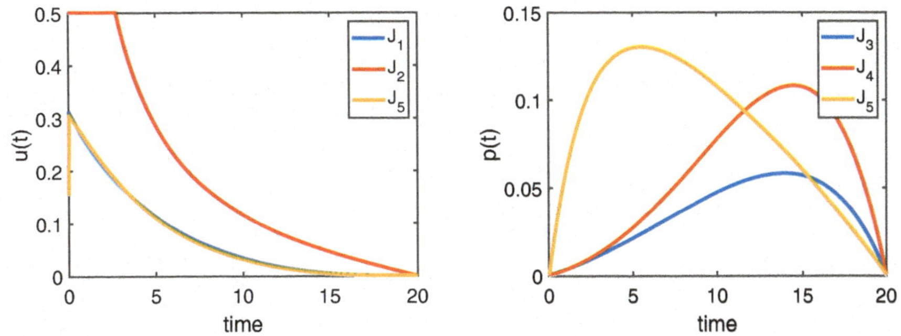

(a) (b)

Fig. 11 Evolution of vaccination and plasma transfusion controls, during 20 time units. **a** Vaccination control $u(\cdot)$. **b** Plasma transfusion control $p(\cdot)$

5 Discussion and Conclusion

The *seir* model (1) was solved numerically in both uncontrolled and controlled conditions. Of the controls employed, the combined action of vaccination and plasma transfusion seems to have the higher impact in reducing the fraction of infectious individuals. Moreover, the plasma transfusion acquires a more important role as the fraction of individuals in the recovered state increases, which explains why whether joining the vaccination or increasing the duration of the simulations leads to an higher peak of the plasma transfusion rate. In fact, by joining the vaccination, one can not only increase the plasma transfusion rate peak but also anticipate it.

To sum up, controls can act at different timings of the epidemics dynamics and one control can be more adequate in the beginning of the epidemic whilst other might be more appropriated in a later state.

Code availability

The code is available from the authors on request.

Acknowledgements This research was partially supported by the Portuguese Foundation for Science and Technology (FCT) within "Project n. 147 – Controlo Ótimo e Modelação Matemática da Pandemia Covid-19: contributos para uma estratégia sistémica de intervenção em saúde na comunidade", in the scope of the "RESEARCH 4 Covid-19" call financed by FCT. The work of Silva and Torres was also partially supported within project UIDB/04106/2020 (CIDMA). Moreover, Silva is also supported by national funds (OE), through FCT, I.P., in the scope of the framework contract foreseen in the numbers 4, 5 and 6 of the article 23, of the Decree-Law 57/2016, of August 29, changed by Law 57/2017, of July 19. The authors are grateful to two anonymous reviewers for helpful comments and suggestions.

References

1. Brauer, F., Castillo-Chavez, C.: Mathematical Models in Population Biology and Epidemiology. Texts in Applied Mathematics. Springer, New York (2011)
2. Murray, J.D.: Mathematical Biology. Springer, Berlin Heidelberg (2013)
3. Silva, C.J., Torres, D.F.M.: On SICA models for HIV transmission. In: Hattaf, K., Dutta, H. (eds.) Mathematical Modelling and Analysis of Infectious Diseases. Springer Nature, Switzerland, 155–179 (2020). https://doi.org/10.1007/978-3-030-49896-2_6
4. Kermack, W.O., McKendrick, A.G.: A contribution to the mathematical theory of epidemics. Proc. Roy. Soc. Lond. A **115**, 700–721 (1927)
5. Kermack, W.O., McKendrick, A.G.: Contributions to the mathematical theory of epidemics I. Bltn Mathcal Biology **53**, 33–55 (1991)
6. COVID-19 Projections Using Machine Learning, https://covid19-projections.com
7. SEIR Model for the COVID-19 Epidemic, https://www.comsol.pt/model/seir-model-for-the-covid-19-epidemic-86511
8. Carcione, J.M., Santos, J.E., Bagaini, C. and Ba, J.: A Simulation of a COVID-19 Epidemic Based on a Deterministic SEIR Model, Front. Public Health 8:230 (2020)
9. López, L., Rodó, X.: A modified SEIR model to predict the COVID-19 outbreak in Spain and Italy: simulating control scenarios and multi-scale epidemics. https://doi.org/10.2139/ssrn.3576802
10. Ng, K.Y., Gui, M.M.: COVID-19: Development of a robust mathematical model and simulation package with consideration for ageing population and time delay for control action and resusceptibility. Phys. D **411**, 132599 (2020)
11. Prem, K. et. al.: The effect of control strategies to reduce social mixing on outcomes of the COVID-19 epidemic in Wuhan, China: a modelling study. Lancet Public Health **5** (5), e261–e270 (2020)
12. Cesari, L.: Optimization—Theory and Applications. Problems with Ordinary Differential Equations, Applications of Mathematics 17, Springer-Verlag, New York (1983)
13. Pontryagin, L., Boltyanskii, V., Gramkrelidze, R., Mischenko, E.: The Mathematical Theory of Optimal Processes. Wiley Interscience (1962)
14. Area, I., Ndairou, F., Nieto, J.J., Silva, C.J., Torres, D.F.M.: Ebola Model and Optimal Control with Vaccination Constraints. J. Ind. Manag. Optim. **14**(2), 427–446 (2018)
15. Lemos-Paião, A.P., Silva, C.J., Torres, D.F.M., Venturino, E.: Optimal control of aquatic diseases: a case study of yemen's cholera outbreak. J. Optim. Theory Appl. **185**(3), 1008–1030 (2020)
16. Silva, C.J., Maurer, H.: Optimal control of HIV treatment and immunotherapy combination with state and control delays. Optim Control Appl. Meth. **41**, 537–554 (2020)
17. Silva, C.J. and Torres, D.F.M.: A TB-HIV/AIDS coinfection model and optimal control treatment, Discrete Contin. Dyn. Syst., 35, no. 9, 4639–4663 (2015)
18. Schättler, H., Ledzewicz, U.: Optimal Control for Mathematical Models of Cancer Therapies. An Application of Geometric Methods. Springer-Verlag, New York (2015)
19. American Society of Hematology, COVID-19 and Convalescent Plasma: Frequently asked questions, https://www.hematology.org/covid-19/covid-19-and-convalescent-plasma
20. Jung, E., Lenhart, S., Feng, Z.: Optimal control of treatments in a two-strain tuberculosis model, Discrete Contin. Dyn. Syst. Ser. B 2 (4), 473–482 (2002)
21. Silva, C.J., Torres, D.F.M.: Optimal control for a tuberculosis model with reinfection and post-exposure interventions, Math. Biosci. 244, no. 2, 154–164 (2013)
22. Campos, C., Silva, C.J., Torres, D.F.M.: Numerical optimal control of HIV transmission in Octave/MATLAB. Math. Comput. Appl. **25**(1), 20 (2020)
23. Nemati, S., Lima, P.M., Torres, D.F.M.: A numerical approach for solving fractional optimal control problems using modified hat functions. Commun. Nonlinear Sci. Numer. Simul. **78**, 14 (2019) (Art. 104849)

24. Salati, A.B.; Shamsi, M.; Torres, D.F.M. Direct transcription methods based on fractional integral approximation formulas for solving nonlinear fractional optimal control problems. Commun. Nonlinear Sci. Numer. Simul. 67 (2019) 334–350
25. Fourer, R., Gay, D.M., Kernighan, B.W.: AMPL: A Modeling Language for Mathematical Programming. Duxbury Press, Brooks-Cole Publishing Company (1993)
26. Wächter, A., Biegler, L.T.: On the implementation of an interior-point filter line-search algorithm for large-scale nonlinear programming, Math. Program. 106, 25–57 (2006)
27. NEOS Interfaces to Ipopt, https://neos-server.org/neos/solvers/nco:Ipopt/AMPL.html
28. Silva, C.J., Maurer, H., Torres, D.F.M.: Optimal control of a tuberculosis model with state and control delays, Math. Biosci. Eng. 14, no. 1, 321–337 (2017)
29. Shampine, L.F., Reichelt, M.W.: The MATLAB ODE Suite, SIAM Journal on Scientific Computing 18, 1–22 (1997)

Fractional Diffusion Equation as a Mathematical Model of the Incidence of Coronavirus Disease Covid-19

Ludmila Kirianova, Temirkhan Aleroev, and Vladimir Griguletskiy

Abstract In present paper we provide the statistical analysis of the numerical indicators of the incidence in Russian Federation in 2020 of Covid-19. These were consructed corresponding histograms and theoretical distribution densities, and found estimates of the distribution parameters by the maximum likelihood method. Based on the statistical analysis of the data, were verified the parameters of the differential equation containing fractional differentiation operator in Caputo sense. In connection with the spread of coronavirus infection Covid-19, it seems helpful to build a mathematical model of the number of infected persons to predict the spread of infection.

Keywords Fractional diffusion equation · Difference scheme · Model of the spread of infectious diseases

1 Introduction

This paper is devoted to mathematical modeling of the spread of the coronavirus infection Covid-19. As it known, the coronavirus infection Covid-19 spreads through all the world and has serious clinical consequences. So, the subject of our paper will undoubtedly attract attention.

L. Kirianova · T. Aleroev (✉)
National Research Moscow, State University of Civil Engineering (NRU MGSU), Yaroslavskoe Shosse 26, Moscow 129337, Russia
e-mail: aleroev@mail.ru

L. Kirianova
e-mail: ludmilakirianova@yandex.ru

V. Griguletskiy
Gubkin Russian State, University of Oil and Gas (National Research University), Leninskiy Prospekt 65, Moscow 119991, Russia
e-mail: GVG-TNC@mail.ru

P. Agarwal et al. (eds.), *Analysis of Infectious Disease Problems (Covid-19) and Their Global Impact*, Infosys Science Foundation Series,
https://doi.org/10.1007/978-981-16-2450-6_24

There are some methods of modelling the process of the infections, for example, the kinetic equations constructed according to the law of mass action. This approach unambiguously suggests the "quick mixing" of the reactants. It is justified when the diffusive processes are proceeding much faster than the reaction kinetics. There are hundreds of such kinetic models in population and epidemic dynamics. We formulated an coronavirus spread model as a differential equation of fractional order (the basic equation of a mathematical model of a random walk of a point particle over a self-similar fractal set) with natural initial conditions and numerically solve this problem. It is important to note that proposed model is adequate for any the population size. It is obvious, therefore, that the technique of the theory of fractional differential equations can be applied to the study model's dynamics (analytically or numerically). We do not see the need to prove the theorems, such as those on the existence and uniqueness of the solution because such theorems do not have significant mathematical content in this particular case. In our opinion, the relevance of the article could refer to epidemiology, such as to the forecast of the any infection propagation and possible impact of medicines and social limitations. To approach reality, we attempted to take into account the interplay of different organisms involved into Covid-19 propagation.

2 Main Results

In connection with the spread of coronavirus infection Covid-19, it seems relevant to build a mathematical model of the number of infected people to predict the spread of infection.

Ronald Ross, a British physician and parasitologist, in 1911 was one of the first who investigate the problem of the spread of malaria on Earth [1] and define the basic equations that, with sufficient accuracy for practice, described the process of the spread of malaria. These equations were later used by A. Lotka (1925), G. Gause (1931), V. Volterra (1926–1932) for developing a general theory of the struggle for existence for different physical and biological systems [2–4].

According to Ross, the spread of malaria is determined by two continuous and simultaneously occurring factors: the number of new diseases depends on the total number of people in a given area and the total number of people already infected: thus, it is assumed that the rate of increase in diseases among people is equal to the number of new diseases per unit time minus the number of recoveries per unit of time.

A detailed analysis of Ross equations was carried out by Vito Volterra, who proposed a more realistic definition of the growth rate (increment per unit time) through the value of the potential increase in diseases and the degree of potential increase in diseases. The experiments of G. Gause and A. Lotka confirmed the theoretical studies of V. Volterra.

Note that V. Volterra used the following mathematical model: the growth rate of infected persons is proportional to the potential increase of number of healthy persons and the degree of potential increase of number of infected persons, and the growth rate of number of healthy persons is proportional to the potential increase of number of infected persons and the degree of potential increase of number of healthy persons.

So, Volterra's general theory of the struggle for existence uses a system of two ordinary differential equations:

$$\begin{cases} \frac{dX_1}{dt} = b_1 X_1 \frac{K_1-(X_1+uX_2)}{K_1} \\ \frac{dX_2}{dt} = b_2 X_2 \frac{K_2-(X_2+vX_1)}{K_2} \end{cases} \tag{1}$$

Here

X_1—the number of infected persons;

X_2—the number of healthy persons in the mixed population at a given time;

$b_1,\ b_2$—possible constant positive coefficients of increase of number of infected (b_1) and healthy (b_2) persons;

$K_1,\ K_2$—the maximum possible values of the number of sick (K_1) and healthy (K_1) persons with free growth;

$\frac{dX_1}{dt},\ \frac{dX_2}{dt}$—the growth rates, of infected (N_1) and healthy (N_2) persons at a given moment (t) in a mixed population respectively;

$u,\ v$—"coefficients of the struggle for existence" (according to R. Ross).

The coefficients of the struggle for existence (u, v) in the system of equations (1) are easily determined from the experimental data $\{\widetilde{X}_1(t_1), \widetilde{X}_1(t_2), \widetilde{X}_2(t_1), \widetilde{X}_2(t_2)\}$, known for two values time t_1 and t_2 according to the formulas below:

$$\begin{cases} u = \frac{1}{\widetilde{X}_2(t_1)} \left(K_1 - \widetilde{X}_1(t_1) - \frac{\widetilde{X}_1(t_2)}{b_1 \widetilde{X}_1(t_1)} K_1 \right) \\ v = \frac{1}{\widetilde{X}_1(t_1)} \left(K_2 - \widetilde{X}_2(t_1) - \frac{\widetilde{X}_2(t_2)}{b_2 \widetilde{X}_2(t_1)} K_2 \right) \end{cases}$$

Changes in the coefficients of the struggle for the existence of two species in a mixed population characterize the change in the nature of the interaction between infected and healthy persons under anaerobic conditions: the number of infected persons per unit time is determined by the number of new diseases minus the number of recovered persons per unit time, and the number of healthy persons per unit time is determined by the number all healthy persons minus the number of deaths per unit of time.

In the general case, the rate of growth (or decline) in the number of infected and healthy persons depends on the potential increase in each number and the unused opportunity for growth (or decline) of each type of infected (or healthy) persons.

Such a model is not determined only by a rigorous calculation of the growth rate (or decline) of persons of different species, therefore, a diffusion definition of the distribution of coronavirus infection is used below.

The main disadvantage of system (1) is the fact that the basic ordinary differential equations of the first order do not determine the conditions of equilibrium between the number of infected and healthy persons: by definition, there should be a complete displacement of healthy persons, or complete displacement of infected by healthy persons, which does not correspond to the experimental and actual data. To substantiate this thesis, we pass from the system of differential equations to one equation, introducing one more variable: M is the population size. Then

$$M = X_1 + X_2. \tag{2}$$

Substituting (2) into (1) and use the first equation of the system, then we have

$$\frac{dX_1}{dt} = b_1 X_1 \left(1 - \frac{X_1 + u(M - X_1)}{K_1}\right).$$

Let's denote

$$a_1 = b_1(1 - \frac{uM}{K_1})\ a_2 = \frac{b_1\{u - 1\}}{K_1}).$$

We obtain a special case of the Riccati equation with constant coefficients (or the Bernoulli equation):

$$\frac{dX_1}{dt} = a_1 X_1 + a_2 (X_1)^2. \tag{3}$$

Assuming that someone got sick first to start the epidemic, we have the initial condition:

$$X_1(0) = 1. \tag{4}$$

The solution of the problem (3)–(4) for $a_1 \neq 0,\ a_2 \neq 0$ is

$$X_1(t) = \left((1 + \frac{a_2}{a_1})e^{-a_1 t} - \frac{a_2}{a_1}\right)^{-1}.$$

For $a_1 > 0, a_2 > 0$ the limit value of the function $X_1(t)$ at the ∞

$$\lim_{t\to\infty} X_1(t) = -\frac{a_1}{a_2}.$$

Since the coefficients are of the same sign, the limiting value of the function turns out to be negative, which does not correspond to the meaning of the problem being solved.

For $a_1 > 0,\ a_2 < 0$ the limit value of the function $X_1(t)$ at infinity

$$\lim_{t\to\infty} X_1(t) = -\frac{a_1}{a_2} = \frac{K_1 - uM}{1 - u}.$$

That is, if the "coefficient of the struggle for existence" u is equal to 0, we obtain that the entire population is infected in a rather distant future. So, the indicated signs of the coefficients have a practical meaning.

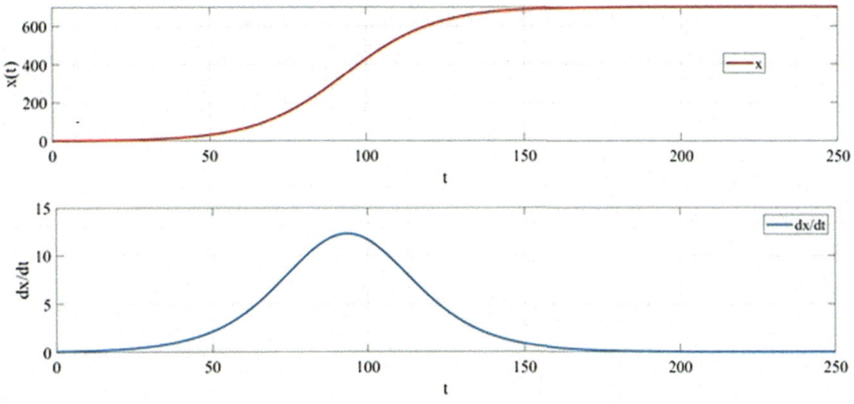

Fig. 1 Figures of the $X_1(t)$ and $X_1'(t)$ for $a_1 = 0.07, a_2 = 0.0001$

For $a_1 < 0$ and any sign of a_2, the limiting value of the solution to problem (3)–(4) at infinity

$$\lim_{t\to\infty} X_1(t) = 0$$

This value does not correspond to the meaning of the problem being solved.

Thus, the signs of the constants in Eq. (3) are justified.

The increase in the number of cases in this model with $a_1 \neq 0,\ a_2 \neq 0$ has the following expression:

$$\frac{dX_1}{dt} = a_1\left((1+\frac{a_2}{a_1})e^{-a_1 t} - \frac{a_2}{a_1}\right)^{-1} + a_2\left((1+\frac{a_2}{a_1})e^{-a_1 t} - \frac{a_2}{a_1}\right)^{-2}$$

Figure 1 shows an example of graphs of functions $X_1(t)$ - solutions of the problem (3)–(4) and its derivative $X_1'(t)$ for $a_1 = 0.07,\ a_2 = 0.0001$.

In addition, there are two more "extreme" cases of solving problem (3)–(4): for $a_1 = 0,\ a_2 \neq 0$

$$X_1(t) = \frac{1}{1 - a_2 t}.$$

In this case, we have a decreasing function, which does not make sense in the context of the problem under consideration. for $a_1 \neq 0,\ a_2 = 0$

$$X_1(t) = e^{a_1 t}.$$

In the latter case, we have an exponential growth in the number of cases without restrictions, which is at odds with common sense.

Analyzing the kinetics of growth of homogeneous populations of G. Gause in 1931, he established that under anaerobic conditions in two independent experiments in a mixed population, there is an "extremely slow growth" of the volume of yeast. One might think that this is how the spread of coronavirus infection in the human population occurs: at a very low rate.

Experimental growth (decline) curves of yeast volume separately and in a mixed population are usually reflected by logistic curves, which are graphs for solving equations of the form:

$$\frac{dY}{dt} = bY - \frac{b}{K}Y^2$$

where

Y - volume of yeast; b, K - constants; t - time.

In such case, we have the problem (3)–(4) again.

To build a more accurate mathematical model, we shall to give up ordinary differential equations and use methods of fractional calculus.

It is assumed below that the process of coronavirus disease disease has a diffusion mechanism and is determined by a differential equation of a fractional order.

Let's consider the process $N(t)$ -the increase in the number of cases of illness during the epidemic by time t. We will use the basic equation of a mathematical model of a random walk of a point particle over a self-similar fractal set [1] to model the process $N(t)$, using the considerations detailed in one of author's papers:

$$D_{0x}^{\alpha} N(t) = \eta(t) N(t) \tag{5}$$

$D_{0x}^{\alpha} N(t)$- fractional derivative (fractional differentiation operator) according to Caputo [3] of order $\alpha \in [0, 1]$:

$$D_{0x}^{\alpha} N(t) = \frac{1}{\Gamma(1-\alpha)} \int_0^t (t-\tau)^{-\alpha} N'(\tau) d\tau.$$

The multiplier $\eta(t)$ known argument function of t. We establish the natural initial condition:

$$N(0) = 1 \tag{6}$$

We solve problem (5)–(6) numerically, assuming that $\alpha \in [0, 1]$. Let's divide the interval $[0; T]$ to n equal parts:

$$t_0 = 0;\ t_k = kh;\ k = 1, ..., N;\ h = \frac{T}{n};$$

h - uniform grid step.

Denote $N_k = N(t_k)$, assume $N_k' = \frac{N_k - N_{k-1}}{h}$ and consider the operator of fractional differentiation, as well as in [4]:

$$D_{0t_1}^{\alpha}N(t) = \frac{1}{\Gamma(1-\alpha)}\left[\int\limits_{t_0}^{t_1} N'(\tau)(t_1-\tau)^{-\alpha}d\tau\right] \approx \frac{[N_1-N_0]}{h\Gamma(1-\alpha)}\int\limits_0^h (h-\tau)^{-\alpha}d\tau =$$

$$\frac{[N_1-N_0]}{h\Gamma(1-\alpha)}\frac{-(h-\tau)^{-\alpha+1}}{-\alpha+1}\Bigg|_h^0 = \frac{[N_1-N_0]}{h^{\alpha}\Gamma(2-\alpha)}$$

Similarly,

$$D_{0t_1}^{\alpha}N(t) = \frac{1}{\Gamma(1-\alpha)}\left[\sum_{k=1}^{m}\int\limits_{t_{-1}}^{t_k} N'(t)(t_n-\tau)^{-\alpha}d\tau\right] \approx$$

$$\approx \frac{1}{h^{\alpha}\Gamma(2-\alpha)}\sum_{k=1}^{m}[N_k-N_{k-1}][(m-k+1)^{1-\alpha}-(m-k)^{1-\alpha}].$$

So,

$$D_{0t_m}^{\alpha}N(t) = \frac{1}{h^{\alpha}\Gamma(2-\alpha)}\sum_{k=0}^{m} a_{mk}N_k. \tag{7}$$

Here,

$$a_{mk} = [(m-k+1)^{1-\alpha} - 2(m-k)^{1-\alpha} + (m-k-1)^{1-\alpha}];,\ 1 \le k \ge m-1;$$

$$a_{m0} = -m^{1-\alpha} + (m-1)^{1-\alpha};\ a_{mm} = 1.$$

Further, from (5), (6) and (7), denoting $\eta_m = \eta(t_m)$ we get the system

$$\begin{cases} N_0 = 1, \\ \frac{1}{h^{\alpha}\Gamma(2-\alpha)}\sum\limits_{k=0}^{m} a_{mk}N_k = \eta_m N_m, \\ m = 1, 2, ..., n. \end{cases}$$

Or resolving respectively N_m

$$\begin{cases} N_0 = 1, \\ N_m = \frac{1}{h^{\alpha}\Gamma(2-\alpha)\eta_m - 1}\sum\limits_{k=0}^{m-1} a_{mk}N_k, \\ m = 1, 2, ..., n. \end{cases} \tag{8}$$

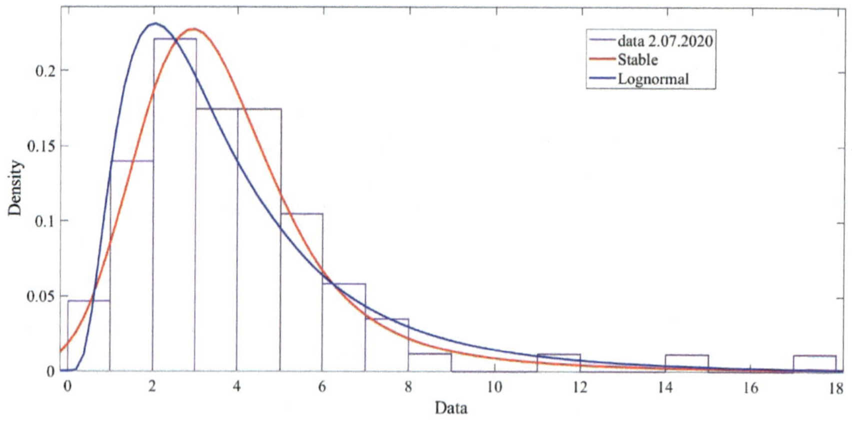

Fig. 2 A histogram of the number of cases per 1000 population in Russia on July 2, 2020

System (4) is easily solved with known α and η.

To verify the proposed model (5)–(6), we analyze the statistical information available in open sources [5] on the spread of Covid-19 in Russian Federation. Figure 2 shows a histogram of the number of cases per 1000 population in Russia at t = July 2, 2020.

The agreement with a stable distribution is much better than with a lognormal one. Due to the asymmetry of the histogram, it makes no sense to check any symmetric distribution, in particular, the normal one. Due to the statistical analysis, the distribution of the number of cases can be considered stable. Sustainable distribution with parameters $\alpha, \beta, \gamma, \delta$ has a characteristic function:

$$\varphi(z) = \begin{cases} exp\left(-\gamma^{\alpha}|z|^{\alpha}\left[1 + i\beta sign(z) tan\frac{\pi\alpha}{2}((\gamma|z|^{1-\alpha} - 1)\right] + i\delta z\right), \ \alpha \neq 1 \\ exp\left(-\gamma|z|\left[1 + i\beta sign(z) tan\frac{2}{\pi} ln(\gamma|z|)\right] + i\delta z\right), \ \alpha = 1 \end{cases}$$

Sustainable distribution parameters have the following meaning:

α—The characteristic indicator of the decrease of the "tails"ž of the distribution;

β—Asymmetry parameter;

γ—Scale parameter;

δ—Position parameter.

For $\alpha = 2$ the stable distribution coincides with the normal, and at $\alpha = 1$ with Cauchy distribution. Estimates of the parameters of the stable distribution of the number of cases per 1000 population were carried out using the built-in fitdist function of the Matlab application package $\alpha = 1.5$, $\beta = 1$, $\gamma = 1.2$, $\delta = 3.1$.

It is known [6] that stable distributions with the corresponding normalization are fundamental solutions of the diffusion equation containing a fractional derivative. Since we are considering an increase in the number of cases, we take in (1) the order of the fractional derivative, $\alpha = 0.536$.

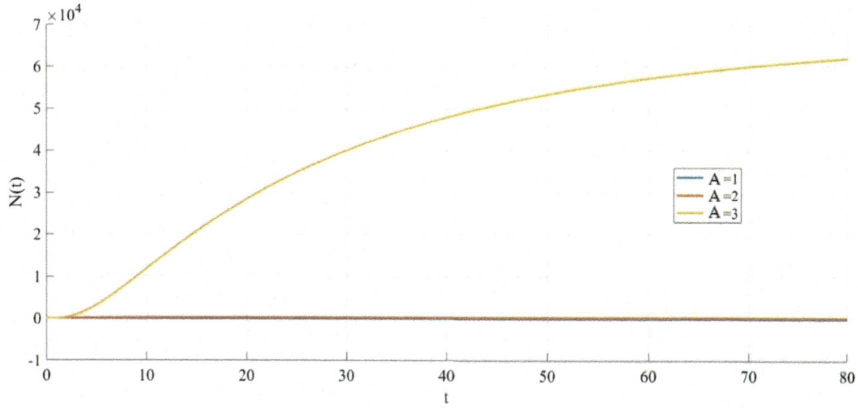

Fig. 3 Graphs of solving problem (5)–(6) for $\alpha = 0.5$ and $\eta(t) = \frac{1}{(1+t)^{0.85}}$ for $A{=}1,\ A{=}2,\ A{=}3$

Note that for $\alpha = 1$ and $\eta(t) = A$, the problem (5)–(6) has solution

$$N(t) = exp(At)$$

and the proposed model gives an exponential growth of the investigated function. For the numerical solution, we set the factor on the right-hand side in a decreasing power-law manner:

$$\eta(t) = \frac{1}{(1+t)^B}$$

Figure 3 shows graphs of the solution to problem (5)–(6) for $\alpha = 0.5$ and

$$\eta(t) = \frac{1}{(1+t)^{0.85}}$$

and for three parameters $A = 1,\ A = 2,\ A = 3$. Obviously, parameter A can be interpreted as an "infection spread index" and it has a stronger effect at the initial stage of spread (the graphs of the solution for two values of the parameter $A = 1$ and $A = 2$ seem to be the same due to their large difference from the graph of the solution for the value $A = 3$. The parameters differ by equal values, i.e. taken with a unit step, while the solutions differ unevenly from each other. This fact is demonstrated in Fig. 3).

Figure 4 shows graphs of the solution to problem (5)–(6) for $\alpha = 0.5$ and

$$\eta(t) = \frac{1}{(1+t)^B}$$

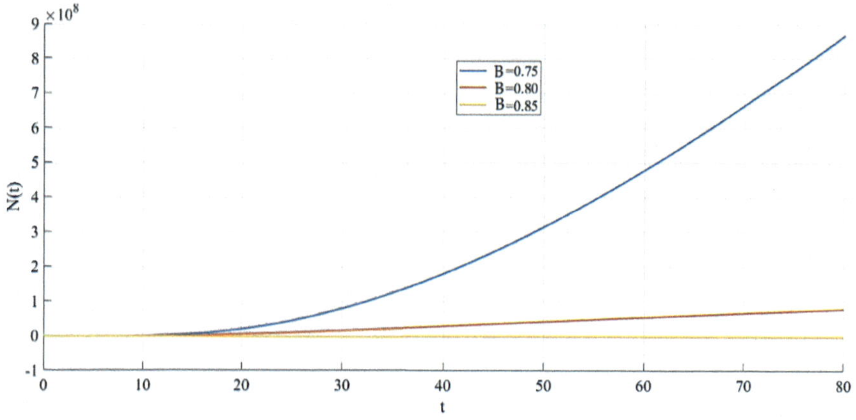

Fig. 4 Graphs for solving problem (1)–(2) for $\alpha = 0.5$ and $\eta(t) = \frac{1}{(1+t)^B}$ for $B = 0.75$; $B = 0.80$; $B = 0.85$

and three parameter values $B = 0.75,\ B = 0.8,\ B = 0.85$. Obviously, parameter B can be interpreted as an "index of the effectiveness of measures taken to contain" and it has a stronger effect on the second (final) stage of distribution.

Exact selection of the values of parameters A and B can be carried out by the nomographic method. Based on the analysis of numerically found solutions to problem (5)–(6), we can conclude that the proposed model is flexible enough to model the spread of an infectious disease.

References

1. Ross, R.: The Prevention of Malaria. London (1911)
2. Lotka, A.J.: Elements of Physical Biology. Baltimore (1925)
3. Gause, G.F.: Ecology of populations. Q. Rev. Biol. **7** (1932)
4. Volterra, V.: Lecons sur la theorie mathematique de la lutte pour la Vie. Paris (1931)
5. Aleroev, T.S., Zveriaev, E.M., Larionov, E.A.: Fractional calculus and its applications. Keldysh Institute preprints (2013), 037, 26 p. http://library.keldysh.ru/preprint.asp?id=2013-37
6. Caputo, M.: Linear models of dissipation whose Q is almost frequency in-denpendent. Geophys. J. R. Astr. Soc. **13**, 529–539 (1967)
7. Kirianova, L.: The Begley-Torvik model difference scheme matrix eigenvalues. Model. Methods Struct. Anal. IOP Conf. Ser. J. Phys. Conf. Series (2020) 012111. (2019 Dec, 1425). https://doi.org/10.1088/1742-6596/1425/1/012111
8. Official statistic of the COVID-19 spread in Moscow, Russia https://coronavirus-monitor.info/country/russia/moskva/
9. Handbook of Fractional Calculus with Applications. Series edited by J.A.Tenreiro Machado, De Gruyter GmbH, Berlin/Boston, Vol. 1–8 (2019)
10. Mainardi, F.: Fractional Relaxation-Oscillation and fractional Diffusion wave Phenomena. Chaos, Solutions Fractals **7**(9), 1461–1477 (1996)

11. Kekharsaeva, E.R., Aleroev, T.S.: The model of deformation and strength characteristics of the chlorine–containing polyesters based on derivatives of fractional order. Plasticheskiye Massy (3), 35 (2001)
12. Erokhin, S.V.: Mathematical modeling of stress-strain state of viscoelastic bodies using fractional calculus methods. PhD doctor's Thesis, Penza (2016)
13. Aleroev, T.S.: Boundary value problems for differential equations with fractional derivatives. Doctor's math. degree, MSU (2000)
14. Aleroev, T.S., Kirane, M., Tang, Y.F.: The boundary value problem for a differential operator of fractional order. J. Math. Sci. **194**(5), 499–512 (2013)
15. Popov, A.Y., Sedletskii, A.M.: Distribution of roots of Mittag–Leffler functions, Theory of functions. CMFD, 40, PFUR, M. 3–171 (2011)

An SEIR Epidemic Model of Fractional Order to Analyze the Evolution of the Covid-19 Epidemic in Argentina

Juan E. Santos, José M. Carcione, Gabriela B. Savioli, and Patricia M. Gauzellino

Abstract A pandemic caused by a new coronavirus (Covid-19) has spread worldwide, inducing an epidemic still active in Argentina. In this chapter, we present a case study using an SEIR (Susceptible-Exposed-Infected-Recovered) diffusion model of fractional order in time to analyze the evolution of the epidemic in Buenos Aires and neighboring areas (Región Metropolitana de Buenos Aires, (RMBA)) comprising about 15 million inhabitants. In the SEIR model, individuals are divided into four classes, namely, susceptible (S), exposed (E), infected (I) and recovered (R). The SEIR model of fractional order allows for the incorporation of memory, with hereditary properties of the system, being a generalization of the classic SEIR first-order system, where such effects are ignored. Furthermore, the fractional model provides one additional parameter to obtain a better fit of the data. The parameters of the model are calibrated by using as data the number of casualties officially reported. Since infinite solutions honour the data, we show a set of cases with different values of the lockdown parameters, fatality rate, and incubation and infectious periods. The different reproduction ratios R_0 and infection fatality rates (IFR) so obtained indicate the results may differ from recent reported values, constituting possible alternative solutions. A comparison with results obtained with the classic SEIR model is also

J. E. Santos (✉) · J. M. Carcione
School of Earth Sciences and Engineering, Hohai University, Nanjing 211100, China
e-mail: santos@purdue.edu

J. E. Santos
Universidad de Buenos Aires, Facultad de Ingeniería, Instituto del Gas y del Petróleo, Av. Las Heras, 2214 Piso 3 Buenos Aires, Argentina

Department of Mathematics, Purdue University, West Lafayette, IN 47907, USA

J. M. Carcione
National Institute of Oceanography and Applied Geophysics-OGS, Trieste, Italy

G. B. Savioli
Universidad de Buenos Aires, Facultad de Ingeniería, Instituto del Gas y del Petróleo, Av. Las Heras 2214 Piso 3, Buenos Aires, Argentina

P. M. Gauzellino
Facultad de Ciencias Astronómicas y Geofísicas, Universidad Nacional de La Plata, La Plata, Argentina

P. Agarwal et al. (eds.), *Analysis of Infectious Disease Problems (Covid-19) and Their Global Impact*, Infosys Science Foundation Series,
https://doi.org/10.1007/978-981-16-2450-6_25

included. The analysis allows us to study how isolation and social distancing measures affect the time evolution of the epidemic.

Keywords 34A08 Fractional Differential Equations · 65L07 Numerical investigation of stability of solutions · 92C20 Medical epidemiology · 34A55 Inverse problems

1 Introduction

We present an SEIR subdiffusion model of fractional order ν, with $0 < \nu \leq 1$ to analyze the time evolution of the Covid-19 epidemic in Buenos Aires and neighboring areas (Region Metropolitana de Buenos Aires, (RMBA)) with a population of about 15 million inhabitants. RMBA consists of Ciudad Autónoma de Buenos Aires (CABA) plus forty municipalities covering an area of about thirteen thousand square kilometers, where some of these municipalities have rural areas. Thus, RMBA has an average population density of 1100 people/km^2, but in CABA and many of its neighboring cities this number increases significantly. For example, CABA has a population density of about 14000 people/km^2. In this work, we consider that RMBA has a uniform population distribution.

The epidemic started officially on March 9th with the number of cases and deaths still increasing at the day of writing (September 22th, 2020). The classical SEIR model ($\nu = 1$) has been used by Carcione et al. [1] and Santos et al. [2] to model the Covid-19 epidemic in Italy and Argentina, respectively.

Fractional calculus has been used to define diffusion and wave propagation models in biological and viscoelastic materials [3–10]. One important property of the fractional-order SEIR model is that incorporates memory and hereditary properties, a behavior exhibited by most biological systems. The use of fractional order derivatives affects the duration of the epidemic, peaks of infected and dead individuals per day and number of number casualties.

Among other authors that have applied fractional calculus to obtain solutions of the SEIR model, we mention Scherer et al. [11], that used a Grünwald-Letnikov time-discrete procedure, introduced by Ciesielski and Leszczynski [12] (CL method). Besides, Zeb et al. [13] presented an analysis of several numerical methods to solve the SEIR model of fractional order. For general works on fractional calculus including numerical methods, we refer to Podlubny [14] and Li and Zeng [15].

We first formulate an initial-value problem (IVP) for the classical SEIR model ($\nu = 1$) and the SEIR subdiffusion equations of fractional order ν at the continuous level using the Caputo definition of the fractional derivative [6]. Existence and uniqueness of the solution of this IVP, with positive values, is demonstrated in [13]. The numerical solutions of the continuous IVP are computed by using the time-explicit algorithm of Gorenflo-Mainardi-Moretti-Paradisi (GMMP method) [16, 17]. The conditional stability of the time-explicit GMMP method (and also of the CL method) was demonstrated by Murillo et al. [19] [see their equation (19)]. The validation of the GMMP method is performed by comparison of its results against those of the classic SEIR model and those of the fractional Adams-Bashford-Moulton method (ABM method) as defined in [15].

The parameters of the SEIR model are the birth and death rates, infection and incubation periods, probability of disease transmission per contact, fatality rate and initial number of exposed individuals. These parameters, together with the order of the fractional derivative, are obtained by fitting the number of fatalities officially reported. This is an inverse problem with an infinite number of solutions (local minima) honouring the data, which is solved by using a quasi-Newton technique for nonlinear least squares problem with the formula of Broyden-Fletcher-Goldfarb-Shanno [20]. The numerical simulations give an effective procedure to study the spread of the evolution of virus, analyze the effects of the lockdown measures and predict the peak of infected and dead individuals per day.

2 The Caputo Derivative and Initial Value Problems

For $0 < \nu \leq 1$, the time fractional Caputo derivative $D_c^\nu(u(t)$ is defined as [3, 6, 16, 17]

$$D_c^\nu(f(t) = \frac{1}{\Gamma(1-\nu)} \int_0^t \left[\frac{\partial}{\partial f(\tau)}\right] \frac{d\tau}{(t-\tau)^\nu}, \tag{1}$$

where $\Gamma(\cdot)$ denotes the Euler's Gamma function.

Note that the Caputo derivatives of constant functions $f(t) = 1$ vanish and those of powers of t, $f(t) = t^k$ are

$$\frac{\Gamma(k+1)}{\Gamma(k-\nu+1)} t^{k-\nu}.$$

The advantage of using the Caputo derivative in Caputo-type IVP's is that the initial conditions are the same as those of the classical ordinary differential equations. For details on the Caputo derivative and its relation with the Riemann-Liouville fractional derivative we refer to [6].

To approximate the time-fractional Caputo derivative, we use a backward Grünwald-Letnikov approximation at time $t_n = n\Delta t, n = 0, 1, \cdots,$ with $f_n = f(n\Delta t)$, Δt being the time step, as follows [16, 17]:

$$D_c^\nu(f(t)|_{t_{n+1}} \approx \frac{1}{(\Delta t)^\nu} \sum_{j=0}^{n+1} (-1)^j c_j^\nu \binom{\nu}{j} f_{n+1-j}. \tag{2}$$

The coefficients

$$c_j^\nu = (-1)^j \binom{\nu}{j}$$

can be obtained in terms of Euler's Gamma function using the recurrence relation

$$\binom{\nu}{j} = \frac{\Gamma(\nu+1)}{\Gamma(j+1)\Gamma(\nu-j+1)} = \frac{\nu-j+1}{j}\binom{\nu}{j-1}, \quad \binom{\nu}{0} = 1. \tag{3}$$

The work by Abdullah et al. [18] presents an analysis of the fractional-order SEIR model formulated in terms of the Caputo derivative and its GMMP time discretization.

3 The Classical and Fractional-Order SEIR Models

The IVP for the classic SEIR system of nonlinear ordinary differential equations is

$$\begin{aligned}
\dot{S} &= f_1(S,E,I,R)(t) = \Lambda - \mu S(t) - \beta S(t)\frac{I(t)}{N(t)}, \\
\dot{E} &= f_2(S,E,I,R)(t) = \beta S(t)\frac{I(t)}{N(t)} - (\mu+\epsilon)E(t), \\
\dot{I} &= f_3(S,E,I,R)(t) = \epsilon E(t) - (\gamma+\mu+\alpha)I(t), \\
\dot{R} &= f_4(S,E,I,R)(t) = \gamma I(t) - \mu R(t),
\end{aligned} \tag{4}$$

with initial conditions $S(0)$, $E(0)$, $I(0)$ and $R(0)$. A dot above a variable indicates the time derivative, while $N(t)$ is the number of live individuals at time t, i.e., $N = S + E + I + R \leq N_0$, N_0 being the total initial population. In (4), S is the number of individuals susceptible to be exposed while E is the number of exposed individuals, in which the disease is latent; they are infected but not infectious. Individuals in the E-class become infected (I) with a rate ϵ and infected become recovered (R) with a rate γ. People in the R class do not move back to the S class since lifelong immunity is assumed. Furthermore, $1/\gamma$ and $1/\epsilon$ are the infection and incubation periods, respectively, Λ is the birth rate, μ is the natural per capita death rate, α is the average fatality rate, and β is the probability of disease transmission per contact. All of these coefficients have units of 1/time. Given the short period of the epidemic in Argentina (6 months at the time of writing), and that the average life expectancy is about 76 years, it is reasonable to assume that $\Lambda = \mu N$, so that the deaths balance the newborns.

Dead individuals $D(t)$ are computed as $D(t) = N_0 - N(t)$, so that the dead people per unit time $\dot{D}(t)$, can be obtained as [21]:

$$\dot{D}(t) = \alpha I(t). \tag{5}$$

Next, we reformulate the system (4) into a fractional-order system by using the Caputo derivative in (1):

$$\begin{aligned} D_c^\nu S(t) &= f_1^\nu(S,E,I,R)(t) = \mu^\nu N - \mu^\nu S(t) - \beta^\nu S(t)\frac{I(t)}{N(t)}, \\ D_c^\nu E(t) &= f_2^\nu(S,E,I,R)(t) = \beta^\nu S(t)\frac{I(t)}{N(t)} - (\mu^\nu + \epsilon^\nu)E(t) \\ D_c^\nu I(t) &= f_3^\nu(S,E,I,R)(t) = \epsilon^\nu E(t) - (\gamma^\nu + \mu^\nu + \alpha^\nu)I(t), \\ D_c^\nu R(t) &= f_4^\nu(S,E,I,R)(t) = \gamma^\nu I(t) - \mu^\nu R(t). \end{aligned} \tag{6}$$

The reproduction ratio, R_0, indicates the number of cases induced by a single infectious individual. When $R_0 < 1$, the disease dies out; when $R_0 > 1$, an epidemic occurs. Al-Sheikh [22] analyzes the behavior of the SEIR models in terms of R_0. For the SEIR model, R_0 is given by [23]

$$R_0 = \frac{\beta^\nu \epsilon^\nu}{(\epsilon^\nu + \mu^\nu)(\gamma^\nu + \alpha^\nu + \mu^\nu)}. \tag{7}$$

The infection fatality rate (IFR) is defined as

$$\text{IFR } (\%) = 100 \cdot \frac{\alpha^\nu}{\alpha^\nu + \gamma^\nu} \approx 100 \cdot \frac{\alpha^\nu}{\gamma^\nu}, \tag{8}$$

where this relation holds at all times, not only at the end of the epidemic.

3.1 Time Discretization

An explicit conditionally stable GMMP algorithm for the fractional order system (6) is formulated as follows [16, 17]:

$$S_{n+1} = -\sum_{j=1}^{m+1} c_j^\nu S(m+1-j) + S_0 \sum_{j=0}^{m+1} c_j^\nu + (\Delta t)^\nu f_1(S_n, E_n, I_n, R_n) \tag{9}$$

$$E_{n+1} = -\sum_{j=1}^{m+1} c_j^\nu E(m+1-j) + E_0 \sum_{j=0}^{m+1} c_j^\nu + (\Delta t)^\nu f_2(S_n, E_n, I_n, R_n) \tag{10}$$

$$I_{n+1} = -\sum_{j=1}^{m+1} c_j^\nu I(m+1-j) + I_0 \sum_{j=0}^{m+1} c_j^\nu + (\Delta t)^\nu f_3(S_n, E_n, I_n, R_n) \tag{11}$$

$$R_{n+1} = -\sum_{j=1}^{m+1} c_j^\nu R(m+1-j) + R_0 \sum_{j=0}^{m+1} c_j^\nu + (\Delta t)^\nu f_4(S_n, E_n, I_n, R_n) \tag{12}$$

The results of the GMMP method (9)–(12) will be validated against the solution of the classical SEIR model ($\nu = 1$) and the Adams-Bashford-Moulton (ABM) time-explicit scheme as defined in [15] and included in the Appendix.

4 Numerical Results

4.1 Validation of the GMMP Algorithm

The results of the GMMP algorithm are cross-checked with those of the ABM solver for the classical SEIR model ($\nu = 1$) and SEIR models of fractional orders $\nu = 0.9$ and 0.8.

We use the following parameters, given in Chowel et al. [24] and used by Carcione et al. [1] to perform a parametric analysis of the model. Average disease incubation $1/\epsilon = 3$ days, infectious period $1/\gamma = 8$ days, induced fatality rate $\alpha = 0.006$/day, $\beta = 0.75$/day, and $\Lambda = \mu = 0$. The initial conditions are $E(0) = 1$, $S(0) = N(0) - E(0) - I(0)$, $I(0) = 1$ and $R(0) = 0$. The time step is $dt = 0.01$ day and $N_0 = 10$ million. This case corresponds to a high reproduction ratio $R_0 = 5.72$.

Figures 1, 2, 3, 4, 5 and 6 show the results of the four classes, S,E,I,R, and the dead and dead per day individuals computed by using the GMMP and ABM algorithms. First, an excellent agreement between the results of the two algorithms is observed for all values of the fractional order derivative ν. To quantify this agreement, we compute a mean squared relative error between the estimations of both methods. For example, in the computation of infected individuals, the following errors are obtained: 1.512×10^{-5} for $\nu = 1$, 9.880×10^{-6} for $\nu = 0.9$ and 1.053×10^{-5} for $\nu = 0.8$. In particular, the results for $\nu = 1$ agree with those of Figs. 1 and 2 in [1]. Figure 1 shows that decreasing the order of the fractional derivative causes a delay and an increase in the number of susceptible individuals. While for the classical model the number of infectious individuals vanish at long times, this is not the case for the orders $\nu = 0.8$ and $\nu = 0.9$ (Fig. 3). We run the simulator up to a very long time but the individuals do not vanish, so that the epidemic never ends (in theory). This happens because $R_0 \geq 1$. We run other examples with different parameters such that $R_0 < 1$ and as expected the number of infectious individuals vanish and the epidemic dies out. For brevity these plots are not shown. The case $R_0 < 1$ is analyzed in Sect. 4.2, when simulating the evolution of the epidemic in the RMBA using fractional derivatives. This value of R_0 is associated with the strict lockdown imposed by the government, with a corresponding decrease in the number of infected individuals.

Regarding the exposed infected classes (Figs. 2 and 3), a decrease in ν causes delays and reduces the amplitude of the peaks of these classes. Furthermore, as ν decreases the number of casualties increase as seen in Fig. 4 while Fig. 6 shows a delay and increase of the peak in the number of dead individuals per day. Also, note

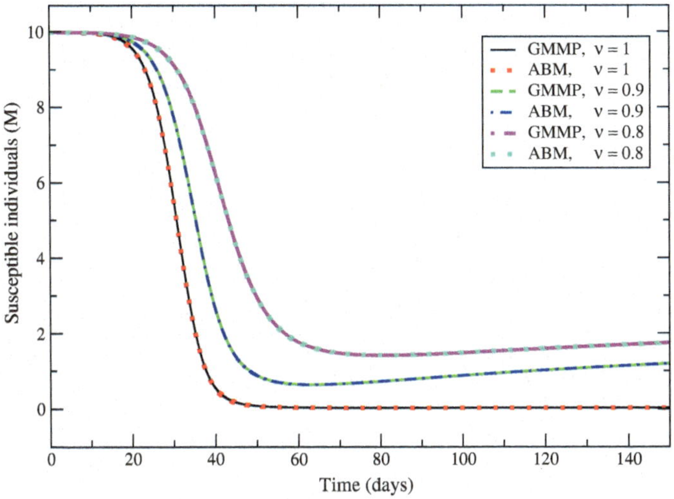

Fig. 1 Susceptible individuals for the classical SEIR model ($\nu = 1$) and fractional-order derivatives $\nu = 0.8$ and 0.9

that Fig. 5 shows a delay and decrease in the number of recovered individuals as the order of the fractional derivative decreases.

These simulations consider a single value of β, the lockdown parameter. In a realistic case, β is a function of time and the procedure is that every time β changes, the algorithm has to be fully initialized from the beginning. Changing β in the same time loop yields wrong results. This fact has been verified by cross-checking different algorithms and several fractional orders.

4.2 Analysis of the Covid-19 Epidemic in the RMBA

We model the Covid-19 epidemic in the RMBA, with a population $N_0 = 14839026$ individuals according to the 2010 Census (https://www.indec.gob.ar/indec/web/Nivel4-Tema-2-41-135). The prediction of the time evolution of the epidemic is very difficult due to the uncertainty of the parameters defining the SEIR model. Virus properties such as the infectious and incubation periods (γ^{-1} and ϵ^{-1}) and life expectancy of an infected individual (α^{-1}) lie in certain bounded intervals. Instead, the parameter β is time dependent, due to changes according to the lockdown and social-distance measures imposed by the government. Most authors use the infectious individuals to calibrate the model, e.g., González-Parra et al. [25], who model the AH1N1/09 influenza epidemic in Bogotá, Colombia and in the Nueva Esparta state in Venezuela.

Since the number of asymptomatic, undiagnosed infectious individuals in RMBA is unknown, we choose to calibrate the model with the number of officially reported

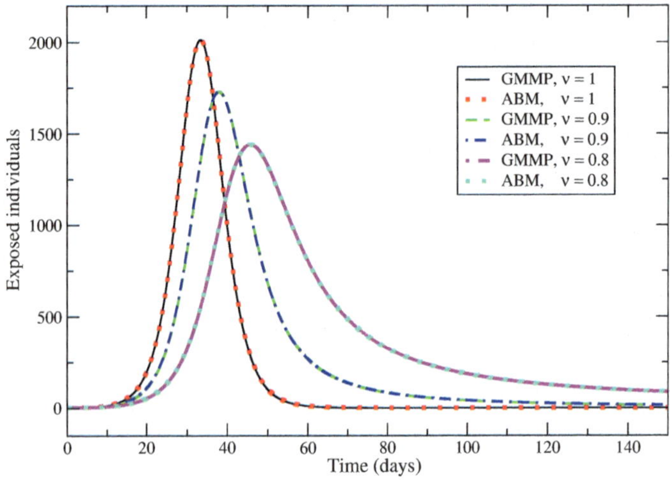

Fig. 2 Exposed individuals for the classical SEIR model ($\nu = 1$) and fractional-order derivatives $\nu = 0.8$ and 0.9

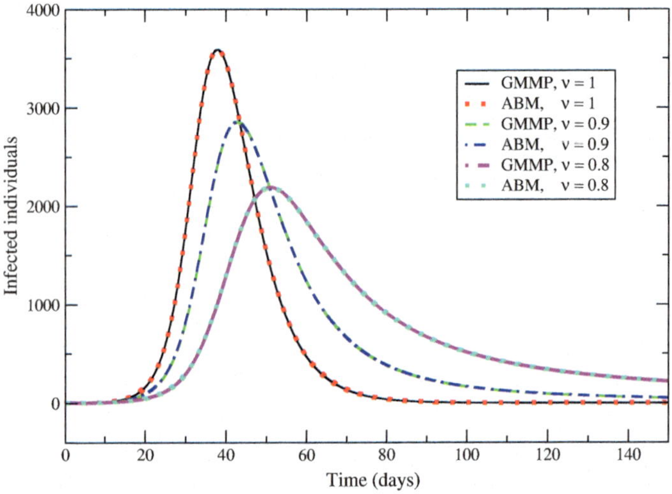

Fig. 3 Infected individuals for the classical SEIR model ($\nu = 1$) and fractional-order derivatives $\nu = 0.8$ and 0.9

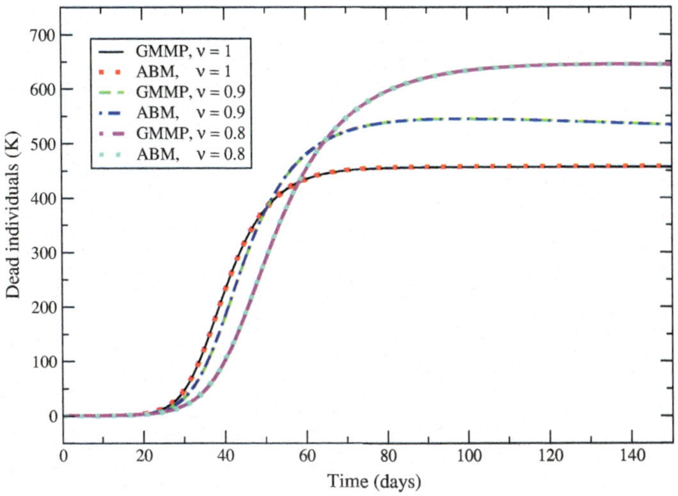

Fig. 4 Dead individuals for the classical SEIR model ($\nu = 1$) and fractional-order derivatives $\nu = 0.8$ and 0.9

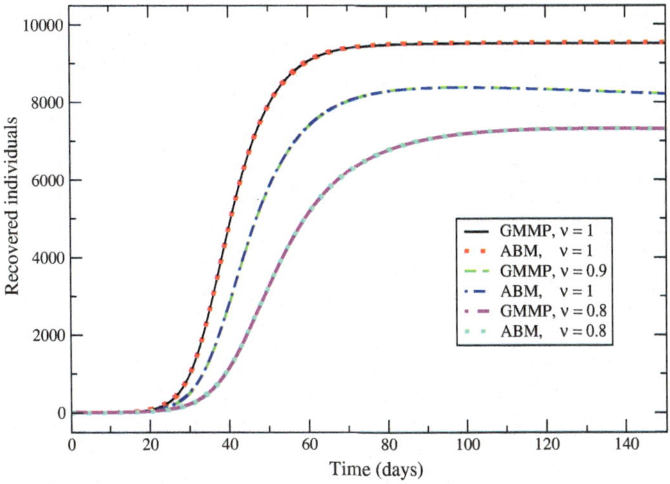

Fig. 5 Recovered individuals for the classical SEIR model ($\nu = 1$) and fractional-order derivatives $\nu = 0.8$ and 0.9

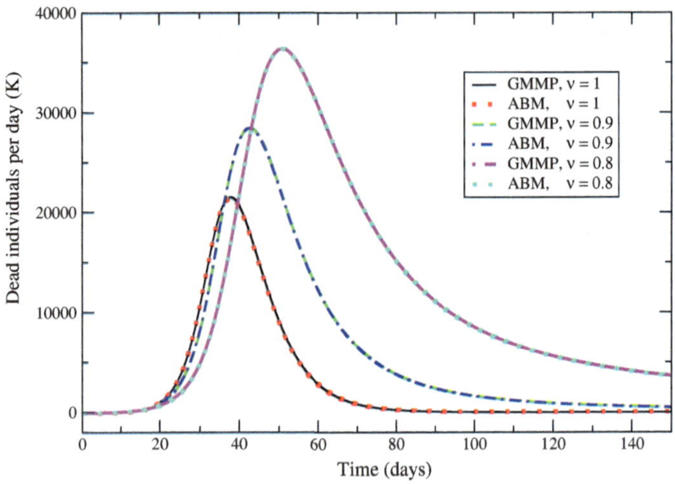

Fig. 6 Dead individuals per day for the classical SEIR model ($\nu = 1$) and fractional-order derivatives $\nu = 0.8$ and 0.9

casualties as the most reliable data, from day 1 (March 9, 2020) to day 198 (September 22th, 2020) (https://www.argentina.gob.ar/coronavirus/informe-diario). Concerning the parameters, fractional order and initial conditions of the model, we assume $\mu = 3.6 \times 10^{-5}/$ day, corresponding to a life expectancy of 76 years. Changes in the β parameter are associated with different measures of lockdown and social distance imposed by the goverment. Thus, we assume that β is a piecewise constant function, where its variations are related to the inflection points observed in the curve of casualties. After the initial time $t_0 = 1$ day, this curve shows two inflection points at times $t_1 = 31$ day and $t_3 = 50$ day. The fractional-order derivative ν, the values of α, β, ϵ, γ and the initial exposed individuals $E(0)$ are estimated by minimizing the L^2-norm between the simulated and actual casualties, which is an inverse problem with an infinite number of solutions due to the existence of local minima. The estimation is also performed for the classical case $\nu = 1$. This inverse problem is solved by using a quasi Newton approximation technique for nonlinear least-squares problems, based on the formula of Broyden-Fletcher-Goldfarb-Shanno [20]. Application of this technique to solve inverse problems in reservoir engineering can be found in [26]. Table 1 shows ranges of the fractional derivative ν, of the parameters $\alpha, \beta, \epsilon, \gamma$ and the initial exposed individuals $E(0)$ used in the inversion procedure. Table 2 displays the initial values and results of four outputs (Cases) of the fitting procedure.

Let us analyze four cases, resulting from the minimization algorithm. We obtained the SEIR parameters, the fractional order and the initial exposed humans values fitting the data. In all the cases, the initial number of infected individuals is assumed to be $I(0) = 100$.

Figures 7 and 8 show the dead individuals and dead individuals per day for Case 1. The inflection point at $t_1 = 30$ day, related to a change of R_0 from 3.178 to

Table 1 Constraints and ranges of the estimation procedure

Variable →	ν	α day^{-1}	β day^{-1}	ϵ^{-1} day	γ^{-1} day	$E(0)$
Lower bound	0.8	10^{-5}	0.1	3	3	10^2
Upper bound	1.0	10^{-1}	0.9	9	9	10^4

Table 2 Initial values and results of the estimation procedure

Variable →	ν	α day^{-1}	β_1 day^{-1}	β_2 day^{-1}	β_3 day^{-1}	ϵ^{-1} day	γ^{-1} day	$E(0)$
Case 1								
Initial	0.9	6.00×10^{-3}	0.5	0.2	0.3	5.0	4.0	500
Optimum	0.919	2.130761×10^{-4}	0.66090	0.12507	0.34002	8.976007	5.335143	1623
R_0 IFR =0.197			3.178	0.688	1.725			
Case 2								
Initial	0.85	6.00×10^{-3}	0.4	0.2	0.3	5.0	4.0	1000
Optimum	0.812	4.179268×10^{-4}	0.77273	0.47231	0.56801	8.121503	3.022527	1138
R_0 IFR =0.444			1.982	1.329	1.539			
Case 3								
Initial	1	6.00×10^{-3}	0.5	0.2	0.3	5.0	4.0	500
Optimum	1	2.822018×10^{-4}	0.49040	0.10396	0.27568	8.975264	6.212071	2821
R_0 IFR =0.175			3.041	0.645	1.710			
Case 4								
Initial	0.9	6.00×10^{-3}	0.4	0.2	0.3	5.0	4.0	1000
Optimum	0.929	2.787611×10^{-4}	0.47289	0.10168	0.31122	8.244641	5.751017	4110
R_0 IFR =0.254			2.526	0.606	1.713			

0.688, shows a decay in the simulated curves, because of the effect of the lockdown. After $t_1 = 50$ day, the curves exhibits a continuous increase in casualties due to the relaxation of the lockdown measures with $R_0 = 1.725$. Figure 9 shows the behavior of all classes, with a a peak of 555 thousand infected individuals at day 188 (September 12th, 2020) while Fig. 10 exhibits a death toll of 19000 people after 800 days (May 17th, 2022) and a peak of 234 casualties at day 188.

The parameters of Cases 2 and 3 in Table 2 also fit the data, with graphs similar to those in Figs. 7 and 8. Case 2 estimates peaks of 309 deaths and 285 thousand infected individuals at day 222 (October 16th, 2020). At day 800 (May 17, 2022), there are 34 thousand deaths and 7457 thousand recovered humans. This increase in the number of casualties is due to the higher infection fatality rate IFR and higher reproduction ratios R_0 as compared with those of Case 1 (see Table 2).

Case 3, which corresponds to the classical SEIR model ($\nu = 1$), exhibits a peak of 171 casualties at day 184 (September 8th, 2020) and 607 thousand people infected.

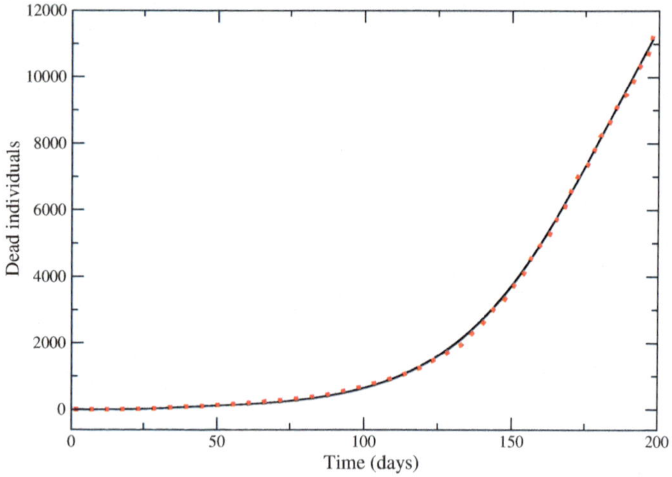

Fig. 7 Dead individuals. The red dots represent the data and the solid line the fit using the SEIR model of fractional order with $\nu = 0.919$

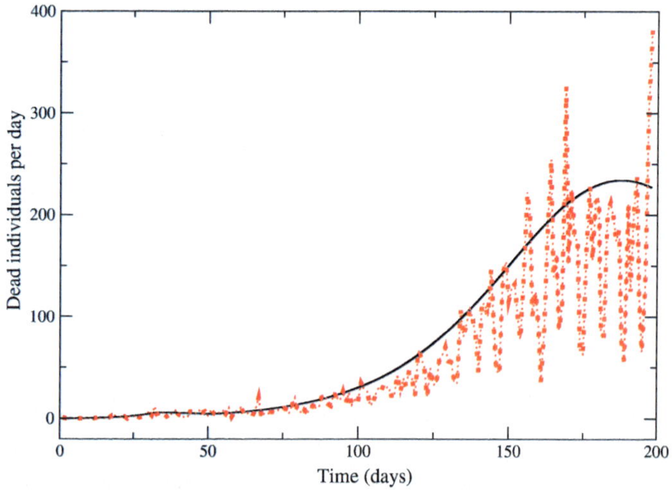

Fig. 8 Dead individuals per day. The red dots represent the data and the solid line the fit using the SEIR model of fractional order with $\nu = 0.919$

The end of the epidemic is consider the day at which the number of infected individuals is smaller than 1, which is day 594 (October 24th, 2021) for this case. At this day, the total number of recovered and dead individuals are 10157 thousand and 18 thousand, respectively, so that the total number of infected people at the end of the epidemic is 10175 thousand individuals. This is the case predicting the smallest number of casualties.

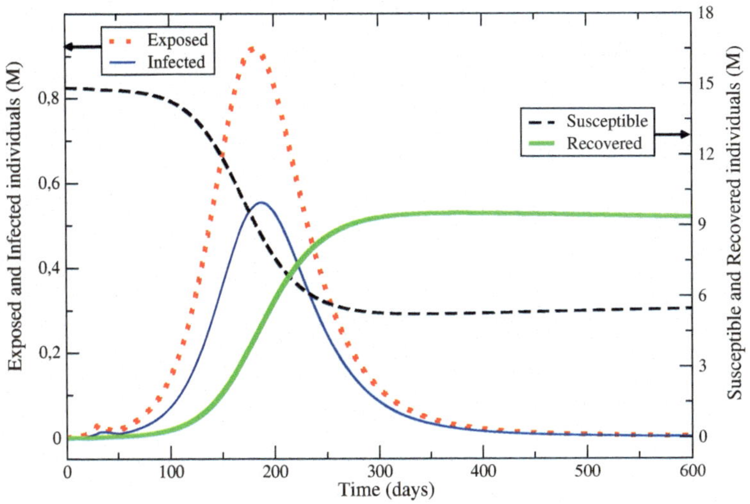

Fig. 9 Number of individuals in all classes (millions) for the SEIR model of fractional order with $\nu = 0.919$

Finally, since the reported number of deceased people could possibly be underestimated due to undeclared cases and delays in the upload of official data, we also consider a case with 30 % more casualties to date (Case 4 in Table 2), giving IFR = 0.254 % and values of the parameters similar to those of Case 1. Besides, the peak occurs almost at the same day of Case 1 (day 187: September 11th, 2020) with 592 thousand infected individuals and 296 casualties. This peak of casualties and the death toll of 24400 individuals are approximately 30 % higher than those of Case 1.

In the following, we compare the behavior of all classes for the different orders of the fractional derivative used in this analysis, i.e., $\nu = 1, 0.919$ and 0.812. Figure 11 displays the number of infected individuals, where there is a delay and decrease of the peak values as the order of the fractional derivative decreases. This behavior is consistent with that observed in Fig. 3. Figure 12 shows an increase in the number of casualties by decreasing the order of the fractional derivative, with a 47 % increase between $\nu = 1$ and $\nu = 0.812$. Moreover, it can be seen that the curves stabilize at later times as the fractional order decreases. Finally, Figs. 13 and 14 exhibit the estimated recovered and susceptible individuals for the three values of ν. Recovered individuals increase and, consequently, susceptible individuals decrease as the order of fractional derivative increases. The curves exhibit asymptotic values at later times as ν decreases, and the lower the value of ν the later individuals recover from the virus infection. Note that the general trends of Figs. 11, 12, 13 and 14 are similar to those of the figures in Sect. 4.1, in spite of the fact that parameters obtained from the adjustment are different for the three cases.

In the four cases described above, we consider that the initial number of infected individuals is $I(0) = 100$. Nevertheless, we tested other values: if $I(0)$ belongs to the interval [10, 150] a reasonable adjustment is obtained, with similar values to those

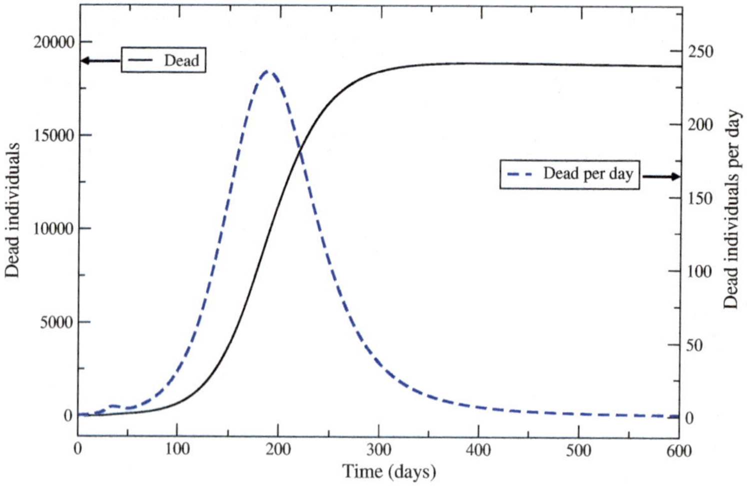

Fig. 10 Total number of deaths and deaths per day for the SEIR model of fractional order with $\nu = 0.919$

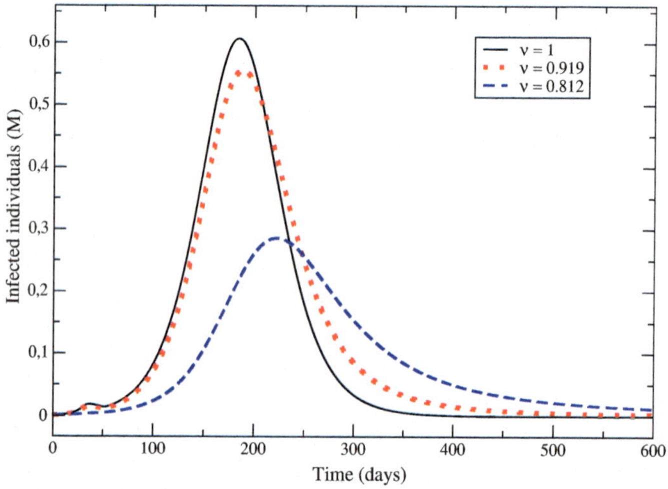

Fig. 11 Infected individuals for the SEIR model of fractional orders $\nu = 1, 0.919$ and 0.812

shown in Table 2 and a slight delay on the infected individuals peak as $I(0)$ decreases. Outside this interval, the fit is poor and the results have no physical meaning.

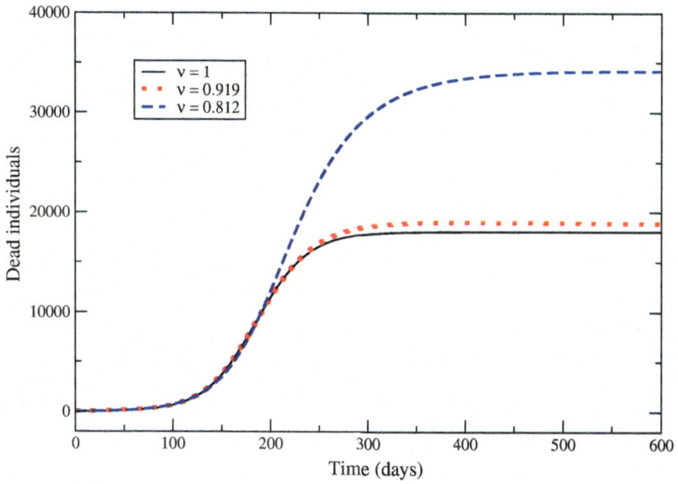

Fig. 12 Dead individuals for the SEIR model of fractional orders $\nu = 1, 0.919$ and 0.812

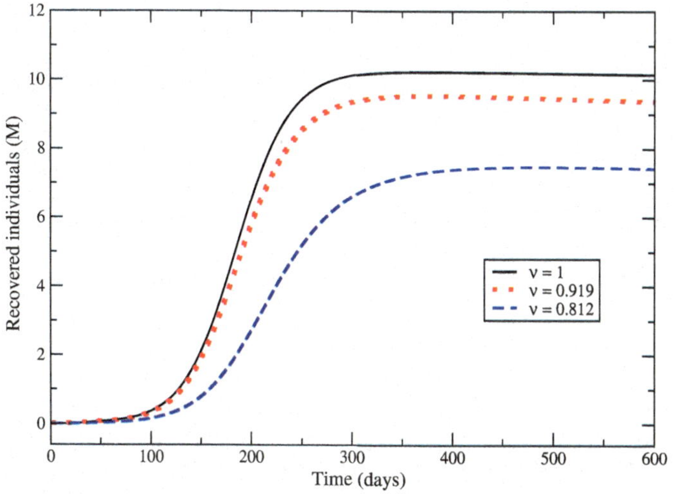

Fig. 13 Recovered individuals for the SEIR model of fractional orders $\nu = 1, 0.919$ and 0.812

5 Conclusions

We use a fractional SEIR (Susceptible, Exposed, Infected, Recovered) diffusion model to analyze the evolution of the Covid-19 epidemic in Argentina, particularly in the Region Metropolitana de Buenos Aires (RMBA), where a significant number of the population is concentrated.

We solve the SEIR system of fractional order $\nu, 0 < \nu < 1$ and the classical ($\nu = 1$) SEIR model by using a time-explicit Gorenflo-Mainardi-Moretti-Paradisi

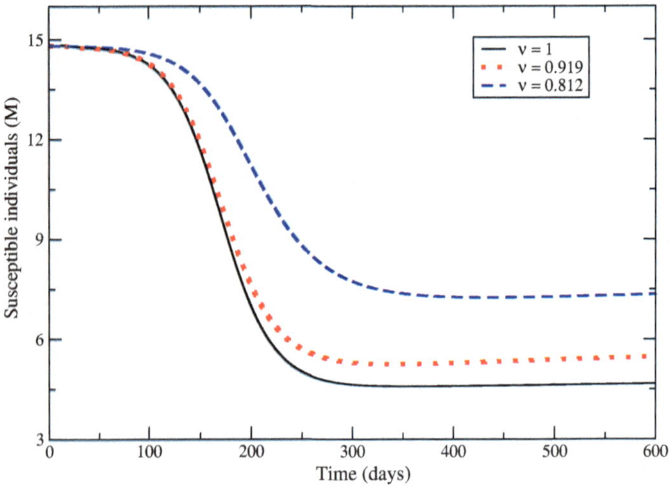

Fig. 14 Susceptible individuals for the SEIR model of fractional orders $\nu = 1, 0.919$ and 0.812

(GMMP) method. To validate this method, the results were cross-checked with those of the time-explicit fractional Adams-Bashford-Moulton (ABM) method, obtaining an excellent agreement between the two schemes.

Assuming that the birth and death rates are balanced, the parameters that characterize the model are the infection and incubation periods, the probability of disease transmission per contact, the fatality rate and the initial number of exposed individuals. These parameters and the orderν of the fractional derivative are estimated by fitting the number of casualties officially reported. This inverse problem is solved by using a quasi-Newton technique for non-linear least-squares problem with the Broyden-Fletcher-Goldfarb-Shanno formula.

In all the simulations we used three lockdown parameters (denoted by β), associated with the different measures taken by the government during the evolution of the epidemic. One important conclusion related with this time-dependent parameter is that both the fractional GMMP and ABM algorithms need to be fully initialized from the beginning in order to obtain correct results.

Different cases have been analyzed since the inverse problem has an infinite number of solutions. We observe a similar behavior in all the cases, with a fatality rate IFR varying in the range, $[0.175, 0.444]$. After the 50th day of lockdown, it is observed a continuous increase in casualties due to the relaxation of the preventive social isolation and community circulation of the virus.

The numerical simulations in RMBA show that when the order of the fractional derivative decreases, i.e., higher subdiffusion of the virus, the duration of the epidemic is extended, and the peak of infected individuals and number of casualties increase. Furthermore, the classical SEIR model yield a smaller number of casualties and infected individuals with associated peaks located at earliest times as compared with those of the fractional-order cases.

Appendix

The Adams-Bashford-Moulton explicit scheme for the fractional order SEIR equations is formulated as follows [15]

Predictor

$$S^p_{n+1} = ((n+1)\Delta t)S_0 + \sum_{j=0}^{n} b_{j,n+1)} f_1^{\nu}(S_j, E_j, I_j, R_j) \tag{13}$$

$$E^p_{n+1} = ((n+1)\Delta t)E_0 + \sum_{j=0}^{n} b_{j,n+1)} f_2^{\nu}(S_j, E_j, I_j, R_j)$$

$$I^p_{n+1} = ((n+1)\Delta t)I_0 + \sum_{j=0}^{n} b_{j,n+1)} f_3^{\nu}(S_j, E_j, I_j, R_j)$$

$$E^p_{n+1} = ((n+1)\Delta t)R_0 + \sum_{j=0}^{n} b_{j,n+1)} f_4^{\nu}(S_j, E_j, I_j, R_j)$$

$$N^p_{n+1} = S^p_{n+1} + E^p_{n+1} + R^p_{n+1} + I^p_{n+1}.$$

Corrector

$$S_{n+1} = ((n+1)\Delta t)S_0 + \sum_{j=0}^{n} a_{j,n+1} f_1^{\nu}(S^p_{n+1}, E^p_{n+1}, I^p_{n+1}, R^p_{n+1}) \tag{14}$$

$$E_{n+1} = ((n+1)\Delta t)E_0 + \sum_{j=0}^{n} a_{j,n+1} f_2^{\nu}(S^p_{n+1}, E^p_{n+1}, I^p_{n+1}, R^p_{n+1})$$

$$I_{n+1} = ((n+1)\Delta t)I_0 + \sum_{j=0}^{n} a_{j,n+1} f_3^{\nu}(S^p_{n+1}, E^p_{n+1}, I^p_{n+1}, R^p_{n+1})$$

$$R_{n+1} = ((n+1)\Delta t)R_0 + \sum_{j=0}^{n} a_{j,n+1} f_4^{\nu}(S^p_{n+1}, E^p_{n+1}, I^p_{n+1}, R^p_{n+1})$$

$$N_{n+1} = S_{n+1} + E_{n+1} + R_{n+1} + I_{n+1}.$$

In (13)-(14) the coefficients $b_{j,n+1}, a_{j,n+1}$ are

$$b_{j,n+1} = \frac{1}{\Gamma(1+\nu}\left[(n-j+1)^{\nu} - (n-j)^{\nu}\right]$$

$$a_{j,n+1} = \frac{1}{\Gamma(2+\nu)} = \begin{cases} (n)^{\nu+1} - (n-\nu)(n+1)^{\nu}, & j = 0, \\ (n-j+2)^{\nu+1} + (n-j)^{\nu+1} - 2(n-j+1)^{\nu+1}, & 1 \le j \le n-1 \\ 1, & j = n+1. \end{cases}$$

Concerning the error of the numerical scheme ABM, Abdullah et al. [18] give a bound in terms of the time step size Δt. On the other hand, Li and Zeng [15] and Li et al. [27] show that the fractional forward Euler and ABM methods are stable and convergent of order one in Δt.

References

1. Carcione, J.M., Santos, J.E., Bagaini, C., Ba, J.: A simulation of a COVID-19 epidemic based on a deterministic SEIR model. Front. Public Health (2020). https://doi.org/10.3389/fpibh.2020.00230, abs:2004.035752004
2. Santos, J.E., Carcione, J.M., Savioli, G.B., Gauzellino, P.M., Ravecca, A., Moras, A.: A numerical simulation of the COVID-19 epidemic in Argentina using the SEIR model. Lat. Am. Appl. Res. (2020) (submitted to)
3. Caputo, M.: Linear models of dissipation whose Q is almost frequency independent, Part II. Geophys. J. R. Astr. Soc. **13**, 529–539 (1967) [Reprinted in Fract. Calc. Appl. Anal. 11, 4–14 (2008)]
4. Mainardi, F.: The fundamental solutions for the fractional diffusion-wave equation. Appl. Math. Lett. **9**, 23–28 (1996)
5. Carcione, J.M., Cavallini, F., Mainardi, F., Hanyga, A.: Time-domain seismic modeling of constant Q-wave propagation using fractional derivative. Pure Appl. Geophys. **159**, 1719–1736 (2002)
6. Mainardi, F.: Fractional Calculus and Waves in Linear Viscoelasticity. Imperial College Press, London (2010)
7. Caputo, M., Carcione, J.M., Cavallini, F.: Wave simulation in biological media based on the Kelvin-Voigt fractional-derivative stress-strain relation. Ultrasound Med. Biol. **37**(6), 996–1004 (2011)
8. Caputo, M., Carcione, J.M.: Hysteresis cycles and fatigue criteria using anelastic models based on fractional derivatives. Rheologica Acta **50**, 107–115 (2011)
9. Kochubei, A.N.: General fractional calculus evolution equations and renewal processes. Integral Equ. Fract. Order Theory **71**, 585–600 (2011)
10. Carcione, J.M., Mainardi, F.: On the relation between sources and initial conditions for the wave and diffusion equations. Comput. Math. Appl. **73**, 906–913 (2017)
11. Scherer, R., Kalla, S.L., Tang, Y., Huang, J.: The Grünwald-Letnikov method for fractional differential equations. Comput. Math. Appl. **62**, 902–917 (2011)
12. Ciesielski, M., Leszczynski, J.: Proceedings of the 15th Conference on Computer Methods in Mechanics (Wisla, Polonia) (2003) arXiv:math-ph/0309007v1
13. Zeb, A., Khan, M., Zaman, G., Momani, S., Ertürk, V.S.: Comparison of numerical methods of the SEIR epidemic model of fractional order. Z. Naturforsch. **69**, 81–89 (2014). https://doi.org/10.5560/ZNA.2013-0073
14. Podlubny, I.: Fractional Differential Equations. Academic Press, San Diego (1999)
15. Li, C., Zeng, F.: Numerical Methods for Fractional Calculus. CRC Press, Taylo & Francis Group, Boca Raton (2015)
16. Gorenflo, R., Mainardi, F., Moretti, D., Paradisi, P.: Time fractional diffusion: a discrete random walk approach. Nonlinear Dyn. **29**, 129–143 (2002)
17. Gorenflo, R., Abdel-Rehim, E.A.: Convergence of the Grünwald-Letnikov scheme for time-fractional diffusion. J. Comput. Appl. Math **205**, 871–981 (2007)
18. Abdullah, F.A., Liu, F., Burrage, P., Burrage, K., Li, T.: Novel analytical and numerical techniques for fractional temporal SEIR measles model. Numer. Algor. **79**, 19–40 (2018). https://doi.org/10.1007/s11075-017-0426-6
19. Murillo, J.Q., Bravo Yuste, S.: On three explicit difference schemes for fractional diffusion and diffusion-wave equations. Phys. Scripta T136 014025, 6 (2000)

20. Gill, P., Murray, W., Wright, M.: Practical Optimization. Academic Press, London (1981)
21. De la Sen, M., Ibeas, A., Alonso-Quesada, S., Nistal, R.: On a new epidemic model with asymptomatic and dead-infective subpopulations with feedback controls useful for Ebola disease. Discrete Dyn. Nature Soc. (2017) https://doi.org/10.1155/2017/4232971
22. Al-Sheikh, S.: Modeling and analysis of an SEIR epidemic model with a limited resource for treatment. Glob. J. Sci. Front. Res. Math. Decis. Sci. **12**(14) (2012)
23. Zhang, L.J., Li, Y., Ren, Q., Huo, Z.: Global dynamics of an SEIRS epidemic model with constant immigration and immunity. WSEAS Trans. Math. **12**, 630–640 (2013)
24. Chowell, G., Fenimore, P.W., Castillo-Garsow, M.A., Castillo-Chavez, C.: SARS outbreak in Ontario, Hong Kong and Singapore: the role of diagnosis and isolation as a control mechanism. J. Theor. Biol. **224**, 1–8 (2003)
25. González-Parra, G., Arenas, A.J., Chen-Charpentier, B.M.: A fractional order epidemic model for the simulation of outbreaks of influenza A(H1N1). Math. Meth. Appl. Sci. **37**, 2218–2226 (2014)
26. Savioli, G.B., Bidner, M.S.: Comparison of optimization techniques for automatic history matching. J. Pet. Sci. Eng. **12**(1), 25–35 (1994)
27. Li, C.P., Zhao, Z.G., Chen, Y.Q.: Numerical approximation of nonlinear fractional differential equations with subdiffusion and superdiffusion. Comput. Math. Appl. **62**, 855–875 (2011)

Modeling Effectiveness of Partial Lockdown in Breaking Covid-19 Transmission Chain in Malaysia

Su Yean Teh, Hock Lye Koh, and Katia S. Joo

Abstract The Coronavirus Disease 2019 (Covid-19) was first reported in Wuhan, China in early December 2019. On 11 March 2020, the World Health Organization declared Covid-19 a worldwide pandemic. Within six months, this highly infectious disease has rapidly spread over 200 countries in six continents, infecting more than 12 million and killing more than 560,000. Malaysia recorded as of July 12, a total of 8718 persons tested positive for Covid-19, with 122 deaths, and 8519 fully recovered, out of a population of 32.4 million. Unprecedented public health and socio-economic policy have been formulated by the Malaysian government to control the catastrophic pandemic spread and to resolve deep socio-economic disruptions and uncertainties. For Malaysia, a major pandemic control policy measure is the Movement Control Order (MCO) over a period of 24 weeks from March 18 to August 31, 2020. This MCO decision is facilitated by the use of epidemiology models such as SIR (Susceptible-Infected-Recovered) model. This MCO has resulted in major socio-economic disruptions and uncertainty. To overcome these immense economic disruptions and uncertainty, several major economic stimulation packages amounting to RM 250 billion, equivalent to 17% of Malaysia 2019 GDP, are formulated to revitalize Malaysia's economy. Epidemiology models are widely used worldwide to formulate socially acceptable policy measures for breaking the infection transmission chain and for enhancing economic resilience. Since the start of Covid-19 outbreak in Malaysia, we use and continuously calibrate the existing SIR-based in-house FluSiM@USM model to examine the effectiveness of various

S. Y. Teh (✉)
School of Mathematical Sciences, Universiti Sains Malaysia, 11800 USM, Pulau Pinang, Malaysia
e-mail: syteh@usm.my

H. L. Koh
Jeffrey Sachs Center on Sustainable Development, Sunway University, Jalan Universiti, 47500 Bandar Sunway, Selangor, Malaysia
e-mail: hocklyek@sunway.edu.my

K. S. Joo
School of International and Public Affairs (SIPA), Columbia University, New York, NY 10027, USA
e-mail: ksj2126@columbia.edu

P. Agarwal et al. (eds.), *Analysis of Infectious Disease Problems (Covid-19) and Their Global Impact*, Infosys Science Foundation Series,
https://doi.org/10.1007/978-981-16-2450-6_26

intervention and mitigation measures in reducing the pandemic burden, the result of which is presented in this chapter. Our epidemic model analysis suggests that MCO has managed to effectively control the spread of Covid-19 by significantly reducing the effective reproduction number R_t, from 3.5 to 0.2 over a period of 12 weeks. The constantly evolving knowledge of Covid-19 transmission dynamics requires regular data updates and model enhancements. Collaboration and communication between modelers and public health authorities are essential to formulating and supporting complex public health policy decision. This chapter highlights the effectiveness of MCO in controlling Covid-19 spread. It discusses major socio-economic disruptions and uncertainties caused by Covid-19 and MCO to the Malaysian and world economy. Guided by the Sendai Framework for Disaster Risk Reduction developed by the United Nations, this chapter will focus the deliberation on the trade-offs between saving life and saving the economy.

Keywords Covid-19 · SIR model · Pandemic control · Socio-economic impacts

1 Introduction

The Coronavirus Disease 2019 (Covid-19) first emerged in Wuhan city, China in early December 2019. On January 23, 2020, China imposed a total lockdown in Wuhan and other cities in Hubei to take effect through April 8 for a total of 76 days. The lockdown involved suspension of all public transport, and imposed strict control of movement within and out of the city of 11 million. The lockdown appeared to have halted the spread of Covid-19 in Wuhan and China. By mid-February 2020, it was obvious from model simulations that Covid-19 would soon become a global pandemic. To confront the pandemic, Malaysian government was urged to be adequately prepared in advance, including the preparation for lockdown to break the infection transmission chain [1]. On March 11, 2020, the World Health Organization declared Covid-19 a worldwide pandemic. On 16 March 2020 the Malaysian Prime Minister announced the first two-week Movement Control Order (MCO) to take effect beginning 18 March 2020 to contain the spread of Covid-19 [2]. Within six months, the highly infectious disease has rapidly spread over 200 countries in six continents. By 12 July 2020, the total global confirmed cases have exceeded 12 million cases, with deaths of over 560,000. The United States alone contributed a total of 3,163,581 infections, resulting in 133,486 deaths [3].

In this introductory section, a brief description of the timeline of Covid-19 control measures in Malaysia, known locally as the Movement Control Order (MCO), is presented. This timeline allows model simulations to be performed to evaluate and improve on the effectiveness of MCO in containing Covid-19. The in-house FluSiM@USM model simulations performed throughout March-July 2020 indicated that MCO is effective in containing community transmission. Further, model simulations indicate that MCO is absolutely necessary over an extended duration of 12 weeks to reduce the effective reproduction number R_t from 3.5 to around 0.2 in order to prevent the resurgence of a second wave [4, 5].

1.1 MCO Timeline in Malaysia

Initiated by its first case on January 25, Covid-19 cases in Malaysia increased gradually to a total of 22 by February 26. The subsequent big wave was triggered by infections linked to the clusters who recently travelled overseas, and to those who attended a tabligh gathering from Feb 27 to March 1 at Masjid Jamek Sri Petaling. The religious event was attended by about 16,000 people including 1,500 foreigners. On March 15, a staggering 190 new cases was reported, triggering the imposition of a nationwide Movement Control Order (MCO) to take effect from March 18 to March 31. Throughout the various MCOs, contact tracing to find and contain infected persons has been a key containment strategy, following the guideline stipulated by CDC [6]. During MCO1, schools, universities and non-essential businesses were closed, while essential businesses such as banks, petrol stations and non-sit-in restaurants were allowed within reduced hours. Only one person per family was allowed to leave home to get daily essentials. Inter-state or inter-district travels were banned. The number of infections continued to increase throughout MCO1, reaching a total of 2,320 cases by March 28. The short two-week MCO1 had only limited impact because the infections were already prevalent among certain clusters spread over large areas. Hence, MCO1 was extended to MCO2 from April 1 to April 14, with stricter restrictions imposed. A 10-km movement restriction was imposed to limit the movement of people to within 10 km radius. Districts were categorized by four color codes: Green, Yellow, Orange and Red according to the number of active cases respectively (0, 1–20, 21–40, more than 40). In red districts, very strict enhanced MCO (EMCO) was enforced to stop people from leaving or entering. The infection curve began to show preliminary signs of flattening during MCO2, with reduction in R_t from 3.5 to slightly more than 1.0 (Figs. 1 and 2). However, the persistent 3-digit daily new cases throughout MCO2 prompted the extension of MCO2 to MCO3, spanning from April 15 to 28, with tighter control measures imposed. During this period of MCO3 certain concern arose regarding undetected Covid-19 infections particularly among high-risk groups, such as the elderly in old folk's homes and foreign migrant workers living in cramped and unhygienic dormitories. This concern was further highlighted by the persistent large surges of new cases in Singapore, exceeding 1000 daily cases among migrant workers living in crowded quarters. The lesson learned is that populations living in close contact with each other under unhygienic environment such as migrant workers living in cramped dormitories can indeed be an efficient source of Covid-19 transmission. The strict EMCO imposed on the identified clusters consisting of migrant workers helped to contain the spread of Covid-19 in Malaysia and Singapore. However, issues regarding humanitarian treatment of migrant workers remain unresolved. This is a critical concern as there are close to five million foreign workers in Malaysia.

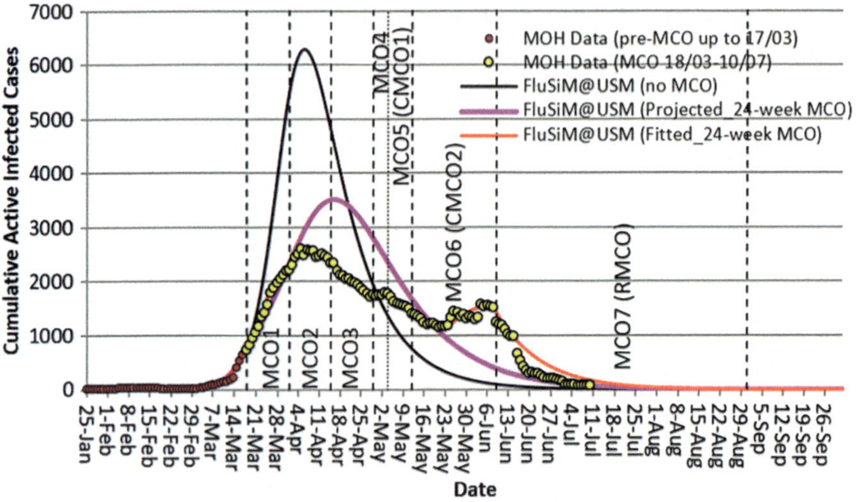

Fig. 1 FluSiM@USM projected cumulative active cases (black line) based on MOH data up to March 17, 2020 without partial lockdown enforce-ment. FluSiM@USM projected a flattened epidemic curve (pink line) as a result of 24-week partial lockdown using a reduced simulated using a constant contact rate $\beta = 0.19\,\text{day}^{-1}$. To estimate R_t, FluSiM@USM result (red line) is fitted to MOH data up July 10, 2020 using a piecewise-linear $\beta(t) \in [0.1, 0.22]$ within the various MCO periods. The horizontal axis is in weekly interval

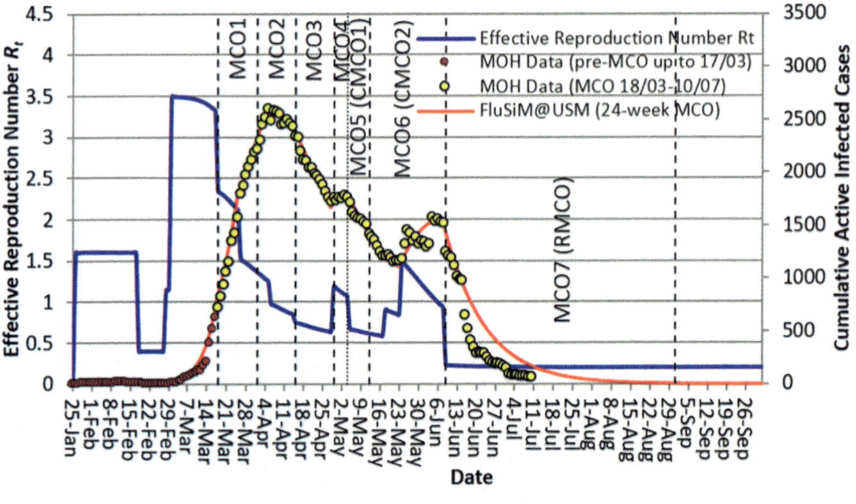

Fig. 2 Estimated R_t based on the fitting of FluSiM@USM result to MOH data up July 10, 2020

1.2 Economic Repercussions of MCOs

With the announcement of MCO4 (Apr 29 to May 12), emotional exhaustion and economic anxiety had started to set in, particularly among low-income workers. As nations close borders and enforce lockdowns, global trade could potentially shrink by USD1.7 trillion to USD2.6 trillion or about 1.9 to 2.9% of global GDP [7]. Output losses could reach between USD5.8 trillion to USD8.8 trillion (6.4 to 9.7% of global GDP) under a 3 to 6-month containment scenario [7]. The impact on the Malaysian economy is profound. The pandemic may cause a contraction of 2.6 to 6.9% of Malaysia 2020 GDP [8]. With many non-essential businesses forced to close, layoffs are inevitable, resulting in 1 to 2 million unemployment, out of which 68% are low-skill jobs [8]. Small and medium enterprises (SMEs) provide jobs to 66% of the nation's workforce, and contribute to 40% of GDP. For SMEs, crowded working spaces and limited online business platforms are not conducive to working remotely and practising social distancing. SMEs are particularly vulnerable to the malaise caused by the MCOs; hence assisting SMEs to enhance their resilience is crucial to the nation's economy recovery. About five million foreign migrant workers fill employment gaps available in the low and middle skilled job sectors in Malaysia [9] Their well-being is intimately connected to the overall health and wealth of the nation. As part of the MCO containment strategy, all migrants will be provided with free testing and treatment for Covid-19 during the MCOs [10].

1.3 Further Relaxations After MCO4

During the MCO4, the R_t values computed by FluSiM@USM dropped from 3.5 to slightly below 1.0, but it was still significantly above 0.0. It was still not advisable to abruptly abandon MCO altogether. Such an approach might trigger an unpredictable resurgence of infections, given the uncertainty over infection clusters that lurk around the corners. The trade-off between socio-economic recovery and epidemic control dominated the debate over the continuation and protocol beyond MCO4. To stimulate short-term and medium-term economic growth, the Government initiated the economic stimulation measures and initiatives [2]. A major goal is to encourage confidence of the people and to empower the investors on the Malaysian economy resilience. The downward trend of daily new cases, now mostly of lower 2-digit figures, throughout MCO4 empowered the government decision to further relax some MCO4 measures. The relaxation of MCO4 is critical to stimulating economic recovery and promoting social equity. Interstate travel was allowed to permit workers trapped in their respective hometowns to return to the city where they work. About 100,000 students from public and private universities were permitted to return home, from their university hostels where they had been stranded since MCO1. The degree of relaxation of the standard operating procedures (SOPs) of MCO in each color-coded district would depend on the infection status of the respective district, be it green, yellow or red. This approach of flexible and humanitarian pandemic containment MCO is commendable. It helps to narrow the conflict between saving life and saving the economy, while leaving no one behind. It conforms to basic principles enshrined in the Sendai Framework for Disaster Risk Reduction (SFDRR) developed by the United Nations [11, 12]. However, the persistent global sharp surges in Covid-19 in the US, Brazil and India, mandates vigilance to prevent a local resurgence from hidden infection clusters originating from overseas. The time is ripe to cautiously move on to the economic recovery phase with implementation of a business-friendly recovery MCO to stimulate social economic growths.

2 Business-Friendly Recovery MCO

To promote economic recovery, MCO4 was replaced by a more business friendly form of MCO, known as the conditional movement control order (CMCO). This CMCO1 or MCO5 (May 4 to 12), witnessed the re-opening of almost all sectors of the economy and businesses, albeit still under strict control conditions. Individual travel between states was allowed with police permit. CMCO1 was extended to CMCO2 or MCO6 with further business-friendly restrictions from May 13 to June 9. At this point, only four districts across the country were still classified as red zones. It is important to avoid high risk and still banned activities, such as visiting bars and night clubs, and to remain vigilant to potential infection clusters. Model simulations by FluSiM@USM will continue to provide a numerical approach to track the infection progress via the R_t values, and to be readily adaptable to any sudden resurgence of new infections. On June 10, the Recovery Movement Control Order (RMCO) was implemented to take effect until Aug 31 to further spur economic growths while saving life.

2.1 Spurring Economy Growth and Saving Life

The variations in MCO protocols has gradually evolved over time in the effort to maintain a delicate balance between spurring economy growth and saving life. The resurgence of renewed infections in Melbourne on July 7, however, would serve a potent reminder regarding the constant need to be vigilant during the RMCO. Abrupt reversal of RMCO containment policy might be possible. The abrupt resurgence of Covid-19 cases in Melbourne on July 7 prompted the Victoria state government to reimpose a six-week second lockdown starting from July 10. Abrupt resurgence after lifting of lockdown is not an isolated event as many resurgences have emerged in many other cities, such as in Hong Kong, Miami, Seoul and Tokyo. For the months of June to July, many US states including Arizona, Florida, Georgia, Louisiana and Texas recorded alarming resurgences in renewed infections. Seven US states reported record increases in cases on July 10: Alaska, Georgia, Louisiana, Montana, Ohio,

Utah and Wisconsin. These continuing resurgences are cogent reminder to maintain vigilant, particularly in cities where R_t hovers at levels around or above 1.0.

Sporadic spikes in Malaysian Covid-19 new cases associated with localized clusters regularly emerged during the MCOs. It is essential to document these localized clusters in order to properly assess the effectiveness and adaptation of the various forms of MCOs. Amongst these clusters, the Sri Petaling tabligh cluster remained the largest cluster with five generations of infection recorded. As of June 22, out of 42,002 samples taken from the Sri Petaling tabligh cluster, 3375 were tested positive, representing an infection rate of 8%. Fortunately, this cluster infection has been eliminated with proper medical treatment and effective infection containment. Seventeen weeks after the first confirmed case of the Sri Petaling tabligh cluster, this largest cluster in Malaysia is officially declared to have ended on July 9. With a total of 647 positive cases detected by June 22, the Bukit Jalil Immigration Detention Depot (BJ IDD) cluster was the second-largest Covid-19 cluster in Malaysia. The Pedas cluster with 316 positive cases detected by June 22 was the third-largest Covid-19 cluster in Malaysia. The source of this cluster was an infected local who subsequently spread the infection to the foreign workers at the chicken factory in Negeri Sembilan. The persistence of Covid-19 cases among migrant workers highlights the importance of resolving the humanitarian treatment of crowded accommodation, unsatisfactory practices of personal hygiene and unsanitary living environment among migrant workers. Fortunately, the limited socializing and mixing between Malaysians and these migrant workers prevented the spread of Covid-19 between the two population sectors. It is important to combat the transmission among these migrant workers in humanitarian terms without sidelining and stigmatizing them, following the SFDRR framework guidelines for disaster risk reduction applied to pandemics [1]. After 15 weeks of MCOs, Malaysia has finally achieved a first zero local transmission case on July 1, 2020, prompting the cautious optimism to re-open schools in phases starting July 15, 2020. However, sporadic spikes prevented the infection R_t from quickly levelling down to 0.0 (Fig. 2).

This chapter aims to simulate the evolution of Covid-19 epidemic curve for Malaysia using the SIR model. An important task is to provide an early warning signal to any potential surge of large-scale community transmissions. The epidemic curve is first calibrated with the number of Covid-19 active cases from January 25 up to March 17. The reported number of Covid-19 daily active cases in Malaysia from March 17 to 28 was used to validate the model results. The classical SIR model is able to satisfactorily represent the disease progression in Malaysia from January 25 to July 10, as shown in Fig. 1. Simulations were performed to investigate the effectiveness of the two-week MCO1 (March 18–31), the result of which indicated that the first two-week MCO1 was not sufficient to significantly reduce the spread of Covid-19, due to its short duration and relaxed social and business restrictions. Based on the SIR model simulation, the authors opined early on that the MCOs were absolutely necessary and should be further extended, with more strict restriction rules imposed, to further reduce the infection rate [5]. This chapter documents the mathematical modelling performed to address two critical issues: (1) How effective is this

MCO and (2) What additional mitigation and adaptation measures can be employed to prevent resurgence of infections.

3 Epidemiology Models

An overview of epidemiology models is presented in this section followed by the introduction of FluSiM@USM.

3.1 *Brief Literature Review*

Epidemiology models have been successfully used to track and control the evolution of Covid-19 in China recently [13–15]. The ultimate objective of these modelling studies is to provide a framework for understanding how Covid-19 could spread across the population and for informing local infection control measures and policy. A brief literature review of epidemiological modelling of Covid-19 would provide the scientific basis to formulate an appropriate modelling framework for this study, and to inform current and future pandemic mitigation and adaptation measures and policies in Malaysia. For this, a good knowledge on the transmission dynamics of Covid-19 is essential for focusing on the critical factors that govern the disease spread.

An age-structured SIR model was recently used by Singh and Adikari [16] to study the impact of the most common social distancing measures that have been initiated to contain the epidemic in India. Both morbidity and mortality rates for the Covid-19 infection have significant differences across age-groups, with mortality increasing rapidly among the elderly. An age-structured SIR model was proposed to enable the assessment of age-structured impacts of social distancing measures. However, much is unknown about the true age-specific susceptibility and transmissibility of Covid-19. Hence, such age-structured models with copious number of unknown processes and ill-defined parameters are considered not reliable, as reliable estimates of age-structured contact structures including susceptibility and transmissibility are not available. Because of these shortcomings, the said authors candidly acknowledged the high uncertainties in all the parameters used in their age-structured SIR model. These uncertainties would ultimately translate into uncertainties in parameter estimates and infection forecasts [16]. Further, the asymptomatic component in their model could not be used due to the paucity of data on the prevalence of asymptomatic cases. Their desktop study mainly suggested that prolonged and sustained periods of lockdowns with periodic relaxations are required to substantially reduce the prevalence of cases to levels where individualized social contact tracing and quarantine may become feasible. With $R_0 = 2.10$, their model projected 900 million infections for India, which is equivalent to 69% of India population of 1.3 billion. Such astonishing projection, without any supporting evidence, is truly beyond imagination, given that India currently has less than one million cases.

Wu et al. [15] nowcasted and forecasted the Wuhan outbreak size of Covid-19 back in January 2020 when the reported cases were rising exponentially. Their intention was to provide useful insights for public health planning and control, both domestically and internationally. Their model incorporated an "exposed" compartment into their SEIR model to simulate the epidemic in Wuhan. To account for infections among diverse populations across mega cities, they subsequently extended the model to SEIR-Metapopulation to simulate the epidemics across all major cities in China. The one-month data (31 Dec 2019 to 28 Jan 2020) of internationally-exported cases was used to infer the R_0 using Markov Chain Monte Carlo methods. The inferred R_0 value was used in their SEIR model to simulate the outbreak in Wuhan. Then the number of cases that had been exported from Wuhan to other major cities in mainland China was estimated. The probable course of spread domestically and internationally was forecasted. They assumed similar disease transmissibility as in the initial phase in Wuhan. They then accounted for the potential mitigation impact of the various social and personal non-pharmaceutical interventions that have been progressively and quickly implemented since 23 January 2020. Based on the simulation results, it was inferred that the epidemics were already growing exponentially in multiple major cities of China with a lag time of about 1 to 2 weeks behind the Wuhan outbreak. Their study suggested that other major Chinese cities, which are global transport hubs with huge numbers of both inbound and outbound passengers, were probably sustaining localized outbreaks. Most importantly, the study highlighted that large cities overseas with close transport links to China could become outbreak epicenters, unless substantial public health interventions at both the population and personal levels are implemented immediately. To succeed in containment of the spread of infection, draconian measures that severely restrict population mobility should be seriously and immediately implemented in affected areas. At the same time, strategies were required to drastically reduce within population contact rates through cancellation of mass gatherings, through school closures, and through instituting work-from-home arrangements [17]. Their findings are highly relevant to the implementation of MCO in Malaysia beginning on March 18, 2020. However, several limitations in their study were noted, namely (i) traveling behavior was not affected by disease status and that all infections eventually show symptoms, (ii) estimate of transmissibility and outbreak size was somewhat sensitive to the assumption regarding the zoonotic mechanism that initiated the epidemic at Wuhan, (iii) epidemic forecast was based on inter-city mobility data from 2019 that might not necessarily reflect actual mobility patterns in 2020, and (iv) little was known regarding the seasonality of coronavirus transmission.

To lay a foundation for further modelling studies on the transmission of Covid-19 in Wuhan, China, Lin et al. [13] adopted a Susceptible-Exposed-Infectious-Removed (SEIR) model. The authors demonstrated the different effects of individual reaction and governmental action and estimated the magnitude of these effects. Two additional classes were incorporated into their SEIR framework, i.e. (i) the class D mimicking the public perception of risk regarding the number of severe and critical cases and deaths and (ii) the class C representing the number of cumulative cases (both reported and not reported). In their model, the transmission (contact) rate $\beta(t)$ is given by $\beta(t) = \beta_0(1-\alpha)(1-D/N)^{\kappa}$, which incorporated the impact of governmental action (α), and of the decreasing contacts among individuals responding to the proportion of deaths (D). This model was conceptualized to address the individual reaction (controlled by κ) and governmental action (controlled by α), as well as time-varying reporting rate. The parameters in $\beta(t)$ were largely unknown and hence assumptions and curve fitting were used to estimate them. For example, β_0 is derived by assuming that $R_0 = 2.8$ when $\kappa = 0$. It is noted that Lin et al. [13] reported a delay of 14 days between symptom onset and laboratory confirmation of Covid-19. This is consistent with our modeling findings that there is a noticeable time delay of about 10 days between the reported number of infected individuals and the reported number of recovered individuals [5]. It was also noted that disease transmission from asymptotically infected cases was reported but the contribution of asymptomatic transmission was unclear (presumably small). Their study concluded that both individual reaction and governmental action need to be considered in the model to match the observed data in Wuhan. This observation is clearly reflected in our model study.

The SEIR model was also used by Prem et al. [14] to estimate the effects of physical distancing measures on the progression of the Covid-19 epidemic. Social mixing patterns vary across locations, across households, workplaces, and schools. But these patterns were largely unknown. Their modelling study used synthetic location-specific contact patterns in Wuhan and adapted these to account for school closures, workplace closures, and social distancing in the general community. The SEIR model used was age-structured with the population divided into 16 age classes. The infectious properties of asymptomatic were largely unknown. Hence, the asymptomatic cases were incorporated in the model using the probability coefficient $(1-p)$, indicating the probability of an infected case being asymptomatic. It was further assumed that younger individuals were more likely to be asymptomatic and were less infective. The values of the parameters used in their model were estimated from literature. Consistent with our preliminary findings [4], they reported that sustained social distancing measures will delay the time to peak and reduce the height of the peak, thereby giving healthcare systems more time and better resources to adapt and respond. Their model also suggested that the effects of the physical distancing strategies vary across age categories. The reduction in mixing incidence was the highest among school children and among older individuals and was the lowest among working-age adults. The implication is that schools and universities should remain closed for longer period during the MCO social distancing duration. Premature and sudden lifting of interventions could lead to an earlier secondary peak. This observation provided valuable insights to the implementation of MCO in Malaysia. Hence, relaxation of the social distancing measures should be performed gradually and in stages, based upon the infection curve and the computed R_t. Similarly, staggered return to work should be implemented at the end of the intense control period to prevent resurgence should the disease have a longer duration of infectiousness. Prem et al. [14] admitted limitations to their analysis, including large uncertainties around estimates of R_0 and the duration of infectiousness.

3.2 SIR Model: FluSiM@USM

The brief literature review on Covid-19 transmission modelling outlined in the previous section provides the justification for the selection of the SIR model in this study. The "exposed" compartment is not included in our SIR model because the exposed compartment would entail several unknown parameters. Further, their inclusion is not likely to improve model performance. Complex models contain many unknown processes and often ill-defined parameters, with unreliable estimations, leading to difficulty in interpretation of simulation results. The transmission dynamics of an infectious disease such as the Covid-19 within a population, can be effectively described by a system of differential equations known as the SIR (Susceptible-Infectious-Recovery) epidemic model. In this SIR model, the population is divided into three groups: the susceptible group, denoted by S, the infected group, denoted by I, the recovered group, denoted by R. In the normalized SIR model (1), we use $s = S/N$, $i = I/N, r = R/N$ to denote fraction in each group. For a short period of outbreak time, the total population is constant with $N = 1$. Table 1 lists the definition and unit of the parameters in SIR model.

$$\frac{ds}{dt} = -\beta si\ , \qquad \frac{di}{dt} = \beta si - \gamma i\ , \qquad \frac{dr}{dt} = \gamma i\ . \tag{1}$$

Epidemiology models such as the SIR model can provide the important concept of infection transmission thresholds, such as the basic reproduction number R_0, which is used to determine if the disease can cause an epidemic outbreak. A key issue in epidemiology modelling is to determine what can be done to ensure the outbreak will die out quickly. The most important epidemic threshold is known as the basic reproduction number typically denoted by R_0. For the SIR model in (1), the basic reproduction number R_0 is a ratio between contact rate β and infectious rate γ as shown in (2). The value of R_0 reveals how fast the disease will spread by measuring the expected number of cases generated by one case. For an epidemic to grow, the basic reproduction number R_0 must exceed 1. If R_0 is less than 1, the disease will die out.

$$R_0 = \frac{\beta}{\gamma} = \beta T \tag{2}$$

To assess the effectiveness of intervention measures such as MCO, it is more relevant to estimate the time-dependent variations of this transmission potential of Covid-19, referred to as the effective reproduction number R_t. For this purpose, an in-house simulation model known as FluSiM@USM that solves SIR equations numerically using Runge-Kutta 4 was developed and applied [18]. The number of

Table 1 Definition and unit of the parameters in SIR model (1)

Parameter	Definition	Unit	Value	Source
β	Contact rate	Per day	0.3045	Curve fitting
T	Mean infective period	Day	11.5	Lauer et al. [21]
γ	Rate at which infective individual recovers	Per day	$= 1/T = 0.087$	–
s	Susceptible fraction of population	Dimensionless	–	–
i	Infectious fraction of population	Dimensionless	–	–
r	Recovered fraction of population	Dimensionless	–	–
N	Total population	Dimensionless	1.0	–

confirmed infected cases in Malaysia [19], up to March 17, 2020, was used for calibrating the epidemic curve. Subsequent confirmed cases up to July 10 were used to estimate the time evolution of R_0, also referred to as the effective reproduction number R_t (3) [20].

$$R_t = \frac{\beta s}{\gamma} = R_0 \times s \tag{3}$$

The SIR model simulations indicated that R_t started with 3.5 around March 10 but was reduced gradually to 0.2 around July 10. As indicated in earlier sections. the MCOs were regularly adjusted to achieve two major mutually conflicting goals: (i) To break the Covid-19 transmission chain as quickly as possible by increasing the duration and severity of MCO restrictions and (ii) To maintain good socio-economic activities as much as possible by reducing the duration and severity of MCO restrictions. The estimation of R_t would help guide the decision towards the form of MCO, particularly its duration and severity.

4 Simulation Results

Three important parameters must be estimated, namely R_0, β and γ. This is performed by fitting simulated results from FluSiM@USM to the actual data of confirmed and active Covid-19 cases reported by the Malaysian Ministry of Health (MOH). Based on 181 confirmed cases, Lauer et al. [21] estimated that 95% of them developed symptoms within 5.1 days of infection, while 97.5% developed symptoms within 11.5 days. Therefore, it is reasonable to assume conservatively that the effective infectious period T is 11.5 days, implying $\gamma = 1/T = 0.087$ per day. A good fit of FluSiM@USM simulation result to the MOH data up to July 10, 2020, is shown in Fig. 1. The best fitted epidemic curve is obtained by choosing the calibration parameters: $\gamma = 0.087$ per day, $\beta = 0.3045$ per day and $R_0 = 1.5$ at the onset of the disease on January 25, 2020. For Covid-19, R_0 is largely reportedly between 2.00 and 3.00 [15, 22–24] while some studies reported $R_0 > 3.00$ [25]. FluSiM@USM predicted a higher peak of active cases that would arrive earlier around mid-April if no MCO measures were taken. From March 18, the first day of MCO the number of active cases was tracked and included in Fig. 1 for continuous curve fitting to obtain the estimate of time dependent R_t.

The classical SIR model FluSiM@USM is able to adequately provide insights on the effectiveness of MCOs in reducing the disease progression in Malaysia. As illustrated in Fig. 1, if no MCO measures were taken, FluSiM@USM predicted that the cumulative active infected cases could exceed 6000 cases around mid-April. This large number of active cases would overwhelm the capacity of Malaysian public health system. Subsequent simulation is performed to examine the effectiveness of the 24-week MCOs, namely MCO1 (March 18–31), MCO2 (April 1–14), MCO3 (April 15–28), MCO4 (April 29-May 3), CMCO1/MCO5 (May 4–12), CMCO2/MCO6 (May 13-June 9) and RMCO (June 10-Aug 31). For this purpose, the pre-MCO contact rate $\beta = 0.3045\ d^{-1}$ is reduced to $\beta = 0.19\ d^{-1}$ during the MCO periods. Model projection demonstrated that the MCO is effective in managing to delay the time to peak to around mid of April, with a sharp flattening of the curve (pink line, Fig. 1). This delay in peak time and flattening of curve gave healthcare systems much needed time to prepare and adapt. Further, this simulation allows the estimation of the length of MCO needed for the disease to die off. The simulations performed allow us to address two critical issues: (i) How effective is MCO and (ii) What additional soft mitigation measures can be employed to further reduce the number of infections and to prevent resurgence of infections. FluSiM@USM result is also fitted to the MOH data up to July 10, 2020 (red line, Fig. 1) by varying $\beta(t) \in [0.1, 0.22]$ within the MCO period to allow the estimate of R_t. The estimated value of R_t based upon the current trajectory of the disease is shown in Fig. 2. At the onset of the second wave of Covid-19 in Malaysia, the R_t is estimated to be 3.5. The R_t declined to below 2.5 upon implementation of MCO1 and continued to decline throughout MCO2 and MCO3 to below 1.0 at the end of MCO3. The R_t slightly increased to above 1.0 during the brief period of MCO4 due to the emergence of new clusters, consisting of migrant workers living in crowded and unhygienic accommodations. Throughout MCO5 and MCO6, R_t stayed below 1.0 most of the time, with occasional spike due to cases from migrant clusters. This is not yet the time to abandon the MCO altogether to prevent resurgence. Subsequently during RMCO period R_t consistently maintained at value below 1.0 and ultimately being reduced to 0.2. This suggests that the decision of the Malaysian Government to implement MCO starting March 18 and continue with various forms of MCOs is wise and timely. Public confidence in and adherence to the SOPs imposed by the Government are vital for the success in curbing the spread of Covid-19.

5 Discussion

Epidemiology models are frequently used to forecast epidemic progression and to investigate the effectiveness of intervention strategies. Subject to unpredictable human social behavior during a pandemic, detailed forecasts are unlikely due to the evolving complexity and uncertainty in the dynamics of pandemic transmission. However, the general pattern of a local outbreak can be identified if the behavioral uncertainties can be minimized by the imposition of effective MCOs as in the case in Malaysia. The major goal of the MCO is to maintain a delicate balance between the desire to prevent resurgence of infections and the wish to achieve quick and sustainable socio-economic recovery to prevent massive financial calamity across a wide spectrum of the economy. At the time of the submission of this chapter, MCOs have enabled Malaysia to successfully progress to the stage of epidemic recovery phase, having reduced R_t to around 0.2 from 3.5. It is hopeful that this recovery would be sustainable to allow a predictable and sustained socio-economic rehabilitation. However, we are mindful of potential pitfalls, having witnessed recent resurgences of infections in many cities and nations worldwide, such as Melbourne in Australia, and many major cities in the US, Brazil and India. These resurgences were the immediate repercussion of reopening the economy prematurely in attempts to rehabilitate the economy from potential financial calamity. Tens of millions in the US alone have lost their jobs. More will follow if a second wave was to resurge. Model simulations performed in conjunction with integrated holistic approach may be a useful analytical tool for mitigating and adapting to evolving pandemic scenarios such as resurgence.

5.1 *Resurgence of Infections*

To curb Covid-19 spread, Australia quickly and vigorously enforced travel and movement restrictions early in the coronavirus outbreak compared to most other countries. Slow and lethargic in response, the US has recorded more than three million infections and deaths of more than 133,000, with daily new infection exceeding 64,000 cases. Conversely, Australia has escaped a high number of casualties from the new coronavirus, with just under 8900 infections and 106 deaths as of July 8. Australian states and territories, other than Victoria, have recorded few or zero cases in recent weeks and are continuing to reopen their economies. Australia began to ease its lockdown in May to revive its economy after a significant slowdown in infection rates. However, a flare-up in daily cases beginning July 6 forced the state of Victoria to reimpose stay-at-home restrictions in metropolitan Melbourne and one regional area of the state. On July 8, alarmed by abrupt 191 new infections within 24 h, Melbourne went back into lockdown again for six weeks. Five million residents in Melbourne will have to stay at home for all except essential business for the next six weeks, beginning July 9. Three neighboring Australian states, i.e. Queensland, New South Wales and South Australia have imposed a hard border lockdown with the state of Victoria, of which Melbourne is the capital, after a resurge in infections. The state of Queensland will ban non-residents from Victoria from entering Queensland from July 10. Queensland residents were urged to avoid travelling to Victoria, and they would have to quarantine in a hotel for 14 days at their own expense on their return from Victoria. Similar preventive measures are imposed by New South Wales and South Australia state to close their border with Victoria. There is anecdotal evidence of gross negligence of pandemic prevention measures, such as blatantly inadequate enforcement of quarantine that generated a major source of this abrupt resurgence. Another main source of this resurgence is the lifting of premature lockdowns for a quick economic recovery to prevent certain sectors such as tourism, hospitality and aviation from financial calamity.

5.2 *Recovery from Financial Calamity*

The Covid-19 has caused large financial losses and stresses to many sectors, such as the aviation, tourism, hospitality and retail industry, with abundant examples of business failures and bankruptcy. The biggest low-cost carrier AirAsia Group reported an 804 million-ringgit (USD188 million) first-quarter 2020 (January to March) loss, with no sight of quick recovery. Technically, it is now classified under the PN 17 status, with implied risk of being delisted. AirAsia market conditions deteriorated abruptly beginning in February as the outbreak began to spread rapidly, resulting in collapsed demand for air travel in February and March as domestic and international routes were halted. The Covid-19 crisis has resulted in border closures in AirAsia's key markets including Malaysia, Thailand, Indonesia, the Philippines, China and India. It remains unclear if AirAsia is able to fully recover, as it is generally anticipated that the travel industry will need extraordinary multi-sector coordinated efforts to recover.

Similarly, Singapore Airlines reported on May 14 a net loss of 732 million SGD (USD512 million) in the fourth quarter of the financial year, dragging the whole year performance into the red, its first annual net loss in its 48-year history. The loss was attributed to the plunge in air travel demand. In response, the Singapore Airlines have imposed management pay cuts, voluntary and compulsory no-pay leave schemes, and a shorter work month for ground staff. Due to the sharp decline in flight movements because of the Covid-19 pandemic, terminal operations at Singapore Changi Airport will be consolidated, including the suspension of operations in Terminals 2 and 4 for 18 months. Manpower from the avian industries affected by Covid-19 are re-deployed to take on new roles in the hospitals, as care ambassadors, by providing administrative support and attending to patients, under the close supervision of nursing staff. Another major EU airline Lufthansa will be rescued by the German government with a bailout of nine billion euros (USD9.8 billion). Burdened by high debts and large losses from cancelled flights, Virgin Atlantic Airways and Virgin Australia have entered voluntary administration, the UK's equivalent to Chapter 11 bankruptcy to restructure the airlines. Thai Airways International will submit a rehabilitation plan and an application for restructuring proceedings to a bankruptcy court, the Thai equivalent of the US Chapter 11 bankruptcy rule. Retailers J Crew and JC Penney filed for Chapter 11, to seek bankruptcy protection in the wake of the Covid-19 crisis. Can more sectors and corporations be saved from failures and bankruptcy by a quick return to normal by reopening of the economy? Will premature reopening risk resurgences of new infections? Finding a clear, unequivocal answer to these questions remains a challenge.

6 Conclusion

A key objective in this study is to examine the effectiveness of the Malaysian MCO in breaking the infection transmission chain in Malaysia. The aim of the MCO is to bring the infection basic reproduction number R_0 to 0.0 as soon as possible, in such a manner as not to harm the economy excessively. For the SIR model, the basic reproduction number is given by $\mathrm{R}_0 = \beta T$, where β is the contact rate and T is the mean infective period. While we cannot reduce T, we certainly can and must do everything possible to cut down the contact rate β, by effective implementation of MCO by maintaining good social distancing, by self-isolation of Covid-19 positive persons, by contact tracing and containment of infected persons and by good personal hygiene. In this chapter, we use daily infected cases from January 25 to July 10 provided by MOH to calibrate and validate the FluSiM@USM model. For the first phase between January 25 and March 7, R_t was about 1.6, allowing the infection to grow slowly. But soon after March 8, R_t quickly skyrocketed to 3.5, pushing the infection to grow very quickly with 3-digit new cases daily. Simulation result revealed that two months of MCO is needed to reduce R_t from 3.5 to 1.0. An additional one and a half months of MCOs is required to bring R_t to 0.2, a level considered as safe to vigilantly reopen the economy in stages, with the guarded hope that resurgence would not occur.

In a highly interconnected globalized world, will premature reopening of the economy plunge the world back into another more severe round of pandemic, with potentially more destructive calamity? Will the US degrade into a deep and sustained recession should the current rampant pandemic turn catastrophic as predicted by some prominent epidemiological experts? In the absence of effective vaccines and pharmaceutical treatments, sustained vigilant and social distancing is urgently needed to prevent an escalation of infections in a highly interconnected world. America should lead by providing genuine support to the global coordinated efforts to contain the pandemic by avoidance of risky actions and by demonstrating convincingly good social distancing behavior.

We acknowledge some limitations of this modelling study. Premised upon several assumptions such as homogeneous mixing, the deterministic SIR model is a simplification of reality. Deterministic models do not fully reflect the uncertainty and stochasticity in disease transmission dynamics. Modelers need to fit models to observed data to project the evolution of an epidemic and to estimate key parameters as in the case of FluSiM@USM. Temporal variation in R_0 is adjusted to reflect social adaptations induced by MCOs and to fit evolving pandemic outcomes.

Acknowledgements This study was funded by USM RUI grant #1001/PMATHS/8011018. KHL acknowledges Jeffrey Sachs Center on Sustainable Development of Sunway University for providing a conducive environment to conduct this research.

References

1. Koh, H.L., Fan, A., Chong, K.B.: Malaysia must be ready to confront an epidemic. The Malaysian Insight (2020) Available via The Malaysian Insight. https://www.themalaysianinsight.com/s/220503. Accessed 11 July 2020
2. Md Shah, A.U., Safri S.N.A., Thevadas R., et al.: COVID-19 outbreak in Malaysia: actions taken by the Malaysian government. Int. J. Infect. Dis. **97**, 108–116 (2020)
3. WHO: Coronavirus disease (COVID-19) Situation Report-172. World Health Organization (2020) Available via WHO. https://www.who.int/emergencies/diseases/novel-coronavirus-2019/situation-reports. Accessed 13 July 2020
4. Koh, H.L., Teh, S.Y.: Covid-19 Simulation in Malaysia for Assessing Effectiveness of MCO: Implications on Social Economy. In: Joint 10th ICEII2020 International Conference on Environment and Industrial Innovation, and 7th ICCOE International Conference on Coastal and Ocean Engineering, Nanyang Technological University, Singapore, 22–24 Apr 2020
5. Teh, S.Y., Koh, H.L., Lutfi, A.A.M.: MCO is absolutely necessary: Mathematics of Covid-19. MalaysiaKini (2020) Available via MalaysiaKini. https://www.malaysiakini.com/news/518244. Accessed 11 July 2020
6. CDC: Case investigation and contact tracing: Part of a multipronged approach to fight the COVID-19 pandemic. Centers for Disease Control and Prevention (2020) Available via CDC. https://www.cdc.gov/coronavirus/2019-ncov/php/principles-contact-tracing.html. Accessed 11 July 2020
7. ADB: An updated assessment of the economic impact of COVID-19. In: Asian Development Bank Briefs, No. 133 (2020) Available via Asian Development Bank. https://www.adb.org/sites/default/files/publication/604206/adb-brief-133-updated-economic-impact-covid-19.pdf. Accessed 11 July 2020
8. MIER: The economic impacts of Covid-19. Malaysia Institute of Economic Research (2020) Available via MIER. https://www.mier.org.my/the-economic-impacts-of-covid-19/. Accessed 11 July 2020
9. Lee, H.A., Khor, Y.L.: Counting migrant workers in Malaysia: A needlessly persisting conundrum. In: Perspective of Institute of Southeast Asian Studies (ISEAS), No. 25 (2020) Available via ISEAS. https://www.iseas.edu.sg/images/pdf/ISEAS_Perspective_2018_25@50.pdf. Accessed 11 July 2020
10. Sandanasamy, F., Paavilainen, M., Baruah, N.: COVID-19: Impact on migrant workers and country response in Malaysia. International Labor Organization: Regional Office for Asia and the Pacific (2020) Available via ILO. https://www.ilo.org/asia/publications/issue-briefs/WCMS_741512/lang--en/index.htm. Accessed 11 July 2020

11. UNISDR: Sendai framework on disaster risk reduction 2015-2030. In: United Nations Office for Disaster Risk Reduction, Geneva (2015). Available via UNISDR. https://www.unisdr.org/files/43291_sendaiframeworkfordrren.pdf. Accessed 2 July 2020
12. Koh, H.L., Teh, S.Y.: Disaster risk reduction and resilience through partnership and collaboration. In: Leal Filho, W., et al. (eds.) Encyclopedia of the UN Sustainable Development Goals. Partnerships for the Goals. World Sustainability Series. Springer, Cham (2019)
13. Lin, Q., Zhao, S., Gao, D., et al.: A conceptual model for the outbreak of Coronavirus disease 2019 (COVID-19) in Wuhan, China with individual reaction and governmental action. Int. J. Infect. Dis. **93**, 211–216 (2020)
14. Prem, K., Liu, Y., Russell, T.W., et al.: The effect of control strategies to reduce social mixing on outcomes of the COVID-19 epidemic in Wuhan, China: a modelling study. Lancet Public Health **5**, E261-270 (2020)
15. Wu, J.T., Leung, K., Leung, G.M.: Nowcasting and forecasting the potential domestic and international spread of the 214 2019-nCoV outbreak originating in Wuhan, China: a modelling study. The Lancet **395**, 689–697 (2020)
16. Singh, R., Adikari, R.: Age-structured impact of social distancing on the COVID-19 epidemic in India. e-prints in arXiv (2020). Available via arXiv. https://arxiv.org/pdf/2003.12055.pdf. Accessed 11 July 2020
17. Saidan, M.N., Shbool, M.A., Arabeyyat, O.S., et al.: Estimation of the probable outbreak size of novel coronavirus (COVID-19) in social gathering events and industrial activities. Int. J. Infect. Dis. (2020) https://doi.org/10.1016/j.ijid.2020.06.105
18. Koh, H.L., Teh, S.Y.: FluSiM simulation for Malaysia: towards improved pandemic surveillance. Int. J. Chem. Eng. Appl. **2**, 53–59 (2011)
19. MOH: Situasi semasa pandemic COVID-19 di Malaysia. In: Malaysian Ministry of Health (2020). Available via MOH. http://covid-19.moh.gov.my. Accessed 12 July 2020
20. Susanto, H., Tjahjono, V.R., Hasan, A., et al.: How many can you infect? Simple (and naive) methods of estimating the reproduction number. Commun. Biomath. Sci. **3**, 28–36 (2020)
21. Lauer, S.A., Grantz, K.H., Bi, Q., et al.: The incubation period of Coronavirus disease 2019 (COVID-19) from publicly reported confirmed cases: estimation and application. Ann. Intern. Med. **172**, 577–582 (2020)
22. WHO: Report of the WHO-China Joint Mission on Coronavirus Disease 2019 (COVID-19). World Health Organization (2020) Available via WHO. https://www.who.int/docs/default-source/coronaviruse/who-china-joint-mission-on-covid-19-final-report.pdf. Accessed 11 July 2020
23. Zhang, S., Diao, M., Yu, W., Pei, L., Lin, Z.: Estimation of the reproductive number of novel coronavirus (COVID-19) and the probable outbreak size on the Diamond Princess cruise ship: A data-driven analysis. Int. J. Infect. Dis. **93**, 201–204 (2020)
24. Zhao, S., Ran, J., Musa, S.S., et al.: Preliminary estimation of the basic reproduction number of novel coronavirus (2019-nCoV) in China, from 2019 to 2020: A data-driven analysis in the early phase of the outbreak. Int. J. Infect. Dis. **92**, 214–217 (2020)
25. Liu, Y., Gayle, A.A., Wilder-Smith, A., Rocklöv, J.: The reproductive number of COVID-19 is higher compared to SARS coronavirus. J. Travel Med. **27**, taaa021 (2020)

An Extensive Time Series Analysis of Covid-19 Data Sets on the Indian States

J. V. N. Lakshmi and Vandana Bhagat

Abstract Pandemic influenza coronavirus is causing a great loss to mankind. It is creating a chaos on the global economy. Fight against this unseen enemy is affecting all the sectors of the global economy. Mankind is quivering with fear and scared to do something. This study gives a detailed presentation of the current position of virus escalation in India. Sentiment analytics from Twitter data is evaluated on sentiment, emotions and fear opinions are analyzed in the study. The analysis is on red, orange and green zones in several states of India and also gave a comprehensive interpretation on various phases of lockdown. Confirmed, active, recovered and deceased cases in all states are modeled to predict the increase of number of cases. Textual, geographical and graphical analytics are extensively described in the research study. Time series analysis is broadly elaborated as a case study till July 22, 2020, forecasting the impact of virus on Maharashtra, Kerala, Gujarat, Delhi and Tamil Nadu. This study will favor the administrative system to control the disease spread across the nation.

Keywords Covid-19 · SIR model · Pandemic control · Socio-economic impacts

1 Introduction

The research article focuses on significant critical issues: (1) sentiment analysis indicating the status of Covid-19 in India (2) Twitter data is used of sentiment analysis (3) textual analysis and data visualization of various statewise progress of Covid-19 in India and (4) textual classification by evaluating the association between the various tweets using machine learning techniques. Rapid increase of coronavirus has paved a way for extensive analytics for interpreting the textual information from masses in pandemic situation. Sentiment data from tweets articulates on care, health, vaccine, preventive, masks, recovery, social distancing, agriculture, migration, lock-

J. V. N. Lakshmi (✉)
JAIN (Deemed to be University), Bangalore, India

V. Bhagat
CHRIST (Deemed to be University), Bangalore, India

P. Agarwal et al. (eds.), *Analysis of Infectious Disease Problems (Covid-19) and Their Global Impact*, Infosys Science Foundation Series,
https://doi.org/10.1007/978-981-16-2450-6_27

down, economic, financial, trade and network information. This data emphasizes on swift increase of the virus and also association among the various sectors. World Health Organization (WHO) discusses on handling the situation in pandemic, managing the industry, economy and financial sectors becomes a tedious task for the government to manage.

Natural language processing, data analytics, visualization, artificial intelligence and deep learning are the various tools for analyzing the data in research and development. Tokenization, stemming, frequency, association, classification, categorization and polarity matching are various techniques for exploratory textual analytics. Descriptive, statistical, prescriptive and predictive mechanisms are applied for the current research study. Preventive measures, use of sanitization, wearing masks, vaccine invention, lockdown and hot zones are a frequently used terms from the Twitter analysis. Behavioral study of electronic data, modeling the market trends and mining the outcomes from extracted insights of complex information are typical machine learning applications using textual analytics.

In the current scenario of pandemic Covid-19, sentiment analytics is collected from Twitter data in the first stage of analysis fear sentiment which is visualized in Fig. 1.

Many numbers of open-source communication platforms are rightly available for expressing the opinions, moods, views, positive comments and negative texts with respect to any phenomenon. The text posted in such communication platforms is spontaneously available for textual analytics and performs rapid research on the post available. Experiences, reviews, advertisement and personal associations are playing an important source for research insights. Wide-ranging research study is executed on text analytics gathered from social media data on product reviews, political polls, stock market trend analysis and public emotions.

Fear Lowess curve in Fig. 1 represents the textual sentiment data visualization to analyze the trend of change in people's behavior from the tweets posted in India which were gathered. From January 1, 2020, to June 15, 2020, there is an increasing trend line of tweets posted on the Twitter, as the month on month increase of fear

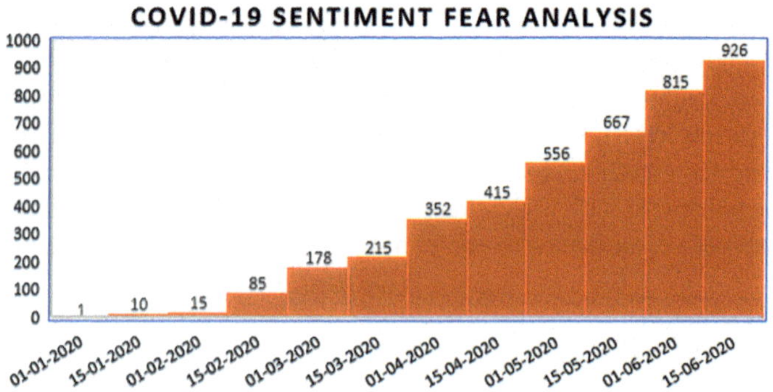

Fig. 1 Fear sentiment analysis in India since January 2020

Fig. 2 Word cloud from tweets collected worldwide

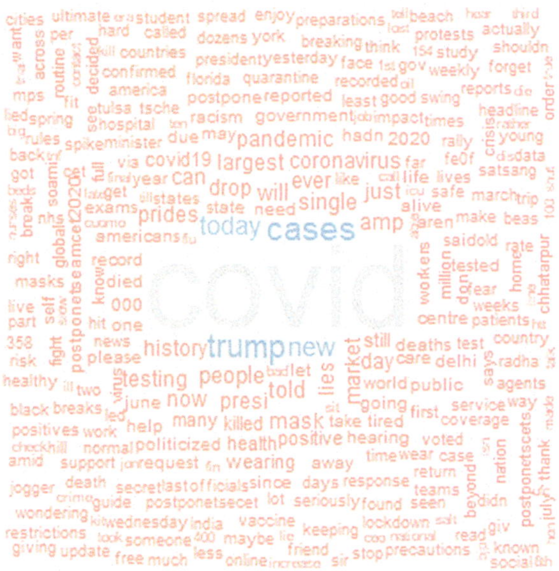

sentiment tweets indicates the threat of fast spread of disease. In the month of January, hardly only a few people are fearful about the dreadful disease as the months pass, and in the month of June the increase of tweets on fear was rapid.

The current research study focuses on spread of coronavirus and from the textual analysis conducted, and the fear building in the mind of people's view is being tracked. Keywords associated with the phenomenon are represented using the data visualization with a communicative word cloud. Word clouds are popular communicators indicating the term frequency iterating over several words. Hence, Fig. 2 represents the word cloud representing the term frequency.

Ten thousand tweets were analyzed for representing, as shown in Fig. 2, word cloud. These tweets were collected from all over the world. The most repetitive terms are Covid, cases, Trump, new, died and many more. Size of the term indicates the frequency of the word from the given tweets. Hence, the association can be easily trailed from the word clouds.

From Fig. 3, tweets are taken by giving the geocode mentioning the latitudinal and longitudinal degrees of India. Postponement of Eamcet exams, vaccine, mask, home, quarantine and test are some of the special terms that can be identified from the word cloud in Fig. 3. The classification of textual data into positive and negative sentiment categories. The analytics also includes sentiment analysis of the textual component of Twitter data.

Exploratory analysis conducted on the tweets reveals exciting truths, complex relations and unknown facts can be drawn. From Table 1, use of certain words from different Indian states has been interpreted. The number of tweets using these words in Telangana, Kerala, Maharashtra, Delhi, Tamil Nadu and Andhra Pradesh narrates a story behind each word frequency. Maharashtra state has higher tweet frequency

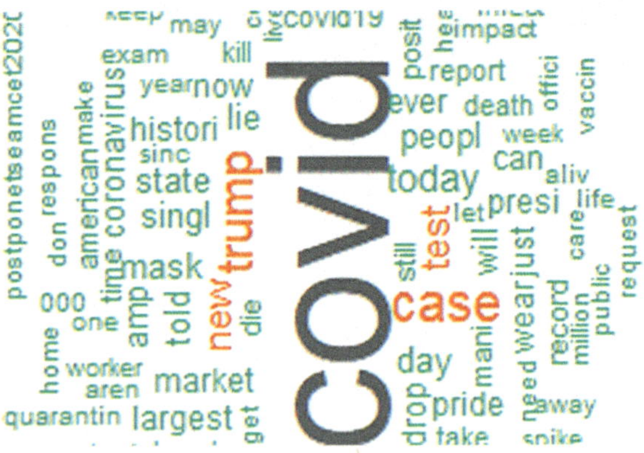

Fig. 3 Word cloud from tweets collected India wide

Table 1 Tweet features summarized by source category

Source	Corona	Flu	Bear	Vaccine	Test
Telangana	14	75	17	17	10
Kerala	78	50	10	5	8
Maharastra	112	90	80	20	87
Delhi	85	74	74	15	21
Tamil Nadu	0	0	54	14	54
Andhra Pradesh	0	0	14	13	4

on corona, flu, vaccine and test word. As the number of cases is more in this state and initially the test was conducted vigorously in this state, hence the frequency was more. Vaccine research is dynamically progressing in IIT Bombay and in IIT Hyderabad, henceforth the table shows the tweets frequency in those states.

2 Literature Review

Exponential raise of Covid-19 cases all over the world created fear. Using the descriptive sentiment analysis and data visualization for textual data is implemented to evaluate the fear sentiment in this paper [1]. The paper also focuses on crucial machine learning techniques for classifying the varied length tweets as a part of textual analytics. The observations from the paper are Naïve Bayes classification method gives 91% accuracy if the tweets are short and 74% accuracy from the logistic regression for shorter length tweets. Both these algorithms are showing poor performance for lengthier tweets.

EM inverse exponential exponential (EMIEE) model is introduced in Table 2 [2] fit data of confirmed Covid-19 cases in Pakistan from March 21 to May 29,

Table 2 EMIEE model analysis on Covid-19 confirmed cases in Pakistan

• Provide a precise estimation for some measures of interest related to Covid-19 cases in Pakistan (mean of cases, probability to have a certain number of cases and so on)
• Compare the repartitions of the number of Covid-19 cases in Pakistan with those in other countries
• Propose an efficient strategy for fitting data on Covid-19 cases in other countries
• Model the distribution of the number of cases for any pandemic with similar features and under a similar environment (with comparable populations, comparable climate, sanitary system, etc.)

2020. The proposed model was compared with the Weibull exponential (WE), Lomax exponential (LE), gamma exponentiated exponential (GaE), beta Weibull (BW), Kumaraswamy exponential (KE), Burr X exponential (BXE), exponentiated exponential (EE), CS transformation of exponential (CE), standard exponential (E), alpha power inverse Weibull (AIW), Gompertz inverse exponential (GomIE), Weibull inverse exponential (WIE), inverse Weibull inverse exponential (IWIE), inverse exponential (IE) and the 'unexponentiated' version of the proposed EMIEE model. The proposed model was answering the questions in Table 2.

An extensive research on outbreak of Covid-19 has been conducted solving six research survey questions to control the spread of disease in this paper [3].

A statistical model is created for analyzing the rapid increase of Covid-19 cases in India. A wide range of research is conducted as a study of reported cases in India till April 22, 2020. Exploratory data analysis implemented examines the impact of coronavirus on daily and weekly basis. A comparative study analyzing other country's pandemic situation and health structures is drafted in article [4] (Table 3).

Social media and communication media play a significant role in such pandemic scenarios. An interactive dashboard CO. ME. T. A. has been introduced to perform the lexical analysis on social and mass media content. Text mining, textual networking, latent topic modeling and sentiment analysis are merged together as a unique feature of the dashboard. CO. ME. T. A. dashboard displays demographics of health, finance, socialization and economic variances of the nation [5].

Topological segmentation of text helps researchers to systematize the knowledge in a vast amount of textual information available right now. While performing the segmentation and analyzing each segment, the whole volume of data gets split into clusters, which simplifies the analysis and understanding of the data.

Susceptible infectious recovered dead (SIDR) model estimates were computed by considering the infection mortality and recovery percentage per day in the first phase of analysis. In the first phase as the asymptomatic courses were higher than the actual, there is a requirement of updating the computations. Hence in the second scenario, 20 times the infected cases and 40 times the recovered cases were taken into consideration. This second scenario was resulting to be average leaving the number of deaths neutral. Therefore, SIRD model was suggested to slow down the outbreak of pandemic in Hubei [6].

Table 3 Research questions on Covid-19 outbreak in India

Research question	Survey queries
RQ1	How has the situation changed in post-lockdown period in India, i.e., what is the outbreak situation after March 22, 2020, in India as compared to pre-lockdown period?
RQ2	What are the short-term predictions for the number of infected cases in India for the next 3–4 weeks based on current situation?
RQ3	Has the lockdown been followed by the Indian citizens after March 22, 2020? Has the social distancing worked for Indian citizens? What are the mobility changes in the various regions of India?
RQ4	Whether the community outbreak spread started in India with the conduct of a religious event in Delhi? How is the outbreak different for citizens related to event and for citizens not related to the event?
RQ5	Which are the prominent clusters which were formed in the last few weeks with respect to Covid-19 outbreak in India? Does network analysis provide influential points in the infected patient network?
RQ6	Whether the national lockdown should be opened after April 14, 2020, in India or should it continue? Are there any partial regions for which lockdown can be removed? Which all essential services should be opened in India after one week under restricted lockdown?

Analyzing the present scenario to handle the spread of the disease plays a keen role. From the available literature, running the regression model on the data resulted in prediction [7]. ARIMA time series models, exponential smoothing technique, pattern mining and network modeling are various models applied in various countries comparing the several parameters with that of India [8]. These models discussed in time series and could not accommodate the parameters associating the patient information.

Mathematical models were developed for trend analysis on the outbreak of Covid-19 in India. A model described the impact of implementing the social distance, wearing masks and avoiding the use of contaminated items. Another research model elaborates the necessary precautions with respect to various ages and gender [9]. Some structures from the literature discussed the entry of foreign national's impact in the spread of the disease. Death rate and recovery rate are analyzed in comparison with many countries based on the medical and infrastructural resources [10].

With respect to vaccine, all over the world, many countries are striving hard to for its invention [11]. China, USA, Italy, Russia and India scientists are involved in generating a hardcore antidote to control the spread of disease [12]. A research model also described the effect of low immunity is the initial cause of infection and its various with respect to age groups [13].

A network model was used to observe the other peculiar clusters formed and also predicts the confirmed cases in a nation [14]. The model considered foreign nationals coming to India. In another research paper, analysis was conducted on medical practitioners, laboratories, testing equipment and infrastructure for the increase of cases in various countries [15]. Based on the resource availability, the required arrangements are taken care.

In another paper by Lixiang analyses, the existing data of Hubei epidemic situation, corresponding model implemented and the simulation carried out is illustrated in detail. The main factors affecting the spread of Covid-19, such as the number of basic regenerations, the incubation period and the average number of days of cure were analyzed under this research. Predicting the evolution trend of the existing epidemic data and found that imposing controls would have important impact on the epidemic. In addition, according to the existing data abroad, strong predictions of the epidemic development trends in South Korea, Italy and Iran, pointing out the possible outbreaks and the corresponding control time and tracing the earliest transmission dates of countries, were described in this article [16].

A research on quarantine facilities, equipment, medical resources and health workers is to monitor the patients in various regions [17]. Accommodating massive groups in quarantine and providing all the services is again a challenging task. Hospital beds are not sufficient for the large groups. Hence, area wise quarantine locations are identified [18]. Government schools, colleges and private buildings are used as quarantine locations by government [19].

From Table 4, it is evident that available facilities such as physicians, beds and health expenditure are comparatively very low per 1000 persons. GDP and per capita are considerably minimum in comparison with other neighboring countries. In terms of poverty lines, individual health expenditure is remarked all citizens cannot afford medical facilities and government hospitals are not equipped with the required facilities and physicians to [20].

Throughout the world, researchers have developed mathematical models to reveal the spread of disease and analyzed country wise report discussing on the country's readiness in tackling the virus in order to get a down trend line. Research needs to be reviewed and continuously monitored to examine the phases of the virus and also in developing a vaccine. Therefore, current analysis attempts to give an absolute level to report on Covid-19 in India. Various government strategies are analyzed both at central and state level.

Table 4 Health VS poverty in India

Health and Poverty	India
Population	1352.6
Physicians (per 1000 persons)	0.8
Hospital beds (per 1000 population)	0.7
Current health expenditure (% of GDP)	3.5
Current health expenditure per capita ($)	253.3
General government expenditure (% health Expenditure)	27.1
Individual average expenditure (% Health Expenditure)	62.4
Poverty headcount ratio at national poverty lines	21.9
GDP per capita ($)	6888.2

3 Sentiment Analysis

For textual analysis, determining the sentiments from the text plays a substantial insight. Extracting the associated text and reviewing the relations from the emotions, opinions, feedback and ideas in an extant study. Computing the polarity score from the sentiments and assigning these scores to the respective categories assess the positive, negative or neutral features of the content. Open-source statistical software R also has standardized polarity sentiment score method for customized lexicons. Anger, anticipation, disgust, fear, joy, negative, positive, sadness, surprise and trust are few of the sentiment classes taken into the current study. Five thousand tweets are classified under the above sentiment classes as shown in Fig. 5. The sentiment score ranges between -1 and $+1$. $+1$ indicates the positive opinion, 0 indicates neutral, and -1 indicates the negative polling (Fig. 4).

4 Textual Analytics

Various representations have been implemented using analytics based on theme of textual data. Emotional analysis and text frequency are analyzed from the collected tweets of 5000. Use of the words trust, fear, anticipation and sadness is emotionally associated with the tweets. Fear in the people's mind due to the increase of coronavirus is clearly visible from Fig. 5. People's anticipations toward life expectation, vaccine invention, immunity boosting and health care are significant parameters of thought process; hence, these elements are categorized under anticipation. Hope for tomorrow, life is achievement, stay home and stay healthy are some of the positive

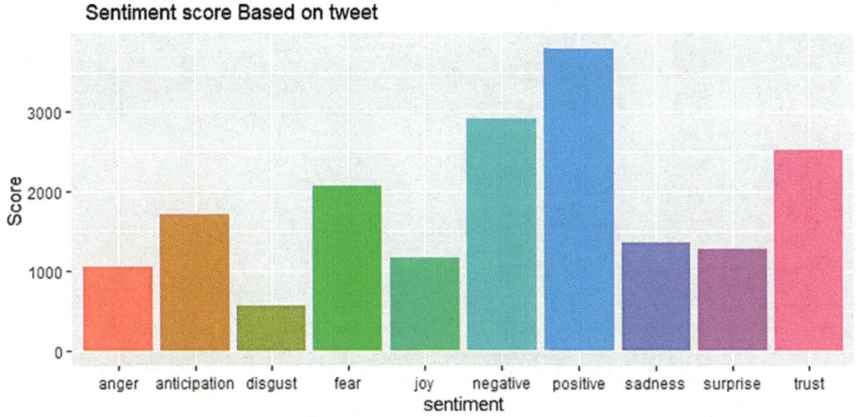

Fig. 4 Sentiment analysis score based on tweets in regard to pandemic

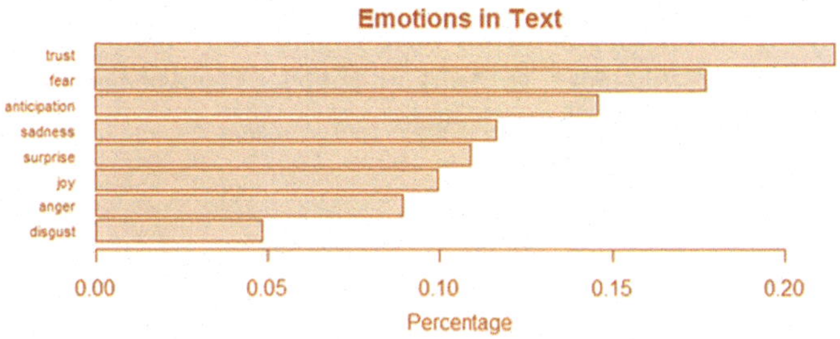

Fig. 5 Emotion percentages from the tweets

tweets representing the trust emotions. From Fig. 5, 5000 tweets are categorized into various emotions as shown below.

Twitter data analysis assesses the person's habits, likes, interests and relations by evaluating human communication through tweets. Content selection, product positioning, information retrieval and psychological assessment are analyzed from emotions of past research of social media.

This research also analyzed coronavirus tweet texts for potential association with other variables, in addition to endogenous analytics. Words such as Covid, people positive, doctors, test and cases are frequently repeated terms from the tweets. Elaborate study applied using time-aware knowledge extraction (TAKE) technique demonstrates acquittance of significant information from massive data of social media. This study gives a classified approach in summarizing the Twitter data to produce quality outcome.

Figure 6 is another word frequency graph representing high-frequency terminology from the 5000 tweets associated with the coronavirus. Among 5000 tweets, 3363 tweets were based on Covid, and remaining tweets indicate the other sensitive issues prevailing in the country. 'Positive cases are increasing rapidly', 'people are trem-

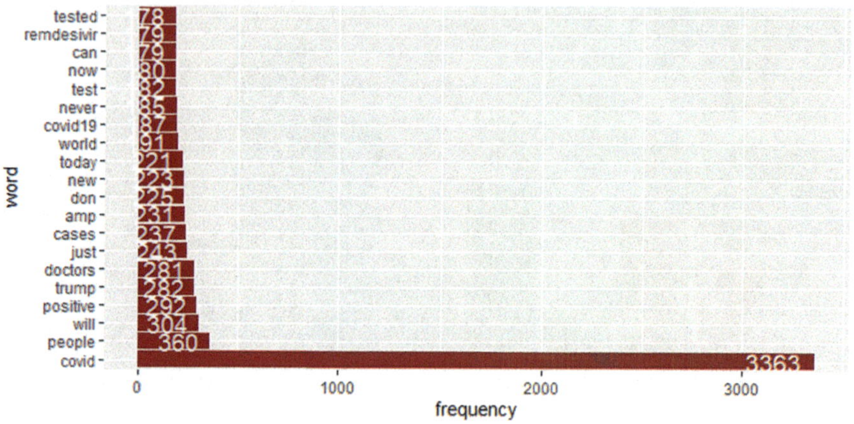

Fig. 6 Word frequency from the tweets

bling with fear' and 'Scientists are working hard for new vaccine invention' such tweets are depicting other word frequencies.

5 Geographical Analytics

Hot spots are regions in India that recorded higher rate of confirmed Covid cases. Detected people do not belong to same family, hence the possibility of transmission is more in those areas. In order to prevent spreading, Indian government has recognized and sealed those areas to restrict the people from unwanted moment. Many districts of Indian states are recognized as hot spots by enforcing the harsh lockdown. States have issued regulations during the lockdown to curb blowout of the coronavirus. Maharashtra, Delhi, Punjab, Odisha, Meghalaya, West Bengal, Tamil Nadu and Telangana states have extended lockdown beyond the date announced.

Government has taken a crucial step in identifying the hot spots and categorizing as red zone, green zone and orange zones. Escalating cases and high severity is represented as red zone, recovery rate is high, and recorded few cases are considered as orange zone. Non-restricted areas are recognized as green zones. The zonal wise categorization is represented in Fig. 7.

Zonal wise division of states is categorized into three representations red, orange and green zones in Table 5 considering the months April and May 2020. In Fig. 7a, green zones are represented in Madhya Pradesh, Chhattisgarh, Assam, Arunachal Pradesh and Uttar Pradesh having fewer number of cases. In Fig. 7b, Uttar Pradesh, Rajasthan, Bihar, Gujarat, Telangana and Tamil Nadu are represented as orange zones. Finally, Delhi, Maharashtra, Uttar Pradesh and Tamil Nadu are darker representing the red zones in Fig. 7c. The observations from this are Maharashtra, Delhi,

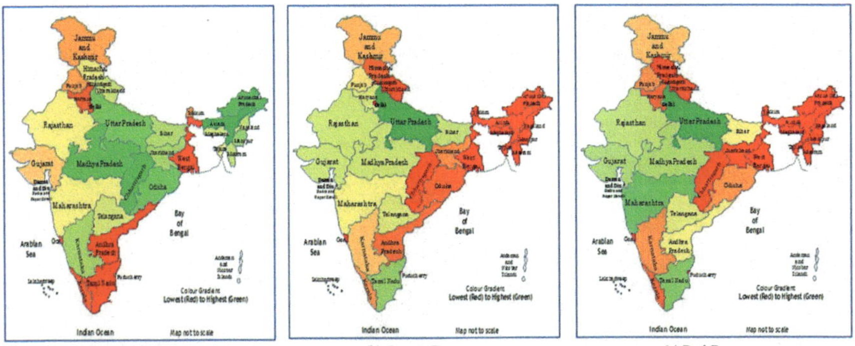

(a) Green Zone (b) Orange Zone (c) Red Zone

Fig. 7 Statewise zonal division based on the spread of coronavirus

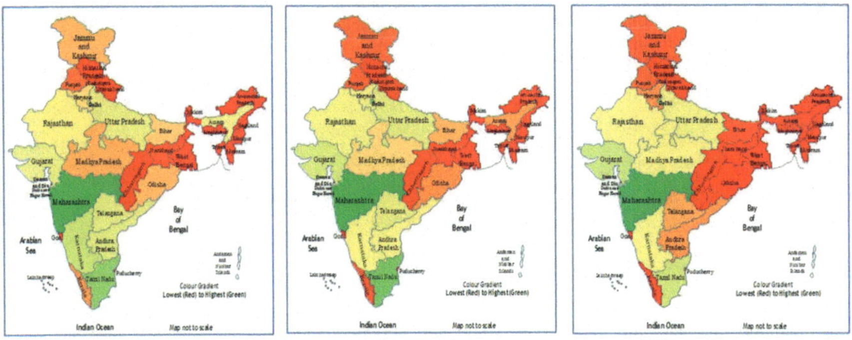

(a) Active (b) Recovered (c) Deceased

Fig. 8 Georepresentation of cases in India

Rajasthan, Gujarat and Tamil Nadu that are the critical states rapidly becoming serious and spreading extensively.

As the statewise cases are increasing exponentially, an comprehensive analysis is conducted on confirmed, active, recovered and deceased cases. From March 15 to July 15, all the cases have been tracked and scrutinized. Following Table 5 gives a detailed statewise report. Table 5 shows the color scales depicting the regions with red, yellow and green shades. Dark red displays higher number of cases, lighter shades of red illustrate the relative less number of cases, and yellow shades exemplify fewer cases than red shades. Finally, green shades demonstrate the safer zones.

In Fig. 8, Indian map is representing active, recovered and deceased cases from March 15 to July 15. Active cases are recorded in Maharashtra, Tamil Nadu, Delhi, Karnataka, Telangana, Andhra Pradesh, Gujarat and Uttar Pradesh. Recovered cases are more in Maharashtra, Delhi and Tamil Nadu. Maharashtra, Gujarat, Delhi and Tamil Nadu have recovered more number of death cases.

Table 5 Regions in India indicating red, orange and green zones

States	Red	Orange	Green	States	Red	Orange	Green
Andaman and Nicobar	1	0	2	Ladakh	0	2	0
Andhra Pradesh	5	7	1	Lakshadweep	0	0	1
Arunachal Pradesh	0	0	25	Madhya Pradesh	9	19	24
Assam	0	3	30	Maharashtra	14	16	6
Bihar	5	20	13	Manipur	0	0	16
Chandigarh	1	0	0	Meghalaya	0	1	10
Chhattisgarh	1	1	25	Mizoram	0	0	11
West Bengal	10	5	8	Nagaland	0	0	11
Daman and Diu	0	0	2	Odisha	3	6	21
Delhi	11	0	0	Puducherry	0	1	3
Goa	0	0	2	Punjab	3	15	4
Gujarat	9	19	5	Rajasthan	8	9	16
Haryana	2	18	2	Sikkim	0	0	4
Himachal Pradesh	0	6	6	Tamil Nadu	12	24	1
Jammu and Kashmir	4	12	4	Telangana	6	18	9
Jharkhand	1	9	14	Tripura	0	2	6
Karnataka	3	13	14	Uttar Pradesh	19	36	20
Kerala	2	10	2	Uttarakhand	1	2	10

6 Graph Analysis

An interactive graph analysis on various Indian states is represented in Fig. 9. From Fig. 9, the highest red zone regions are recorded in Maharashtra. Later Tamil Nadu, Delhi, Gujarat and Madhya Pradesh are other states having more red zones. Uttar Pradesh has the highest number of orange zone. Assam has the more number of green zones.

Figure 10 shows the statewise analysis of confirmed, recovered, active and deceased cases that are illustrated in detail. The time span of data set is from March 23 to July 22, 2020. The highest number of recovered cases recorded on Maharashtra, Delhi and Tamil Nadu are 1,00,000, 87,692 and 67,345 respectively. 43,000 active cases are recorded in Tamil Nadu. 11,000 are the highest confirmed cases from Maharashtra. Joint plots using the seaborn package are divulged in Fig. 11. Four joint plots are showing the confirmed, active, recovered and deceased cases efficiently.

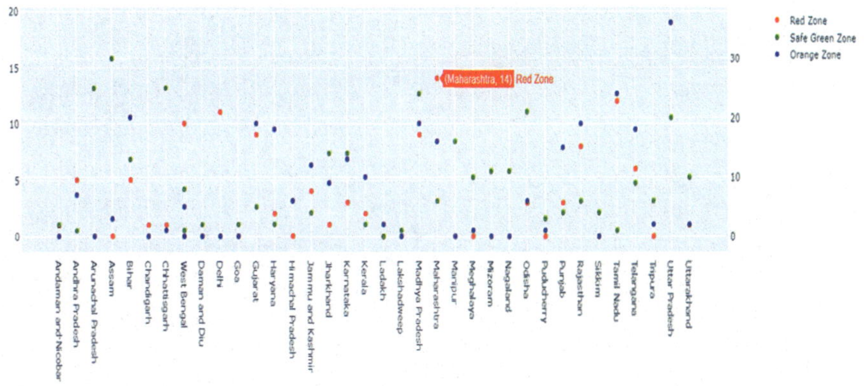

Fig. 9 Interactive graph representing zonewise cases in India

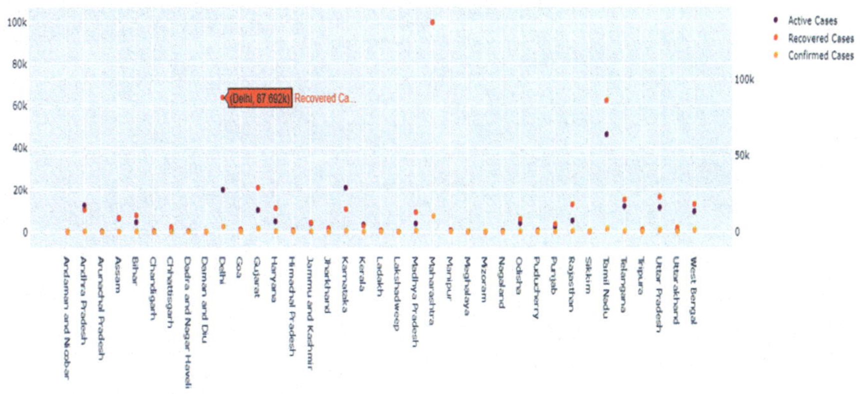

Fig. 10 Interactive graph representing statewise cases in India

- Active and Recovered Cases—Plot 11 (a) describes the number of recovered cases is more than the active cases. By observation, it shows that there are high chances of recovery.
- Active and Deceased Cases—Plot 11 (b) explains the number of death cases is very less compared to the active cases. For 1,00,000 cases, there are 10,000 death cases.
- Confirmed and Recovered Cases—Plot 11 (c) displays 1,40,000 recovered cases out of 2,50,000 confirmed cases. It records more than 60% recovery rate.
- Confirmed and Death Cases—Plot 11 (d) elucidates 10,000 death cases out of 2,50,000 confirmed cases. Death rate is comparatively low showing a positive analysis.

This paper presented a time series model in Sect. 8 and predicted number of infected cases and the turning point where the spread is at peak. Feasibility analysis of controlling Covid-19 spread is by isolating infected cases and quarantine. Simulation

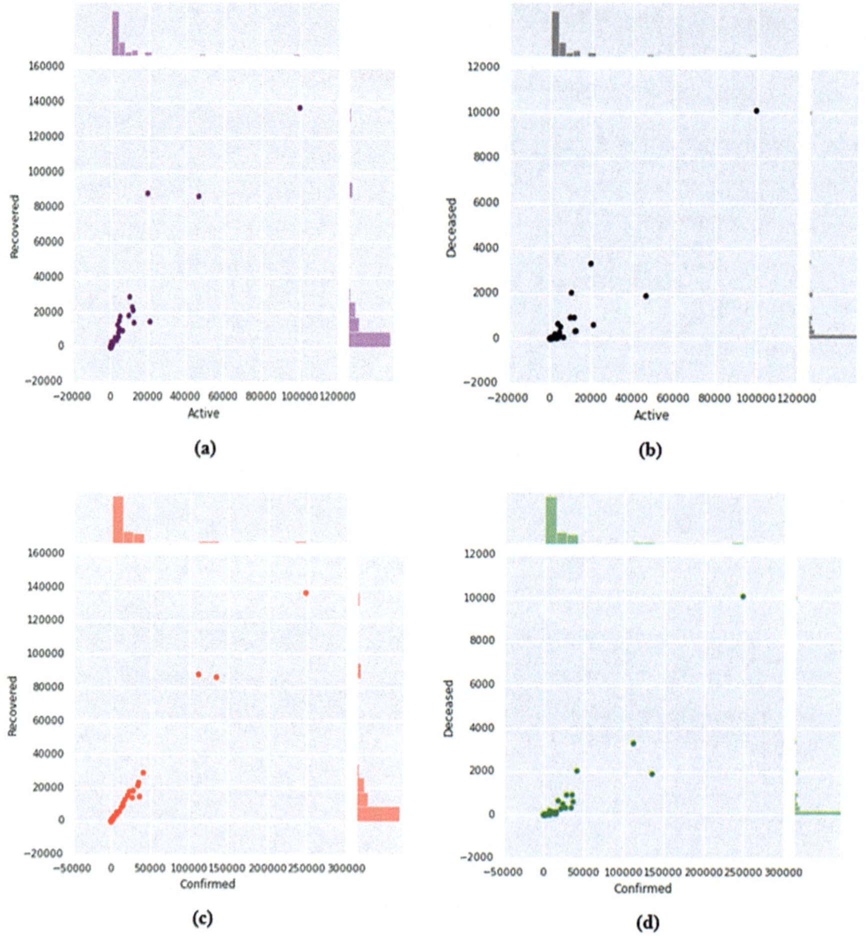

Fig. 11 Join plots for scenario analysis in India

results show that if the restrictions would have been applied one week before, then there would have been significant reduction in the number of infected cases. This research aims to present statistical framework for combining various estimates of this reproductive number into growth, interval and dispersion. The results generated from this framework show that all estimates of reproductive number are not accurate.

7 Results and Discussions Using Time Series Analysis

The recent data is used for analysis is taken from 'Covid-19 India API'. This site contains the recent data related to Covid-19 in various formats. This section puts more focus on time series analysis and forecasting of Covid-19 data starting from March 14, 2020, till July 21, 2020. Time series analysis can help to analyze the overall spread and recovery of the pandemic during given time period. It helps to analyze the impact of actions taken by government to decrease the spread and increase recovery cases. This section is divided into time series analysis and forecasting.

- Time Series Analysis

This section contains time series analysis of specifically five states, namely Maharashtra, Kerala, Gujarat, Delhi and Tamil Nadu. These five states are taken into consideration, because these states come in the list of hights ten states of Covid-19 detected cases.

The analysis concentrates two types of cases, i.e., confirmed cases and recovered cases. These parameters are taken into consideration to check the spread and recovery of the pandemic in specific area.

Figure 12 shows the time series analysis for Maharashtra state. From the graph, following observations can be drawn:

1. Due to lockdown From March till mid of May, the pandemic spared was in control but after that the spread started increasing and after June 20 and the spread went beyond 75 percentiles of the data. The overall trend is upward. It can be also observed that the spread is very high and crossed the highest percentile.

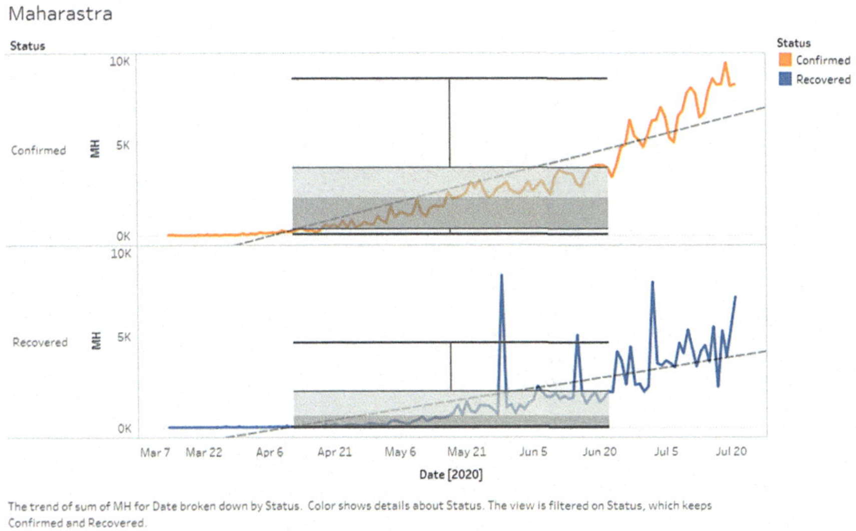

Fig. 12 Time series analysis for Maharashtra state

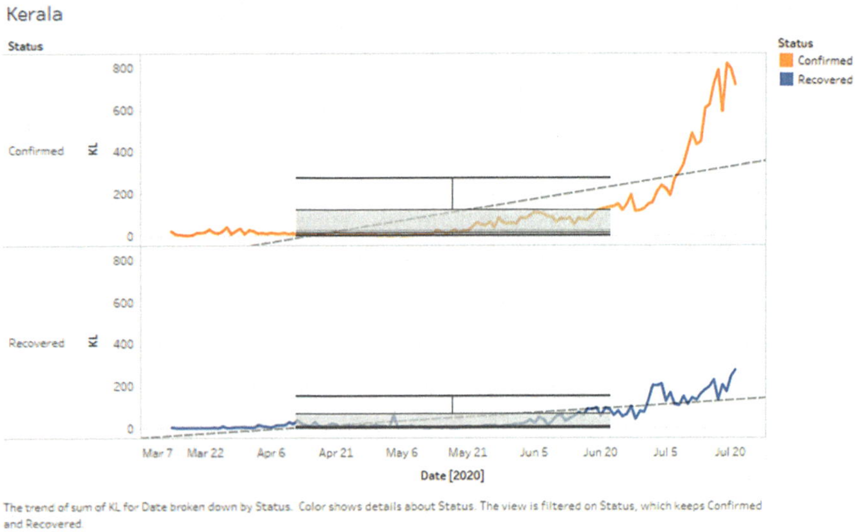

Fig. 13 Time series analysis for Kerala state

2. The recovery rate also shows upward trend in Maharashtra. The graph displays some peaks which shows there are a greater number of recoveries on certain days. The recovery rate is less compared to spread, but it is gradually increasing with spread rate.

Figure 13 shows the time series analysis for Kerala state. From the graph, following observations can be drawn:

1. In Kerala state, Covid-19 spread is very high from the month of July. Till then, the spread was very slow. After July 10, the spread has reached to the highest percentile.
2. Compared to spread, the recovery rate in Kerala state is very low. The recovery has just crossed the 75 percentiles of data.

Figure 14 shows the time series analysis for Delhi state. From the graph, following observations can be drawn:

1. From the graph, it can be observed that in mid of June, Covid-19 spared in Delhi was at the peak during mid of June. After that it started coming down, and now it has become less than 50 percentiles of the data.
2. In Delhi, recovery rate was also in the peak in mid of June, and it became stable after that till date.

Figure 15 shows the time series analysis for Gujarat state. From the graph, following observations can be drawn:

1. Gujarat state shows upward trend where it can be observed that there was a sudden increase in the spread on mid of May 2020. That time the spread has reached to

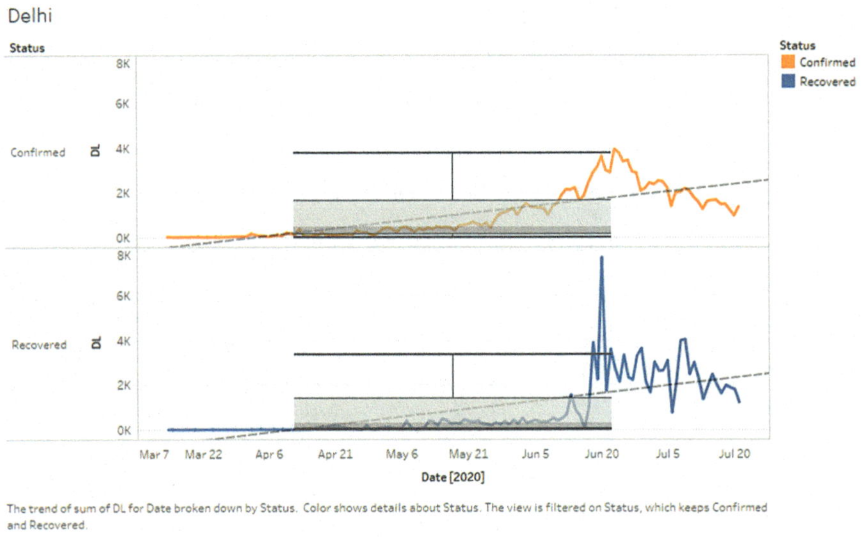

Fig. 14 Time series analysis for Delhi state

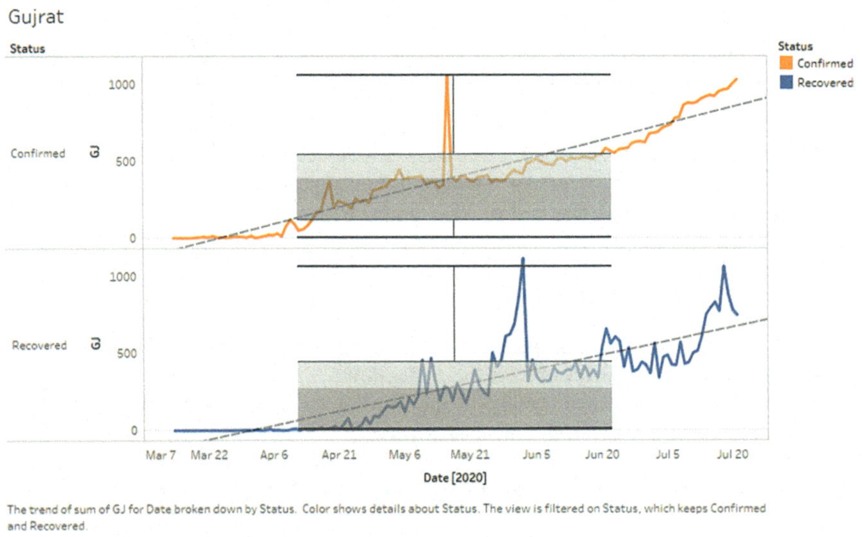

Fig. 15 Time series analysis for Gujarat state

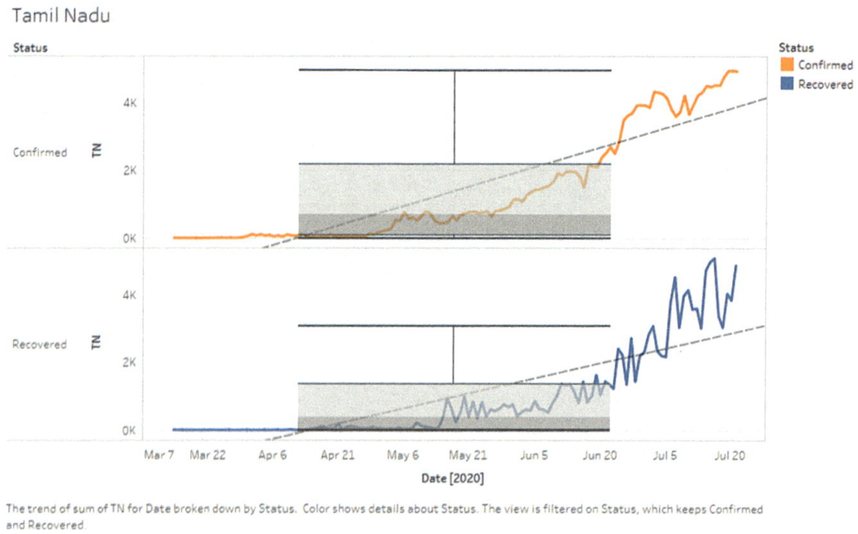

Fig. 16 Time series analysis for Tamil Nadu state

the highest percentiles but after that it has decreased and again started growing gradually. The cases are increasing and again started reaching to the highest percentile.

2. Recovery cases in Gujarat are showing equal upward trend like the spread. The number of recoveries is almost equal to the number of spared. There is a considerable recovery during the end of May and starting of June.

Figure 16 shows the time series analysis for Tamil Nadu state. From the graph, following observations can be drawn:

1. After lockdown, in Tamil Nadu state, the spread is increasing gradually till date. It has crossed the highest percentile of the data.
2. The recovery rate shows upward trend similar to spread. With the spread, the recovery rate is also high in Tamil Nadu state.

- Comparative weekly analysis of spread and recovery rate of Covid-19

The weekly analysis was done for confirmed and recovery rate of five states as shown in Fig. 17. The graph shows interesting insights as follows:

1. Maharashtra has gradually increased the spread and recovery over the time period, while the growth was very high from 25th week of the year.
2. In Delhi, cases started increasing from 23rd week and reached to the peak on 26th week. But after that there is a gradual drop in spread and recovery rate.
3. In Tamil Nadu, there was increased number of confirmed cases from 25th week, and then it came down after 29th week.

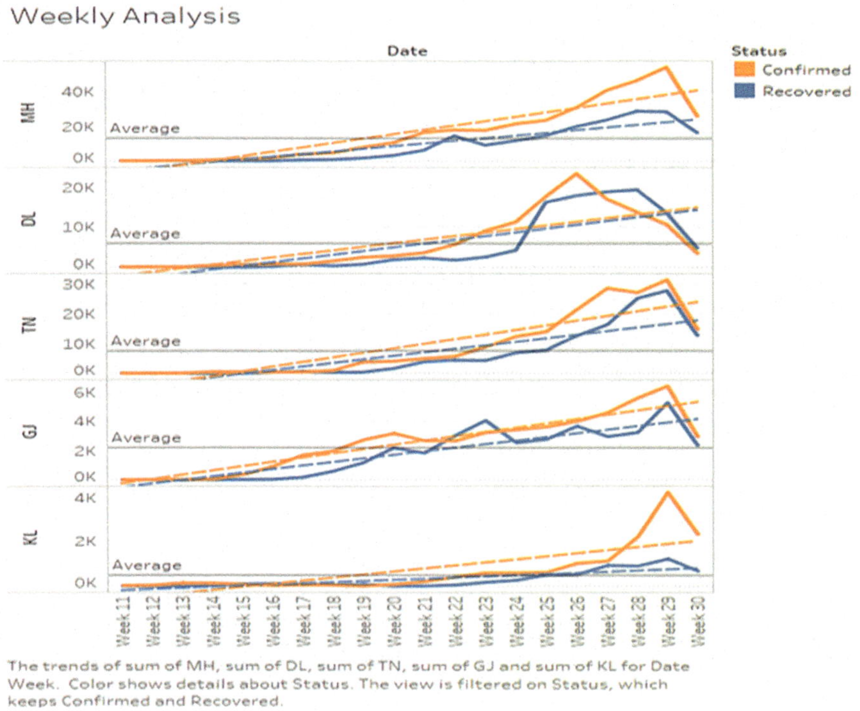

Fig. 17 Pandemic weekly time series analysis for Maharashtra, Delhi, Tamil Nadu, Gujarat and Kerala state

4. In Gujarat till 27th week, the spread was quite gradual but after that confirmed cases started increasing.
5. Similar to Gujarat, late in 27th week, the confirmed case number has increased
6. All the states have decreased number of confirmed cases after 29th week.
7. In all the states, the recovery rate is almost going parallel to the spread rate.

- Comparative daily analysis of spread and recovery rate of Covid-19

The daily analysis was done for confirmed and recovery rate of five states as shown in Fig. 18. The graph shows following observations:

1. There is a gradual spread of Covid-19 in four states such as Maharashtra, Tamil Nadu, Gujarat and Kerala, but there is a considerable drop of cases in Delhi.
2. In Maharashtra, frequently recovery rate has gone to the peak, but overall rate is going parallel with confirm cases with little less number.
3. In Tamil Nadu and Gujarat state, the confirmed and recovery rates are going parallel.
4. In Kerala, the number of confirmed cases is increasing gradually, but recovery rate is stable with less number.

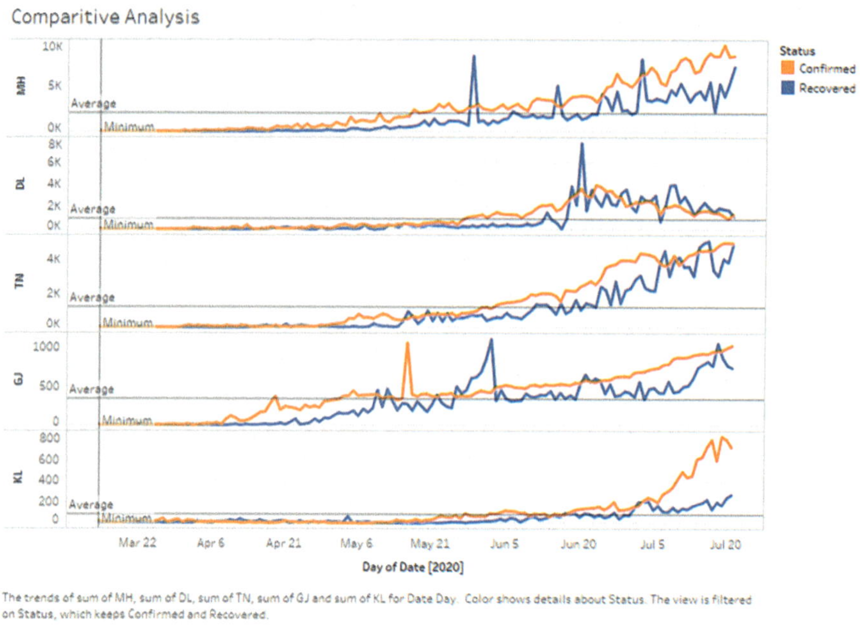

Fig. 18 Pandemic daily time series analysis for Maharashtra, Delhi, Tamil Nadu, Gujarat and Kerala state

8 Forecasting of Covid-19 on Five States

This section contains the forecasting of the confirmed and recovery cases of Covid-19 in five states. Forecasting helps to understand the future activity of Covid-19 spread and recovery. It can also help government to take corrective action as per the observation. Figure 19 has shown the graphical representation of forecast of Covid-19 for next two weeks after July 21, 2020.

From Fig. 19 graph, it can be observed from the following insights:

1. There will be considerable increase in spread and recovery in Maharashtra, Gujarat and Tamil Nadu states.
2. In Delhi, spread will drop down, while recovery rate will increase in next two weeks.
3. Reverse to Delhi, in Kerala spread rate will increase drastically while recovery rate will be stable with a smaller number of recoveries. These observations will illustrate the necessity of the state and requirements the government has to initiate in the states. Series strategy has to be implemented to control the spread of virus. In the view of above-mentioned related issues, we should promote ecumenical and interfaith collaboration and peaceful coexistence during the Covid-19 pandemic, ensuring that the accurate information is shared with communities and misinformation is addressed through ICT [21].

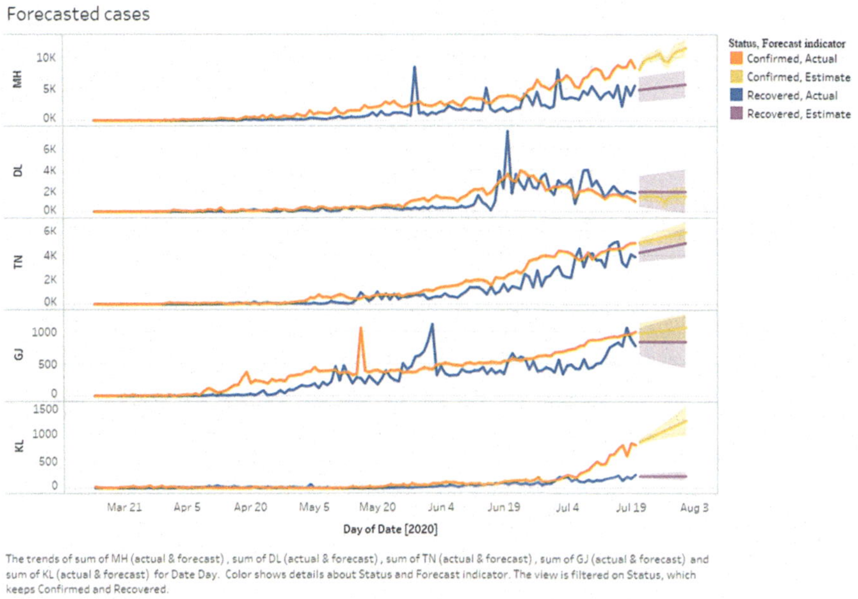

Fig. 19 Pandemic daily time series analysis for Maharashtra, Delhi, Tamil Nadu, Gujarat and Kerala state

9 Conclusion

Exponential spread of coronavirus has affected entire individual globally. It is an immediate need to mitigate the virus and its spread by executing the scientific and technical models on the Covid-19 cases. An elaborate study of literature describes mathematical models for analyzing the medical perspective to empower the predictions. Sophisticated analyses using Twitter data, geographical analysis, sentiment analysis and time series analysis are various assessments conducted to analyze people's opinions and interpret the forecasts on five crucial states having high rate of confirmed cases. Simulation outcome displays the critical situation that there are 2,60,000 confirmed cases in India. There is a sudden increase in the spike from May to June. Hence, the research analysis conducted in this paper would help government, pharmaceutical companies and the scientist to manufacture vaccine in a rapid mode. Hope produced vaccine will help us to live coexisting.

References

1. Samuel, J., Ali, N.M.: COVID-19 public sentiment insights and machine learning for tweets classification 1–23 (2020). http://arxiv.org/abs/2005
2. Bhatan, R., Chesneau, C.: On the Analysis of New COVID-19 Cases in Pakistan Using an Exponentiated Version of the M Family of Distributions. MDPI 953–968 (2020)
3. Rajan, G., Saibal, P.K., Gaurav, P.: A comprehensive analysis of COVID-19 outbreak situation. medRxiv 1–17 (2020). https://doi.org/10.1101/2020.04.08.20058347.t
4. Sarvam, M.: An Exploratory data analysis of COVID-19 in India. Int. J. Eng. Tech. Res. 580–587 (2020)
5. Emma, Z., Maria, G., Marina, M.: CO.ME.T.A.—covid-19 media textual analysis. A dashboard for media monitoring 748–757 (2020). http://arxiv.org/abs/748--757
6. Anastassopoulou, C.: Data-based analysis, modelling and forecasting of the COVID in Hubei. PLOS 845–856 (2020)
7. Kucharski, A., Russell, T., Diamond, C., Liu, Y.: Early dynamics of transmission and control of COVID-19: a mathematical modelling study. The Lancet Infect. Dis. 1–24 (2020)
8. Myers, J.: India is now the world's 5th largest economy, World Economic Forum. Retrieved from weforum. https://www.weforum.org/agenda/2020/02/india-gdp-economy-growthuk-france. Accessed 15 March 2020
9. Tanne, J.H., Hayasaki, E., Zastrow, M., Pulla, P., Smith, P., Rada, A.G.: Covid-19: how doctors and healthcare systems are tackling coronavirus worldwide. BMJ 368–384 (2020)
10. Organization, W.H.: Coronavirus disease (COVID-19) Pandemic. Retrieved from WHO. https://www.who.int/emergencies/diseases/novel-coronavirus-2019. Accessed 31 March 2020
11. University, J.H.: Novel Coronavirus (COVID-19) cases, provided by. Retrieved from John Hopkins University. https://github.com/CSSEGISandData/COVID-19. Accessed 6 Apr 2020
12. Sohrabi, C., Alsafi, Z., O'Neill, N.: World Health Organization declares global emergency: a review of the 2019 novel coronavirus (COVID-19). Int. J. Surg. 1–20 (2020)
13. Sahasranaman, A., Kumar, N.: Network structure of COVID-19 spread and the lacuna in India's testing strategy 1–8 (2020)
14. Sharma, N.: India's swiftness in dealing with Covid-19 will decide the world's future. Retrieved from Quartz, India. https://qz.com/india/1824041/who-saysindias-action-on-coronavirus-critical-for-the-world. Accessed 25 March 2020
15. Singh, R., Adhikari, R.: Ge-structured impact of social distancing on the COVID-19 epidemic in India 1–12 (2020)
16. Lixiang, L., Zihang, Y., Meng, C.: Propagation analysis and prediction of the COVID-19. Infect. Dis. Model. 282–292 (2020)
17. Worldometer: Worldometer. Retrieved from Worldometer. https://www.worldometers.info/coronavirus/country/india/. Accessed 31 May 2020
18. Singhal, T.: A review of coronavirus disease-2019 (COVID-19). The Indian J. Pediatr. 1–6 (2020)
19. Gupta, R., Pal, S.: Trend analysis and forecasting of COVID-19 outbreak in India. MEDRXIV 1–15 (2020)
20. thewire.: the wire. Retrieved from the wire. https://thewire.in/health/in-south-asia-lanka-leads-and-india-lags-in-infrastructure-medical-response-to-covid-19. Accessed 25 May 2020
21. Parikshit, M., Nilesh, S.: Predictive analytics of COVID-19 using information, communication and technologies. Corona Anal. NLP 12–24 (2020)
22. Jim, S., Nawaz, A.: COVID-19 public sentiment insights and machine 1–23 (2020). http://arxiv.org/abs/1--23

Modeling the Spread of Covid-19 Pandemic in Morocco

Houssine Zine, El Mehdi Lotfi, Marouane Mahrouf, Adnane Boukhouima, Yassine Aqachmar, Khalid Hattaf, Delfim F. M. Torres, and Noura Yousfi

Abstract Nowadays, coronavirus disease 2019 (Covid-19) poses a great threat to public health and economy worldwide. Unfortunately, there is yet no effective drug for this disease. For this, several countries have adopted multiple preventive interventions to avoid the spread of Covid-19. Here, we propose a delayed mathematical model to predict the epidemiological trend of Covid-19 in Morocco. Parameter estimation and sensitivity analysis of the proposed model are rigorously studied. Moreover, numerical simulations are presented in order to test the effectiveness of

H. Zine
Department of Mathematics, Center for Research and Development in Mathematics and Applications (CIDMA), University of Aveiro, 3810-193 Aveiro, Portugal
e-mail: zinehoussine@ua.pt

E. M. Lotfi · M. Mahrouf · A. Boukhouima · N. Yousfi
Faculty of Sciences Ben M'sik, Laboratory of Analysis, Modeling and Simulation (LAMS), Hassan II University of Casablanca, P.B 7955 Sidi Othman, Casablanca, Morocco
e-mail: lotfiimehdi@gmail.com

M. Mahrouf
e-mail: marouane.mahrouf@gmail.com

A. Boukhouima
e-mail: adnaneboukhouima@gmail.com

N. Yousfi
e-mail: nourayousfi.fsb@gmail.com

Y. Aqachmar
World Health Organization (WHO), Country Office, Rabat, Morocco
e-mail: aqachmary@who.int

K. Hattaf
Centre Régional des Métiers de l'Education et de la Formation (CRMEF), P.B 20340 Derb Ghalef, Casablanca, Morocco
e-mail: k.hattaf@yahoo.fr

D. F. M. Torres (✉)
Center for Research and Development in Mathematics and Applications (CIDMA), Department of Mathematics, University of Aveiro, 3810-193 Aveiro, Portugal
e-mail: delfim@ua.pt

P. Agarwal et al. (eds.), *Analysis of Infectious Disease Problems (Covid-19) and Their Global Impact*, Infosys Science Foundation Series,
https://doi.org/10.1007/978-981-16-2450-6_28

the preventive measures and strategies that were imposed by the Moroccan authorities and also help policy makers and public health administration to develop such strategies.

Keywords Covid-19 · Coronavirus · Mathematical modeling · Basic reproduction number · Prediction

1 Introduction

Coronavirus disease 2019 (Covid-19) is an infectious disease that appeared in China at the end of 2019. It is caused by a new type of virus belonging to the coronaviruses family and recently named *severe acute respiratory syndrome coronavirus 2* (SARS-CoV-2) [1]. On March 11, 2020, Covid-19 was reclassified as a pandemic by the World Health Organization (WHO). The disease spreads rapidly from country to country, causing enormous economic damage and many deaths worldwide. The first case of Covid-19 in Morocco was confirmed on March 2, 2020, in city of Casablanca. It involved a Moroccan expatriate residing in Italy and who came from Italy on February 27, 2020. As of April 17, 2020, the confirmed cases reached 2564 and the number of recoveries reached 281 with a total number of 135 deaths [2].

Moroccan authorities have implemented multiple preventive measures and strategies to control the spread of disease, such as the closing of borders, suspension of schools and universities, closing coffee shops, the shutdown of all mosques in the country, etc. Further, Morocco has declared a state of health emergency during the period from March 20 to April 20, 2020, to avoid the spread of Covid-19. During this period, movement during the day should be limited to work, shopping, medical care, purchasing medicine, medical supplies and emergency situations only. In addition, and from April 6, 2020, the wearing of a mask became compulsory for all persons authorized to move.

Mathematical modeling of Covid-19 transmission has attracted the attention of many scientists. Tang et al. [3] used a susceptible–exposed–infectious–recovered (SEIR) compartmental model to estimate the basic reproduction number of Covid-19 transmission based on data obtained for the confirmed cases of the disease in mainland China. Wu et al. [4] provided an estimate of the size of the epidemic in Wuhan on the basis of the number of cases exported from Wuhan to cities outside mainland China by using a SEIR model. In [5], Kuniya applied the SEIR compartmental model for the prediction of the epidemic peak for Covid-19 in Japan by using the real-time data from January 15 to February 29, 2020. Fanelli and Piazza [6] analyzed and forecasted Covid-19 spreading in China, Italy and France by using a simple susceptible–infected–recovered–death (SIRD) model. The authors of [7] present a mathematical model and study the dynamics of Covid-19 that emerged recently in Wuhan, China. For a fractional (non-integer order) model, see [8].

In the models cited above, the transmission of the disease was assumed to be instantaneous, and therefore, they are formulated by ordinary differential equations

(ODEs), without time delays. In this study, we propose a mathematical model governed by delay differential equations (DDEs) to predict the epidemiological trend of Covid-19 in Morocco and taking into account multiple preventive measures and strategies implemented by Moroccan authorities, related to the confinement period between March 2 and June 20, 2020, in order to control the spread of disease. To do this, Sect. 2 deals with the formulation of the model. Section 3 is devoted to parameters estimation and sensitivity analysis. Forecast of Covid-19 spreading in Morocco is presented in Sect. 4. We end with a discussion of the results in Sect. 5.

2 Formulation of the Model

Around the world, all the countries that are attacked by the Covid-19 have imposed several strategies, with different degrees, to fight against it, namely the reduction of some rights by adopting the quarantine method in order to prevent contacts between vulnerable and infected individuals, closing the geographical borders of the countries and enforcing the capacity of the sanitary system. Similarly, the Kingdom of Morocco quickly followed all of the previous strategies when the pandemic was in its early stages.

Remark 1 The terms "susceptibility" and "vulnerability" are often used interchangeably for populations with disproportionate health burdens [9]. The distinction between vulnerability and susceptibility marks the difference between being intact but fragile–vulnerable and being injured and predisposed to compound additional harm–susceptible [10]. Here, we refer to "the potential to contract the Covid-19" as vulnerability, to emphasize the environmental nature of the disease.

After the first reported positive case in Morocco, March 2, 2020, the closing of schools and universities is done at March 16, 2020; the state of health emergency (containment) is imposed to contain the outbreak from March 20, 2020; and the closure of the borders is performed at March 24, 2020. Additionally, the face mask is obligatory used in the general population at April 6, 2020. Based on these preventive measures and strategies, we model the dynamics of the transmission of Covid-19 in Morocco by extending the classical SIR model. Precisely, the population is divided into eight classes, denoted by V, I_s, I_a, F_b, F_g, F_c, R and D, where V represents the vulnerable subpopulation, which is not infected and has not been infected before, but is susceptible to develop the disease if exposed to the virus; I_s is the symptomatic-infected subpopulation, which has not yet been treated, it transmits the disease, and outside of proper support it can progress to spontaneous recovery or death; I_a is the asymptomatic-infected subpopulation who is infected but does not transmit the disease, it is not known by the health system and progresses spontaneously to recovery; F_b, F_g and F_c are the patients diagnosed, supported by the Moroccan health system and under quarantine and subdivided into three categories: benign, severe and critical forms, respectively. Finally, R and D are the recovered and died classes. The schematic diagram of our extended model is illustrated in Fig. 1.

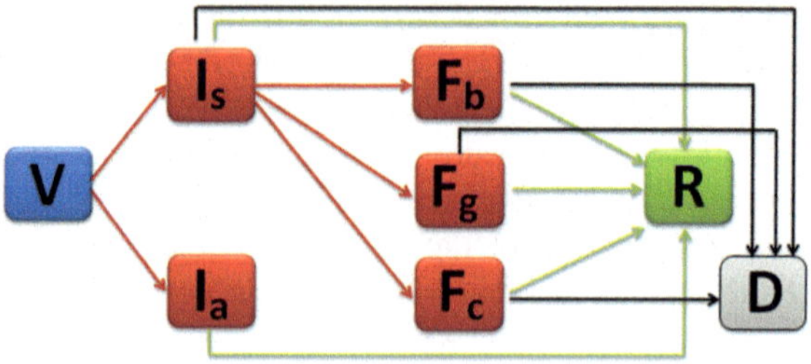

Fig. 1 Schematic diagram of our extended model

Therefore, the extended model can be governed by the following system of DDEs:

$$\begin{cases} \dfrac{dV(t)}{dt} = -\beta(1-u)V(t)I_s(t), \\ \dfrac{dI_s(t)}{dt} = \beta\epsilon(1-u)V(t-\tau_1)I_s(t-\tau_1) - \big(\mu_s + \eta_s + \alpha(\gamma_b + \gamma_g + \gamma_c)\big)\, I_s(t), \\ \dfrac{dI_a(t)}{dt} = \beta(1-\epsilon)(1-u)V(t-\tau_1)I_s(t-\tau_1) - \eta_a I_a(t), \\ \dfrac{dF_b(t)}{dt} = \alpha\gamma_b I_s(t-\tau_2) - \big(\mu_b + r_b\big)F_b(t), \\ \dfrac{dF_g(t)}{dt} = \alpha\gamma_g I_s(t-\tau_2) - \big(\mu_g + r_g\big)F_g(t), \\ \dfrac{dF_c(t)}{dt} = \alpha\gamma_c I_s(t-\tau_2) - \big(\mu_c + r_c\big)F_c(t), \\ \dfrac{dR(t)}{dt} = \eta_a I_a(t) + \eta_s I_s(t) + r_b F_b(t) + r_g F_g(t) + r_c F_c(t), \\ \dfrac{dD(t)}{dt} = \mu_s I_s(t) + \mu_b F_b(t) + \mu_g F_g(t) + \mu_c F_c(t), \end{cases} \tag{1}$$

where u represents the level of control strategies on the vulnerable population. We adopt the bilinear incidence rate to describe the infection of the disease and use parameter β to denote the transmission rate. It is reasonable to assume that the infected individuals are subdivided into individuals with symptoms and others without symptoms, for which we employ the parameter ϵ to denote the proportion for the symptomatic individuals and $1-\epsilon$ for the asymptomatic ones. The parameter α measures the efficiency of public health administration for hospitalization. Diagnosed symptomatic-infected population moves to the three forms: benign, severe and critical, by the rates γ_b, γ_g and γ_c, respectively. The mean recovery periods of these forms are denoted by $1/r_b$, $1/r_g$ and $1/r_c$, respectively. The later forms die also with the rates μ_b, μ_g and μ_c, respectively. Symptomatic-infected population, which is not diagnosed, moves to the recovery compartment with a rate η_s or dies with a rate μ_s. On the other hand, asymptomatic-infected population moves to the recovery compartment with a rate η_a. The times delay τ_1 and τ_2 denote the incubation period and the period time needed before hospitalization, respectively.

For biological reasons, we assume that the initial conditions of system (1) satisfy the following:

$$\begin{array}{lll} V(\theta) \ = \phi_1(\theta) \geq 0, & I_s(\theta) = \phi_2(\theta) \geq 0, & I_a(\theta) = \phi_3(\theta) \geq 0, \\ F_b(\theta) = \phi_4(\theta) \geq 0, & F_g(\theta) = \phi_5(\theta) \geq 0, & F_c(\theta) = \phi_6(\theta) \geq 0, \\ R(\theta) \ = \phi_7(\theta) \geq 0, & D(\theta) = \phi_8(\theta) \geq 0, & \theta \in [-\tau, 0], \end{array}$$

where $\tau = \max\{\tau_1, \tau_2\}$. Let $\mathcal{C} = C([-\tau, 0], \mathbb{R}^8)$ be the Banach space of continuous functions from the interval $[-\tau, 0]$ into $\mathbb{R}^8$, equipped with the uniform topology. It follows from the theory of functional differential equations [11] that system (1) with initial conditions $(\phi_1, \phi_2, \phi_3, \phi_4, \phi_5, \phi_6, \phi_7, \phi_8) \in \mathcal{C}$ has a unique solution.

On the other hand, the basic reproduction number is an important threshold parameter that determines the spread of infection when the disease is introduced into the population [12]. This number is defined as the expected number of secondary cases produced, in a completely susceptible population, by a typical infective individual. By using the next-generation matrix approach [13], the basic reproduction number $\mathcal{R}_0$ of system (1) is given by

$$\mathcal{R}_0 = \rho(FV^{-1}) = \frac{\beta\epsilon(1-u)}{\eta_s + \mu_s + \alpha(\gamma_b + \gamma_g + \gamma_c)}, \tag{2}$$

where ρ is the spectral radius of the next-generation matrix FV^{-1} with

$$F = \begin{pmatrix} \beta\epsilon(1-u) & 0 \\ 0 & 0 \end{pmatrix} \quad \text{and} \quad V = \begin{pmatrix} \eta_s + \mu_s + \alpha(\gamma_b + \gamma_g + \gamma_c) & 0 \\ 0 & \eta_a \end{pmatrix}.$$

3 Parameter Estimation and Sensitivity Analysis

Based on the daily published Moroccan data [14], we estimate the values of some parameters of the model. The proportion of asymptomatic forms can vary from 20.6% of infected population to 39.9% [15]. Then, $\epsilon \in [0.61, 0.794]$. The progression rates γ_b, γ_g and γ_c from symptomatic-infected individuals to the three forms are assumed to be 80% of diagnosed cases for benign form, 15% of diagnosed cases for severe form and 5% of diagnosed cases for critical form, respectively [16]. The true mortality of Covid-19 will take some time to be fully understood. The data we have so far indicate that the crude mortality ratio (the number of reported deaths divided by the reported cases) is between 3 and 4% [16]. As the Moroccan health system is not overloaded at the moment, it is assumed that deaths mainly come from critical cases with a percentage of 40% for an average period of 13.5 days [16]. Since the mortality rate of symptomatic individuals differs from country to country [6], we assume that 1% of symptomatic individuals die for an average period of 21 days, whereas the recovery rate for asymptomatic cases is 100% and is the same for severe and benign forms if a proper medical care is taken with an average period of 21 days. We employ a least-square procedure with Poisson noise as in [5] to estimate the transmission rate. The incubation period is estimated to be 5.5 days [17, 18] while the time needed

Table 1 Parameter values for our model (1)

Parameter	Value	Source
β	0.4517 (95%CI, 0.4484–0.455)	Estimated
u	0–1	Varied
ϵ	0.794	Mizumoto et al. [15]
γ_b	0.8	WHO [16]
γ_g	0.15	WHO [16]
γ_c	0.05	WHO [16]
α	0.06	Assumed
η_a	$1/21$	Calculated
η_s	$0.8/21$	Calculated
μ_s	$0.01/21$	Calculated
μ_b	0	Assumed
μ_g	0	Assumed
μ_c	$0.4/13.5$	Calculated
r_b	$1/13.5$	Calculated
r_g	$1/13.5$	Calculated
r_c	$0.6/13.5$	Calculated
τ_1	5.5	[17, 18]
τ_2	7.5	[19–21]

before hospitalization is estimated to be 7.5 days [19–21]. The estimation of the above parameters is given in Table 1.

Sensitivity analysis is commonly used to determine the robustness of model predictions to some parameter values. It is used to discover parameters that have a high impact on $\mathcal{R}_0$ and should be targeted by intervention strategies. The main objective of this section is to examine the sensitivity of the basic reproduction number $\mathcal{R}_0$ with respect to model parameters by the so-called *sensitivity index*.

Definition 1 [22, 23] The normalized forward sensitivity index of a variable ν, that depends differentially on a parameter ρ, is defined as

$$\Upsilon_{\rho}^{\nu} := \frac{\partial \nu}{\partial \rho} \times \frac{\rho}{\nu}.$$

According to Definition 1, we derive the normalized forward sensitivity index of $\mathcal{R}_0$ with respect to β, ϵ, η_s, μ_s, γ_b, γ_g, γ_c and α, which is summarized in Table 2. As we observe in Table 2, the most sensitive parameters, which have a higher impact on $\mathcal{R}_0$, are β and ϵ, since $\Upsilon_{\beta}^{\mathcal{R}_0}$ and $\Upsilon_{\epsilon}^{\mathcal{R}_0}$ are independent of any parameter of system (1) with $\Upsilon_{\beta}^{\mathcal{R}_0} = \Upsilon_{\epsilon}^{\mathcal{R}_0} = +1$. In addition, the parameter α has a middle negative impact on $\mathcal{R}_0$, while $\mathcal{R}_0$ is slightly impacted by the rest of the parameters.

Table 2 Normalized forward sensitivity index of $\mathcal{R}_0$

Parameters	Sensitivity index of $\mathcal{R}_0$	Value
β	$\Upsilon_{\beta}^{\mathcal{R}_0} = +1$	+1
ϵ	$\Upsilon_{\epsilon}^{\mathcal{R}_0} = +1$	+1
η_s	$\Upsilon_{\eta_s}^{\mathcal{R}_0} = -\dfrac{\eta_s}{\eta_s + \mu_s + (\gamma_b + \gamma_g + \gamma_c)\alpha}$	−0.3864
μ_s	$\Upsilon_{\mu_s}^{\mathcal{R}_0} = -\dfrac{\mu_s}{\eta_s + \mu_s + (\gamma_b + \gamma_g + \gamma_c)\alpha}$	−0.0048
γ_b	$\Upsilon_{\gamma_b}^{\mathcal{R}_0} = -\dfrac{\alpha\gamma_b}{\eta_s + \mu_s + (\gamma_b + \gamma_g + \gamma_c)\alpha}$	−0.487
γ_g	$\Upsilon_{\gamma_g}^{\mathcal{R}_0} = -\dfrac{\alpha\gamma_g}{\eta_s + \mu_s + (\gamma_b + \gamma_g + \gamma_c)\alpha}$	−0.0913
γ_c	$\Upsilon_{\gamma_c}^{\mathcal{R}_0} = -\dfrac{\alpha\gamma_c}{\eta_s + \mu_s + (\gamma_b + \gamma_g + \gamma_c)\alpha}$	−0.0304
α	$\Upsilon_{\alpha}^{\mathcal{R}_0} = -\dfrac{\alpha(\gamma_b + \gamma_g + \gamma_c)}{\eta_s + \mu_s + (\gamma_b + \gamma_g + \gamma_c)\alpha}$	−0.687

4 Prevision of Covid-19 in Morocco

In this section, we present the forecasts of Covid-19 in Morocco relating to different preventive measures and strategies implemented by Moroccan authorities on the confinement period between March 2 and June 20, 2020. Then the parameter u can be defined as follows:

$$u = \begin{cases} u_1, \text{ on (March 2, March 10]}; \\ u_2, \text{ on (March 10, March 20]}; \\ u_3, \text{ on (March 20, April 6]}; \\ u_4, \text{ after April 6}, \end{cases}$$

where $u_i \in (0, 1], i = 1, 2, 3, 4$ measures the effectiveness of applying the multiple preventive interventions imposed by Moroccan authorities presented in Table 3.

To make a better illustration of the different strategies, we test the four decisions made at the government level in Fig. 2.

We see in Fig. 2 the evolution of the number of diagnosed infected positive individuals with different sets of measures: low, middle, high and strict interventions. Up to April 15, the curves corresponding to the first three sets of measures increase exponentially, while the curve corresponding to the fourth set of measures has lost its initial exponential character and tends to flatten over time. In addition, the last daily reported cases in Morocco from March 2 to April 17 confirm the biological tendency

Table 3 Summary of non-pharmaceutical interventions considered

Policies	Control values
Without any intervention measures	$u = 0$, after March 2
First set of measures	$u = 0.2$, after March 2
Second set of measures	$u = 0.2$, (on March 2, March 10] and $u = 0.3$, after March 10
Third set of measures	$u = 0.2$, (on March 2, March 10], $u = 0.3$, (on March 10, March 16] and $u = 0.4$, after March 16
Fourth set of measures	$u = 0.2$, (on March 2, March 10], $u = 0.3$, (on March 10, March 16] and $u = 0.4$, (on March 16, April 6] and $u = 0.8$, after April 6

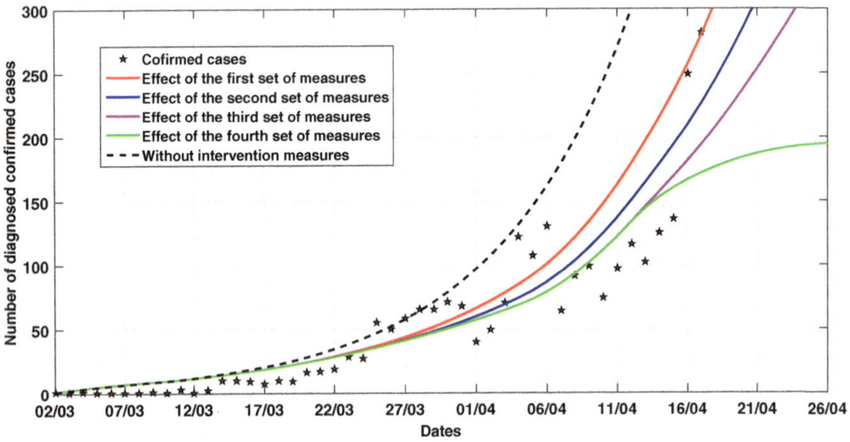

Fig. 2 Comparison of the non-pharmaceutical interventions considered and the daily reported cases of Covid-19 in Morocco from March 2 to April 17, 2020

of our model. Thus, our model is efficient to describe the spread of Covid-19 in Morocco. However, we note that some clinical data are a little far from the values of the model due to certain foci that appeared in some large areas or at the level of certain industrial areas.

Next, we give the graphical results related to delays parameters to prove their biological importance.

We observe in Fig. 3 a highly impact of delays on the number of diagnosed positive cases, thereby the plot of model (1) without delays ($\tau_1 = \tau_2 = 0$) is very far from the clinical data.

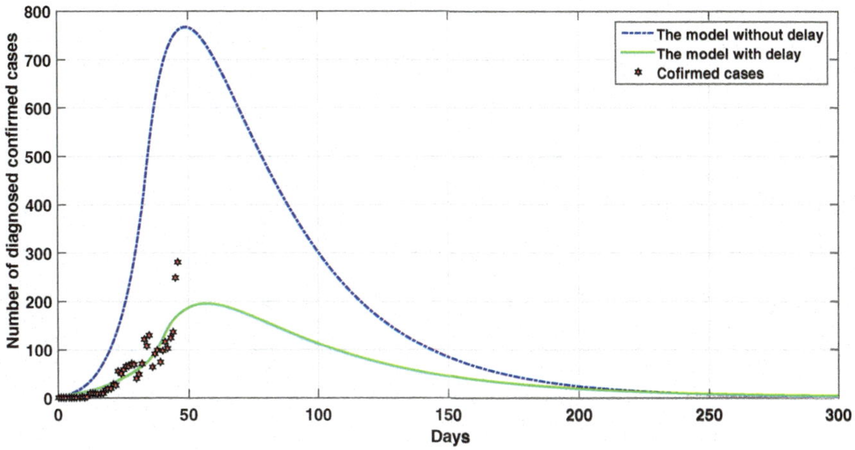

Fig. 3 Effect of delays on the diagnosed confirmed cases

4.1 *Peak Prediction*

Now, we indicate the predicted relative impact of the model and especially the diagnosed infective individuals with and without interventions applied progressively in Morocco.

Before finding the first positive-infected case in Morocco, the authorities have begun with a suspension of international air lines to and from China and installed health control checkpoints at the borders but without any interventions into the Moroccan population. For this, we simulate model (1) in the case $u = 0$, which is illustrated in Figs. 4 and 5.

We remark from Fig. 4 that the estimated epidemic peak is $t^* = 142$ ($95\%CI$, 141–143), that is, starting from March 2, 2020 ($t = 0$), the estimated epidemic peak is July 21, 2020 ($t = 142$).

In the absence of any government intervention, the disease persists strongly and almost all of the vulnerable population will be reached by the infection (Fig. 5).

After the first imported positive-infected case, Moroccan authorities began to establish some preventive interventions between March 2 and 10, namely isolation of positive cases, contact tracing, hygiene measures, prevention measures in workplaces and ban of mass gathering events. For this reason, we have selected in this period $u = 0.2$. From March 10 up to March 20, 2020, additional preventive measures were established: gradual suspension of all international sea, ground and air lines (including with Spain, Italia, Algeria, France, Germany, Netherlands, Belgium and Portugal), closure of coffees, restaurants, cinemas, theaters, party rooms, clubs, sport centers, hammams, game rooms and sport fields, closure of mosques, schools and universities, disinfection of public transportation means, reduction of the carrying capacity of taxis, buses and tramways, movement/travel restrictions and containment measures of the general population. These measures correspond to the choice of the

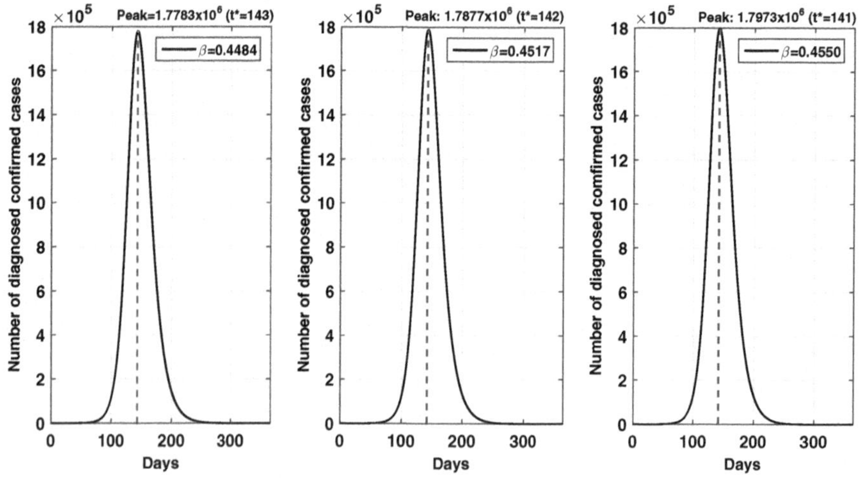

Fig. 4 Time variation of the diagnosed infective individuals without any intervention on the Moroccan population with different values of β ($95\% CI$, 0.4484–0.455)

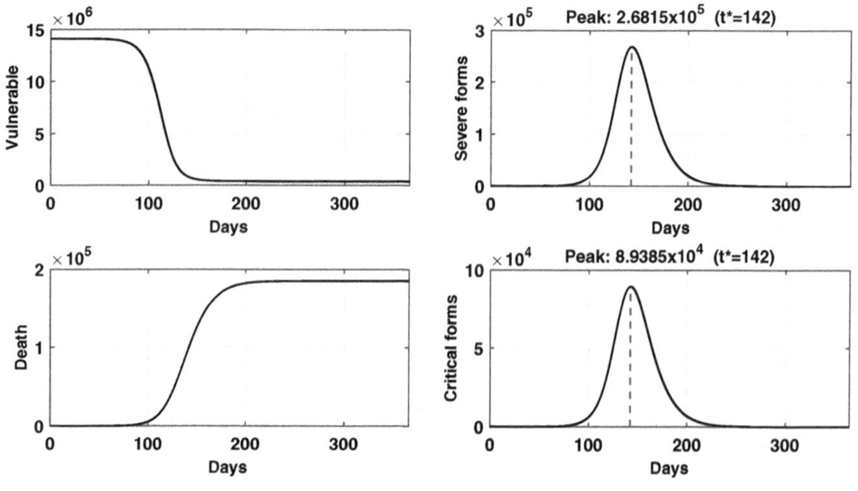

Fig. 5 Time variation of the model with $\beta = 0.4517$ and $\mathcal{R}_0 = 3.6385$

control $u = 0.3$. From March 20 up to April 6, the Moroccan authority declared a state of emergency with a complete lockdown, nighttime curfew, movement restrictions 24/24, ban of human movements between cities, suspension of railway lines, streets disinfection and extensive cleaning and disinfection of port and airport facilities. For this, we assume that $u = 0.4$. From April 6, the authority decided compulsory wearing of masks in public spaces, which implies a significant positive influence on the above interventions and an increase of their efficiency level. In this case, we

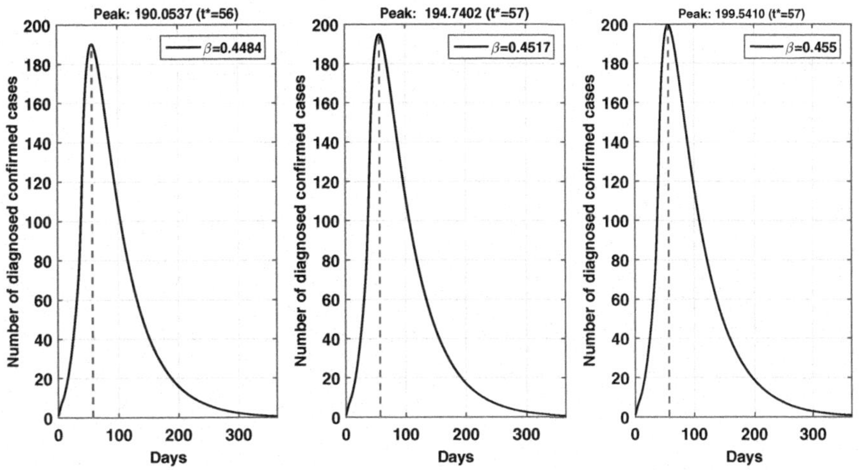

Fig. 6 Time variation of the diagnosed infective individuals with high-level respect of measures for different values of β (95%CI, 0.4484–0.455)

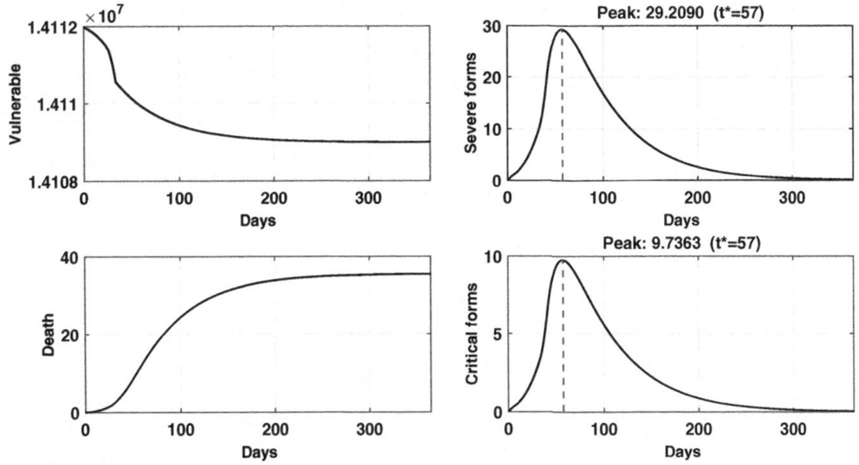

Fig. 7 Time variation of the model with $\beta = 0.4517$ and $\mathcal{R}_0 = 2.9108$ (March 2–10), $\mathcal{R}_0 = 2.5469$ (March 10–20), $\mathcal{R}_0 = 2.1831$ (March 20–April 6), $\mathcal{R}_0 = 0.7277$ (from April 6, 2020)

assume that $u = 0.8$. Tacking into account all these policies, we present Figs. 6 and 7.

We remark from Fig. 6 that the estimated epidemic peak is $t^* = 57$ (95%CI, 56–57), that is, starting from March 2 ($t = 0$), the estimated epidemic peak is April 28, 2020 ($t = 57$).

From Fig. 7, we see that all the measures taken into this second strategy have a significant impact on the number of new positive diagnosed cases per day. Compared to Fig. 5, the time required to reach the peak is reduced by 85 days, avoiding globally

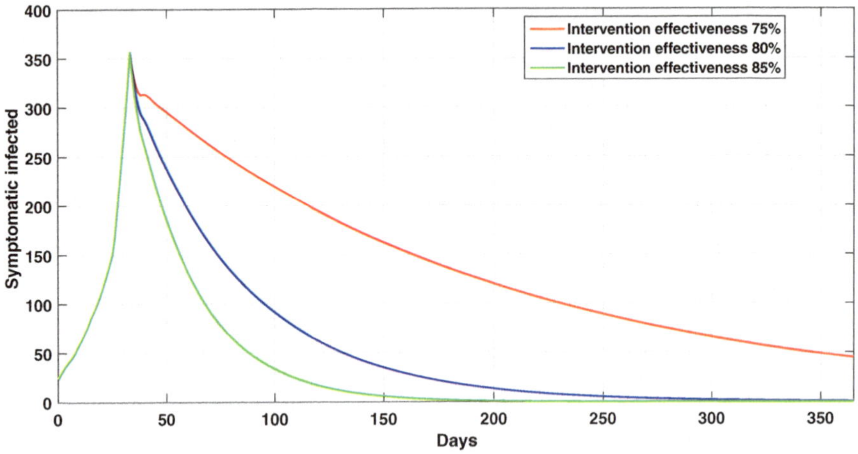

Fig. 8 Evolution of the symptomatic individuals with different effectiveness degrees

Table 4 Cumulative diagnosed cases, severe forms, critical forms and deaths, after 150 days of the start of the pandemic in Morocco

Effectiveness	75%	80%	85%
Diagnosed	42834	29116	21432
Severe forms	6419	4361	3209
Critical forms	2139	1453	1069
Deaths	1500	993	661

an interesting number of new infections and new deaths. Furthermore, the computed basic reproduction number $\mathcal{R}_0$ is less than 1, which means the extinction of the disease if the measures cited above are strictly implemented.

4.2 *Intervention Effectiveness*

Here, on one hand, we compare the impact of different degrees of effectiveness on the evolution of the number of positive-infected diagnosed individuals, symptomatic individuals and deaths (see Figs. 8 and 9). In addition, we present the cumulative cases in Fig. 10, and we summarize it in Table 4. We remark that the effectiveness of the policies plays an important role to reduce, or not, the human damage and ensure the eradication of the illness. However, mitigation measures must be strictly respected to maintain a good level of control over the spread of the virus.

On the other hand, we are carrying out a statistical study on a national scale, and we note that the trend at the beginning was exponential and will undergo a break due to the multiple interventions of the government, which is globally a good sign (see

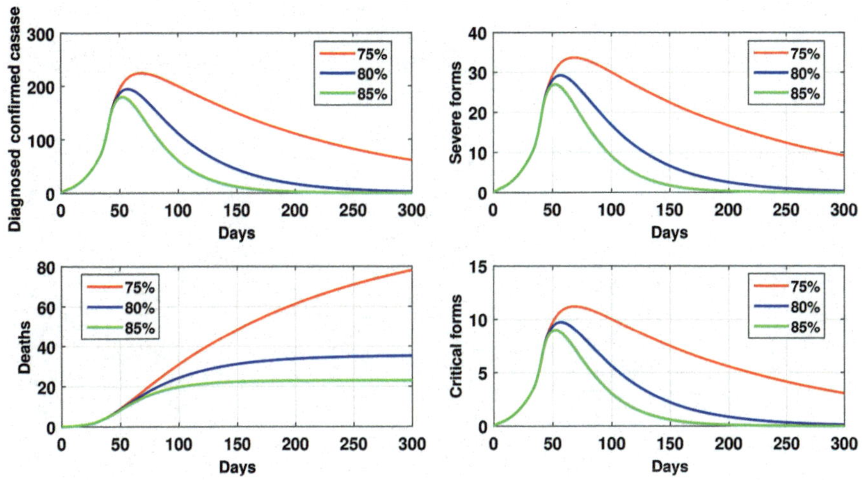

Fig. 9 Evolution of the positive-infected diagnosed individuals and deaths with different effectiveness degrees

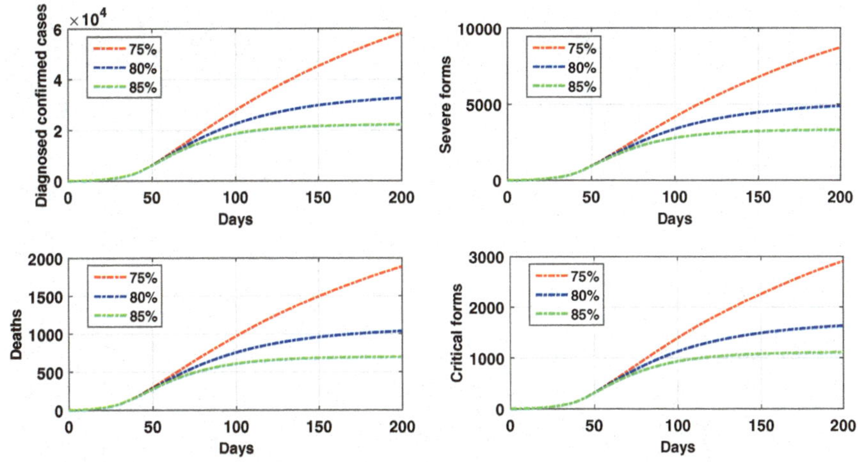

Fig. 10 Cumulative diagnosed cases, severe forms, critical forms and deaths, with different effectiveness degrees

Fig. 11), whereas it is needful to pay attention at the evolution of the curves in the different regions in Morocco. Since the clinical data of Covid-19 were not available on a daily basis at the start of the spread of the epidemic in Morocco, we proceeded with a choice of unit of three days. We also remark that almost all the regions have a homogeneous tendency with the national one, except Tangier–Tetouan–Al Hoceima (TTA), Oriental, Marrakech–Safi (MS), and Casablanca–Settat (CS), which show a mitigation of the epidemic that does not seem very stable (see Figs. 12 and 13).

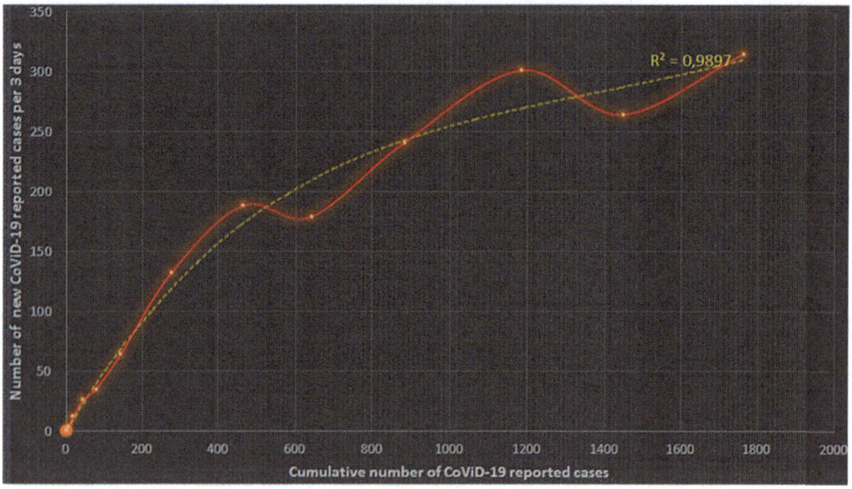

Fig. 11 Trends in the number of new Covid-19 reported cases per three days in Morocco, compared to the cumulative number of Covid-19 reported cases with correlation coefficient $R^2 = 0.9897$

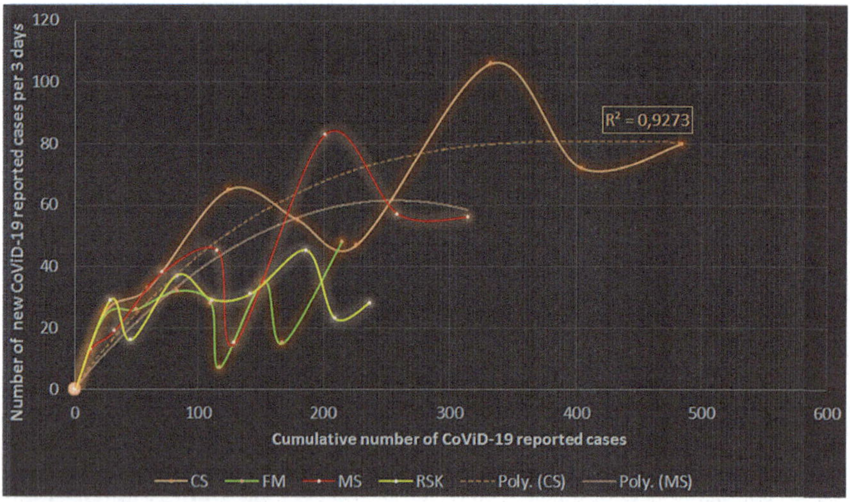

Fig. 12 Trends in the number of new Covid-19 reported cases per three days in Morocco, by regions, compared to the cumulative number of Covid-19 reported cases (CS: Casablanca–Settat; FM: Fes–Meknes; MS: Marrakech–Safi; RSK: Rabat–Sale–Kenitra)

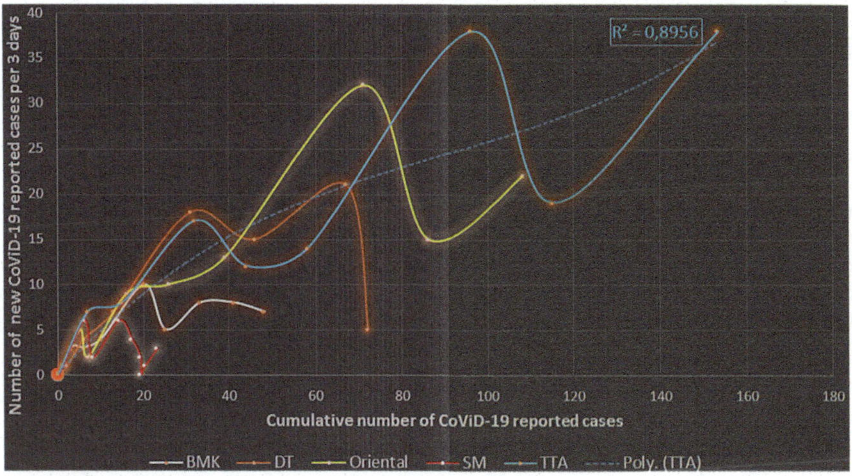

Fig. 13 Trends in the number of new Covid-19 reported cases per three days in Morocco, by regions, compared to the cumulative number of Covid-19 reported cases (BMK: Beni Mellal–Khenifra; DT: Daraa–Tafilalet; SM: Souss–Massa; TTA: Tetouan–Tangier–Assillah)

5 Discussion

Our work followed several steps. First of all, we have formulated an adequate mathematical model to describe the evolution of the Covid-19 disease epidemic in Morocco. This model allows us to have an idea on the number of resuscitation beds to prepare for severe forms and intensive care units for critical forms. Second, we have estimated the corresponding parameters based on the daily Moroccan data. Furthermore, we have applied the least-square method to determine the confidence interval of the transmission rate β, which is given by $(95\%CI, 0.4484–0.455)$. Third, we have computed the basic reproduction number $\mathcal{R}_0$ with the next-generation matrix method, for which we have studied the sensitivity analysis in order to examine the robustness of the model. We have observed that the transmission rate β and the proportion of individuals with symptoms ϵ are the most sensitive parameters and have a high impact on $\mathcal{R}_0$. By performing some numerical simulations, we have represented the effect of measures taken by the government, step by step, with the control u. In the first period, the appropriate basic reproduction number for $u = 0.2$ is $\mathcal{R}_0 = 2.9108$. In the second period, $\mathcal{R}_0 = 2.5469$ for $u = 0.3$. Thirdly, $\mathcal{R}_0 = 2.1831$ for $u = 0.4$. In the last period, $\mathcal{R}_0 = 0.7277$ for $u = 0.8$. Based on all strategies taken by the Moroccan authorities, we affirm that the best one is to increase considerably the level of the lockdown accompanied by the general use of the face masks. In this case, the estimated endemic peak will take place around April 28. Finally, through an analysis of regional data, we have shown that the evolution of the pandemic is consistent with the general epidemiological tendency at the national level.

We finish by mentioning that the used historic data and the different preventive measures and strategies implemented by Moroccan authorities and considered in our study are related to the confinement period in Morocco, between March 2 and June 20, 2020, whereas the use of historic data and other measures and strategies, linked to the deconfinement phase, are left to another research work.

Acknowledgements HZ and DFMT were supported by FCT within project UIDB/04106/2020 (CIDMA). YA brought his expertise in the realization of this work, but this does not, in any way, reflect an opinion of the World Health Organization (WHO). The authors would like to express their gratitude to the anonymous reviewers for their constructive comments and suggestions, which helped them to enrich the work.

References

1. Gorbalenya, A.E., Baker, S.C., Baric, R.S., de Groot, R.J., Drosten, C., Gulyaeva, A.A., Haagmans, B.L., Lauber, C., Leontovich, A.M., Neuman, B.W., Penzar, D., Perlman, S., Poon, L.L.M., Samborskiy, D.V., Sidorov, I.A., Sola, I., Ziebuhr, J.: The species Severe acute respiratory syndromerelated coronavirus: classifying 2019-nCoV and naming it SARS-CoV-2. Nat. Microbiol. **5**, 536–544 (2020)
2. Ministry of Health of Morocco: The official portal of Corona virus in Morocco. http://www.covidmaroc.ma/pages/Accueil.aspx
3. Tang, B., Wang, X., Li, Q., Bragazzi, N.L., Tang, S., Xiao, Y., Wu, J.: Estimation of the transmission risk of the 2019-nCoV and its implication for public health interventions. J. Clin. Med. **9**(2), 462 (2020)
4. Wu, J.T., Leung, K., Leung, G.M.: Nowcasting and forecasting the potential domestic and international spread of the 2019-nCoV outbreak originating in Wuhan, China: a modelling study. The Lancet **395**(10225), 689–697 (2020)
5. Kuniya, T.: Prediction of the epidemic peak of coronavirus disease in Japan, 2020. J. Clin. Med. **9**(3), 789 (2020)
6. Fanelli, D., Piazza, F.: Analysis and forecast of COVID-19 spreading in China, Italy and France. Chaos, Solitons & Fractals **134**, 109761 (2020)
7. Ndaïrou, F., Area, I., Nieto, J.J., Torres, D.F.M.: Mathematical modeling of COVID-19 transmission dynamics with a case study of Wuhan, Chaos Solitons & Fractals **135**, 109846 (2020)
8. Altaf, K.M., Atangana, A.: Modeling the dynamics of novel coronavirus (2019-nCov) with fractional derivative. Alexandria Eng. J. **59**(4), 2379–2389 (2020)
9. Bell, M.L., Zanobetti, A., Dominici, F.: Evidence on vulnerability and susceptibility to health risks associated with short-term exposure to particulate matter: A systematic review and meta-analysis. Am. J. Epidemiol. **178**(6), 865–876 (2013)
10. Kottow, M.H.: The vulnerable and the susceptible. Bioethics **17**(5–6), 460–471 (2003)
11. Hale, J.K., Verduyn Lunel, S.M.: *Introduction to functional-differential equations*, Applied Mathematical Sciences, vol. 99, Springer, New York (1993)
12. Diekmann, O., Heesterbeek, J.A.P., Metz, J.A.J.: On the definition and the computation of the basic reproduction ratio R_0 in models for infectious diseases in heterogeneous populations. J. Math. Biol. **28**, 365–382 (1990)
13. Driessche, P.V., Watmough, J.: Reproduction numbers and sub-threshold endemic equilibria for compartmental models of disease transmission. Math. Biosci. **180**, 29–48 (2002)
14. Ministry of Health, Morocco, Department of Epidemiology and Disease Control. http://www.sante.gov.ma/Pages/Accueil.aspx
15. Mizumoto, K., Kagaya, K., Zarebski, A., Chowell, G.: Estimating the asymptomatic proportion of coronavirus disease 2019 (COVID-19) cases on board the Diamond Princess cruise ship, Yokohama, Japan, 2020. Eurosurveillance **25**(10), 2000180 (2020)

16. WHO: Coronavirus disease 2019 (COVID-19), Situation Report 46, 6 March 2020
17. WHO: Coronavirus disease 2019 (COVID-19), Situation Report 73, 2nd April 2020
18. Baum, S.G.: COVID-19 incubation period: an update. March 13, 2020. https://www.jwatch.org/na51083/2020/03/13/covid-19-incubation-period-update
19. Huang, C., et al.: Clinical features of patients infected with 2019 novel coronavirus in Wuhan, China. Lancet **395**(10223), 497–506 (2020)
20. Wang, D., et al.: Clinical characteristics of 138 hospitalized patients with 2019 novel Coronavirus-Infected pneumonia in Wuhan, China. JAMA **323**(11), 1061–1069 (2020)
21. Haut Conseil de la Santé publique, Morocco, avis relatif aux recommandations thérapeutiques dans la prise en charge du COVID-19 (complémentaire à l'avis du 5 mars 2020), 23 mars 2020
22. Chitnis, N., Hyman, J.M., Cushing, J.M.: Determining important parameters in the spread of malaria through the sensitivity analysis of a mathematical model. Bull. Math. Biol. **70**(5), 1272–1296 (2008)
23. Rodrigues, H.S., Monteiro, M.T.T., Torres, D.F.M.: Sensitivity analysis in a dengue epidemiological model. Conf. Papers in Math. **2013**, 721406 (2013)

Study of Transmission Dynamics of Covid-19 Virus Using Fractional Model: Case of Morocco

M. R. Sidi Ammi and M. Tahiri

Abstract In this paper, a generalized fractional order SEIRP model is proposed in order to study the dynamic behavior of Covid-19 and the effect of lockdown of susceptible population. Some sufficient conditions are supposed to ensure the local asymptotic stability of disease-free and endemic equilibrium points. Our results are applied to the case of Morocco country. The theoretical results are validated by some numerical simulations.

Keywords Mathematical modeling of Covid-19 pandemic · Stability · Numerical simulations · Basic reproduction number · Morocco case study

1 Introduction

Covid-19 (Coronavirus Disease-19) is a respiratory disease caused by an emerging coronavirus, SARS-CoV-2. The epidemic began in the city of Wuhan, China in late December 2019 and quickly spread around the world. The Covid-19 pandemic is the world's biggest health threat. At the time of last revision, according to a WHO report released on September 19, 2020, the cumulative number of confirmed infected cases have risen to 30,863,802 with 958,789 deaths. The global problem of the outbreak has attracted the interest of researchers of different areas, giving rise to a number of proposals to analyze and predict the evolution of the pandemic. In [4] Ndaïrou et al. have proposed a mathematical model consisting of ordinary differential equations with special focus on the transmissibility of super-spreaders individuals. The SEIQRP model with fractional order has been proposed in [13] with an incidence function of type $f(S)g(I)$.

Fractional calculus can be used, among several possibilities, to deal with the memory effect in mathematical modeling. Memory in mathematical modeling makes

M. R. Sidi Ammi (✉) · M. Tahiri
FST Errachidia,MAIS Laboratory, Moulay Ismail University of Meknes, AMNEA Group, Meknes, Morocco
e-mail: rachidsidiammi@yahoo.fr; m.sidiammi@fste.umi.ac.ma

P. Agarwal et al. (eds.), *Analysis of Infectious Disease Problems (Covid-19) and Their Global Impact*, Infosys Science Foundation Series,
https://doi.org/10.1007/978-981-16-2450-6_29

important what happened in the past to explain the present [7]. In [10], a system of fractional differential equations is used to study the effect of memory on epidemic evolution. To illustrate the potential of fractional differential equations in epidemiological processes with memory, we investigate the evolution of Covid-19 in a population with effect of lockdown of susceptible population. Therefore, a SEIRP model, considered as a generalized SEIR epidemic model, is proposed in this paper. However, due to the fact that this disease is little known and underreported, parameters such as speed of propagation and recovery and contact rates are difficult to estimate. Consequently, its modeling using classical differential equations can be inappropriate to represent the dynamics of the populations involved. Thus, it is possible to adjust the order of the differential equation to the real data of the spread of the disease.

The manuscript is organized as follows. In Sect. 2, we propose a new model for Covid-19. A qualitative analysis of the model is investigated in Sect. 3. First, we show that our model is well posed. We then compute the basic reproduction number R_0 of the Covid-19 system model. In Sect. 4, we study the existence of equilibria and their local stability in terms of R_0. The sensitivity of the basic reproduction number R_0 is given in Sect. 5. In Sect. 6, the usefulness of our model is then illustrated by numerical simulations, where we use real data from Morocco. We end with Sect. 7 of conclusion, and possible future research.

2 Proposed Covid-19 Model

We propose a new epidemiological compartment fractional model with general incidence function, taking into account the effect of the lockdown of susceptible Individuals. The total population of size N is subdivided into the following epidemiological classes:

- Susceptible class $S(t)$: the number of uninfected individuals at the time t.
- Exposed class $E(t)$: the number of infected individuals at the time t but still in incubation period (without clinical symptoms).
- Infected class $I(t)$: the number of infected individuals at the time t (with obvious clinical symptoms).
- Recovered class $R(t)$: the number of recovered individuals at the time t.
- Insusceptible class $P(t)$: the number of susceptible individuals who are not exposed to the external environment at the time t.

Our fractional model takes the following form:

Table 1 Values of the model parameters corresponding to the situation of Morocco, as discussed in Sect. 6

Name	Description	Value	Unit
Λ	Birth density of susceptible	6.00×10^5	dimensionless
β_1	Transmission coefficient due to infected individuals	0.87	day^{-1}
δ	Isolation rate of infected	0.26	day^{-1}
λ	Protection rate of susceptible	0.04	day^{-1}
β_2	Transmission coefficient due to exposed individuals	0.90	day^{-1}
μ	Natural death rate	1.00×10^{-4}	day^{-1}
ξ	Rate at which exposed people become infected	0.74	day^{-1}
ρ	Recovery rate coefficient	0.64	day^{-1}
d	Death rate coefficient due to infected	15.00×10^{-3}	day^{-1}

$$\begin{cases} {}_0^C D_t^\alpha S(t) = \Lambda - \beta_1(1-\delta)(1-\lambda)f(S(t), I(t)) - \beta_2 g(S(t), E(t)) - \lambda S(t) - \mu S(t), \\ {}_0^C D_t^\alpha E(t) = \beta_1(1-\delta)(1-\lambda)f(S(t), I(t)) + \beta_2 g(S(t), E(t)) - \xi E(t) - \mu E(t), \\ {}_0^C D_t^\alpha I(t) = \xi E(t) - (\rho\delta + d\delta)I(t) - \mu I(t), \\ {}_0^C D_t^\alpha R(t) = \rho\delta I(t) - \mu R(t), \\ {}_0^C D_t^\alpha P(t) = \lambda S(t) - \mu P(t), \end{cases} \tag{1}$$

where the fractional derivative is considered in the sense of Caputo. For biological reasons, we consider system (1) with the following initial conditions:

$$S(0) \geq 0, \quad E(0) \geq 0, \quad I(0) \geq 0, \quad R(0) \geq 0, \quad P(0) \geq 0. \tag{2}$$

Different parameters intervening in the model are presented in the following table.

The number of death due to the disease at each instant of time is given by

$$D(t) := d\delta I(t). \tag{3}$$

The first four equations in system (1) do not depend on the last equation. Then, the system (1) can be rewritten as

$$\begin{cases} {}_0^C D_t^\alpha S(t) = \Lambda - \beta_1(1-\delta)(1-\lambda) f(S(t), I(t)) - \beta_2 g(S(t), E(t)) - \lambda S(t) - \mu S(t), \\ {}_0^C D_t^\alpha E(t) = \beta_1(1-\delta)(1-\lambda) f(S(t), I(t)) + \beta_2 g(S(t), E(t)) - \xi E(t) - \mu E(t), \\ {}_0^C D_t^\alpha I(t) = \xi E(t) - (\rho\delta + d\delta) I(t) - \mu I(t), \\ {}_0^C D_t^\alpha R(t) = \rho\delta I(t) - \mu R(t). \end{cases} \tag{4}$$

The incidence functions $f(S, I)$ and $g(S, E)$ are assumed to be positive, continuously differentiable in the interior of $\mathbb{R}_+^2$ and satisfies the following hypotheses:

(H1) $f(0, I) = g(0, E) = g(S, 0) = 0$ for all S, E and I non-negative,
(H2) $\partial_S f(S, I) > 0, \partial_I f(S, I) > 0, \partial_S g(S, E) > 0, \partial_E g(S, E) > 0$ for all S, E and I positive,
(H3) $\phi_1(S, I) = \frac{f(S,I)}{I}$ and $\phi_2(S, E) = \frac{g(S,E)}{E}$ are bounded and monotone increasing functions of $I > 0$ and $E > 0$ respectively, for any fixed $S \geq 0$.

$(H1)$ explains that when the number of susceptible, infected or exposed equals to zero then there are no incidences and there is no transmission of the disease. $(H2)$ reflects that when the number of susceptible, infected or exposed individuals increases then the transmission of disease also increases. $(H3)$ translates that when the number of infected increases then the incidence between susceptible and infected increases more quickly. The same is occurred for susceptible and exposed individuals.

3 Qualitative Analysis of the Model

3.1 Existence of Non-negative Bounded Solution

We assume that the functions S, E, I, R and their Caputo fractional derivatives are continuous at $t \geq 0$.

Theorem 1 *The solution of system* (4) *are bounded and non-negative, and the closed set* $\Omega = \{(S, E, I, R) \in \mathbb{R}_+^4 : S + E + I + R \leq N(0) + \dfrac{\Lambda}{\mu}\}$ *is a positive invariant set of system* (4).

Proof The existence of the solution is obtained by applying [3, Theorem 3.1]. By virtue of [3, Remark 3.2], we prove the uniqueness. It remains to prove that the solution is non-negative. Observe first that:

$$\begin{aligned} &{}_0^C D_t^\alpha S(t)|_{S=0} = \Lambda, \\ &{}_0^C D_t^\alpha E(t)|_{E=0} = \beta_1(1-\delta)(1-\lambda) f(S(t), I(t)), \\ &{}_0^C D_t^\alpha I(t)|_{I=0} = \xi E(t), \\ &{}_0^C D_t^\alpha R(t)|_{R=0} = \rho\delta I(t). \end{aligned}$$

Using [1, Lemma 1] and a similar argumentation as used in the proof of [1, Theorem 2], we prove the desired result.

Let $N(t) = S(t) + E(t) + I(t) + R(t)$. By adding the equations of system (4), one can deduce

$$\begin{aligned} {}_0^C D_t^\alpha N(t) &= \Lambda - \mu N(t) - \lambda S(t) - d\delta I(t) \\ &\leq \Lambda - \mu N(t). \end{aligned}$$

By applying the fractional order comparison theorem, one has

$$N(t) \leq N(0) E_\alpha(-\mu t^\alpha) + \frac{\Lambda}{\mu}(1 - E_\alpha(-\mu t^\alpha)).$$

Because $0 \leq E_\alpha(-\mu t^\alpha) \leq 1$, we have $N(t) \leq N(0) + \frac{\Lambda}{\mu}$. This completes the proof. □

3.2 *Basic Reproduction Number*

The system (4) has always a disease-free equilibrium point of the form $E_f = (S_f, 0, 0, 0)$, where $S_f = \frac{\Lambda}{\lambda+\mu}$. Using the next generation matrix approach outlined in [11] to our model (4), the basic reproduction number can be computed by considering the generation matrices F and V given hereafter. Namely, the Jacobian matrices associated to the rate of appearance of new infections and the net rate out of the corresponding compartments, respectively,

$$F = \begin{bmatrix} \beta_2 \partial_E g(S_f, 0) & \beta' \partial_I f(S_f, 0) \\ 0 & 0 \end{bmatrix} \;\; ; \;\; V = \begin{bmatrix} -(\xi + \mu) & 0 \\ \xi & -(\rho\delta + \mu + d\delta) \end{bmatrix},$$

where $\beta' = \beta_1(1 - \delta)(1 - \lambda)$. The basic reproduction number is then

$$R_0 = -F \cdot V^{-1} = \frac{\xi(\beta_1(1 - \delta)(1 - \lambda))\partial_I f(S_f, 0)}{(\xi + \mu)(\rho\delta + \mu + d\delta)} + \frac{\beta_2 \partial_E g(S_f, 0)}{\xi + \mu}. \quad (5)$$

4 Existence of Equilibria and Local Stability

In this section, we firstly discuss the existence of equilibria for model (4).

Theorem 2 *Assume that the hypotheses* (H_1), (H_2) *and* (H_3) *hold. The fractional* $SEIR$ *model* (4) *has at most two equilibrium points:*

1. *a disease free equilibrium* $E_f = (S_f, 0, 0, 0)$, *where* $S_f = \frac{\Lambda}{\lambda+\mu}$.
2. *an endemic equilibrium point* $E_e = (S^*, E^*, I^*, R^*)$ *if* $R_0 > 1$, *where* $S^* = \frac{\Lambda-(\xi+\mu)E^*}{\lambda+\mu}$, $I^* = \frac{\xi E^*}{\rho\delta+\mu+d\delta}$, $R^* = \frac{\rho\delta\xi E^*}{\mu(\rho\delta+\mu+d\delta)}$.

Proof 1. For $E = 0$, it's clair that E_f is the unique steady state of system (4) .
2. By using the following system

$$ {}_0^C D_t^\alpha S(t) = {}_0^C D_t^\alpha E(t) = {}_0^C D_t^\alpha I(t) = {}_0^C D_t^\alpha R(t) = 0, $$

we get the equation

$$ \beta_1(1-\delta)(1-\lambda) f\Big(\frac{\Lambda - (\xi + \mu)E}{\lambda + \mu}, \frac{\xi E}{\delta + \mu + d}\Big) + \beta_2 g\Big(\frac{\Lambda - (\xi + \mu)E}{\lambda + \mu}, E\Big) = (\xi + \mu)E $$

for $E \neq 0$. The fact that $S = \frac{\Lambda-(\xi+\mu)E}{\lambda+\mu} \geq 0$ yields to $E \leq \frac{\Lambda}{\xi+\mu}$. Hence, there is no positive equilibrium point if $E > \frac{\Lambda}{\xi+\mu}$. Now, we consider the following function h defined on the interval $\left[0, \frac{\Lambda}{\xi+\mu}\right]$ by

$$ h(E) = \beta_1(1-\delta)(1-\lambda)\frac{f\Big(\frac{\Lambda-(\xi+\mu)E}{\lambda+\mu}, \frac{\xi E}{\rho\delta+\mu+d\delta}\Big)}{E} + \beta_2 \frac{g\Big(\frac{\Lambda-(\xi+\mu)E}{\lambda+\mu}, E\Big)}{E} - (\xi + \mu). $$

According to hypotheses (H_2) and (H_3), h is strictly increasing on $\left[0, \frac{\Lambda}{\xi+\mu}\right]$. Since $h(\frac{\Lambda}{\xi+\mu}) = -(\xi + \mu) < 0$ and $\lim_{E\to 0^+} h(E) = (\xi + \mu)(R_0 - 1) > 0$ for $R_0 > 1$, there exists a unique endemic equilibrium E_e with $0 < E_e < \frac{\Lambda}{\xi+\mu}$. This completes the proof.

Next, we study the local asymptotic stability of disease free equilibrium point E_f and endemic equilibrium point E_e for system (4). The Jacobian matrix of system (4) at any equilibrium $\bar{E}_q = (\bar{S}, \bar{E}, \bar{I}, \bar{R})$ is given by

$$ J_{\bar{E}_q} = \begin{pmatrix} c & -\beta_2\partial_E g(\bar{S}, \bar{E}) & -\beta'\partial_I f(\bar{S}, \bar{I}) & 0 \\ \beta'\partial_S f(\bar{S}, \bar{I}) + \beta_2\partial_S g(\bar{S}, \bar{E}) & \beta_2\partial_E g(\bar{S}, \bar{E}) - (\xi + \mu) & \beta'\partial_I f(\bar{S}, \bar{I}) & 0 \\ 0 & \xi & -\Delta & 0 \\ 0 & 0 & \rho\delta & -\mu \end{pmatrix} $$

where $c = -\beta'\partial_S f(\bar{S}, \bar{I}) - \beta_2\partial_S g(\bar{S}, \bar{E}) - (\lambda + \mu)$ and $\Delta = \rho\delta + \mu + d\delta$. We recall that a sufficient condition for the local stability of $\bar{E}_q$ is

$$ |\arg(\xi_i)| > \frac{\alpha\pi}{2}, \quad i = 1, 2, 3, 4, \tag{6} $$

where ξ_i are the eigenvalues of $J_{\bar{E}}$ (see [6]). We begin by establishing the local stability of E_f.

Theorem 3 *Assume that the condition* (H_1) *holds. Then the disease-free equilibrium* E_f *is locally asymptotically stable if and only if* $R_0 \leq 1$.

Proof The eigenvalues of J_{E_f} are $\xi_1 = -(\lambda + \mu)$, $\xi_2 = -(\xi + \mu)$, $\xi_3 = -\Delta$, and $\xi_4 = -\mu$. Since all eigenvalues are negative, then satisfy condition (6).

We are now concerned with the local stability of E_e.

Theorem 4 *Assume that hypotheses* (H_1), (H_2) *and* (H_3) *are verified. Then the endemic equilibrium* E_e *is locally asymptotically stable, if and only if* $R_0 > 1$.

Proof At equilibrium E_e, the characteristic equation for the corresponding linearised system of model (4) is $\xi^4 + a_1\xi^3 + a_2\xi^2 + a_3\xi + a_4 = 0$, where, if the coefficients a_1, a_2, a_3 and a_4 are positives, from condition 6 in [14, Lemma 5.1] the positive equilibrium point E_e is locally asymptotically stable. □

5 Sensitivity Analysis

The sensitivity analysis for the basic reproduction number (3.2) tells us how each parameter is important to disease transmission. This information is crucial not only for experimental design, but also to data assimilation and reduction of complex models [8]. Sensitivity analysis is commonly used to determine the robustness of model predictions to parameter values, since there are usually errors in collected data and presumed parameter values. It is used to discover parameters that have a high impact on the threshold R_0 and should be targeted by intervention strategies. More accurately, sensitivity indices' allows us to measure the relative change in a variable when a parameter changes. For that purpose, we use the normalized forward sensitivity index of a variable with respect to a given parameter, which is defined as the ratio of the relative change in the variable to the relative change in the parameter. If such variable is differentiable with respect to the parameter, then the sensitivity index is defined as follows.

Definition 1 *(See* [2, 9]*)* The normalized forward sensitivity index of R_0, which is differentiable with respect to a given parameter θ, is defined by

$$\Upsilon_\theta^{R_0} = \frac{\partial R_0}{\partial \theta}\frac{\theta}{R_0}.$$

Note that the sensitivity index may depend on several parameters of the system, but also can be constant, independent of any parameter. For example, $\Upsilon_\theta^{R_0} = +1$ means that increasing (decreasing) θ by a given percentage increases (decreases) always R_0 by that same percentage. The estimation of a sensitive parameter should be carefully done, since a small perturbation in such parameter leads to relevant quantitative changes. On the other hand, the estimation of a parameter with a rather small value for the sensitivity index does not require as much attention to estimate, because a small perturbation in that parameter leads to small changes. The results of this analysis are presented in Table 2.

6 Numerical Simulations

In the following discussion, the standard incidences rate are used to describe the transmission of Covid-19. They are given by $\beta_1(1-\delta)(1-\lambda)f(S,I)=\beta_1(1-\delta)(1-\lambda)SI$, $\beta_2 g(S,E)=\beta_2 SE$. Hence, we get the following system

$$\begin{cases} {}_0^C D_t^\alpha S(t) = \Lambda - \beta_1(1-\delta)(1-\lambda)SI - \beta_2 SE - \lambda S(t) - \mu S(t), \\ {}_0^C D_t^\alpha E(t) = \beta_1(1-\delta)(1-\lambda)SI + \beta_2 SE - \xi E(t) - \mu E(t), \\ {}_0^C D_t^\alpha I(t) = \xi E(t) - (\rho\delta + d\delta)I(t) - \mu I(t), \\ {}_0^C D_t^\alpha R(t) = \rho\delta I(t) - \mu R(t). \end{cases} \tag{7}$$

We perform numerical simulations to compare the results of our model with the real data obtained from worldometers [12]. The system (7) is numerically integrated by using the fractional Euler's method which can be seen as a generalization of the classical Euler's method for the numerical solution of ordinary differential equations [5]. The accuracy of the approximation depends on the step size of discretization. It is worthwhile to mention that Morocco has a population of about 34 million. As for the initial conditions, the following values have been fixed: $S(0) = 33999931$, $E(0) = 20$, $I(0) = 29$, $R(0) = 18$, $D(0) = 2$. We can estimate some parameters'values of Morocco from June 11th to August 9th (see Table 1). One computes the basic reproduction number, we obtain $R_0 = 1.0006$. This epidemiologically means that the disease will persist in the population. During the Covid-19 pandemic, there were restrictions on the movement of individuals due to the lockdown of susceptible population in the country. As a result, disease prevalence was limited. However, starting June 11th, the Moroccan government has relaxed the measures it has taken regarding the epidemic, which led to the increase in the number of infectious cases and death cases as can be seen in the Figs. 1 and 2. We remark also the fitting effect of the fractional order system (7) notably for ($\alpha = 0.7$) is better than that of the integer order system (i.e. $\alpha = 1$). It comes down to the memory effect which represents precautions taken by susceptible individuals. Finally, let's study the effect of the protection rate of susceptible λ on the basic reproduction rate R_0. We note that R_0 decreases when λ increases (see Fig. 3). Hence, we conclude the importance of lockdown of susceptible population to keep the situation stable until a vaccination for this disease is found.

Finally, the values of the sensitivity indices for the parameters values of Table 1, are presented in Table 2.

We conclude that the most sensitive parameters to the basic reproduction number R_0 of the Covid-19 model (7) are Λ and λ. In concrete, an increase of the value of Λ will increase the basic reproduction number by 99.9%. In contrast, an increase of the value of λ will decrease R_0 by 72.2%.

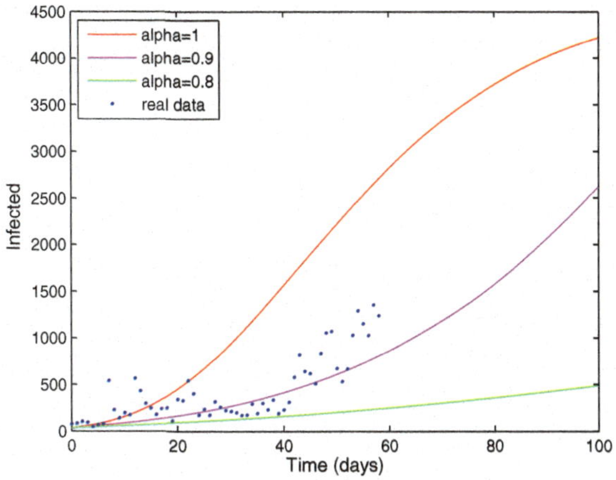

Fig. 1 Number of infected cases per day, by using a Matlab code

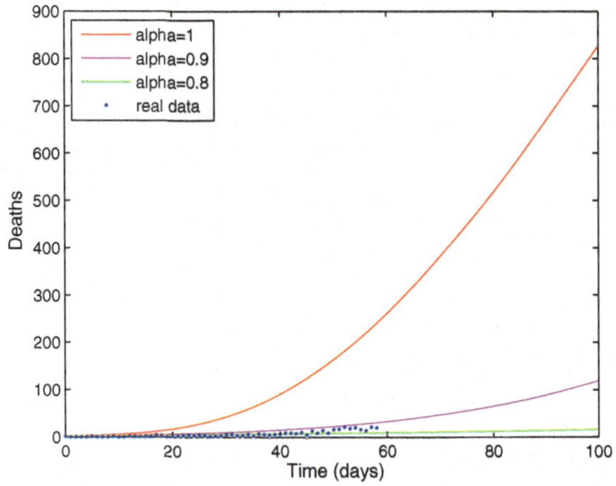

Fig. 2 Number of death cases per day, by using a Matlab code

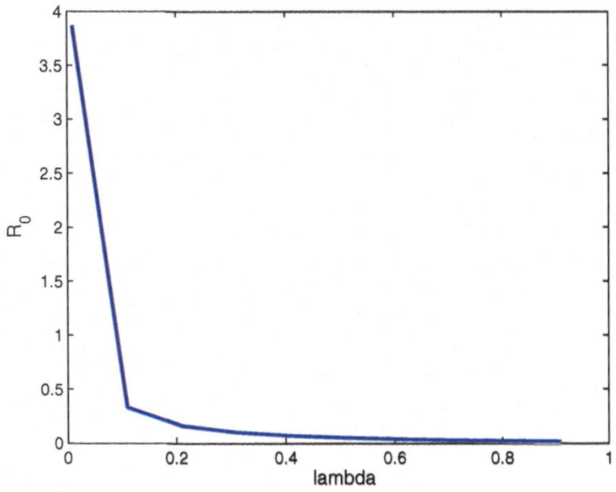

Fig. 3 Variation of R_0 according to the lockdown effect (λ)

Table 2 Sensitivity of R_0 evaluated for the parameter values given in Table 1

Parameter	Sensitivity index
Λ	0.999
β_1	0.542
δ	−0.541
λ	−0.722
β_2	0.180
μ	−0.368
ξ	−0.181
ρ	−0.52
d	−0.012

7 Conclusion

In this work, we presented a new model based on fractional nonlinear differential equations for modelling Covid-19 in Morocco. The aim of our work, at first, is to provide initial ideas and guidelines for a quantitative and qualitative study of our considered model. In particular, the positivity, boundness and the existence of a solution are established. The importance of the effect of lockdown of susceptible population is verified. We also showed that the model can be adjusted to real data, then, we have obtained a good prediction of the evolution of the disease for $\alpha = 0.7$. We hope our work motivates new researchs to give significant improvements, especially the suitable choice of the incidence function which models the transmissibility from asymptomatic individuals.

Acknowledgements The authors wish to thank the reviewers for careful reading and valuable suggestions to improve the quality of the paper. The support from Moulay Ismail University of Meknes (project UMI 2018) and Covid-19 project (Analyse épidémique du Covid-19 au Maroc par modélisation dynamique et intelligence artificielle) jointly funded by CNRST and the Moroccan Ministry of Higher Education and Scientific Research, is acknowledged.

References

1. Almeida, R., Brito da Cruz, A.M.C., Martins, N., Monteiro, M.T.T.: An epidemiological MSEIR model described by the Caputo fractional derivative. Int. J. Dyn. Control **7**, 776–784 (2019)
2. Chitnis, N., Hyman, J.M., Cushing, J.M.: Determining important parameters in the spread of malaria through the sensitivity analysis of a mathematical model. Bull. Math. Biol. **70**, 1272–1296 (2008). https://doi.org/10.1007/s11538-008-9299-0
3. Lin, W.: Global existence theory and chaos control of fractional differential equations. J. Math. Anal. Appl. **332**, 709–726 (2007)
4. Ndairou, F., Area, I., Nieto, J.J., Torres, D.F.M.: Mathematical modeling of COVID-19 transmission dynamics with a case study of Wuhan. Chaos, Solitons & Fractals (2020)

5. Odibat, Z., Momani, S.: An algorithm for the numerical solution of differential equations of fractional order. J. Appl. Math. Inform **26**, 15–27 (2008)
6. Petráš, I.: Fractional-order nonlinear systems: modeling, analysis and simulation. Springer, Berlin (2011)
7. Pinto, C., Tenreiro Machado, J.A.: Fractional dynamics of computer virus propagation. Math. Problems in Eng. (2014)
8. Powell, D.R., Fair, J., LeClaire, R.J., Moore, L.M., Thompson, D.: Sensitivity analysis of an infectious disease model. In: Proceedings of the International System Dynamics Conference. Boston (2005)
9. Rodrigues, H.S., Monteiro, M.T.T., Torres, D.F.M.: Sensitivity analysis in a dengue epidemiological model. In: +Conference Papers in Mathematics, vol. 2013, p. 721406. Hindawi. https://doi.org/10.1155/2013/721406. arXiv:1307.0202
10. Sidi Ammi, M.R., Tahiri, M., Torres, D.F.M.: Global stability of a Caputo fractional SIRS model with general incidence rate. Math. Comput. Sci. (2020)
11. Van den Driessche, P., Watmough, J.: Reproduction numbers and sub-threshold endemic equilibria for compartmental models of disease transmission. Math. Biosci. **180**, 29–48 (2002)
12. https://www.worldometers.info/coronavirus/country/morocco/
13. Xu, C., Yu, Y., Yang, Q. Lu, Z.: Forecast analysis of the epidemics trend of COVID-19 in the United States by a generalized fractional-order SEIR model. *arXiv preprint* arXiv:2004.12541 (2020)
14. Yaro, D., Apeanti, W.O., Akuamoah, S.W., Lu, D.: Analysis and optimal control of fractional-order transmission of a respiratory epidemic model. Int. J. Appl. Comput. Math. **5** (2019)

Printed by Printforce, the Netherlands